S0-AZK-695

Contemporary Hypnosis Research

CONTEMPORARY HYPNOSIS RESEARCH

Edited by
ERIKA FROMM, Ph.D.
University of Chicago

MICHAEL R. NASH, Ph.D.
University of Tennessee

Foreword by John F. Kihlstrom, Ph.D.

THE GUILFORD PRESS
New York   London

#25966182

BF
1141
.C686
1992

© 1992 The Guilford Press
A Division of Guilford Publications, Inc.
72 Spring Street, New York, NY 10012

All rights reserved

No part of this book may be reproduced, stored in a retrieval
system, or transmitted, in any form or by any means, electronic,
mechanical, photocopying, microfilming, recording, or otherwise,
without written permission from the Publisher.

Printed in the United States of America

This book is printed on acid-free paper.

Last digit is print number: 9 8 7 6 5 4 3 2 1

Library of Congress Cataloging-in-Publication Data

Contemporary hypnosis research/edited by Erika Fromm and Michael R. Nash;
  foreword by John F. Kihlstrom.
      p.   cm.
   Includes bibliographical references and index.
   ISBN 0-89862-893-8
   1. Hypnotism. I. Fromm, Erika.   II. Nash, Michael R.
   [DNLM: 1. Hypnosis.   BF 1152 C761]
   BF1141.C686   1992
   154.7—dc20
   DNLM/DLC
   for Library of Congress   92-1570
                                                              CIP

Contributors

ARREED F. BARABASZ, Ed.D., Ph.D., Department of Counseling Psychology, Washington State University, Pullman, Washington

MARIANNE BARABASZ, Ed.D., Department of Counseling Psychology, Washington State University, Pullman, Washington

KENNETH S. BOWERS, Ph.D., Department of Psychology, University of Waterloo, Waterloo, Ontario, Canada

PATRICIA G. BOWERS, Ph.D., Department of Psychology, University of Waterloo, Waterloo, Ontario, Canada

DANIEL P. BROWN, Ph.D., Department of Psychiatry, Harvard Medical School, Cambridge, Massachusetts

JENNIFER BUTTON, B.A., Department of Psychology, Concordia University, Montréal, Québec, Canada

WILLIAM C. COE, Ph.D., Department of Psychology, California State University at Fresno, Fresno, California

JAMES R. COUNCIL, Ph.D., Department of Psychology, North Dakota State University, Fargo, North Dakota

HELEN J. CRAWFORD, Ph.D., Department of Psychology, Virginia Polytechnic Institute and State University, Blacksburg, Virginia

MICHAEL DIXON, Ph.D., Department of Psychology, Concordia University, Montréal, Québec, Canada

ERIKA FROMM, Ph.D., Department of Psychology, University of Chicago, Chicago, Illinois

JOHN H. GRUZELIER, Ph.D., Department of Psychiatry, Charing Cross and Westminster Medical School, University of London, London, England

ERNEST R. HILGARD, Ph.D., Department of Psychology, Stanford University, Stanford, California

JEAN HOLROYD, Ph.D., Department of Psychiatry and Biobehavioral Sciences, Neuropsychiatric Institute, University of California, Los Angeles, Los Angeles, California

SPIRIT LIBRARY

93 v1904

STEPHEN KAHN, Ph.D., Department of Psychology, University of Chicago, Chicago, Illinois

IRVING KIRSCH, Ph.D., Department of Psychology, University of Connecticut, Storrs, Connecticut

JEAN-ROCH LAURENCE, Ph.D., Department of Psychology, Concordia University, Montréal, Québec, Canada

STEVEN JAY LYNN, Ph.D., Department of Psychology, Ohio University, Athens, Ohio

KEVIN M. MCCONKEY, Ph.D., School of Behavioural Sciences, Macquarie University, Sydney, New South Wales, Australia

ROBERT NADON, Ph.D., Department of Psychology, Brock University, St. Catharines, Ontario, Canada

MICHAEL R. NASH, Ph.D., Department of Psychology, University of Tennessee, Knoxville, Tennessee

JONATHAN M. OAKMAN, B.A., Department of Psychology, University of Waterloo, Waterloo, Ontario, Canada

CAMPBELL PERRY, Ph.D., Department of Psychology, Concordia University, Montréal, Québec, Canada

VICTOR A. SHAMES, M.S., Department of Psychology, University of Arizona, Tucson, Arizona

PETER W. SHEEHAN, Ph.D., Department of Psychology, University of Queensland, Brisbane, Queensland, Australia

HARRY SIVEC, M.S., Department of Psychology, Ohio University, Athens, Ohio

NICHOLAS P. SPANOS, Ph.D., Department of Psychology and Laboratory for Experimental Hypnosis, Carleton University, Ottawa, Ontario, Canada

ERIK Z. WOODY, Ph.D., Department of Psychology, University of Waterloo, Waterloo, Ontario, Canada

Foreword

This year and next, hypnosis celebrates its sesquicentennial—or, at least, the sesquicentennial of its naming by James Braid. Since that time, and especially over the past quarter-century, hypnosis has matured as both a fascinating topic for scientific research and an effective technique for clinical application. How fitting, then, that Erika Fromm and Michael Nash should have produced this volume—essentially the third in a series collecting authoritative summaries of research and theory in the field of hypnosis.

The first volume in the series appeared in 1972 *(Hypnosis: Research Developments and Perspectives)*, under the editorship of Erika Fromm and Ronald Shor, and quickly found a place on the bookshelf of everyone interested in hypnosis. Together with Ernest Hilgard's classic *Hypnotic Susceptibility* (1965), its chapters provided a summary of where the field was: the most important empirical and theoretical developments since the revival of hypnosis research in the mid-1950s. Already in 1972, there was a wealth of literature to review: research on imagination and creativity, psychoanalytic and psychophysiological research, the task-motivational and real–simulator paradigms, conditioning, sleep, and much, much more. But that was just the beginning.

The second volume, published in 1979 *(Hypnosis: Developments in Research and New Perspectives*, also edited by Fromm and Shor), overlapped considerably with the first: pretty much the same chapters by pretty much the same authors. But against the background of updating, some new developments were visible: a statement of Hilgard's neodissociation theory, a view of hypnosis based on psychoanalytic ego psychology, and an approach that emphasized the phenomenology of the hypnotic experience as opposed to the description and analysis of hypnotic behavior. It is hard to imagine more essential reading for the scientist or practitioner interested in hypnosis—not just for their constituent chapters, but also for the comprehensive, meticulously verified reference lists found at their backs.

This new volume is not merely a third edition. Almost everything about the book is different. Only a few chapters are carried over from the earlier volumes, and most of these are by new authors, reflecting new approaches to their subject matter. The ego-psychological and neodissociative approaches outlined in 1979 have now generated a large corpus of literature, both supportive and critical. The new technology of home videotape has given us a new vehicle for exploring the phenomenology of hypnosis. Advances in cognitive psychology give us new perspectives on hypnosis, imagery, and creativity. This is all represented here.

More interesting, however, is the simple fact that the majority of chapters are entirely new. We have come a very long way in 20 years. There are three chapters on hypnotizability and its correlates, collectively providing a kind of update of Hilgard's work, but also opening up problems, and hypotheses, that were not imagined 27 years ago. There is a chapter on self-hypnosis, reflecting developments in that area. And the blending of theoretical and practical concerns, the laboratory and the consulting room, which makes hypnosis research so exciting, is represented by three chapters on applied issues in psychopathology, clinical psychology, and forensic uses of hypnosis. The wide range of conceptual approaches to hypnosis is exemplified by two chapters, one approaching hypnosis from the standpoint of social psychology and sociology, the other from the perspective of neuropsychology and psychophysiology. But perhaps the most exciting thing to note, the biggest difference between the present volume and its predecessors, is the pluralism characteristic of these chapters. Most authors move easily between the experimental and the clinical, the social, the cognitive, and the psychodynamic; there seems to be less concern with defending preconceived theoretical positions, and more interest in exploring the peculiar blend of interpersonal influence and altered consciousness that is hypnosis as we know it today.

Like its predecessors, this volume stands as a monumental summary of where hypnosis has been, where it stands today, and where it is heading tomorrow. My own copies of the earlier books were handled so much, by myself and others, they lost their wrappers early in life and their bindings have been terribly stressed (though neither has given way). Even my dictionary has not suffered that fate! What better tribute to the utility of a book?

John F. Kihlstrom, Ph.D.
Amnesia and Cognition Unit
Department of Psychology
University of Arizona
Tucson, Arizona

Preface

In 1972, Erika Fromm and Ronald E. Shor published an edited volume on the then-current development and perspectives of hypnosis research. This book, which became a classic in the field, was updated in a revised second edition in 1979.

We want to continue the Fromm and Shor tradition. But there have been so many changes and advances in the field of experimental hypnosis since 1979 that a simple update of the Fromm and Shor volume would be quite inadequate. New laboratories, new ideas, and new methodologies have transformed the research landscape as familiar theories are further refined, new ones emerge, and some old ones fade away.

The current book thus again is a survey of contemporary hypnosis research, methodology, and theory—a comprehensive reference text. We hope that it will, like the Fromm and Shor volume, be a book that sits on one's shelf and does not collect dust; it should be an eminently usable and comprehensive reference book that is consulted frequently and with confidence when researchers, theorists, and clinicians want to know the current scientific status of hypnosis-related phenomena.

To this end, we have selected our authors very carefully, so that their combined efforts will give readers a survey of the entire range of empirically based theories of hypnosis. We are undeniably more sympathetic to the theoretical orientation of some of our authors than to that of a few others; nevertheless, it is our conviction that dialogue and reasoned debate between our colleagues is furthered by an even-handed and definitive treatment of all prominent theories in one book.

As in the Fromm and Shor volume, we have tried to enhance the usability of this present book by gathering all references into one large bibliography at the end of the book, instead of in separate reference sections at the end of each chapter. The readers of the earlier volume have commented on how helpful it was to have a single listing well suited as a reliable reference and a scholarly tool.

Our book is definitely structured and formatted with the research investigator in mind—both the seasoned veteran and the newcomer to the field. For the veteran, we hope that our chapters on theoretical paradigms and programmatic research are informative and challenging. For the young and aspiring researcher, we intend this book to be a hands-on tool, providing the conceptual underpinnings, methodological perspectives, and scholarly documentation necessary to begin disciplined investigation.

But we remind the reader that both of us coeditors and many chapter authors are clinicians. It still is especially true in hypnosis that clinicians continue to pose many of the most interesting and complex questions facing the field. We hope that clinicians will profitably seek answers or guidelines for their own work among all the chapters in our book, in the best tradition of science's informing practice. Certainly clinicians will find the chapters on ego psychology, psychological regression, memory, and clinical efficacy quite relevant.

ERIKA FROMM
MICHAEL R. NASH

Contents

PART THREE
Surveys of Broad Areas

A Conceptual Analysis of Hypnotic Responsiveness: Experience, Individual Differences, and Context

ERIK Z. WOODY
KENNETH S. BOWERS
JONATHAN M. OAKMAN

Theories usually succeed by leaving out a great deal—namely, all those phenomena that seem at the time to be "inessential." Indeed, Lewis Carroll once satirized the objective of seeking a truly thorough theory by likening it to an idealized map:

> "We actually made a map of the country, on the scale of *a mile to the mile!*"
> "Have you used it much?" I enquired.
> "It has never been spread out, yet," said Mein Herr: "the farmers objected: they said it would cover the whole country, and shut out the sunlight! So we now use the country itself, as its own map, and I assure you it does nearly as well." (Carroll, 1893/1989, pp. 556–557)

Although there is as yet no 1:1 map of the realm of hypnosis, there are two widely employed, contrasting, incomplete maps—the social-psychological and special-trait theories. Most recent writing in hypnosis has proceeded by fitting one or the other of them to data in a forceful "top-down" fashion, such that the preferred explanation has had clear priority over observation. There is nothing wrong with this approach, which has been carried out very persuasively in the past, and which doubtless finds expression in some of the other chapters of the present book.

However, here our aim is somewhat different: It is, as it were, to "use the country itself, as its own map." Specifically, in our discussion of theoretical issues in hypnosis research, we want to take more of a "bottom-up" approach—one that begins by reasserting the basic interest of some of the observed phenomena, lawless and perplexing as they may seem at times, and then works upward by reconsidering some of the problems of fitting *any* kind of theoretical explanation to them. Eventually, of course, we will arrive "at the top" with the two prominent theoretical perspectives, but we hope that we will have illuminated them from a novel angle, thereby providing some fresh insights.

Three Crucial Kinds of Phenomena in Hypnosis

Things that are easy to explain are usually not very interesting, and the fact that hypnosis is quite intriguing to most people suggests that much about it seems to fall outside of our everyday explanations of behavior. In particular, there are three kinds of phenomena in hypnosis that seem to capture much of its intrigue and, as well, seem to us to provide its principal explanatory challenges; each of them is introduced briefly below.

First, what is striking about hypnosis is usually not its effect on overt behavior. Despite occasional claims to the contrary, hypnotized subjects do not leap over tall buildings at a single bound, run faster than a speeding bullet, or anything like that (Orne, 1977). Rather, even when the overt behavior of hypnotized subjects is impressive—as, for example, when a subject wrinkles his or her brows and stammers over a suggested "negative hallucination"—it is because the behavior suggests a striking and unusual alteration in subjective experience (Orne, 1966).

The chief problem with experiential alterations is not that they are somehow less important than changes in things that may be overtly observed. Indeed, William James (1896/1979, pp. 108–109) engagingly argued just the opposite: "Whence this piece of matter comes and whither that one goes, what difference ought that to make to the nature of things, except so far as with the comings and goings our wonderful inward conscious harvest may be reaped?" Rather, the issue is that to index much of the most germane parts of this subjective realm, we seem forced to rely on subjects' verbal self-reports of their experience. The problem of how to construe these verbal reports is unfortunately quite vexing, as we shall soon see.

Second, a widely accepted and critically important observation about hypnosis is that some subjects seem to be far more capable hypnotic subjects than others. Indeed, it is not too much of an exaggeration to claim that individual differences in hypnotizability have come to serve as the axle around which turns the entire modern enterprise of hypnosis research. Specifically, a study of hypnosis that takes no account of such individual differences has become nearly inconceivable. Nonetheless, attempting to explain what these individual differences may represent raises a host of as yet only very partially solved problems. For example, are highly responsive hypnotic subjects different from their less responsive counterparts in one way or in several? Are highly responsive subjects all achieving suggested effects via the same mechanism or via different ones? Is it some kind of ability that is central, or some other sort of propensity?

Third, the hypnotic circumstance or context itself seems crucial for eliciting hypnotic responses. This circumstance usually consists of explicitly labeling the situation as "hypnosis" and administering some kind of formal or semiformal induction. To the layperson, whether subject or observer, the effects of such an induction ritual can sometimes seem little short of magical. Why these preliminaries seem to have such potency is not at all self-evident, and attempts to explain the effect of such contextual factors on the expression of hypnotic ability quickly run into formidable interpretive ambiguities. For example, how could we hope to reconcile the phenomenon of "waking suggestibility" (hypnotic-like responsiveness in the absence of any formal induction) with the fact that, if there is no hint that hypnosis is investigatively relevant, suggested effects may not occur (e.g., Weitzenhoffer, Gough, & Landes, 1959)? Are large context effects inconsistent with certain trait- and ability-like explanations of hypnotic responsiveness? And so forth.

Let us turn now to a more detailed account of how each of these kinds of phenomena poses problems for explanation—problems we might characterize as lying at a "middle level," between the basic phenomena themselves and the high-level theoretical perspectives that characterize current research.

Introspective Reports of Hypnotic Phenomena

The first issue to be addressed concerns the nature of various self-reported hypnotic experiences and their relationship to one another. In particular, we examine the relationship among reports of three distinct kinds: (1) reports that demonstrate or express a suggested effect (e.g., analgesia, amnesia, hallucinations); (2) reports of nonvolitional experiences that regularly accompany hypnotically suggested effects; and (3) reports of various cognitive images, fantasies, and the like that often accompany (and may help engender) suggested effects. For example, a hypnotized subject may report reduced sensitivity to a normally painful stimulus, feelings that this attenuation is taking place "by itself" without any volitional effort, and accompanying fantasies and images. How might we go about making sense of such a complex set of self-reports?

First, reports of hypnotic experience are subject to the general limitations of introspective reports. These limitations have been especially well addressed by Nisbett and Wilson (1977), K. S. Bowers (1984a), and Lyons (1986). Essentially, what is common to these critical accounts is this: *There is a fundamental difference between reports of experience on the one hand, and understanding of how reported experiences are produced on the other.* In other words, introspective reports are not direct readouts of the underlying cognitive–environmental causes of one's reported experience. A sensible account of one's experience needs to be informed by some understanding of how the mind works, and by a sophisticated appreciation of how various influences can subtly and even unconsciously determine thought, feeling and behavior (K. S. Bowers, 1984a,b, 1987a,b). Whether an account of a specific behavior or experience has some claim to validity thus depends on the sophistication of one's theory of mind and behavior. This is as true for first-person attempts to account for one's own behavior and experience as it is for attempts to understand the behavior and reported experience of another person. As Lyons (1986) puts it,

> If, for various reasons, someone else's account of my cognitive activities is based on a better model than mine or on a better interpretation of the modeling—which is not merely conceivable in respect of all of us but highly likely if I am a child or just poor at such perceptual model building and interpreting— then he or she is in a position to correct my report of my cognitive activity. (p. 132)

Reports of "Raw Feels"

This model of introspection implies a distinction between one's subjective experience—what Feigl (1958) called "raw feels"—and an informed interpretation of this raw experience. *I* am the expert on where the pain is in my stomach, whether it is a deep ache or a sharp pain, whether it is unremitting or intermittent, and so forth. My physician, by virtue of training and experience, is in a much better position to provide a valid account of the pain—whether it is due to appendicitis, gallstones, peritonitis, ulcers—and how best to treat it. Similarly, a psychologist can presumably provide a more valid account of specific sensations, perceptions, emotions, and so on (as revealed in first-person accounts of them) than can the relatively unsophisticated person who reports these experiences.

However, there can often be profound differences in the theoretical position of various psychologists regarding subjective experiences (e.g., associationistic and gestalt interpretation of the "Aha!" experience in problem solving; K. S. Bowers, Regehr, Balthazard, & Parker, 1990)—and so it is in the realm of hypnosis. To illustrate, a skeptical understanding of hypnotic analgesia for many years implied that in reports of attenuated pain, surgical patients simply falsified their actual experience (G. Rosen, 1946; T. X. Barber, 1963; cf. Perry & Laurence, 1983a). This claim was buttressed by the fact that physiological indices often continued to register the occurrence of a painful stimulus, even though subjects reported a much reduced experience of pain (T. X. Barber & Hahn, 1962; Sutcliffe, 1961). However, the *experience* of pain and its psychophysiological concomitants are not one and the same thing; thus, the fact that physiological responses to painful stimuli often persist in the face of hypnotically suggested reductions in pain (e.g., Halliday & Mason, 1964b; E. R. Hilgard, 1969) does not necessarily mean that the analgesia is faked. The attenuation of pain may simply occur *after* physiological indices have registered the presence of an (ordinarily) painful stimulus. Moreover, there is growing evidence that various indices of brain activity are in fact responsive to the suggested state of affairs, such as negative hallucinations (D. Spiegel, Cutcomb, Ren, & Pribram, 1985; D. Spiegel, 1989).

Over the last 20 years, there has been a growing consensus that even though hypnotized subjects could intentionally misreport their internal experience, they are unlikely to do so—barring some special reason or motivation to malinger (K. S. Bowers, 1983; E. R. Hilgard, 1969). This consensus has emerged despite T. X. Barber's (1963, 1970) claim that suggestions for hypnotic analgesia, for example, motivate people to under report their experience of pain in order to please the hypnotist/clinician (see also Wagstaff, 1981a, 1986). For the most part, however, even investigators who are otherwise skeptical about traditional views of hypnosis now argue that hypnotically suggested effects represent genuine alterations in perception. For example, Spanos (1987) asserts that "the controversies in this area are not about whether hypnotic phenomena exist or are 'real.' Instead, they revolve around disagreement about the most useful ways of conceptualizing these phenomena and about which variables are thought to mediate hypnotic responding" (p. 778). Our hunch is that the success of other, nonhypnotic but psychological procedures for reducing pain (see, e.g., Turk, Meichenbaum, & Genest, 1983; Zimbardo, Cohen, Weisenberg, Dworkin, & Firestone, 1969) has made hypnotic analgesia—and other hypnotically suggested phenomena, such as amnesia, hallucinations, and so on—more credible.

In general, then, current investigators of hypnosis tend to view first-person direct reports of "raw feels" as correspondent to internal experience, unless there is some extrahypnotic reason to question the honesty or motives of the subject (see, e.g., Orne, Dinges, & Orne, 1984). Thus, the "expert status" of hypnotized subjects who report suggested alterations in pain, visual and auditory experience, memory, and so forth, is more or less intact; however, their expert status regarding how these suggested alterations come about is very much in doubt, and properly so. Accordingly, the fact that hypnotized subjects typically report that suggested effects are experienced as nonvolitional, or that they are accompanied by various imaginings or cognitive strategies, does not automatically imply that the behaviors in question are truly nonvolitional on the one hand or strategically enacted on the other. Just where the truth lies on these matters is something to be thrashed out among investigators of hypnosis. So it is to reports of nonvolition and of various imaginings and related cognitive strategies that we now turn.

Reports of Nonvolitional Experience and of Cognitive Strategies

According to Weitzenhoffer (1978, 1980), the "classic suggestion effect" is the transformation of a suggested idea into a suggested effect that is experienced as nonvolitional. A classic suggestion effect is exemplified when hypnotized subjects receive suggestions for their extended hands to approach each other more and more closely as if they were magnets, and then experience their hands coming together "by themselves"—that is, without the usual experience of initiative or intention. Although this experience of nonvolition is by no means an invariant feature of hypnotically suggested responses (Spanos, Rivers, & Ross, 1977; K. S. Bowers, 1981; P. G. Bowers, 1982), it is sufficiently characteristic that the Stanford Hypnotic Susceptibility Scales, Forms A and C (SHSS:A and SHSS:C; Weitzenhoffer & Hilgard, 1959, 1962), have been criticized for not specifically assessing the experience of nonvolition (Spanos, Salas, Menary, & Brett, 1986; Weitzenhoffer, 1989). The fact that hypnotic responses are frequently experienced nonvolitionally has often been viewed as indexing an alteration in the underlying control processes by which the hypnotic response is generated (E. R. Hilgard, 1977a; K. S. Bowers, 1991a; K. S. Bowers & Davidson, 1991), but others have strongly contested this view (Spanos, Cobb, & Gorassini, 1985; Lynn, Rhue, & Weekes, 1990) in ways that we examine later.

The other frequent accompaniments of hypnotically suggested responses are subjects' reports of various fantasies, images, and related cognitions that seem consistent with and conducive to the production of the suggested state of affairs. Accordingly, when hypnotized subjects report that their outstretched hands feel as though they are attracted to each other like magnets, the strong implication is that the hands came together *because* of the associated imagery. Such imagery was dubbed "goal-directed fantasy" (GDF) by Spanos (1971), who hypothesized that GDFs are an important determinant of successfully enacted suggestions. Although this hypothesis has not been sustained well by subsequent research (e.g., Buckner & Coe, 1977), GDFs do tend to accompany subjects' reports of nonvolitional experience. Consequently, Spanos and others (Lynn, Rhue, & Weekes, 1990) have argued that reports of nonvolition represent not so much an alteration in control processes as a misattribution of active, goal-directed behavior to accompanying GDFs and related mental processes—a misattribution that helps the subject regard the hypnotically enacted behavior as nonvolitional.

Hypnotic patter often implies or explicitly mentions that the experience of nonvolition and the various mental images will subsequently accompany the suggested state of affairs. For instance, the suggestion that a hypnotized subject's outstretched hands will attract each other like magnets includes both an explicit reference to magnets, and an implication that the hands will therefore be attracted to each other automatically—without the subject's volition or initiative. In other words, both the experience of nonvolition and the "hands as magnets" image are suggested along with the specific target behavior. The inclusion of such collateral suggestions in the hypnotic patter doubtless flows from a conviction that they will increase the probability of a successful response to the target suggestion. This assumption may be correct, but it is not validated simply by the suggested co-occurrence of the target behavior, the reported experience of nonvolition, and a magnet fantasy.

The neodissociation and social-psychological models of hypnosis have decidedly different views of how reports of nonvolition and reports of various cognitive events (e.g., images and related coping strategies) relate to the suggested target behavior. People working within the neodissociation model of hypnosis, as proposed and elaborated by E. R. Hilgard (1973b, 1977a), tend to view reports of nonvolition as prima facie evidence that high-level executive initiative and effort are minimally involved in the production of hypnotically suggested behavior. Instead, they assume that hypnotic suggestions more or less directly activate subsystems of control. Insofar as the experience of volition is closely linked with executive initiative and ongoing effort, and insofar as the production of hypnotic responses tends to circumvent the need for such initiative and effort, it is not surprising that hypnotically suggested effects are often experienced and reported as occurring nonvolitionally (K. S. Bowers, 1990, 1991a).

How then do advocates of a neodissociation model regard reports of cognitive imagery and related events that often accompany the hypnotically suggested response? Perhaps the best answer is "somewhat variably and ambivalently, depending on the investigator." Within the ranks of neodissociationists, one can certainly find support for the view that imagery does not simply accompany suggested events, but at least in part mediates them (e.g., E. R. Hilgard, 1977a). Our own views on this matter are elaborated in due course, but we can anticipate a bit by saying that the importance of imagery and related cognitions to the production of hypnotic responding probably varies both within and between persons, depending on a variety of factors (including most prominently the level of hypnotic ability, and the specific suggestion involved). However, we argue that in many cases, the imagery and related cognitive events may simply be suggested experiences that co-occur with but do not mediate the suggested target behavior.

In contrast to the neodissociation model, the social-psychological model of hypnosis regards a host of person and demand variables as entirely sufficient to account for hypnotic responding. The person variables include a variety of factors (i.e., not just imagery or GDF), such as expectations, positive attitudes toward hypnosis, motivations to please the hypnotist, the tendency to view hypnotic suggestions as something to be actively achieved, and so on (Spanos, 1986b). What is *not* required—indeed, is specifically proscribed as an important variable in the production of hypnotic responses—is the "special process" of dissociation.

Given that the social-psychological model views hypnotic responses as actively and purposely achieved, there has to be some way for it to handle the commonplace observation that subjects often report hypnotically suggested effects to be experienced as nonvolitional. As we have already seen, the social-psychological model views these nonvolitional reports as misattributions—as errors in interpreting one's own behavior as nonvolitional when in fact it is strategically enacted, goal-directed behavior. The basis for this misattribution derives from the fact that hypnotized subjects are motivated to respond in accordance with suggestion; since part of the suggestion typically implies that the behavior will be experienced as nonvolitional, and since the suggested behavior can be (falsely) attributed to the accompanying imagery, GDFs, and so on, the subject has a convenient "hook" on which to hang attributions of nonvolition.

What should be stressed at this point is that there is no *a priori* reason to accept strategy reports as valid indicators of how hypnotic responses are generated, while rejecting for this purpose nonvolitional reports. But there is also no *a priori* reason to regard reports of nonvolition as valid indications of how hypnotic responses are achieved, while rejecting for this purpose reports of strategies and other related cognitions. Indeed, as we have already indicated, reports of both kinds—insofar as they represent attempts by hypnotized subjects to explain their own suggested behavior—are subject to the general and very serious limitations of introspection to provide a valid account of behavior and experience. Although the reports of "raw feels" (of reduced pain, of visual alterations, etc.) have the authority of first-person experience, first-person accounts or explanations of these experiences have little or no evidential authority. Nevertheless, it is clear that the neodissociation model of hypnosis is theoretically disposed to invoke nonvolitional reports as evidential, and that the social-psychological model is disposed to invoke reports of strategic enactment in the same way. To reiterate, however, neither preference can be authorized on *a priori* grounds.

The principal way of investigating the relationship between suggested target behaviors on one hand, and reports of cognitive strategies and nonvolition on the other, has been to create various experimental manipulations of the conditions to which subjects of varying hypnotic ability are exposed. Unfortunately, these studies, with their nonmanipulated subject variable (hypnotic ability) and retrospectively reported dependent variables, do not yield causal interpretations that even approach the hypothetical clarity of the classic "true experiment." Spanos has reported a number of such studies concerned with hypnotic analgesia (e.g., Spanos, Hodgins, Stam, & Gwynn, 1984; Stam & Spanos, 1980; Spanos, Kennedy, & Gwynn, 1984), and has regularly found that the extent of cognitive coping as retrospectively reported seems to covary with the degree of pain reduction. However, subjects also indicate that their responses to suggestions occur nonvolitionally (e.g., Spanos, Rivers, & Ross, 1977). In summarizing these two different kinds of findings, Stam and Spanos (1980) ask the following question:

> Is hypnotic responding automatic and nonvolitional, or is it strategic and mediated by subjects' cognitive responses to treatment generated expectations? The answer is that hypnotic responding is often both strategic and automatic—as long as it is understood that terms such as automatic and nonvolitional refer not to a quality of behavior but to an attribution of causality made by subjects about their own behavior. . . . For example, Spanos . . . found that many subjects whose postexperimental testimony indicated the use of coping strategies insisted nonetheless that they had done nothing to reduce pain. Despite engaging in suggestion-induced coping cognitions, these subjects defined their pain reductions as effortless occurrences instead of activities brought about by their own efforts. (p. 760)

Given a commitment to a social-psychological model of hypnosis, nothing could be more sensible than to interpret the results of Spanos's work on hypnotic analgesia in this fashion.

However, it is important to note that when subjects who have been hypnotized report both reduced pain and the use of coping strategies, both effects have for the most part been part and parcel of the initial analgesia suggestion. Hence, the finding that hypnotically analgesic subjects who report the most pain reduction typically report the most use of coping strategies may simply be result of the fact that these are both suggested effects. It does not follow (except from a prior commitment to a social-psychological model of hypnosis) that the suggested pain reduction is mediated by the suggested coping strategies; they can instead be independent, co-occurring responses to suggestion. And of course, the more hypnotizable people are, the more responsive they will be to both suggestions.

However, Spanos also includes nonhypnotic conditions in many of his investigations of analgesia, and in these groups there is typically no correlation between hypnotic ability and the amount of pain reduction. In fact, in these nonhypnotic conditions, low hypnotizables often demonstrate as much pain reduction as high hypnotizables in receipt of hypnotic suggestions for analgesia. Moreover, it is evident that in these nonhypnotic conditions lows report using coping strategies as often as highs do, adding credence to the idea that these coping strategies are what mediate the analgesic effects. There is no question that active attempts to cope with pain are often quite effective; this is the message of an important nonhypnotic literature concerned with cognitive-behavior modification programs of pain control (Turk et al., 1983). Indeed, Spanos has invoked this literature in support of his contention that "analgesia suggestions exert their effects by modifying the cognitions subjects engage in during noxious stimulation (Meichenbaum, 1977)" (Stam & Spanos, 1980, p. 760).

An alternative possibility, however, is that in hypnotic conditions, reduced pain is a specifically suggested effect that results more from dissociative mechanisms than from coping strategies per se. According to this view, the degree of pain reduction and hypnotic ability are correlated because individual differences in the latter are typically important for the magnitude of suggested effects. However, in nonhypnotic interventions, coping strategies doubtless mediate reduced pain, and as much for low as high hypnotizables. The fact that lows in nonhypnotic conditions reduce pain as much by coping strategies as hypnotized highs do in response to suggestions for analgesia is an interesting finding, to be sure, but does not tell against the neodissociation model of *hypnotically* induced analgesia—repeated claims by Spanos to the contrary notwithstanding (e.g., Spanos, Perlini, & Robertson, 1989).

The situation came to a head with the publication of an article by M. E. Miller and Bowers (1986), in which it became evident that cognitive-behavior modification of pain control (in particular, stress inoculation techniques) were not the basis for hypnotic analgesia. They concluded from their findings that

> pain reductions occurring in hypnotic and nonhypnotic treatments are brought about by different means. The use of cognitive strategies and one's hypnotic responsiveness each play a powerful role in the potentiating treatment effects, but they seem to operate quite distinctly and independently from one another. Cognitive strategy use leads to pain reductions only in nonhypnotic treatments, whereas hypnotic ability potentiates pain reduction only in the hypnotic treatment. (p. 12)

Needless to say, Spanos has tendered vigorous objections to this investigation (Nolan & Spanos, 1987; Spanos & Katsanis, 1989). His concerns have been addressed in a recent chapter (K. S. Bowers & Davidson, 1991) and in another study (M. E. Miller & Bowers, 1992). Suffice it to say here that relying entirely on subjects' verbal reports of nonvolition and of various cognitive strategies has not been decisive in discriminating the relative merits of the two major models of hypnosis as they attempt to account for various suggested target behaviors. Indeed, this continuing impasse may be regarded as more or less of a restatement of our argument that introspective reports of suggested effects, of nonvolitional experience, and of various cognitive events (strategies, imaginings, etc.) do not in and of themselves authorize any particular model or explanation of hypnosis.

A rather different approach is possible, however. Rather than tending to regard such verbal reports of nonvolition or of strategy use as valid explanations of the enactment of suggested target behaviors, we might instead view them as first-person reports of "raw feels," thereby giving them the same epistemological status as reports of suggested hallucinations, amnesia, analgesia, and so on. Our job would then be to see how these three different kinds of report relate to one another under various conditions, *within*—as well as across—low, moderate, and high levels of hypnotizability. By looking at the larger patterns of interrelationships so revealed—perhaps, eventually, with structural modeling techniques (e.g., Dwyer, 1983)—we might have a broader basis for developing (rather than simply presuming) a model of hypnosis that provides coherence to the observations.

This strategy may be illustrated, at least in a relatively simple form, by an investigation recently completed at the University of Waterloo. Hughes (1988; see also K. S. Bowers, 1991a), in her doctoral dissertation, examined the impact of neutral and fear imagery on heart rate responding. She chose heart rate as a dependent variable, because it had earlier been shown to index either cognitive effort (Lacey, 1967) or emotional arousal (Bauer & Craighead, 1979), depending on the specific nature of the stimulus conditions. Presumably, under conditions of neutral imagery, heart rate increases over a nonimagery baseline should largely be sensitive to the amount of cognitive effort required to produce the imagery. However, fear imagery might well produce additional heart rate increases, proportional to the amount of emotional reaction engendered by the imagery.

Consider, however, the possibility that the mechanisms underlying the production of hypnotically suggested effects may differ from low to high hypnotizables. Such differences should express themselves in a different pattern of correlates with heart rate change. Suppose, for example, that low hypnotizables have to initiate and effortfully maintain the suggested imagery; then, regardless of whether the imagery is neutral or fearful, heart rate should increase in proportion to the amount of cognitive effort involved in the production of the suggested imagery. Suppose, on the other hand, that high hypnotizables become effortlessly absorbed in imagery that is more or less directly activated by hypnotic suggestion; then heart rate increases should be less an index of cognitive effort required to generate the imagery than of its emotional impact. In that case, only fearful imagery should engender heart rate increases proportional to the amount of experienced fear.

The results were in accordance with this model. Thirty low hypnotizable subjects (scores of 0–4 on a group adaptation of the SHSS:C) demonstrated a positive correlation of heart rate increase with ratings of cognitive effort involved in producing neutral ($r = .52$) and fear ($r = .49$) imagery. The 30 high hypnotizable subjects (scores of 8–12), however, demonstrated a *negative* correlation (–.52) between heart rate increase and ratings of cognitive effort required to produce fear imagery; there was essentially no relationship between these two variables in the neutral-imagery condition. Evidently, for the high hypnotizables, the less cognitive effort involved in producing the imagery, the more heart rate increased. Other analyses suggested that for high hypnotizables, heart rate indicated not cognitive effort involved in producing the imagery, but its emotional impact: The correlation between retrospective fear ratings and heart rate increase was .59 (for low hypnotizables, the correlation was only .11).

All in all, the findings from Hughes's dissertation suggest that relatively low hypnotizable subjects work cognitively to produce the suggested state of affairs, just as the social-psychological model predicts; however, relatively high hypnotizables seem to become effortlessly absorbed in the suggestion-activated imagery, just as the neodissociation model predicts. Such findings begin to suggest that the eventual resolution of the theoretical debate might incorporate both kinds of explanations, but perhaps with each restricted to certain ranges of hypnotic ability. Hence we now turn to a re-examination of the nature and role of these individual differences in hypnotic ability.

Explaining Individual Differences in Hypnotic Responsiveness

The content of hypnosis scales has evolved for a period of over 100 years, and the items comprising these scales are a highly representative sample of a domain that was already established by the late 19th century (Balthazard, 1990). By now, hundreds of empirical studies have made it abundantly clear that summing across the rather heterogeneous items on such scales results in an overall score that is powerfully *predictive* of a wide variety of other hypnotic performances.

However, the task of explanation is more difficult than that of prediction. In explaining why the overall score is predictive, the usual assumption, however implicit, is that the score for the most part represents a person's level on a *single* underlying dimension or construct. Researchers typically label this inferred construct, rather circularly, as "hypnotic susceptibility," "hypnotic ability," or "hypnotizability," and interpret it as if it were the only determinant of the subject's hypnotic performance. This assumption seems necessary because if, on the contrary, researchers were to regard the overall score on hypnosis scales as measuring a grab bag of different but undifferentiated characteristics, then the possibilities for any sort of coherent explanation would appear to be bleak indeed—despite good prediction.

One way of trying to assess whether the hypnosis scales actually do mainly measure just one characteristic is to factor-analyze the items of the scale in question and see if they appear to be unidimensional. Although factor analysis of hypnosis scales raises a number of vexing methodological problems, careful review of this work leads to the conclusion that the domain tapped by these scales is not unidimensional (see Balthazard & Woody, 1985, for a review). There appear to be at least two major, distinct characteristics measured by these scales (cf. Tellegen, 1978–1979).

Balthazard and Woody (1992) have argued that the essential factor-analytic result is a fan-shaped distribution of items in the two-dimensional factor space. The position of an item in this fan or "spectrum" is closely related to the item's difficulty level: The more difficult the item, the higher its correlation with one of the two underlying dimensions of hypnotic ability, and the lower its correlation with the other dimension. The relative contribution of these two dimensions to hypnotic performance thus shifts gradually with item difficulty (as indexed by the proportion of subjects who pass the item); difficult items would be more dependent on one latent characteristic, and easy items more dependent on the other characteristic. Items in the middle range of difficulty would tend to confound the two characteristics.

It is interesting that over the years a number of authors have advanced two-component formulations similar to this one (e.g., E. R. Hilgard, 1977a; Shor, Orne, & O'Connell, 1962; Spanos, Mah, Pawlak, D'Eon, & Ritchie, 1980; Tellegen, 1978–1979; Tellegen & Atkinson, 1976); nonetheless, it does not seem to be widely recognized how much such a pattern complicates the task of explanation. To a considerable extent, researchers tend to invoke a preferred mechanism to explain any and all hypnotic performances, *as if scores at all levels of hypnotic ability represented only the one thing the researcher had in mind.* In addition, once the researcher has taken this step, it appears sensible to believe that there is no "room" in the scores for some other mechanism that competing theories posit. In truth, however, the researcher has no assurance that a favored mechanism is the one that procured the result in question, or that a rival mechanism is ruled out; only the misguided assumption of unidimensionality suggests, wrongly, that the explanatory situation is unmuddled.

Perhaps a parallel conceptual example will help clarify this problem. Imagine a test of mathematical ability in which people are given the correct answers to problems, and then asked whether they can solve them. Clearly, such a test would tend to measure two things: To the extent that a subject is being forthright and honest, it would measure mathematical ability; but it might also measure some social-desirability-like characteristic, such as the tendency to claim that one has solved problems that are in fact beyond one's capability. Convincing oneself or others that a problem has actually been solved would perhaps be more feasible with easier items than with the harder ones. If that were the case, social desirability would have more impact on easy items, and its role might be very responsive to situational pressures, such as high motivation to do well. Conversely, mathematical ability would have a purer and more consistent role vis-à-vis hard items.

Now imagine two researchers, both thinking unidimensionally, but with opposing theoretical views. One researcher, finding that scores on the test are highly reactive to situational pressures, concludes that the test does not measure *any* ability per se. It is only a short step beyond this, if all such tests happened to be of this nature, to assert that mathematical ability does not exist! The other researcher, finding that the scores are reasonably predictive of other ability-based performances, cannot imagine what the first researcher is fussing about—and concludes that his or her point must perforce be very trivial. Yet it is actually such a major confound that such a test of mathematical ability would probably be regarded as having rather little validity.

Unfortunately, hypnosis scales are rather like this hypothetical test, in that hypnosis items inescapably suggest their own "correct" responses. And by assuming unidimensionality in such a test, hypnosis researchers may readily be led astray in their theoretical inferences, rather like our two hypothetical researchers.

Some Consequences of Multidimensionality in Hypnotic Performance

In the hypothetical test we have used as an example, the obvious solution is to change the item format so as to eliminate the role of the nonability component. This is readily done by presenting the math problem without its accompanying solution. However, there is reason to believe that matters are not so simply resolved in the assessment of hypnotic ability. First, it is difficult to imagine how one could "purify" hypnosis items so as to give hypnotic suggestions without clearly suggesting what the "correct" performances are. Second, if we accept the idea that the items of the hypnosis scales are a highly representative sampling of the classically appropriate domain, then the spectral or fan-shaped pattern of these items in the factor space indicates that in most hypnotic performances, the two latent characteristics are in some way inherently mixed together or confounded. Only the very hardest and the very easiest items approach being factor-pure. In other words, over a broad range of scores, hypnotic performance itself would appear to be intrinsically complex.

The breadth of the spectral or fan-shaped pattern of items in the factor space implies that no one theoretical view or hypothesized mechanism is likely to explain the whole spectrum. Indeed, items at the two extreme ends of the spectrum are nearly uncorrelated (Balthazard & Woody, 1989)—*even though each item of the scale correlates well with the entire scale, minus the item* (E. R. Hilgard, 1965a, p. 216). It seems quite likely that researchers of different theoretical persuasions have been exploring and working at explaining different parts of the spectrum: The social-psychological theorists have been examining the relatively easy-performance range, and the special-trait theorists the difficult-performance range (Balthazard & Woody, 1992). The spectrum is certainly wide enough to accommodate two such different views of underlying mechanism, and an understanding of performances on the middle-difficulty items may well require a simultaneous consideration of both mechanisms.

Unfortunately, as optimistic as the foregoing rapprochement sounds, the multidimensionality of the hypnosis scales still poses some serious problems for the interpretation of research. In particular, how does a researcher know which kind of underlying mechanism was responsible for a given result? The scores earned on a standardized scale of hypnotic ability offers no such discrimination. For example, the true underlying nature of some social-psychological studies of hypnosis, which manipulate expectancies and the like, may actually be quite indeterminate. Many expectancies, beliefs, and implicit or explicit ideas or demands could in fact influence hypnotic performance in the manner proposed by special-trait theorists. That is, such information may be received and acted upon *qua* suggestion, despite the fact that neither the hypnotist nor the subject realizes it. This is the implication of Mesmer's crises, which were not explicitly suggested, but which surely were implicitly anticipated by par-ticipants in his treatment. It is also the implication of Orne's (1959) classic demonstration of dominant-arm catelepsy, which demonstrated how mis-information regarding such catelepsy could, on a subsequent occasion, engender a suggested response of catelepsy (K. S. Bowers, 1984b). Neither does the special-trait camp escape from this dilemma of interpretative indeterminacy. Spanos, for instance, has shown considerable resourceful-ness in reinterpreting "neodissociationist" findings in terms of various social-psychological influences (expectation, compliance to experimental demands, etc.). Thus, the social-psychological position has had notable success in showing how reports of nonvolitional experience are subject to various instructional manipulations (e.g., Spanos, 1986b; Lynn, Rhue, & Weekes, 1990).

In sum, we are arguing that the success of each theoretical camp in reinterpreting the preferred observations of the other camp is largely a result of the interpretive indeterminacy engendered by the multi-dimensional nature of hypnosis scales. In other words, subjects' total scores on a hypnosis scale cannot unequivocally specify whether a "true" ability or some other kind of more socially oriented propensity is responsi-ble for the results.

Our consideration of the spectral pattern of multidimensionality in hypnosis scales has thus indicated three things: (1) This multidimensionality might well be considered an intrinsic property of a wide range of hypnotic performances, rather than some readily curable artifact; (2) there is "room" in the spectrum for at least two quite different views of underlying mechanism, and indeed the spectrum is wide enough that it is improbable that any one theoretical view would take in its full sweep; and (3) this multidimensionality generates an interpretative indeterminacy that readily permits findings to be understood in terms of a favored underlying mechanism.

Does Two plus Two Equal Four? Or Two? Or Six? How Two Latent Characteristics Might Act Together

Given that hypnosis scales tap more than one latent characteristic, how might these latent characteristics together engender hypnotic performances? For purposes of illustration, let us assume the model outlined above, in which a latent attribute allied with social-psychological effects is particularly associated with the easy range of performances, and a latent attribute allied with absorption/dissociation-based effects is particularly associated with the difficult range of performances (cf. Balthazard & Woody, 1992; Shor et al., 1962; Tellegen, 1978–1979; Nadon, Laurence, & Perry, 1987). This is clearly the sort of possibility that Kihlstrom (1985a) has in mind when he argues that

> the behavior of hypnotic "virtuosos," who make extreme scores on the scales of hypnotic susceptibility, may best be analyzed in terms of underlying dissociative changes in the cognitive system. For the remainder (arguably the greater portion of the population at large), it may be more profitable to focus on the cognitive strategies that they deploy to construct responses to hypnotic suggestions, and the situation factors that lead them to do so. (p. 409)

Consider, however, moderately high scorers on a hypnosis scale; the same overall score may be obtained by individuals with rather different latent profiles. The performance of some of these individuals may solely reflect a high level of the latent "special-trait" attribute, and a low level of the other attribute. Conversely, the performance of other moderately high scorers may solely reflect a high level of the latent "social-psychological" attribute, and a low level of the special-trait attribute. Already, the lesson here is that unless the cutoff score for a group of high hypnotizables is set very high indeed, the researcher would wind up with a grab bag of at least two quite different kinds of subjects, the happenstance proportions of which could play havoc with attempts to replicate either dissociative or social-psychological effects.

However, the situation may be even more complex than this. Among the moderately high scorers may be subjects whose performance reflects a combination of at least moderate levels of *both* attributes, and we are faced with the interesting problem of how these two attributes might work together. One possibility is that the two are simply additive: They both aid in the production of hypnotic performances, but in a way that is not more than the simple sum of their parts. Or the two attributes might interact in the statistical sense, giving us two additional possibilities. Their combined effect may be synergistic—that is, each potentiating the other and yielding more than the simple sum of their respective parts. In this case, really high performers would tend to be at least moderately high in levels of both the latent attributes, so that someone with just moderate levels of both attributes might be expected to perform better than those high in one but low in the other. On the other hand, the combined effect of the two attributes might instead be disjunctive, in which case being high on both yields no better performance than being high on either one. For example, suggestions might be enacted via either one mechanism *or* the other, but not both at the same time.

These three models of performance—additive, synergistic, and disjunctive—would clearly have quite different implications for our explanation of hypnotic performance. It is the additive model that is generally presumed (cf. Tellegen, 1978–1979). This model suggests that socialpsychological and special-trait effects are in principle separable, but in practice, on hypnosis scales, simultaneously coexisting. By contrast, the synergistic model would suggest that the essence of hypnotic performance may inhere in the holistic combination of the two kinds of mechanisms. Finally, the disjunctive model would suggest that a substantial proportion of subjects—namely, those possessing at least moderate levels of both attributes—can enact a given suggestion in either a social-psychological fashion or a dissociative one, depending, presumably, on situational factors. (Examples of other conceptual schemes that suggest nonadditive models of hypnotic performance are provided in Balthazard & Woody, 1985.)

Unfortunately, just as scores on a hypnosis scale do not specify the underlying mechanisms that produced them, neither do they allow us to track down how these mechanisms work together. Although nonadditive models can be pursued readily enough with multiple regression, their evaluation would most likely require unconfounded measures of the two latent characteristics. However, this requirement may well necessitate obtaining such measures outside of the classical hypnotic context. But if we had ready access to unconfounded measures of these latent characteristics, surely we would have solved long ago the problem of what mechanisms in what proportions produce specific hypnotic effects. So the question remains: How can we proceed with the task of explaining hypnotic behavior with hypnosis scales that seem inseparably multidimensional?

Possible Methods for Advancing Our Understanding of Individual Differences

Having raised so many problems that complicate the task of explaining what underlies individual differences in hypnotic responsiveness, we here wish to suggest two possible approaches for moving beyond what may presently seem to be an impasse. We do so by raising two new considerations: (1) The items of the hypnosis scales may contain useful information about individual differences that is concealed by the overall score; and (2) it may be productive to put somewhat more reliance on what has been called a "result-centered" strategy of research (Greenwald, Pratkanis, Leippe, & Baumgardner, 1986).

Putting Items to Work: Spectral Analysis

Given that the total score on hypnosis scales fails to distinguish the various individual-difference components that may underlie performance, it seems attractive to try some less aggregated analysis. However, interpreting correlations of a variable with individual items appears distinctly problematic on the face of it, because such analyses would be confounded with item difficulty level; in addition, even individual items would still tend to involve blends of the two (or more) latent attributes (i.e., the items, for the most part, are not at all factor-pure). To deal with these problems, Balthazard and Woody (1992) have proposed a method they call "spectral analysis."

This method, capitalizing on the spectrum notion discussed earlier, is essentially a systematic way of investigating whether an external variable correlates differently with hypnotic performance at different levels of performance. One looks for a consistent pattern in the latent (biserial) correlations between such an external variable and individual hypnosis items when these items are arranged according to their position in the spectrum, which is indicated by item difficulty. From differential patterns of correlation, one may be able to make inferences about the mechanisms underlying a particular range of performances—namely, the range that yields elevated latent correlations with the external variable.

Using this technique, Balthazard and Woody (1992) were able to show that the Absorption Scale of Tellegen (1980) is differentially related to the hardest hypnotic performances, indicating that absorption is closely allied with what has been termed "true" hypnotic responsiveness. Indeed, they went so far as to suggest, only a little facetiously, "that if one wants to measure true 'hypnotic susceptibility,' one might be better off using the absorption scale than one of the standard hypnosis scales." Interestingly, in a precocious adoption of this recommendation, Isaacs (1982) selected the 10 of 102 subjects who scored 8–10 on a shortened, 10-item version of the SHSS:C, and then used absorption as "the best measure of the remaining variation in hypnotic responsiveness" (p. 139). He found a correlation of .89 between absorption and imagery vividness—dramatically higher than the .46 correlation between these two variables found across the entire range of hypnotic ability.

Athough they were not guided by the more sophisticated spectral analysis suggested by Balthazard and Woody, several earlier reports showed findings broadly consistent with its intent (viz., a higher correlation of hypnotic ability with external variables for high hypnotizable subjects than for subjects across the entire range of hypnotic ability, or for subjects low in hypnotic ability. For example, K. S. Bowers (1971) found that in women (but not in men), scores of 7 and above on the SHSS:C (Weitzenhoffer & Hilgard, 1962) correlated .55 ($p < .01$) with a composite measure of creativity test performance; however, across the entire range of hypnotic ability, the correlation was only .25 (n.s.). In the same study, correlations between hypnotic ability (as assessed on the Harvard Group Scale of Hypnotic Susceptibility; Shor & Orne, 1962) and the intensity of unusual experiences in everyday life (as assessed on Shor's [1960] Personal Experiences Questionnaire, or PEQ) increased dramatically from low (less than 0) to moderate (about .40) to high (.63) in women low, moderate, and high in hypnotizability, respectively (see K. S. Bowers, 1971, Figure 1). Similarly, Shor et al. (1962) showed that among eight high hypnotizable subjects, the correlation between hypnotic ability and PEQ scores was .84, though across the entire range of hypnotic ability, the correlation was only .44. Notice that in all these cases, restricting the range of hypnotic ability to the very highest scorers should have *decreased* the size of correlations if hypnotic ability were in fact unidimensional. The fact that correlations increased within the restricted range of highly hypnotizable subjects is basically consistent with what has already been implied by several considerations—that people who achieve high hypnotic ability scores simply tend to be arrayed on a different dimension than do subjects with low to moderate scores.

Balthazard and Woody (1992) also suggested that spectral analysis might be used to illuminate mechanisms operating in the easier range of hypnotic perfomance, a topic to which we shall return in a moment. Earlier, we have pointed out that further elucidation of the processes in hypnotic performance may require purer indicators of the individual differences underlying these processes, possibly obtained outside the classic hypnotic context. It should be evident that spectral analysis may be a promising technique in the search for such external variables, because the multidimensionality of the hypnosis scales may obscure correlations with the total score.

A More "Result-Centered" Approach

We hope that our earlier discussion of the spectrum of hypnotic performance has made clear why the seemingly implacable opposition of social-
psychological and neodissociationist views has become somewhat stag-
nant, if not counterproductive. In addition, the danger in such a highly
charged atmosphere is of a kind of theory-induced myopia, a problem
addressed in a paper by Greenwald and his colleagues entitled "Under
What Conditions Does Theory Obstruct Research Progress?" These authors make the following comments:

> There is typically a great deal of wasted effort in the competitive resolution of
> an empirical controversy. This inefficiency is largely due to researchers' sup-
> pressed attention to results that did not come out as hoped. The consequence
> is that valuable information—about conditions under which a predicted effect
> fails to occur—is not available to the community of interested researchers.
> (Greenwald et al., 1986, p. 225)

The authors argue that to counteract such theory-driven tendencies, researchers should be actively interested in the conditions that qualify the
generality of their theoretically favored effects, even to the point of seeking
them out. They term this type of research strategy "result-centered."

We need not embrace the totality of the view expressed by Greenwald
and his colleagues to draw a potentially useful inference or two. As they
point out, to progress beyond established theoretical views, it is necessary
to be sensitive to disconfirming data and to look for the limits of generality
of these views. A partial or complete failure to obtain an expected finding
might be profitably regarded not just as a botched study, but rather as a
potentially informative message about as yet unacknowledged complexity.
We would urge researchers to take a close look at those within-cell
heterogeneities, apparently anomalous results, and conditions under
which an expected effect seems not to occur. In these temporary embar-
rassments may lie the future of our understanding, rather than in the
ability to marshal unbroken forces against a current opposing view.

In closing, let us give a brief example to illustrate three themes of this
section: (1) the shift from unidimensional to multidimensional thinking
about individual differences; (2) the use of the items on a hypnosis scale as
a source of information, rather than simply summing them to achieve a
total score; and (3) a "result-centered" approach, in which blemishes in the
overall findings are inspected for their potential informativeness.

One of us, in citing a classic study by Moore (1964), has written that
"hypnotic responsiveness is not the same as conformity, gullibility, per-
suasibility, or other forms of compliance. . . . These forms of compliance
. . . simply lie outside the domain of hypnosis" (K. S. Bowers, 1976/1983, p.
86). First, it is worth noting that this rather hard-line position (compared,
say, to that of Tellegen, 1978–1979) is eminently sensible if one is

at least implicitly assuming a unidimensional conception of hypnotic susceptibility. That is, if hypnotic susceptibility is all *one* thing, it had better not be the "wrong" thing; and correlations indicating otherwise would need to be very compelling in magnitude. However, if we adopt a multi-dimensional conception of what the hypnosis scales measure, there is room for a possibly modest correlation of a compliance-like measure with the hypnosis scales to be informative, rather than troubling.

Now if we turn to the Moore paper itself, we can look more closely at results that seem somewhat inconsistent with its own favored special-trait position. We find that one test of "social influencibility" correlated a statistically significant .21 with the total score on the hypnosis scale (the SHSS:A). This degree of relation may seem rather small; nonetheless, it is about the same magnitude as the much-touted correlation of absorption with this hypnosis scale (e.g., Nadon, Hoyt, Register, & Kihlstrom, 1991). But of even more interest are the correlations between social influencibility and some of the items of the SHSS:A. The correlation between the social influencibility measure and the postural-sway item was a whopping .66. When this correlation is disattenuated, to take account of the limited reliabilities of the single hypnosis item and of the social influencibility measure, the resulting correlation is 1.00! In other words, postural sway would appear to be the *same* thing as social influencibility, and thus arguably is not tapping "true" hypnotic responsiveness at all. Similarly, some other easy SHSS:A items appear to have correlated impressively with social influencibility: .37 for the arm rigidity item, and .39 for the hands-moving item.

How can we make sense of item-related results like these, in light of the fact that the correlation of social influencibility with the total hypnotic ability score is so low ? Here, of course, the notion of spectral analysis readily fits in. Indications are that social influencibility is important in the easy range of hypnotic performance; the total score simply tends to obscure this relation. The social influencibility measure would thus appear to be a promising candidate for a relatively pure indicator of the "social-psychological" component in hypnotic performance. Such an indicator of the low range of hypnotic susceptibility is the counterpart of absorption, which, as mentioned earlier, seems to be a relatively pure indicator of the high range. Together, these indices may be just the kind of measures that we have argued may advance our ability to explain—and not just predict—hypnotic responsiveness. In other words, the measures of social influencibility and absorption are perhaps relatively pure measures of two distinct underlying dimensions of hypnotic ability—and measures that may be relatively free of a hypnotic context, to boot. Finally, these purer measures may offer the possibility of investigating the issues of nonadditivity discussed earlier, and thus of clarifying how multiple components may work together in hypnotic performances.

laboratory (Weitzenhoffer et al., 1959), an attempt was made to evaluate the early physiological view of hypnosis proposed by Braid, to the effect that visual fixation alone induced hypnosis. The laboratory had not yet earned a reputation for investigating hypnosis, so many of the subjects in the experiment had no idea that hypnosis was investigatively relevant. These subjects demonstrated little responsiveness to suggestion even after protracted staring. However, for subjects told that visual fixation was a means of inducing hypnosis, suggestibility was considerably enhanced; indeed, it was similar to the suggestibility attained by the same subjects when they were later hypnotized and administered specific suggestions. Similarly, Barber maintained in his early writing that defining the situation as hypnotic seems crucial to obtaining hypnotic effects (T. X. Barber & Calverley, 1964c).

A series of three studies reported in Rothmar's (1986) doctoral dissertation, conducted at the University of Waterloo, makes this same point with a vengeance. In the first study, subjects were selected who were low, moderate, and high in hypnotic ability as assessed on two standardized scales. These subjects were then called to participate in a study on imagery; no mention was ever made, either on the telephone or upon their arrival in the laboratory, that they had been selected for the study because of their hypnotic ability. Indeed, subjects were led to believe that they had been contacted under the same auspices as other undergraduates participating in various experiments conducted by psychology faculty and graduate students. Furthermore, the experimenter had not been involved in assessment of their hypnotic ability, so a potentially important cue relating subjects' earlier involvement with hypnosis and this first experiment was eliminated. Finally, the experimenter was unaware of subjects' hypnotic ability.

In the actual experiment, subjects were given instructions to vividly imagine various neutral or fear scenes (we focus on the results for the neutral imagery, though the pattern of results was virtually identical for both kinds of imagery). Subjects' heart rate was monitored to see how it responded to imagery, the expectation being that higher hypnotizability would engender higher heart rate change. The rationale for this prediction was based on the previous work of Lacey (1967), who demonstrated that heart rate increased in response to mental work that focused on internal cognitive events and/or reduced the processing of external information. High hypnotizable people tend to become more involved in imagery and fantasy than people who are moderate or low in hypnotic ability (J. R. Hilgard, 1979b), so it seemed reasonable to expect that the higher a person's hypnotic ability, the more heart rate would increase (from a nonimagery baseline). However, this expected result was *not* forthcoming: There was essentially a zero correlation of heart rate increase with hypnotic ability. Thus, in the absence of a hypnotic context, high hypnotic ability was evidently not activated by instructions to become absorbed in imagery.

Nonetheless, when the entire experiment was repeated in a second study, with low, moderate, and high hypnotizable subjects subjected to an actual hypnotic induction and suggestions for neutral imagery, the anticipated relationship between hypnotic ability and heart rate increase did occur ($r = .38$, $p = .01$): The higher the hypnotic ability, the more heart rate increased over a nonimagery baseline. In sum, a hypnotic induction produced the cardiac correlations with hypnotic ability that were completely absent when subjects were unaware of the investigative relevance of hypnosis.

The next question was this: Suppose a similar study were repeated with hypnotically experienced subjects who were selected for their hypnotic ability, and who were informed that hypnosis was investigatively relevant, but who were *not* administered a hypnotic induction? Would a hypnotic context in the absence of a hypnotic induction engender correlations with heart rate increase more like those of the first or the second experiment? This question was examined in a third study, utilizing high and low hypnotizable subjects who had earlier been screened on two standardized scales of hypnotic ability. The hypnotic context was established in two ways: (1) Subjects in the experiment were seen by a person who had been visibly involved in the administration of two standardized scales of hypnotic ability; and (2) when subjects were contacted by telephone to participate in the study, they were "asked to participate in a study on imagery which . . . might or might not involve a hypnotic induction, depending on which group they were assigned to" (Rothmar, 1986, p. 85). Subjects in the experiment were not hypnotized, but were asked to involve themselves in neutral imagery.

The pattern of data in this third study was clearly more like that of the second investigation than that of the first one. For example, the heart rate increase of these high hypnotizables exposed to a hypnotic context with no induction was comparable to the increase demonstrated by *hypnotized* high hypnotizables in the second study; moreover, the high hypnotizables in this final experiment showed a 2.75 times greater increase in heart rate than did highs in the first investigation. Evidently, for high hypnotizable subjects familiar with and experienced in hypnosis, a formal hypnotic induction is not necessary to activate hypnotic potential; however, a hypnotic context is sufficient and its absence insufficient in this regard. On the other hand, low hypnotizables were insensitive to the investigative differences of the three studies: Their heart rate increased to the same relatively small degree, whether they were seen in a hypnosis-free context, in a hypnotic context, or after receiving a hypnotic induction.

Similarly, the importance of subjects' perception of the investigative relevance of hypnosis is also indicated intriguingly in recent findings appearing to indicate that the correlations of hypnotic ability with Tellegen's (1980) Absorption Scale are context-dependent (Council, Kirsch, & Hafner, 1986). In particular, Council and his colleagues found that *only* when the Absorption Scale is administered in a context that conveys its relevance for the *subsequent* assessment of hypnotic ability does the correlation between the two scales emerge; when absorption is assessed in a hypnosis-free context, the correlation disappears. Since the Absorption Scale is the most important and consistent nonhypnotic correlate of the hypnosis scales, this context dependency is rather impressive.

Subsequent research on this context effect has led to a very mixed picture, with some other researchers claiming to corroborate it (e.g., de Groot, Gwynn, & Spanos, 1988) and others claiming to refute it (Nadon, Hoyt, et al., 1991). Research from our own laboratory (E. Z. Woody, Bowers, & Oakman, 1990) has replicated the context effect ($r = .44$ when absorption was assessed in the context of hypnosis, and $r = .04$ when not; the difference between the correlations was significant, $p < .05$). This context effect was found even though absorption was assessed *after* the assessment of hypnotic ability rather than before it—a chronology that reversed the order of assessment employed in the Council et al. (1986) study (the significance of which we return to shortly).

In summary, formal research, like the informal observations presented earlier, indicates that hypnotic performance and its nonhypnotic correlates seem to depend in an important way on subjects' perception that hypnosis is relevant to what they are doing. We turn next to problems in the interpretation of this context sensitivity.

Expectancies and Roles versus Contextualized Traits

Context effects admit of very different explanations, depending on how one views them. First, they lend themselves very readily to interpretation in the light of the social-psychological model. Namely, if subjects are to perform according to their expectancies and understanding of roles in hypnosis, they obviously need to *perceive the situation as hypnosis* in order to know that these particular expectancies and roles are relevant. In this sense, context sensitivity seems absolutely crucial for the social-psychological view. In keeping with this view, subjects unaware of the investigative relevance of hypnosis do not seem to behave hypnotically—and the dependence of hypnotic behaviors on situational cues and demands is closely akin to the logic of research in social psychology generally.

It is at first blush a little more difficult to see how context sensitivity can be squared with the special-trait model. Namely, how can responses that are so context-dependent be indicative of an enduring, bona fide trait? Consider, however, an analogy to a recent game called "Pictionary," in which one player is given a word and makes a drawing, in response to which a second player attempts to guess the word. The game is time-limited, so drawing is in the service of economy; anything but very crude drawing is simply irrelevant. Imagine that a researcher were to collect these drawings and use them in an attempt to measure artistic ability. In these stick figures and simple diagrams, there would be little evidence of meaningful individual differences in artistic ability. However, if the researcher were to call these same people into the laboratory and give them a very similar task labeled as a test of artistic ability, it is not hard to imagine that impressive individual differences would emerge. Indeed, individual differences in artistic ability might be clearly evident *only* when the task is defined as art.

Perhaps the expression of hypnotic ability is in this sense like the expression of artistic ability, as well as many other abilities; that is, its clear manifestation typically depends on appropriate contexts. As Tellegen (1981) has pointed out, the idea that the expression of a trait should be unaffected by situations is actually a misunderstanding of the trait concept, and the interaction of traits with situations has been argued widely in the domain of personality (K. S. Bowers, 1973b; Ekehammer, 1974; Epstein & O'Brien, 1985). The fact that different people pray in church and cheer at football games does not eradicate their pre-existing individual differences in—for example—honesty, obsessiveness, or paranoia; the conditions for expressing these differences have to be present before they are likely to manifest themselves clearly. To illustrate, an apparently unobserved situation in which people can cheat to some advantage will probably distinguish more from less honest individuals, whereas they may all behave honestly when they know they are being observed. Similarly, the fact that hypnotic responsiveness is context-sensitive is consistent with the notion of hypnotic ability as a trait that, like most other traits, expresses itself only in certain relevant circumstances.

It is certainly possible to quibble about some aspects of both the social-psychological and special-trait explanations of context effects. As just one example, consider our own replication of the context dependency of the correlation between absorption and hypnotic ability, mentioned above (E. Z. Woody et al., 1990). Our ability to get the context effect, even though the Absorption Scale was administered *after* the assessment of hypnotic ability, cast some doubt on the main expectancy-based explanation proposed by Council et al. (1986)—namely, that the relevant expectancies are created in the filling out of the Absorption Scale. However, our study left unmolested the other expectancy-based explanation suggested in their paper—namely, one positing the operation of broad, pre-existing expectancies about absorption and hypnotic ability that engender correlations between them. Generally, it has to be admitted that with these context effects, one finds much the same sort of interpretive indeterminacy that we encountered in considering the evidential status of subjective reports. Effects can be interpreted in quite a protean variety of ways, and one senses the lack of any really decisive encounter of the two models in the respective interpretations.

The Hypnotic Context and the Multidimensionality
of Individual Differences

The idea of multiple components underlying individual differences in hypnotic susceptibility, as discussed earlier, offers an interesting vantage point on context effects, but one that is as yet virtually unexplored. There is the intriguing possibility that the two (or more) component attributes may be differentially affected by contextual factors, such that any particular situational manipulation may principally influence the performance of subjects high in one of these components, and not that of those high in the other component.

Two broad, somewhat contrary possibilities seem worth mentioning in this regard. On one hand, "true highs" (i.e., those passing the most difficult hypnotic suggestions) may be especially responsive to contextual factors. This possibility would seem particularly consistent with a special-trait view—for example, recall the virtuoso with poison oak who seemed unable to make use of his talents without the provision of certain simple contextual information. On the other hand, "highly compliant" subjects (i.e., those who readily pass relatively easy items, but not the most difficult ones) may be highly responsive to other contextual factors—namely, those that provide information about what expectancies and roles are relevant. Of course, it is quite possible that both "true highs" and "highly compliant" subjects may respond discriminatively to hypnotic contexts, but for different reasons, and these contrasting reasons may simply have been confounded in previous work based on total scale scores.

Lest we get carried away with this general picture of rather pervasive context dependence, it is interesting to point out that there is growing evidence that some people may spontaneously exploit their high capacity for hypnosis in nonhypnotic contexts. For example, S. C. Wilson and Barber (1983a) have shown that extremely highly hypnotizable women are often fantasy-prone in their everyday lives, such that fantasied alternatives to reality are routinely experienced in a fashion described by them "as real as real," and constitute a considerable source of personal satisfaction. As well, there is growing evidence that some forms of psychopathology (e.g., multiple personality disorder) may have their origin in the development of hypnotic-like dissociative skills for defending against chronic, physically inescapable threat (e.g., childhood abuse) (F. W. Putnam, 1989). Indeed, Bliss (1984b) regards multiple personality as a chronic abuse of self-hypnosis. As adults, such people can continue to use more or less indiscriminate and automatic involvement in hypnotic-like fantasies as a way of escaping traumatic memories and currently unpleasant realities (cf. Bliss, 1984b).

Other people may be more discriminating in their expression of high hypnotic ability, choosing to do so only when it is appropriate—for example, when the circumstances explicitly call for hypnosis. Accordingly, one potentially important individual-difference variable may be represented at one end by the automatic elicitation of hypnotic effects by a wide variety of (threatening) circumstances, and at the other end by its more or less volitional evocation by explicitly hypnotic circumstances. Presumably, the more automatic and less context-sensitive hypnotic-like responding is, the more likely it is to be in the service of psychopathology—an intuition that has earlier been forwarded and found vis-à-vis personality traits generally (e.g., Moos, 1970).

Finally, we close this section with a methodological point. The fact that context effects in hypnosis—as revealed especially well in the three Rothmar (1986) studies—are both subtle and pronounced in their impact mandates special procedural cautions. Simply inviting a person who is already familiar with and practiced in hypnosis to participate as a control subject in a hypnosis study may in fact turn the person into an unintended member of the hypnotized group. The last time we ran a study at the University of Waterloo that did not take this possibility into account, we showed no difference between the level of suggested amnesia by hypnotized subjects and that by people who had received task-motivated suggestions to forget (T. M. Davidson & Bowers, 1991). Moreover, the correlation between hypnotic ability and degree of forgetting was equivalent in both groups. This pattern of outcome no doubt depended in part on the fact that subjects had been hypnotized twice in preparation for the amnesia experiment, and were therefore sensitized to the possibility of responding hypnotically even in the absence of an explicit hypnotic induction. In general, careful efforts need to be taken to sanitize the situation of hypnosis for control subjects, so that no hint of a hypnotic context remains that can convert a high-hypnotizable control subject—one practiced and familiar with hypnosis—into an unintended hypnotized subject.

Summary and Conclusions

The rather considerable range of material covered in this chapter may be summarized in the form of a simple mnemonic diagram (see Figure 1.1). At the left corner of the triangle is "experience"—the realm of subjective self-report so essential to hypnosis, which has been discussed in the first part of this chapter. At the lower corner is the realm of individual differences that underlie hypnotic performance, discussed in the second part of the chapter. And at the right corner is "context"—the realm of situational factors that affect the expression of hypnotic responses, as just discussed. The interconnection of the three corners is meant to represent the idea that hypnosis and hypnotic responsiveness inheres in the mutual transaction among these factors.

However, there are several "conceptual angles" associated with each geometric angle of the triangle. In the realm of experience, there are three

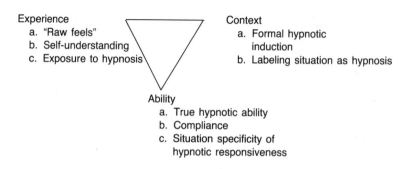

Experience
  a. "Raw feels"
  b. Self-understanding
  c. Exposure to hypnosis

Context
  a. Formal hypnotic
     induction
  b. Labeling situation as hypnosis

Ability
  a. True hypnotic ability
  b. Compliance
  c. Situation specificity of
     hypnotic responsiveness

FIGURE 1.1. The hypnotic triangle.

distinct considerations to keep in mind. First, there are "raw feels"—irreducible elements essential to any meaningful consideration of hypnosis. Indeed, the suggested alteration of experience is the sine qua non of hypnosis, and there is very little serious disagreement among hypnosis investigators about the reality or genuineness of these suggested alterations. Second, there is experience in the sense of self-understanding, including attributions or inferences about one's own mental cause–effect sequences—especially those based on the experience of nonvolition and various cognitive events (images, strategies, etc.) that typically accompany a suggested effect. A great deal of the current dispute between advocates of the neodissociative and the social-psychological views of hypnosis is focused on this issue. Finally, experience also refers to the exposure of subjects to previous hypnotic involvements—both those that are firmly rooted in an explicit hypnotic context, and the self-induced hypnotic-like experiences that characterize the fantasy-prone individual. People who have been exposed to hypnotic-like experiences may require less formal hypnotic procedures to reinduce similar experiences. Indeed, a simple hypnotic context, without a hypnotic induction, is apt to suffice in this regard.

Next is a realm concerned with individual differences in hypnotic responsiveness, which in Figure 1.1 undergirds the other elements, thus representing its pivotal importance for understanding hypnotic responsiveness. It too has several dimensions. First, there is what has been termed "true" hypnotic ability—a dimension that seems particularly associated with absorption and dissociation, and that seems especially represented by the most difficult items of standardized scales of hypnotic ability. A second individual-difference dimension involves the propensity to respond compliantly to social influence—a dimension that may be particularly important for relatively easy items of hypnosis scales, especially when passed by subjects low to moderate in hypnotizability. The tendency for these two dimensions to be inextricably interwoven has generated considerable indeterminacy about how best to conceptualize hypnotic responsiveness. Finally, there may be an important but less noted subsidiary individual-difference variable—represented by the propensity to express one's hypnotic ability in a variety of situations on one hand, or in more situation-specific, explicitly hypnotic contexts on the other. A tendency to express hypnotic responsiveness in a comparatively context-free manner may have implications for psychopathology, especially if the tendency represents a habitual, overdetermined defensive reaction to perceived threat.

The third and last angle to consider is context. Here we must distinguish a formal hypnotic induction (which is surprisingly dispensable under certain circumstances) from the simple labeling of a situation as hypnosis, or as relevant to hypnosis. The labeling of a context as hypnotic (without a hypnotic induction) is a potent contributor to hypnotic responsiveness, especially with highly hypnotizable subjects who have had prior exposure to hypnosis. The context factor can be especially problematic from a methodological point of view. Failure to camouflage the investigative relevance of hypnosis can unwittingly convert a waking, high-hypnotizable control subject—one familiar with and practiced in hypnosis—into a hypnotized subject.

The challenge for future research is to bring these various subcomponents of the "hypnotic triangle" together in meaningful and generative ways, and the chapter has been peppered with suggestions about how this aim might be accomplished. The German philosopher Gadamer made an interesting distinction between a "wrong" question and one that turns out to be answered in the negative: "A wrong question can have no answer, neither false nor true but only wrong, for the answer does not lie in the direction in which the question was asked" (quoted in Palmer, 1969, p. 199). Some of our speculations in this chapter will doubtless turn out to be false, but let us conclude with the hope that the questions we have posed will nonetheless point in the right direction.

CHAPTER TWO

Two Hundred Years of Hypnosis Research: Questions Resolved? Questions Unanswered!

MICHAEL DIXON
JEAN-ROCH LAURENCE

The interest in understanding hypnotic phenomena did not await the advent of contemporary scientific paradigms. It would be as ludicrous to believe such a postulate as it would be to propose that our predecessors knew it all. If such well-known figures as Mesmer, Faria, Liébeault, and even Janet were to come back and reacquaint themselves with the hypnotic literature, whether clinical or experimental, they would probably wonder at the marvelous technological discoveries of the last 40 years; however, they would also probably smile at the constancy of the theoretical conundrum that continues to plague contemporary researchers who seek to explain hypnosis and its related phenomena.[1]

Nevertheless, progress has clearly been made, for certain methodological and statistical developments have allowed us to put to rest some of the most extravagant claims of earlier times. Thus the increased intellectual abilities of Puységur's (1784–1785) somnambulistic patient, or the ability to hear, see, or read with the fingers, toes, or navel documented by Pététin (1787),[2] are no longer the focus of attention of scientific hypnosis. Similarly, the belief that magnetism and hypnosis can be deleterious to the nervous system, or can act as a trigger mechanism for mental disorders, is no longer a serious concern for the contemporary hypnosis practitioner. In addition to these immoderate claims, methodological advances have also laid to rest some of the explanations of hypnotic phenomena that were quite reasonable when considered within the *Zeitgeist* of their era. Magnetic fluids, the spontaneous emergence of analgesia and amnesia upon induction of hypnosis, the increased physical and intellectual abilities of the hypnotized individual, and hypnotizability as an index of a latent hysterical neurosis are all examples of widely held, plausible beliefs about hypnosis that have been proven erroneous by research conducted within the last 50 years.

In reviewing the history of hypnosis research conducted over the last 200 years, it is important to note that our forerunners were not necessarily more naïve than we are, or less gifted observers. In fact, despite the absence of contemporary statistical and methodological weaponry, by the end of the 19th century researchers and clinicians had observed and meticulously described most of the behaviors and experiences seen in hypnotized individuals, and had already espoused most of the contemporary theoretical positions held by current investigators. Debates between opposing factions were fierce, and quite often made the headlines of the written media. Many of those who are today considered to be among the pantheon of early psychological researchers were unable to resist turning their hands toward an explanation of what hypnosis was (Laurence & Perry, 1988).

Even the logic behind contemporary scientific investigations can be found in earlier writings. If Mesmer was incorrect in attributing his clinical and experimental results to the action of a magnetic fluid, he certainly had a point in stating to the Prince-Elector of Bavaria that if he could replicate Gassner's exorcism's results using animal magnetism, it was not necessary to postulate that God (or the Devil, depending upon the behaviors investigated) was doing the work (see Laurence & Perry, 1988). A naturalistic explanation would be sufficient. It is not difficult to recognize the echoes of Mesmer's reasoning in the social-psychological theorists who state that if a behavior or an experience can be demonstrated in a motivated, unhypnotized individual, there is no reason to hypothesize that this behavior or experience is the end result of a specific hypnotic state. Although we have come a long way in our proficiency at demonstrating and testing our assumptions about hypnosis, we should not underestimate the legacy of our predecessors. Nor, as we will see, should we overestimate our own.

Central Issues Then and Now

No matter at which point along the chronological continuum of hypnosis research one chooses to focus, one cannot help being struck by its continuing battle for a scientific status. Mesmer's struggle for recognition is similar to that of the contemporary young researcher striving to put together a research grant on hypnosis that will be acceptable to the scientific jury that will evaluate it![3] The same beliefs, the same preconceptions, the same hesitations still characterize the scientific establishment's position vis-à-vis hypnosis research that were present 200 years ago (E. R. Hilgard, 1971b). Nonetheless, it is to Mesmer that we owe hypnosis's place within the realm of science, for it was his theory of animal magnetism that reclaimed hypnotic phenomena from the penumbra of religion, spiritualism, and magnetic medicine (see Ellenberger 1970; Laurence & Perry, 1988). His brief but significant encounters with Fathers Gassner and Hell succeeded in bringing his movement to the attention of the medical and scientific intelligentsia of the time, as well as to the ordinary physician. Not that Mesmer's theories about the presence of a magnetic fluid pervading the universe were correct, but he certainly was in line with the scientific *Zeitgeist* of his time (for different examples, see Darnton, 1968), and at least for a brief period he established himself as a representative of the Age of Enlightenment.[4]

In addition to the struggle for scientific recognition, another constant factor in hypnosis research from the onset of animal magnetism onward is the continued fascination with two major issues that have intrigued both researchers and clinicians alike. These issues can generally be defined as (1) individual differences in hypnotic responsivity, and (2) the involuntary nature of hypnotic responding.

In terms of the former issue, Laurence and Perry (1988) have pointed out, that what really renders the history of animal magnetism, artificial somnambulism, lucid sleep, nervous sleep, neurypnology, hypnotism, and hypnosis fascinating is the continuous observation of stable individual differences in patients and subjects who undergo an induction procedure. These documented differences not only beg for a scientific explanation, but continue to pit one experimentalist against another in a struggle that is far from being resolved.

Mesmer defined "animal magnetism" not as the magnetic fluid, but as the individual's receptivity to its influence (see Laurence & Perry, 1988; Mesmer, 1779). Mesmer and his followers usually differentiated between the effects attributable to this ability and the more general effect of animal magnetism (see, e.g., Mesmer, 1799). Most of those who have shaped the history of hypnosis not only recognized the major importance of these individual differences in responsivity to suggestions, but also attempted to document them.[5] The Royal Commission of Inquiry led by Benjamin Franklin (Franklin, de Bory, Lavoisier, Bailly, Majault, Sallin, D'Arcet, Guillotin, & Leroy, 1784) was the first to suggest that the behaviors and experiences of the magnetized patient were the end result of three social and/or cognitive factors: imagination, the automatic tendency to imitation found in humans, and sensitivity to the physical touchings of the magnetist. These factors were but the first wave in a host of theories purporting to account for why some individuals were more responsive to suggestions than others. The enigmatic Faria (1819), for example, listed a series of individual differences that he found important in the successful elicitation of "lucid sleep," his way of effecting animal magnetism. For Faria, the important mental attributes possessed by the highly responsive individual were imagination, psychic impressionability, and the ability to restrict attention to some internal or external sensation. Positive beliefs and expectations, as well as a profound confidence in one's ability to experience lucid sleep, were important prerequisites to the activation of these subjective qualities. The rituals surrounding the induction process (the situational components) were considered by Faria to be important contributing factors in the emergence of lucid sleep. Most of these ingredients are still important today,[6] but unfortunately they have been (and still are) all too often ignored, or are investigated in isolation rather than in interaction.

Why such important factors have been so often overlooked can best be understood by looking at the people who were involved with hypnosis. Although certain gifted observers (such as Faria and Mesmer) were cognizant of the importance of individual differences, the majority of hypnosis practitioners were tenacious clinicians, mostly physicians, who struggled to make hypnosis an integral part of the medical armamentarium. For most of them, the sleep-like appearance of the hypnotized subjects, their apparent loss of voluntary control, and (in certain cases) the sensory and perceptual alterations elicited pointed to the physiological origins of magnetism or hypnosis. To have been able to demonstrate such biological roots to such unusual behaviors would not only have been a way of reclaiming hypnosis from the shadows of 18th- and 19th-century mysticism, but would also imply that since humans all share the same biology, individual differences would be of minimal importance. This quest for a physiological model of hypnosis started with Mesmer and continues to this day. Although the technology has changed, what has remained constant is this model's reliance on the conception of hypnosis as a state. Researchers subscribing to this model will therefore talk about the depth of the alleged state achieved by their patients or subjects in a way quite similar to that of a 19th-century research describing the different stages of natural sleep. Depending upon the different suggestions enacted, subjects will be described as experiencing a more or less profound hypnotic sleep in the same way that people can experience a more or less profound sleep. In retrospect, the metaphor of sleep was an unfortunate one, since it led to the tacit acceptance of a hypnotic state per se rather than to the investigation of the abilities underlying the alterations of mood, perceptions, and sensations elicited following a hypnotic induction. This metaphor-driven belief in the "state" of hypnosis has led to an amazing display of physiological research in the last 40 years, once again paralleling the development of medical technology.

Even though Bernheim (1884) stressed that the individual's ability to respond to suggestions in the usual alert state might be crucial in determining hypnotic responsivity, his efforts ultimately failed to focus attention on the importance of individual differences. The alleged state the subject was experiencing at the time of the hypnotic suggestions remained a convenient metaphor on its way to reification. By the end of the 19th century, hypnosis research had largely escaped the attention of European investigators and was solely recognized, if at all, as a clinical tool.[7]

The second important contemporary issue in hypnosis research that has permeated the history of hypnosis involves the concept of nonvolition. We mention it here only briefly, since it is dealt with in more detail later on in this chapter. The subjective report that the hypnotic suggestion is enacted without the subject's conscious and willful participation has been a topic of lively discussion for the last 200 years. It was presented mostly as a moral and legal issue in the early years of animal magnetism; again, Faria was the first one to raise the theoretical conundrum underlying such subjective reports. He wrote in his 1819 book: "Is it not paradoxical to say that we influence our own actions, and that we are not aware of our own influence?" (p. 45). Prior to Faria, practitioners of magnetism did not doubt the physiological effects of the magnetic fluid. After all, how could one doubt the involuntariness of the behaviors and mental states elicited by magnetism, when frogs and canaries could literally be killed by eye fixation alone? Faria explained such a paradox by linking the reports of nonvolition to the subjects' tendency to misattribute the source of their behaviors—an amazingly futuristic explanation at the time. He went even further, stating that for a suggestion to be effective, subjects had to falsely attribute to the operator the power to influence them.

Like reports of differential responsivity to suggestions, reports of nonvolition were to become a characteristic of the successful elicitation of the hypnotic suggestion and, by extension, of the hypnotic sleep. Consequently, few authors sought to answer Faria's question other than via circular reasoning: Subjects report nonvolitional experiences when they are hypnotized, and one knows that subjects are hypnotized because they report nonvolitional experiences.

The observation of the seemingly complete automaticity of response in the highly hypnotizable subject led Liébeault in his 1866 book (followed later on by Bernheim and Liégeois) to describe these subjects as "puppets" in the hands of the hypnotist. This was a quite unfortunate statement, since it would lead to one of the fiercest legal debates surrounding the use of hypnosis in the last 20 years of the 19th century (Laurence & Perry, 1988). It was not, however, a new observation, since Liébeault himself noted that this automaticity of response was linked to the tendency toward imitation found in all humans—a conclusion, as we saw earlier, that the Benjamin Franklin commission had reached in 1784.

The most prominent author (if not the only one) who attempted to tackle this difficult question was Pierre Janet, who would make the investigation of automatisms the basis of his theory of hypnosis, rather than suggestion or suggestibility. This theoretical orientation is best exemplified by his concept of *désagrégation psychologique* seen in some psychopathologies, or the carrying out of a posthypnotic suggestion in the normal individual (Janet, 1889; see also Ellenberger, 1970; Perry & Laurence, 1984; Prévost, 1973). Nonetheless, until the end of the 19th century, and for a good part of the 20th century, these reports of nonvolition were thought to be the end result of some neurological changes happening during hypnosis—an idea that has not been substantiated by contemporary research.

These two major issues, individual differences and the nonvolitional response to hypnotic suggestion, continue to be a major focus of contemporary hypnosis research. Ultimately, if researchers and clinicians alike could finally identify the cognitive, affective, behavioral, and situational factors underlying reports of nonvolition and the ways in which they interact, they would be able to predict *a priori* who will be hypnotizable; they would also be in a better position to understand the multidetermined nature of the hypnotic response.

From Empiricism to Theory-Driven Experimentation

The advent of standardized tests of hypnotic susceptibility in the 1950s marked the beginning of a new era in the experimental investigation of hypnotic phenomena. Scientists employing these tests were finally in a position to empirically validate many of the notions that comprised the scholastic legacy of the 18th- and 19th-century hypnotists. Furthermore, because these tests allowed different laboratories to use a common metric in testing such hypotheses concerning hypnosis, they were able to provide an empirical foundation upon which subsequent hypnosis research could be built. These tests opened up a whole new area of empirical inquiry—the standardized investigation of individual differences in hypnotic susceptibility (for a more detailed look at the measurement of hypnotizability, see Perry, Nadon, & Button, Chapter 17, this volume).

It was over 20 years ago that Fromm and Shor (1972) first documented the amazingly rejuvenating effect that the elaboration of standardized scales of hypnotizability had on the field of hypnosis in the 1950s and 1960s. During this period, many areas of research were beginning to crystallize around new theoretical positions. The nature of hypnosis and its subjective and physiological concomitants, as well as the nature of hypnotizability and hypnotic phenomena, were clearly the central topics of research. Hundreds of papers were published. Almost exclusively, this explosion of research adopted a structural approach to hypnosis, which attempted to demonstrate at all costs that hypnosis was different from the waking state or that certain phenomena elicited during hypnosis were specific to this situation. The plethora of research purporting to support such a position was countered by the research of T. X. Barber (1969) and Sarbin and Coe (1972), whose theories were to severely and dramatically alter the next 20 years, in the same way that Bernheim's demonstrations of the suggested components of Charcot's three stages of hypnosis would lead to a sudden loss of interest in hypnotic research in France.

Whereas the 20 years prior to 1970 saw an outburst of scientific research on hypnosis, the last 20 years have witnessed an amazing shift from a general validation of hypnotic phenomena to a more theory-driven type of experimentation. From hypnosis as a state to hypnosis as a social-psychological phenomenon, hypnotic experimentation has slowly become a means to support one's preferred theory. Researchers currently working in the field of hypnosis still maintain widely divergent views concerning the reasons why some people respond well to hypnotic suggestions while others do not. Although quantitative advances such as analysis of variance (ANOVA) and multiple regression have enhanced the quality of investigations over the last century, research in hypnosis has essentially remained polarized, with separate schools adhering to basically the same theoretical perspectives that were established in the late 19th century. The fundamental principles of these schools of thought have remained virtually unaltered, even though the names have changed. Some of the more recent epithets for these pairs of opposing factions are the "credulous" versus "skeptical" view of hypnosis, and the "social-psychological" versus "special-process" view of hypnosis (see, e.g., Spanos, 1986b; Spanos & Chaves, 1989d).

Although there exist slightly different renditions of the social-psychological interpretation of hypnotic responding, in general this position maintains that the "hypnotized" subject is one who merely reacts to the complex demand characteristics inherent in the hypnotic context. Thus, highly hypnotizable subjects behave in ways that are consistent with their preconceived notions of how a good hypnotic subject is expected to behave. Accordingly, these subjects will use goal-directed strategies designed to produce behaviors that are consonant with the persona of the "good hypnotic subject." That is, rather than actually responding in an involuntary and automatic fashion as suggested by our predecessors, subjects will behave *as if* their responses were involuntary, because such behaviors coincide with their perception of how a hypnotized subject is expected to act (Sarbin, 1984; Spanos, 1986b). As such, the perceptual, sensory, cognitive, and affective alterations that are associated with hypnosis are mere epiphenomena of the social factors embedded in the hypnotic context. Thus, one of the basic premises of the social-psychological position is that there is nothing really special about hypnosis or hypnotic phenomena (Spanos, 1986b). According to this perspective, any behavior that can be elicited in hypnosis can also be elicited outside of hypnosis (Spanos & Chaves, 1989d), and an implicit corollary of this position is that any behavior displayed by highly susceptible subjects can also be elicited from those not capable of experiencing hypnosis, merely by providing the necessary social and cognitive antecedents (Spanos, Cross, Menary, Brett, & de Groh, 1987). This line of reasoning applies both to the observable behavior and to its accompanying subjective response. Individual differences in hypnotizability are thus minimized or sometimes explained away by stating that to the point that subjects are willing to cooperate and go along with a hypnotic role, they will present themselves as mediocre, good, or excellent hypnotic subjects (see Spanos & Chaves, 1989d). That specific individual differences other than attitudes, expectations, and beliefs are linked to differential responses to hypnosis is nonetheless recognized by social-psychological theorists as one of the different ingredients composing the hypnotic response; however, as de Groh (1989) concluded, it may very well be that these individual differences are experimental artifacts created by the method used to induce hypnosis. If we ask subjects to imagine, it may not be too surprising to find that good imagers respond better than bad imagers. Thus, no matter how one looks at it, for social-psychological theorists the emphasis is primarily on the situational as opposed to the dispositional aspects of hypnosis.

A second school of thought, founded primarily by E. R. Hilgard, maintains a very different view of the mechanisms underlying hypnotic behavior. This school of thought, labeled by Spanos as the "special-process view," interprets hypnotic phenomena as reflecting processes that are unique to the hypnotic context and are essentially unrelated to waking behavior. Much of the explanatory power of the special-process view of hypnotic phenomena involves Hilgard's reworking of the concept of dissociation and dissociative abilities proposed earlier by Janet (E. R. Hilgard, 1977a). According to this "neodissociation theory," the structure of cognition consists of a multiplicity of "cognitive subsystems" each of which is capable of carrying out certain specific functions (E. R. Hilgard, 1977a, p. 218). These cognitive subsystems are dominated by what Hilgard has called the "executive ego," a central controlling structure responsible for both planning and monitoring functions—an idea proposed earlier by the psychoanalyst Heinz Hartmann (1939/1958).

Hilgard views hypnosis as a condition in which the normal functioning of the executive ego is temporarily modified so that executive control is divided between the hypnotist and the person being hypnotized (E. R. Hilgard, 1977a, p. 229). In hypnosis, the hypnotized subject turns over some of the functions of the executive ego to the hypnotist. By doing so, the subject allows certain subsystems to be actuated externally by the hypnotist, rather than internally. This external activation creates a unique situation in which the hypnotized subject loses both initiative and the capacity for critical thinking. In this modified condition, certain aspects of the actuated subsystem's activity tend to be dissociated from the resident part of the hypnotized subject's executive ego. Hilgard gives as an example a subject who is told that an extended arm is getting stiffer and stiffer. The subject is able to report, "You said my arm would be stiff and I couldn't bend it; I have tried to bend it and I can't do it." Thus, while certain facets of the situation are monitored, other key elements are dissociated from normal monitoring processes. Among the unmonitored elements is the fact that in trying to bend the arm, rather than merely contracting one set of muscles, the subject voluntarily contracts two antagonistic muscle groups (as occurs when one "makes a muscle"; E. R. Hilgard, 1977a, p. 232). In such a situation rather than regarding the inability to bend the arm as a consequence of his or her own actions, the subject tends to regard the responses to the suggestion as happening "by themselves." Thus, it is because certain facets of the hypnotic response are unavailable to the monitoring aspect of the executive ego that the subject experiences having carried out the hypnotist's instructions in an involuntarily and automatic fashion (E. R. Hilgard, 1977, p. 228). Such a position is quite similar to the one proposed by Faria in 1819. As elegant as Hilgard's rendition of Janet's dissociation theory may be, it is and will remain an exercise in metaphors. Research aimed at substantiating neodissociation theory has at best produced ambiguous results. (see, e.g., the work by Laurence, Perry, and their colleagues on the "hidden-observer" phenomenon: Nadon, D'Eon, McConkey, Laurence, & Perry, 1988; Laurence, Nadon, Nogrady, & Perry, 1986; Laurence, 1984; Laurence, Perry, & Kihlstrom, 1983; Nogrady, McConkey, Laurence, & Perry, 1983; Laurence, & Perry, 1981; Spanos, 1986b).

Thus, whereas the social-psychological position postulates that hypnotic phenomena are the end result of subjects using goal-directed strategies to appear hypnotized, the neodissociation position holds that hypnosis is a condition in which normal cognitive functioning is actually modified. Over the last two decades, these two opposing schools of thought have conducted a plethora of theory-driven experimentation designed to produce data that support one or the other theoretical position. Most often the sequence of events has involved "special-process" researchers' empirically demonstrating hypnotic phenomena (amnesia, analgesia, posthypnotic responses), followed by social-psychological theorists' either demonstrating that similar behaviors can be elicited by means that do not involve hypnosis, or showing that subjects who are incapable of experiencing hypnosis can still demonstrate hypnotic behavior when given "appropriate" instructions. As Nadon, Laurence, and Perry (1991) have noted, this polarization of the field has so tainted the methodologies and the statistical interpretations of these experiments that it is currently impossible to sit comfortably in either of the two camps.

A sampling of studies involving hypnotically induced amnesia provides a good example of this pattern. The first stage was to have both schools agree on the ground rules—that hypnotic amnesia involves the failure to recall items relevant to an amnesic suggestion, as well as the reversal of this amnesia upon being given a cancellation cue (e.g., "Now you can remember everything.") Using this criterion, a number of so-called "special-process" investigators have shown a positive correlation between hypnotic susceptibility and the degree of amnesia demonstrated by subjects (e.g., E. R. Hilgard & Cooper, 1965: Kihlstrom & Evans, 1979a). These authors used these correlations to support the theory that highly hypnotizable subjects were able to cognitively dissociate the material that was to be forgotten, effectively making it inaccessible to conscious awareness until the administration of the cancellation cue.

While "special-process" researchers were devising experiments purporting to demonstrate the ability of some subjects to erect "amnesic barriers" (E. R. Hilgard, 1977a) social-psychological theorists were busy devising their own theory-driven experiments designed to show that amnesia results from nothing more than subjects' voluntarily using strategies to direct their attention away from the material for which they are supposed to be amnesic. For example, in the crucial condition of Spanos and de Groh (1984), subjects of high and low hypnotizability ("highs" and "lows") were neither hypnotized nor given amnesic instructions. Instead, these subjects were given direct instructions about how to focus attention away from target items. Armed with such instructions, both highs and lows performed in a fashion similar to that of highs who in a separate condition had been hypnotized and given amnesic instructions. On the basis of such a finding, and the logic of equivalence, the social-psychological theorists argued that if "amnesic" behavior can be produced using goal-directed strategies, then there is no need to postulate more complicated constructs such as "amnesic barriers" or dissociation between different aspects of memory.[8]

Such a pattern of theory-driven research has been played out time and time again in regard to all manner of hypnotic phenomena. Although the special-process–social-psychological debate has led to some increase in our understanding of hypnotic phenomena, most of the research conducted during the last 20 years has failed to demonstrate in unequivocal terms that any single viewpoint has uniquely captured the essence of the phenomena under study (Nadon, Laurence, & Perry, 1991). Part of the blame resides in the "double-edged sword" quality of the same methodological and statistical tools that have allowed a better understanding of some basic aspects of hypnosis. The use of Martin T. Orne's (1959) hallmark method of separating "genuine" hypnotic responding from social demands—the "real–simulator paradigm"—may best illustrate this point. It was the "real–simulator" paradigm that led to the empirical unveiling of what Orne called "demand characteristics," and simultaneously to the means by which their ramifications could be evaluated.

Simulators are subjects of low hypnotic susceptibility who are told to try and deceive a second experimenter by behaving "as if" they were excellent hypnotic subjects. A double-blind procedure is used, in which the rationale behind the experiment is withheld from both reals and simulators, and the experimenter testing the subjects is unaware of the actual susceptibility level of the subjects being tested. Simulators are used to assess the degree to which intrinsic and extrinsic factors may contribute to determining experimental outcomes. Specifically, simulators are employed to determine whether there are sufficient demands (implicit and explicit) within an experiment to shape the performance of simulating subjects so that they coincide with the predictions of how highly hypnotized subjects behave. If there are insufficient cues for simulating subjects to mimic the performance of reals, then it can (theoretically) be concluded that the behavior of reals is beyond that which can be explained by social factors and is therefore most likely attributable to their responding to hypnotic suggestions.

Thus, the real–simulator paradigm was designed to disqualify the interpretation that demand characteristics could account for the superior performance of highs relative to simulators (and presumably lows). Often, however, the results that are obtained have simulators tending to show greater "hypnotic" effects than reals. For example, several studies have shown that simulators pass a greater number of hypnotic suggestions than "reals" (Spanos, de Groot, Tiller, Weekes, & Bertrand, 1985; Spanos, de Groot, & Gwynn, 1987; McConkey & Sheehan, 1980). A similar pattern of results has held for specific hypnotic phenomena. T. X. Barber and Calverley (1966), F. J. Evans and Thorn (1966), and Williamsen, Johnson, and Eriksen (1965) all report that simulators display greater degrees of amnesia than "reals." Similarly, simulators have been shown to rate their amnesia as being more involuntary than "reals" rate theirs (Spanos, Radtke-Bodorik, & Stam, 1980).

Often, the exaggerated performance of simulators relative to reals is used to buttress the argument that reals and simulators are arriving at their responses by different routes (veridical hypnotic influences for reals, and responding to social cues for simulators). This could well be the case, but the presence of available alternatives weakens the conclusions that can be drawn from studies demonstrating this pattern (see, e.g., Levitt & Chapman, 1979).

Although the real–simulator design is most often employed by researchers aligned with what Spanos has called the "special-process" camp, social-psychological theorists have also sought to support their position by demonstrating that whatever behaviors can be elicited from highly susceptible subjects can also be elicited from subjects who are merely simulating hypnosis. Spanos (1986b), for example, cites numerous studies that show equivalent performance among "reals" and simulators, in order to discredit the special-process position.

In anticipation of such possible uses of his paradigm, Orne (1959, 1972) was careful to stress that simulators should be treated as a *quasi-control* group. He cautioned that if the feigned behavior of simulators does not differ from that of their highly susceptible counterparts, then it can only be concluded that there are sufficient cues within the experimental procedure to allow simulating subjects to successfully mimic the behavior of highly hypnotizable subjects. It cannot, he stressed, be concluded that highly susceptible subjects are simulating hypnosis. As P. G. Bowers (1986, p. 469) eloquently pointed out, "One must not assume that because a person with a headache becomes headache-free after taking aspirin . . . headache-free people secretly take aspirin."[9]

In many ways, the real–simulator paradigm addresses the fundamental problem in hypnosis research. No matter what results experimentation yields, they can be interpreted in many different plausible ways. The logic of equivalence championed by the social-psychological theorists illustrates well the double-edged quality of the experimental approach to hypnosis. The dilemma is that similar behaviors can arise from radically different routes. Time and time again researchers have shown that simulating subjects can behave "as if" they are hypnotized, in such a convincing fashion that they can fool even the most experienced hypnotists.

Researchers who maintain that hypnosis is more than just responding to social-psychological cues must rely on the verbal reports of highly hypnotizable subjects to validate the so-called "special-process" views of hypnosis. Because of the inherent difficulty posed by verbal reports, many researchers have sought to find indicators of hypnosis and hypnotizability that are more amenable to empirical investigation. Such a situation has inevitably led to a re-emergence of the quest for a reliable physiological indicator of hypnosis. Thus, over the last century, researchers have attempted to find an unequivocal physiological indicator that a given subject is experiencing hypnosis; or, alternatively, they have attempted to find some kind of physiological marker capable of distinguishing highly susceptible people from their low susceptible counterparts, particularly with the goal of validating the subjective reports of these subjects.

Physiological Stalemate

Not surprisingly, researchers seeking such physiological indicators have historically aligned themselves with some manifestation of the special-process viewpoint. By definition, the social-psychological viewpoint does not believe in the possibility of a specific physiological indicator of hypnosis. The predictions for each camp are thus clear: The social-psychological camp predicts that because there is nothing really unique about hypnosis per se there cannot be any physiological changes concomitant with hypnosis that cannot be elicited by means of the mechanisms available to waking cognition, or from subjects who are insusceptible to hypnosis. For the special-process camp, on the other hand, a reliable physiological indicator of hypnosis would serve to bolster the theory that hypnosis is a unique state characterized by marked dissociation of cognitive functioning.

As we have already noted, even in the early days of animal magnetism, it was assumed that the physical and psychological transformations seen in the magnetized individual were the end result of the magnetic fluid's action upon the mind and body. Although some authors pointed to the possibility that the phenomena being studied were the direct results of suggestions embedded in the hypnotic rituals, it was generally believed that hallucinations and the various modifications of memory, perception, and sensation were indicative of the physiological effects of the magnetic fluid upon the nervous system. When Braid (1843) rejected the notion of animal magnetism and its reliance on a universal fluid, he nonetheless identified the process of hypnosis as neurological in nature, over and above the role played by suggestion.

The physiological explanations of hypnosis and hypnotic phenomena became the central focus of the work of Charcot and his collaborators at La Salpêtrière in the last 20 years of the 19th century. Hypnosis was seen as a pathophysiological state similar to hysteria and epilepsy. There was no doubt in the minds of these clinicians and researchers that they were dealing with a pathology of the nervous system. From the induction methods used to the different types of physical and psychological phenomena identified, everything pointed to the obvious disturbances of the nervous system of the patients. Inductions, for example, were mostly carried out through the use of mechanical devices that exerted their effects on the sense organs. Intense visual stimuli (e.g., burning a strip of magnesium or introducing a solar lamp into a dark room), sudden auditory stimulation (e.g., the intense noise produced by a Chinese gong), or physical manipulations (e.g., compressing the eyeballs or applying pressure to the head) became common rituals of induction. That these physically invasive procedures triggered such responses as catalepsies, lethargies, and somnambulistic states was seen as proof that hypnosis induced neuropathological aberrations (see, e.g., Binet & Féré, 1888). Physical examinations of the hypnotized or hypnotizable individual also revealed "unmistakable" signs of the neurological underpinnings of the hypnotic state. For researchers of this era, the discovery (?) of hysterogenic, hypnogenic, and erotogenic zones on the patients' bodies was probably the best example of the neurological substantiation of a hypnotic state. In these patients, the hypnotist had only to apply pressure on one of these spots to produce an amazing array of bizarre symptoms, from simple anesthesia to sexual delirium.

When the members of the Nancy school counterattacked and proposed suggestion as the trigger mechanism underlying hypnosis, they did not abandon the notion of physiological state. In fact, when Bernheim (1884) finally demonstrated that responses to suggestion were the same with or without the use of hypnosis, his popularity among his colleagues faded along with the scientific interest in hypnosis (see Laurence & Perry, 1988).

When it became possible to measure neurophysiological functions reliably, researchers renewed their quest for a specific neurological index of hypnosis. With the advent of electroencephalographic (EEG) technology, it became possible to investigate the cortical activity associated with states of consciousness such as waking cognition and sleep. Given the historical association between hypnosis and sleep, researchers attempted to show that hypnosis, like sleep, differed in terms of EEG from waking behavior. The conclusions that could be drawn from this line of inquiry were at best ambiguous. Some researchers found that the records of hypnotized subjects resembled stage 1 sleep (Darrow, Henry, Gill, Brenman, & Converse, 1950). Others found that there was little difference between EEG records of the waking state and hypnosis (Loomis, Harvey, & Hobart, 1936; Dynes, 1947). The greatest difficulty in interpreting such studies is that stage 1 is really a transitional state between sleeping and waking rather than a clearly defined state of sleep (such as stages 2, 3, and 4 and rapid eye movement). As such, the ambiguity between this stage and the waking EEG record may have led to conclusions consonant with the researchers' pre-established views.

Gradually, the lack of confirming evidence caused researchers to realize that the relation between sleep and hypnosis was more metaphorical than biological. After abandoning the notion that hypnosis was a form of sleep, researchers attempted to show that hypnosis was an altered state of consciousness that would be characterized by the prevalence of a specific EEG bandwidth. Ulett, Akpinar, and Itil (1972a), for example, took a pool of 44 subjects and compared the EEG records of the 10 highest and 10 lowest scorers on the Barber Suggestibility Scale (BSS). Their results indicated that the best hypnotic subjects showed a significant increase in alpha and beta waves relative to the poorest subjects. Once again, however, the absence of adequate control groups (i.e. subjects receiving relaxation only, or imagery) makes this evidence impossible to evaluate.

A more adequately controlled study was conducted by Tebecis, Provins, Farnbach, and Pentony (1975), who employed alternating waking–hypnosis conditions and an "imagination-only" control group. This study revealed that of 14 highly hypnotizable subjects, only 1 subject displayed a consistent physiological concomitant of hypnosis. Each time this subject entered hypnosis, his alpha density increased. For the other subjects, no discernible EEG markers were observed.

While these researchers were attempting to show that hypnosis was a physiologically unique state, parallel attempts were being made to demonstrate that the EEG records of (unhypnotized) highly susceptible subjects could be differentiated from the records of (unhypnotized) subjects who were not susceptible to hypnosis. By comparing the EEG records of high- and low-susceptible subjects outside of the hypnotic context, a number of researchers found evidence of a relation between resting baseline alpha and hypnotizability (London, Hart, & Leibovitz, 1968; Nowlis & Rhead, 1968; Engstrom, London, and Hart, 1970a; London, Cooper, & Engstrom, 1974; Morgan, Macdonald, & Hilgard, 1974). As F. J. Evans (1979) noted, however, the data obtained in most of these studies are severely heteroscedastic,[10] with the bulk of the global correlation between hypnotizability and resting baseline alpha being carried by subjects of low rather than high hypnotic ability.

Heteroscedasticity notwithstanding, some researchers failed to demonstrate any correlation between hypnotizability and alpha production. Galbraith, London, Leibovitz, Cooper, and Hart (1970) found a significant correlation between theta activity and Harvard Group Scale of Hypnotic Susceptibility, Form A (HGSHS:A) scores, but no correlation between hypnotizability and alpha production. Similarly, F. J. Evans (1979), Dumas (1976,) and Cooper and London (1976) all failed to obtain a significant correlation between these variables. In a review of the literature that was designed to reconcile these conflicting results, Dumas (1977) concluded that the presence or absence of a significant hypnotizability–alpha correlation depended solely on whether subjects volunteered for experiments, or were invited to participate. In studies using volunteer subjects (Nowlis & Rhead, 1968; Engstrom et al., 1970a; London et al., 1974; Morgan, Macdonald, & Hilgard, 1974), significant correlations were obtained. When selected subjects were asked to participate, no correlation between hypnotizability and resting baseline alpha was observed (Galbraith et al., 1970; F. J. Evans, 1979; Dumas, 1976; Cooper & London, 1976).

Such an interpretation was directly supported by Dumas and Spitzer (1978), who compared resting baseline alpha of 8 volunteers to the EEG records of 12 invited subjects. Volunteer subjects showed a correlation of .72 between hypnotizability and baseline alpha, whereas invited subjects exhibited a correlation of only .02 for these variables. Thus, it seems that a correlation between baseline alpha and hypnotizability can only be found when subjects volunteer for studies, and that among volunteers, the correlation holds primarily for those subjects who are insusceptible to hypnosis. Although the heuristic value of the alpha–hypnotizability correlation is hindered by problems of subject self-selection and heteroscedasticity, it may be even more limited when one considers the failure of studies to control adequately for relaxation and imagic abilities. Such a methodological oversight is potentially serious, for alpha production is known to be related to relaxation ability and imagic thinking (A. F. Barabasz, 1980a).

An alternative avenue of investigation adopted by researchers interested in associating hypnosis with objective physiological indices involved specific hypnotic suggestions. Reasoning that one of the hallmarks of an hypnotic response was an alteration in normal cognitive functioning, researchers attempted to find physiological indicators that would reflect such cognitive alterations for specific hypnotic suggestions. The advent of machines capable of measuring visual evoked responses (VERs) allowed researchers to see whether, for example, the hypnotic suggestion that a flash of light was getting dimmer (or more intense) would alter the VERs for the ensuing target material. Early investigations were conducted on small numbers of subjects, and without the benefit of standardized susceptibility measurements or sophisticated instrumentation for measuring VERs. These studies were variable in their conclusions, with certain studies finding that hypnotic suggestions could significantly alter VER amplitudes (Hernandez-Peon & Donoso, 1959; Clynes, Kohn, & Lifshitz, 1964; N. J. Wilson, 1968), while the majority of studies failed to produce such positive findings (Halliday & Mason, 1964a; Beck & Barolin, 1965; Beck, Dustman, & Beier, 1966; Amadeo & Yanovski, 1975; Andreassi, Balinsky, Gallichio, De Simone, & Mellers, 1976).

One investigation that did measure hypnotic susceptibility and used adequate numbers of subjects was conducted by Galbraith, Cooper, and London (1972). These authors looked at the auditory evoked responses and VERs to stimuli. Subjects were instructed to attend to either the auditory or the visual modality. The results indicated that lows showed greater amplitudes to the nonattended channel, whereas highs showed greater amplitudes to the attended channels, presumably because highs were better able to filter out distracting stimuli. Since subjects were tested outside of the hypnotic context, however, this study does not pertain directly to the question of whether hypnosis can uniquely alter physiological indices such as evoked responses. It does, however, show how these physiological indices can be used to reveal some of the skills used by highly hypnotizable subjects to experience hypnosis.

A study that directly addressed the question of whether hypnosis can alter physiological indices such as evoked responses was conducted by A. F. Barabasz and Lonsdale (1983). They measured the olfactory evoked responses to strong, weak, and odorless stimuli. Results indicated that for both strong and weak odors, highly hypnotizable subjects displayed greater evoked response amplitudes while hypnotized than while awake. These amplitudes were also greater than those emitted by lows either in hypnosis or while awake. The authors concluded that during hypnosis highs paid greater attention to the stimuli, so that they could actively prevent these odors from reaching full awareness. Although compelling, these results cannot be considered unequivocal evidence for a unique physiological concomitant of hypnosis, for the study did not include relaxation and imagination-only conditions. As such, it does not exclude the possibility that such changes in the amplitude of the olfactory evoked response could have been produced by behaviors available to the nonhypnotized subjects.

Another study that considered differences in levels of hypnotic susceptibility was conducted by D. Spiegel, Cutcomb, Ren, and Pribram (1985). In this study, VERs were recorded for lights appearing on a video display terminal. Subjects of high and low hypnotizability were given the hypnotic suggestion that there was a cardboard box in front of the monitor that would prevent subjects from seeing the flashes. This positive hallucination caused a significant suppression of VERs among the highly hypnotizable subjects. Like the A. F. Barabasz and Lonsdale (1983) study, and the Galbraith et al. (1972) study, this study illustrates that physiological indices can distinguish between subjects who differ in hypnotic susceptibility. The results of this experiment, like those of the previously mentioned studies, are consonant with the contention that highly hypnotizable subjects make use of selective attention to filter out sensory stimuli in unattended channels. Unfortunately, once again, these results cannot be considered unequivocal evidence for a unique physiological concomitant of hypnosis, for the study did not include relaxation and imagination-only conditions.

Despite their shortcomings in terms of relaxation and imagination-only control groups, the three studies when considered together suggest that the type of physiological responses emitted by highs depends on the type of hallucination required. For negative hallucinations, such as the suggestion for anosmia administered in the A. F. Barabasz and Lonsdale (1983) study, the stimuli must be actively processed and actively prevented from reaching awareness. Such processing may result in elevations in the evoked response amplitudes. A positive hallucination, such as the cardboard box in the D. Spiegel et al. (1985) study, may allow the highs to selectively attend to something that is perceptually concrete, and thereby to attenuate stimuli attempting to impinge upon consciousness from an unattended channel. The Galbraith et al. (1972) study further emphasizes that selective attention capability may be what distinguishes high, medium, and low susceptible subjects, for only the highs were able to attend primarily to the proper stimulus and attenuate stimuli they were instructed to ignore. But no matter what these studies may be pointing to, the lack of adequate control procedures and the unfortunate but customary lack of replication preclude any conclusion concerning the physiological distinctiveness of an alleged hypnotic state.

To summarize the research concerning the quest for a reliable physiological index of hypnosis, there are to date no reliable EEG indicators that a given subject will enter a state of hypnosis, and no EEG indices that can distinguish subjects of differing levels of hypnotizability. A more promising line of inquiry involves seeing whether specific suggestions can alter physiological indices of cognitive functioning in subjects of differing hypnotizability levels with and without hypnotic induction. Although promising, such studies stand in need of replication and adequate control before they can be considered unequivocal physiological evidence for the ability of hypnotic suggestions to alter the cognition and perception of subjects capable of responding to such suggestions.

In some ways, one has to wonder at the time and effort expended in continuing this quest for physiological correlates of hypnosis. No matter how one looks at hypnosis, it cannot be induced without suggestions, and it always leads to the emergence of individual differences. These two observations point to the importance of investigating the underlying components of hypnotizability rather than a hypothetized general altered state. Thus Sarbin and Slagle's (1979) conclusions still hold: Instead of persevering in the search for an elusive physiological index of hypnosis, researchers should attempt to tackle the more general proposition that physiological indices can be influenced by social-psychological stimuli.

One cannot underestimate, however, the allure of a 200-year-old dream. Many researchers today would still wholeheartedly concur with Binet and Féré (1888), who thought that finding a physiological index of hypnosis would finally eradicate the viability of simulation and expectant attention as explanations of hypnosis. Thus one can certainly predict that the dream will live on, and that the quest not only will continue unimpeded, but will be aided by the inevitable improvements in scientific technology.[11]

Cognitive and Perceptual Correlates of Hypnotizability

Along with the theory-driven social-psychological and special-process research, and all of the experiments conducted in order to reveal physiological markers of hypnosis and hypnotizability, a third branch of inquiry has chronologically paralleled the two approaches reviewed above. This third branch stemmed from the notion that since hypnotizability is so remarkably stable, it should be related to some dimension of personality. Early attempts to correlate hypnotizability with individual personality variables were for the most part in vain (Nadon, Laurence, & Perry, 1987). Hull (1933), for example, attempted to assess the relation between hypnotizability and constructs such as acquiescence, neuroticism, and hysteria, all without success. In subsequent decades, the advent of sophisticated personality measures such as the Minnesota Multiphasic Personality Inventory, led to a resurgence in attempts to correlate hypnotizability and personality characteristics such as extroversion, locus of control, cooperativeness, and influenceability (de Groh, 1989). Like their predecessors, these studies yielded either small, unreliable, or nonsignificant correlations.

As attempts to relate hypnotizability to personality dimensions failed, researchers turned toward individual differences in more cognitively oriented skills, in the hope of ascertaining the factors that allow some people to experience hypnosis. Evidence gleaned over the past 20 years seems to indicate that at least one of these skills involves imaginative abilities. Within this general category are individual differences in the ability to generate and maintain images to suggested external stimuli, and in the degree to which subjects become absorbed in such images (what J. R. Hilgard, 1974a, referred to as "imaginative involvement").

The rationale for proposing a relation between imagery in the mental picture sense and hypnotizability stemmed from some of the more common hypnotic suggestions. For example, subjects are often asked to "imagine" that an arm is getting stiff, as though the arm were in a splint. It makes intuitive sense that the better subjects are at producing mental imagery to accompany this suggestion, the more likely it is that they will subjectively experience the arm as being stiff, and thereby find themselves unable to bend the arm. Similarly, those subjects who can experience visual hallucinations such as the cardboard box in the D. Spiegel et al., (1985) study, are most likely subjects who can produce mental images with such vividness and clarity that they experience the suggested objects as being veridically present (see, e.g. Arnold's [1946] theory of ideomotor action, which links sustained imaginal activities to the experience of "automatic" ideomotor behavior).[12]

Accordingly, a number of researchers have sought to correlate hypnotizability with pencil-and-paper measures of imagery ability. One such instrument is the Vividness of Visual Imagery Questionnaire (VVIQ) of Marks (1973), which assesses the quality of visual images. A number of studies have shown significant correlations between the VVIQ and hypnotic susceptibility (P. G. Bowers, 1978; Coe, St. Jean, & Burger, 1980; t'Hoen, 1978; Crawford, 1978).

In addition, several laboratories (e.g., Sheehan, 1967) have made use of Betts's Questionnaire on Mental Imagery (QMI), which assesses imagery abilities in seven different sensory modalities: visual, auditory, cutaneous, kinesthetic, gustatory, olfactory, and organic. Although the patterns of correlations between the QMI and hypnotic susceptibility are a mixture of significant and nonsignificant correlations, a number of studies have found an inherent heteroscedasticity in the data. For example, Sutcliffe, Perry, and Sheehan (1970) found a significant correlation between the QMI and the Stanford Hypnotic Susceptibility Scale, Form C (SHSS:C) of Weitzenhoffer and Hilgard (1962); however, a closer inspection of the data revealed that good imagers were represented across the entire spectrum of hypnotizability, while poor imagers invariably tended to be low hypnotizable subjects.

This inherent heteroscedasticity of the relation between the SHSS:C and the QMI was replicated by J. R. Hilgard (1979b), who found a small but significant correlation that was largely attributable to the fact that poor imagery ability predicted a lack of hypnotizability. In addition, a study that failed to obtain significant correlations between hypnotizability and the QMI (Perry, 1973) found that while vivid imagers permeated the entire range of hypnotic susceptibility, poor imagers almost always fell within the low susceptibility range. Thus it appears that good imagery ability may be a necessary but not sufficient skill for high hypnotic ability, whereas poor imagery is almost always a predictor of hypnotic insusceptibility.

Finally a number of studies have used the Preference for an Imagic Cognitive Style (PICS) questionnaire of Isaacs (1982), which focuses on imagery preference as opposed to imagery ability. This questionnaire was designed to determine whether subjects prefer a verbal or pictorial style of mentation while thinking about a number of suggested scenes. In two separate experiments, Nadon et al. (1987), using a multivariate framework, found that the PICS was able to contribute uniquely to the ability to predict whether subjects were of high, medium, or low hypnotic susceptibility. This multivariate finding was replicated (M. Dixon, Labelle, & Laurence, in press); in this study the PICS was able to predict unique hypnotizability variance in each of two relatively large ($n = 373$) samples of subjects tested with the HGSHS:A.

Other measures of imagic abilities have been promising in terms of revealing individual differences related to hypnotizability. Individual differences have been observed in voluntary control of sleep processes (F. J. Evans, 1979), in subjective interest in night dreams (Gibson, 1985), and in the ability to control night dreams (Belicki & Bowers, 1982). Gibson (1985) found that women who enjoyed dreaming, arrived at creative ideas while dreaming, and reported having their future foretold in their dreams were more highly hypnotizable than women reporting the opposite pattern. Belicki and Bowers (1982) found that the ability to modify the content of dreams in response to presleep instructions was positively related to hypnotizability.

Furthermore, recent investigations involving the potential relation between hypnotizability and subjective experiences of "paranormal" phenomena have yielded promising results. M. J. Diamond and Taft (1975) reported a significant correlation between hypnotizability and belief in the supernatural. More recently, in an interview study of very highly hypnotizable women, S. C. Wilson and Barber (1983a) found that 92% of their sample considered themselves to possess certain psychic abilities. Many of these subjects further reported experiencing paranormal phenomena, such as telepathy, spiritual apparitions, and precognitions. By contrast, only 16% of low- and medium-hypnotizable subjects reported such beliefs or experiences. Nadon and Kihlstrom (1987) have developed a reliable self-report measure that they call the Paranormal Experiences Questionnaire (PEQ). This questionnaire samples a number of areas that have been labeled as either "paranormal," "psychic," "psi," or "anomalous." These authors report that beliefs in, and subjective experience of, these types of experiences are positively correlated with hypnotizability, a finding that has been replicated repetitively in our laboratory.

Finally, perhaps the most reliable univariate correlate of hypnotizability involves what Tellegen and Atkinson (1974) have referred to as "absorption." The concept of absorption can be defined as the dispositional propensity for having episodes of all-encompassing involvement toward specific attentional objects. These authors indicate that to experience such episodes people must be able to "operate diverse representational modalities synergistically so that a full but unified experience is realized" (Tellegen & Atkinson, 1974, p. 275). The Tellegen Absorption Scale (TAS;

Tellegen, 1982; Tellegen & Atkinson, 1974) is the most widely used measure of such synergistic abilities. In their initial study, Tellegen and Atkinson (1974) reported correlations of .27 and .42 (across two samples) between the TAS and hypnotizability as measured by the HGSHS:A. The finding of a relation between hypnotizability and absorption has been replicated on numerous occasions (e.g., Crawford, 1982a; Finke & Macdonald, 1978; Kihlstrom, Diaz, McClellan, Ruskin, Pistole, & Shor, 1980; Nadon et al., 1987; Roberts, Schuler, Bacon, Zimmerman, & Patterson, 1975; Spanos & McPeake, 1975b [for subjects exposed to favorable information concerning hypnosis]).

Notwithstanding the general reliability of these correlations, a few studies have failed to reveal a significant relation between hypnotizability and TAS scores. For example, Spanos, McPeake, and Churchill (1976) failed to observe a relation between absorption and hypnotizability as measured by the BSS in a sample dichotomized into 36 females and 55 males. These authors indicate, however, that the hypnotizability–absorption relation may depend on the scale that is used to measure hypnotizability. Since the psychometric properties of the BSS are not as well known as the extensively studied Harvard and Stanford scales, this finding may be of secondary importance.

Finally, a study by Spanos and McPeake (1975b) failed to observe the usual positive correlation between absorption and hypnotizability. Subjects in this study were, however, exposed to unfavorable information concerning hypnosis prior to the hypnotic induction. As such, this study related more to the importance of attitudes toward hypnosis than to the relation between hypnotizability and absorption. These isolated failures to replicate, however, point to the importance of taking into account the potential interactive nature of these individual differences with the situational and instructional contexts of testing (for a complete review of this literature, see Roche & McConkey, 1990).

Once again, researchers have used these correlational studies as evidence to bolster their respective theoretical positions. From the special-process perspective, the presence of any reliable correlate of hypnotizability poses a serious threat to the social-psychological camp. The rationale is that if hypnotizability is determined solely by the willingness of subjects to comply with the complex demands of the hypnotic context, and to perform in accordance with what they perceive to be the hypnotist's expectations, then there is no *a priori* reason to predict significant correlations with cognitive attributes that are unrelated to hypnosis per se.

The social psychologists' rebuttal to this argument is that wherever correlations between hypnotizability and cognitive abilities are found, these correlations can be explained by what Council, Kirsch, and Hafner (1986) have referred to as a "context effect." Council et al. (1986) claim that significant correlations occur only when measures of imaginative involvement are obtained prior to the assessment of subjects' level of hypnotic susceptibility. They propose that testing subjects for cognitive abilities in close temporal proximity to the hypnosis sessions allows the subjects to form a logical connection between the two sets of measures, thus permitting them to adjust their degree of hypnotic responsivity so that it is consistent with their previously obtained questionnaire scores. The mechanism by which this context effect operates is that of subjects' expectancies. Council et al. claim that filling out questionnaires on imaginative involvement causes changes in subjects' expectancies about the degree to which they will be hypnotized, and that this change in expectancies results in the active modification of subjects' scores on hypnotizability measures. In other words, proponents of the context effect suggest that subjects look at how they score in terms of absorption, causally link absorption to hypnotizability, derive from this hypothetical relation how they should perform in hypnosis, and adjust their hypnotic responses accordingly.

To substantiate this claim, Council et al. (1986) contrasted the host of studies that showed significant correlations between hypnotic susceptibility and absorption abilities (as assessed with the TAS) with a number of experiments in which failures to obtain significant correlations between the TAS and hypnotizability were observed. According to these researchers, the factor that determined the statistical outcome of the study was the temporal contiguity between testing for absorption and testing for hypnotizability. In all of the positive outcomes, hypnosis testing followed the absorption measure either immediately or within a relatively short period of time. In each of the studies that failed to find significant correlations between hypnotizability and absorption, either the administration of the absorption questionnaire was conducted in a situation removed from the hypnotic context (Buckner & Coe, 1977; Council et al., 1986), or a questionnaire was used in which absorption items were embedded among a large number of filler items (Chiofalo & Coe, 1982; Spanos, McPeake, & Churchill, 1976).[13]

It should be noted that although the context effect has been empirically assessed in terms of absorption, the rationale underlying this effect should hold for all of the cognitive abilities that have been mentioned thus far. Proponents of the social-psychological position could claim that in order for the context effect to operate, the only requirement is that the abilities previously mentioned have at least a face-valid relation with the layperson's conception of hypnosis. Specifically, if subjects can infer the link between hypnosis and the construct being measured by the questionnaire, then they can adjust their hypnotic responsivity to levels that are consonant with their questionnaire performance.[14]

Thus, while followers of the "special-process" camp would argue that reliable cognitive correlates of hypnotizability negate the social-psychological position, it is actually the mechanisms underlying these correlates of hypnotizability that are of paramount importance in choosing among competing explanations of hypnosis and hypnotizability. If subjects of differing hypnotizability actually do differ in terms of non-social-psychological cognitive attributes (such as imaginative involvement or imagery abilities), then the most extreme social-psychological interpretation of hypnosis and hypnotizability must be deemed untenable, as such findings are incompatible with veridical individual differences in cognitive abilities. If, however, correlations are not the results of actual cognitive differences, but are merely artifacts of shifts in expectancies caused by the context effect, then such correlations actually support the social-psychological position.

Thus, what is required to differentiate between the social-psychological and special-process positions are cognitive and/or perceptual tasks that reliably differentiate high and low hypnotizable subjects, yet have no face-valid relation to hypnosis. In general, such tasks involve assessing differences between or among hypnotizability groups in the performance of simple cognitive tasks that are measured outside of the hypnotic context.

One such cognitive task that has proven to be of heuristic value in differentiating the performance of high and low susceptible subjects is the Stroop color-naming task. In the classic Stroop phenomenon, color words (BLUE or RED) or control stimuli (e.g., a series of ×'s) are presented in different colors (Stroop, 1935). Subjects are instructed to ignore the words (or the ×'s) and simply name the physical color of whatever they see as quickly as possible. Despite instructions to ignore the words and concentrate on naming the colors as quickly as possible, however, the color words are processed automatically and involuntarily, evoking faster reaction times for congruent trials than for control trials. More importantly, when the word and the color are incongruent, the automatic and involuntary processing of the word results in much longer reaction times for incongruent trials than for control trials.

A number of recent investigations conducted in our laboratory have shown that highly hypnotizable subjects show greater Stroop effects than their low-hypnotizable counterparts. In our original study, we compared the performance of nine high, nine medium, and nine low subjects (M. Dixon, Brunet, & Laurence, 1990) on a variation of the Stroop task that enabled us to assess both automatic processing and the effect of using different strategies to perform the Stroop task. The data from this experiment indicated that highly susceptible subjects showed significantly greater automaticity in processing the color words, but did not differ from mediums and lows in implementing the suggested strategy.

A second study was conducted to replicate and extend our original findings concerning hypnotizability, automaticity, and strategy (M. Dixon & Laurence, 1992). This follow-up study used a paradigm that more effectively separated automatic and strategic processes. The results of this study showed that highly hypnotizable subjects, were able to implement the given strategy more rapidly than low hypnotizable subjects, indicating that they were better able to implement a performance optimization strategy designed to improve reaction time performance in the Stroop task. More importantly, however, this study replicated the finding that highly hypnotizable subjects processed the color words more automatically than lows did.

The automaticity results of this latter study are important, for they are difficult to reconcile with a purely social-psychological interpretation of why hypnotizability differences may emerge in perceptual experiments involving hypnosis. Although it is possible that subjects could have modified their reaction time performance to coincide with their perceived notions of how a "good" hypnotic subject (or a "poor" hypnotic subject) should perform, a number of factors make this interpretation unlikely. First, in these studies not only was the experimenter unaware of the susceptibility level of the subjects, but also no mention of possible links to hypnotizability was made to subjects until after the experiment was over. Second, in both experiments, despite explicit instructions to name the colors as quickly as possible, highly hypnotizable subjects ("good" hypnotic subjects) showed poorer reaction time performance than lows on incongruent trials. It is doubtful that highly hypnotizable subjects would perceive their role to be one in which they were to show poorer performance than lows on one type of trials but not on another.

Although the automaticity results are incompatible with an extreme version of the social-psychological interpretation of hypnotizability and hypnosis, the finding that highly susceptible subjects are better at implementing performance optimization strategies than low susceptible subjects is consonant with this theory. Thus, the results of these studies indicate the need for a theory of hypnosis that depolarizes the social-psychological and special-process views of hypnosis and hypnotizability into a more unified approach. The integration of these two schools of thought has recently been exemplified by the synergistic view of hypnotic responding (Laurence, 1990; Nadon, Laurence, & Perry, 1991).

Although it acknowledges the role of individual differences that are crucial to the neodissociationist theory, the synergistic position also fully recognizes the importance of social-psychological variables, such as the hypnotic context and the attitudes, beliefs, and expectations of the subject; more importantly, however, it stresses the need to investigate the interactions between these different types of variables. Although the synergistic camp supports the social psychologists' contention that highly susceptible subjects may actively use goal-directed strategies in order to experience the hypnotic suggestion, it differs in suggesting that while such strategies may be necessary for experiencing an hypnotic suggestion, they are not in and of themselves sufficient for hypnotic responsivity. In order for highly susceptible subjects to experience the phenomena suggested during hypnosis, they must make use of certain cognitive abilities that are either less developed or absent in lows. Thus, according to the synergistic view, hypnosis is a situation in which subjects attempt to rally certain cognitive abilities in order to successfully alter normal cognitive functioning in accordance with the given suggestions. The degree to which they are successful depends on the implicit and explicit demands of the hypnotic context, their beliefs and attitudes toward hypnosis and the hypnotist, and the degree to which they utilize certain relevant cognitive skills (see also Balthazard & Woody, 1992; Tellegen, 1978–1979).

Reports of Nonvolition

The experience of nonvolition has traditionally been recognized as the cornerstone of successful hypnotic responsivity, even though research has clearly demonstrated that reports of involuntariness are characteristic of only certain types of hypnotic suggestions and are usually proferred only by highly hypnotizable subjects (P. G. Bowers, Laurence, & Hart, 1988). This single area of research probably provides the best illustration of the inadequacies intrinsic to most current theories of hypnosis.

For the neodissociationists, the experience of nonvolition during hypnosis reflects subjects' diminished conscious control over suggested behaviors and experiences. As E. R. Hilgard (1977a) noted, "one of the most striking features of hypnosis is the loss of control over actions normally voluntary" (p. 115). For Hilgard, this loss of control would be the end result of the dissociation of the cognitive subsystems that are usually at play during conscious experiences. However, it has proven difficult to substantiate the concept of dissociation experimentally, and even more difficult to define it without having to resort to metaphors (e.g., hidden observers, amnesic barriers)—a tendency that tends to send the social-psychological theorists on the warpath.

For the social-psychological theorists, the reports of nonvolition are the results of subjects' misattributing the origins of their behaviors and experiences. This misattribution process (the reader will recognize here the echoes of Faria's ideas) is the result of a number of factors, including preconceptions concerning hypnosis, the structure and wording of suggestions, expectancies, and imaginative abilities. Such a view of nonvolition provides a clear indication of the minimal role attributed to individual differences in the social-psychological explanation of involuntariness. As Lynn, Rhue, and Weekes (1990) have emphasized, subjects' imaginings are not causally related to the experience of involuntariness, but rather serve to reinforce and legitimize subjects' interpretations of their experiences as nonvolitional. In summary, for the tenants of this theoretical position, nonvolition is the result of a chain of goal-directed cognitions guided primarily by situational factors.

It is somewhat ironic that this is probably the area of research where both camps are in fact saying the same thing. A quick perusal of some of the major social-psychological and neodissociationist explanations of involuntariness is quite revealing. For Sarbin and Coe (1972), the experience of nonvolition is explained by subjects' "organismic involvement" in the hypnotic role—that is, the point at which subjects have become so immersed in their role that they have actually become that role. Neodissociationists would say that subjects have dissociated from their normal everyday selves. Lynn, Rhue, and Weekes (1990), on the other hand, have proposed a "creative role engagement" hypothesis of nonvolition, in which "the entire chain of events of imagining or experiencing, responding, and viewing the response as an involuntary occurrence is goal-directed, *even though* subjects may not experience the links of the chain in a deliberate, effortful, or even conscious manner" (p. 172, emphasis added). If subjects are not conscious of the strategies employed to experience their behaviors as involuntary, could we not say that they are dissociated from part of their own cognitive apparatus? Finally, Spanos and Chaves (1989d) have proposed that subjects can apply a range of causal attributions to their own goal-directed enactments, and that the interpretation subjects will adopt will be in line with their understanding of the situation. In the case of hypnosis, subjects will adopt a strategy that will have as an end result the labeling of their responses as involuntary. As Nadon, Laurence, and Perry (1989) have pointed out, to do so, subjects would have to be either unaware of the causal link between strategy and response enactment or simply deceitful.[15] If subjects are unaware of this link, could we not once again describe them as dissociated? What seems to differentiate the two camps is not the actual metaphor of dissociation, but rather the identified source of dissociation. For the neodissociationists, the important triggering mechanisms are mainly internal; the misattribution process is the end result of the cognitive alterations at play during hypnosis. For the social psychologists, the triggering mechanisms are external; the misattribution process is the end result of subjects' interpretations of the situational demands.

Regardless of one's preferred metaphor, the issue of nonvolitional reports remains at the core of an integrated view of hypnosis and hypnotizability. The question remains as follows: By which mechanisms does this occur, and how can we predict *a priori* who will report involuntariness and under what circumstances? Whereas dissociationists have emphasized general cognitive mechanisms and de-emphasized situational factors, social-psychological theorists have emphasized situational variables and de-emphasized individual differences. Given the limitations of both approaches, emphasis will have to be placed not on their continued separation but on their integration, as more and more investigations demonstrate that they clearly interact with each other (see, e.g., Nadon, Laurence, & Perry, 1991).

Questions Resolved? Questions Unanswered!

It should be reasonably clear at this point that many of the basic questions regarding hypnosis still remain unanswered. The phenomenology of hypnosis is certainly well documented, and experiments investigating its multifaceted manifestations are numerous. It is also clear from a review of the literature that the social-psychological models of hypnosis have gained a prominent position over the last two decades. As influential as these models have been, however, they have not succeeded in enticing the researchers of other camps to join their ranks. This may be because, like their predecessors, they have failed to offer an unequivocal explanation of hypnotizability and reports of nonvolition. For the hypnosis researcher, however, they have succeeded in demonstrating very clearly that hypnotic research has to take into account the role played by situational variables. Very few researchers continue to use such words as "trance" or "hypnotic state," although the continuing proliferation of psychophysiological research implicitly suggests that the dream is not yet over!

Still, the last 20 years have seen an amazing theoretical shift in hypnosis research, primarily because of the establishment of social-psychological models as a major force within the current *Zeitgeist* of hypnotic investigations. This reversal of fate should not be too surprising; 19th-century authors had already emphasized the importance of situational and psychosocial variables as determinants of the hypnotic response. The role of external factors in shaping subjects' internal representations of their hypnotic (or magnetic) experiences was noted by Faria (1819) when he wrote that "external procedures in whatever forms are necessary; they must also conform to what *époptes* have been led to expect" (p. 159). Similarly, Bernheim (1884) noticed that he had much less difficulty hypnotizing patients in the hospital setting than in his private practice office. Janet (1889) was probably the author who most emphatically underlined the intricate interactions of heredity, physiology, personality characteristics, and the social context of each individual in shaping their responses to hypnosis and psychopathology. In the spirit of Janet, Nadon, Laurence, and Perry (1991) have suggested that cross-disciplinary studies are needed so that various models of hypnotic response can be pitted against one another within single designs. It may be the only way of resolving the theoretical stalemate that seems to paralyze current hypnotic research.

Along these lines, it is interesting to compare the contemporary theoretical stalemate to the late 19th-century debate between the Nancy and La Salpêtrière schools—a debate that led to the near curtailment of all hypnosis research in Europe (see Laurence & Perry, 1988, for a detailed history of this period). There are many ways of interpreting what happened 100 years ago, but the picture was remarkably similar to today's. For many decades, the notion of a hypnotic state had been rarely questioned by those who used hypnosis in their practice. When Charcot and his colleagues became interested in the similarities between hysteria and the manifestations of hypnosis, hypnotic susceptibility became identified with a pathological state that could be described in ways similar to the nosology of hysteria. The automaticity of the responses elicited through suggestions once a patient had been hypnotized (and, later on, their "spontaneous" manifestations), as well as the restricted number of patients who could demonstrate the full range of hypnotic states, pointed to the specific psychoneurophysiological model eventually championed by Charcot's pupils. It did not take long before clinicians realized that hypnosis was not like a physical illness such as epilepsy, where one can rely on the stability of the symptoms between and within patients. Hypnotized patients were amazingly heterogeneous in their responses to a hypnotic induction. This led to a proliferation of modifications of Charcot's three basic stages, a kind of procrustean race to prove Charcot's theory correct. For physicians like Bernheim who worked in a social circle not influenced by the master's approval, it became clear that suggestions and training were the main ingredients in explaining the behaviors of Charcot's patients. To respond to suggestions was not a pathological symptom, but a natural tendency that could be exacerbated in hypnosis. Bernheim soon demonstrated that suggestion or an individual's suggestibility[16] was a necessary ingredient to the production of an hypnotic response. The blow to Charcot's theory was fatal, for how could a natural process like suggestion be responsible for a pathological (quasi-neurological) state? Similarly, contemporary social psychologists have succeeded in explaining away the notion of state by demonstrating, as Bernheim had done, that most if not all of the hypnotic phenomenology could be produced in subjects by suggestions outside of the hypnotic context.

The parallel, however, does not end here. At the height of the confrontation between the two French schools, hypnosis found its way into the legal arena. Following a series of criminal cases in which hypnosis had been allegedly involved, the two schools once again found themselves on opposite sides of the fence. For La Salpêtrière, only those who had a propensity toward criminality (and hystericals were prime candidates) could be the victims of hypnosis. For the Nancy school, in highly responsive individuals suggestions could lead to criminal behavior. Unfortunately for the Nancy school, it soon became evident that the concept of suggestion was not sufficient in explaining the questions raised by the courts, and Bernheim was forced to recognize that in cases where suggestions had played a role, other dispositional and situational factors were probably more important in the genesis of the reprehensible behaviors. His espousing a too extreme position meant that the baby was thrown out with the bathwater. History may indicate that the same fate is now awaiting contemporary theoretical positions that adopt an extreme stance vis-à-vis the phenomenon of hypnosis.

As if to confirm the adage that history often repeats itself, the last two decades have seen opposing theoretical camps air their divergent viewpoints within the confines of the legal arena. In 1979, Fromm and Shor listed fewer than 10 publications in the area of legal and ethical issues involving hypnosis. Since then, hundreds of theoretical, clinical, and experimental investigations have been undertaken in order to achieve a fuller understanding of the role played by hypnosis in legal issues (for a recent review of this new field, see Laurence & Perry, 1988). In fact, if one had to propose the single most influential development concerning hypnosis research over the last 20 years, it would have to be this one. The forensic use of hypnosis has triggered an amazing amount of research devoted to investigating the role of hypnosis and hypnotizability in memory processes, particularly in hypnotic hypermnesia, confabulation, and the relations between recall and confidence. What seems to come out of this literature is an interesting interaction between hypnosis and hypnotizability, an interaction between the context of testing and certain stable characteristics of the individual—a synergy that none of the traditional theories can comfortably explain.

In briefly summarizing the many investigations concerning the forensic aspects of hypnosis, one can safely say that hypnotizability will differentially influence the recall of correct, incorrect, and neutral information, and that the introduction of hypnosis will also affect recall, but in ways that will depend upon subjects' hypnotizability (see Nadon, Laurence, & Perry, 1991). Furthermore, this synergistic effect will produce a "hardening" of memory that translates into some subjects' being more confident in the accuracy of memories recalled in hypnosis, regardless of whether what they remember actually happened or not.[17]

If nothing else, the explosion of interest in the legal aspects of hypnosis over the last 20 years and the subsequent plethora of important investigations should prompt us to continue to look for new ways of extracting the truth about hypnosis and hypnotizability. Let us hope that this process will transcend the traditional polarization of research and eventually lead to new perspectives in research.

Conclusion

This brief survey of the last 200 years of research and observations on hypnosis and its accompanying phenomena points to the importance of taking advantage of the most recent methodological and statistical advances to achieve a "paradigm shift" in the way we have mapped the hypnotic territory over the last 100 years. Although there are certainly advantages in being guided and informed by past experiences, we must remember that doing more of the same does not necessarily constitute progress, or give us a better understanding of an ensemble of phenomena that still continues to elude satisfactory explanations. The general overview of the research trends concerning the empirical investigation of hypnotic susceptibility indicates a gradual shifting away from polarized views of hypnosis and hypnotizability, to a more synergistic approach acknowledging that social, cognitive, and affective factors all play a part in determining whether a given subject can experience hypnosis. As much as future work certainly needs to be theoretically driven, there is also a crucial need for theoretical flexibility to permit exploration of contingencies that are incompatible or inconsistent with one's particular theoretical orientation. The synergistic model emphasizes the use of a general approach, based on the advantages provided by the fusion of both correlational and experimental methodologies (Nadon, Laurence, & Perry, 1991). Thus far, the univariate approach generally adopted by hypnosis researchers has led to little more than a theoretical stalemate.

History has shown that the polarization of hypnosis research into theoretically divergent camps will eventually lead to a lack of progress in understanding the complex nature of hypnosis, and to a general waning of interest in the phenomenon itself. But perhaps history only repeats itself if we choose to ignore it. If hypnosis research is to grow and ultimately find its place within mainstream psychological research, it will have to begin by integrating the findings of different schools of thought into a unified, more global approach to this fascinating phenomenon.

Notes

1. We would like the reader to keep in mind that the topics we have chosen to discuss represent a very selective as well as subjective choice. Any other colleague would not necessarily believe that these topics are the most important ones in the unfolding history of hypnosis. In the same line, we do not discuss clinical research at any length, since it is the focus of Chapter 16 in the present book.

2. Although not an explicit topic of the present chapter, the uses and abuses of hypnosis in the legal arena have allowed the contemporary researcher to glance— sometimes with amazement, sometimes with total disbelief—at the perpetual transformations and disguises of these early beliefs. For example, although no reasonable scientist, whether experimenter or clinician, would claim today that a conscious individual can see through senses other than the eyes, it is not unusual to find reports of the "subconscious mind" (?) being able to perform similar feats once the individual has been hypnotized (see Laurence & Perry, 1988, for different examples).

3. Mesmer's fate in that regard was also quite similar to that of numerous young colleagues who get their research proposals rejected because hypnosis is not "mainstream" science. Fortunately, he could rely on the clinic to subsidize his projects—a fate that few experimentalists share!

4. A brief survey of the evolution of psychological theories of the mind—or, even more specifically, theories of specific brain functions such as memory and perception—will convince the reader that theories often lag a few steps behind technological discoveries. Whether one wonders at the amazing invisible power of electricity and magnetism and dreams of the human being as the perfect electromagnetic machine (Puységur, 1784–1785), or is baffled by holographic reproduction and builds a memory system on such a principle (M. K. Johnson, 1983), the reasoning is the same. Along similar lines, the somnambulistic patients who could, once magnetized, connect with a source of knowledge that rendered them omniscient (albeit amnesic, once demagnetized) may not be so removed from the contemporary Ericksonian subconscious, which knows what has to be done for the conscious to heal, even though the conscious mind may be unaware of such knowledge.

5. As is the case today, even those who did not emphasize the idea of individual differences in their theoretical explanations of hypnosis nonetheless spent their time and energy looking for a hypnotic virtuoso to demonstrate or refute certain phenomena.

6. As an example of the changing *Zeitgeist* then and now, Faria believed that if subjects did not respond to his usual lucid sleep induction, bleeding them increased their sensitivity to lucid sleep. This observation prompted Faria to conclude that thin blood was probably one agent responsible for the elicitation of the phenomenon. Although we would look at such procedure as a rather intrusive persuasive technique, Faria never mentioned this possibility. Bleeding was a normal, accepted, and frequently used medical technique at the time.

7. It is interesting to note again the recycling nature of hypnosis theorizing. Whereas the last 35 years or so have solidly established the importance of individual differences, the advent of the Ericksonian movement in the world of clinical hypnosis has revived the notion that everyone is hypnotizable. The skilled hypnotist can unleash the subconscious artistry of his or her patient, since humans all possess the ability to experience altered states of consciousness. As Fromm and Shor (1972) noted, little attention has been paid to the correspondences and differences between clinical and experimental research in hypnosis. Unfortunately, the last 20 years have not bridged that gap. Recent articles by Sherman and Lynn (1990) and Kihlstrom (1987a) may pave the way to a new integration of research and clinical work.

8. It is interesting to note that in the specific case of hypnotic amnesia, both "camps" agree that amnesic subjects demonstrate a decrease in temporal and categorical organization of the amnestic stimuli. However, they disagree on the hypothetized mechanisms underlying such replicated findings. The research on hypnotic amnesia illustrates well the limitations that standard ANOVA-type designs place on interpretation when they are guided by rather inflexible theoretical orientations (see Nadon, Laurence, & Perry, 1991, for further examples.)

9. It may not come as a surprise to anyone that subjects asked to simulate hypnosis will outperform their nonsimulator counterparts. Moll (1889/1982) proposed long ago that simulators have a tendency to overrespond during hypnotic testing. It is the best strategy that one can take if asked to perform as an excellent hypnotic subject. Furthermore, the usual hypnotic suggestions are far from being ambiguous; they state clearly what behaviors and experiences are expected from

simulators. In fact, when a behavior or experience seen in highly hypnotizable subjects is counterexpectational or ambiguous, simulators will not enact it as long as they are not specifically informed of what is expected from them (see, e.g., Nogrady, McConkey, Laurence, & Perry, 1983, and Nadon, D'Eon, McConkey, Laurence, & Perry, 1988).

10. "Heteroscedasticity" means that the standard error of estimate is different for different values of the predictors. This type of data is sometimes referred to as "twisted pears." In other words, one may find in correlating imagery with hypnotizability that low imagers are mostly low in hypnotizability, whereas high imagers may span the whole range of hypnotizability.

11. In the end, the physiological quest will certainly triumph. Humans are by nature physiological machines. No matter how one chooses to look at this issue, ultimately everything is physiological. That does not, however, and probably will not, make hypnosis a special state.

12. Although one typically assumes that the link between hypnotizability and imagery was only recently forged by experimental investigators, it should no longer be surprising to discover that clinicians like Braid and Liébeault had already noticed that highly responsive individuals seemed endowed with the power of visualization.

13. Nadon (1989) has correctly pointed out that the significance–nonsignificance distinctions proposed by Council et al. (1986) constitute inappropriate statistical procedures. In order to show a context effect, the correlation obtained in context must be shown to be significantly different from correlations obtained out of context. Because the contextual arguments are representative of the type of approach favored by the social-psychological camp, an attempt was made to disprove such a hypothesis on theoretical rather than statistical grounds.

14. However, in a recent methodological, statistical, and empirical re-evaluation of the context effect, Nadon, Hoyt, Register, and Kihlstrom (1991) concluded that contextual effects, if genuine, are most likely to be small, and pose little if any threat to the validity of past research that has found relations between hypnotic ability and various experiences and processes outside of the hypnotic context. The debate, however, is ongoing; given the propensity for scientists to view debates as more important than the resolution of issues, it may be with us for quite a while. That being said, it must be noted that there are different types of context effects, and it would be impossible at this point to state that there are no context effects at play in hypnosis. However, to state that correlations of hypnotizability with absorption and imagery are completely expectancy-based is not supported by available evidence. Nonetheless, hypnotizability is a context-defined skill, and to expect that undergoing such procedures does not influence subjects' responses would be illogical. A more promising line of research may be the investigation of the influence of situational variables on specific responses. The research on hypnotic hypermnesia, for example, seems to demonstrate that the introduction of hypnosis produces a differential response set among subjects.

15. Certain authors view hypnotic performance in terms of simple social compliance or deceit (Wagstaff, 1981a). For other authors, compliance or deceit may be a useful way of explaining away difficult phenomena. From a social-role stand-point, one does not necessarily assume that subjects' reports are always honest or

that they are dishonest. As Spanos (1986b) has suggested, one has to determine the conditions under which it is theoretically useful to do so. Such a position, however, may very well taint the methodological and statistical strategies used to buttress or reject a particular theoretical stance.

16. Since the late 19th century, there have been innumerable attempts to clarify the distinction between hypnotic susceptibility and suggestibility. As we have mentioned before, the induction of hypnosis cannot proceed without the communication (verbal or nonverbal, explicit or implicit, from the hypnotist or the subject) that it will proceed. The concept of suggestibility per se is the subject of many controversies in research, and nobody agrees on what it represents (Schumaker, 1991). To discuss the similarities and differences between the two constructs at this point is an exercise in futility.

17. These interesting and often replicated results should have a major impact on clinical theories of hypnosis that rely on this procedure to unravel the mysteries of the past. They could lead also to new ways of utilizing hypnosis to restructure clients' memories and ongoing cognitions.

PART TWO

CURRENT EMPIRICALLY BASED THEORIES

CHAPTER THREE

Dissociation and Theories of Hypnosis

ERNEST R. HILGARD

There is nothing especially new about the concept of "dissociation," defined as the splitting off of certain mental processes from the main body of consciousness with various degrees of autonomy. When "association" was the favorite process to describe the binding between two ideas, it was not surprising that a word was selected to represent their separation, or "disassociation." Janet (1889) used the French word *désagrégation*, which might have been better translated as "disaggregation" in English. However, the term "dissociation" became accepted in English, as used by William James in his *Principles of Psychology* (1890), and by Janet himself in his Harvard lectures, *The Major Symptoms of Hysteria* (1907). In Janet's correspondence with James, he admitted that dissociation need not be complete, and supported partial dissociation in the sense that dissociated ideas might still affect the emotional life of the patient (James, 1890, Vol. 2, p. 456, footnote).

Dissociation in Hypnosis

Some Background on Dissociation

My own attraction to the concept of dissociation began in the early years of my writing on hypnosis. In my first hypnosis book (E. R. Hilgard, 1965a), I found "dissociation," particularly "partial dissociation," to be a term more useful than "regression" as an interpretation of hypnotic phenomena (pp. 392–393, 395–396). Following this aroused interest, I delved into the history of the concept of dissociation (E. R. Hilgard, 1973a). In the United States, the term was popularized in the writings of Boris Sidis (e.g., 1902), and Morton Prince (e.g., 1906).

Later, however, the term fell into disuse. Two important papers, one by Bernard Hart (1927) and one by William McDougall (1938), found plausible reasons for the decline in the use of the term. Hart, who was much interested in psychoanalysis, placed some of the blame upon the rise of psychoanalytic thinking. His 1927 paper was delivered as the presidential address before the Medical Section of the British Psychological Society. He accepted the general notion of dissociation, but favored partial dissociations and felt that Janet had overemphasized the complete splitting of parts of the personality.

He wrote later: "Instead of regarding dissociation as the splitting of conscious materials into separate masses, it must be regarded as an affair of gearing, the various elements of the mental machinery being organized into different functional systems by the throwing in of the appropriate gear" (Hart, 1929, p. 163). This use of an automobile analogy is obviously a metaphor and is rather incompletely explained. He went on to say that Freud's notion of the unconscious is an entirely different conceptualization:

> [The unconscious] is not itself a fact of consciousness and its existence cannot be demonstrated in the way in which the existence of Janet's dissociated items can be demonstrated. . . . The subconscious of Janet is a description of phenomenal facts, while the unconscious of Freud is a conceptual construction, an imaginary entity created in order to explain phenomenal facts. (Hart, 1929, pp. 165–166)

Hart explained the lack of interest by psychoanalysts in dissociation on two grounds: (1) The psychoanalytic method is not one under which multiple personalities grow; and (2) dissociative phenomena do not yield the psychodynamic interpretations that psychoanalysts seek. Hart believed that his own position was that of a mediator: He thought analysts *ought* to take more note of dissociation and multiple personality.

The second paper to which I am calling attention was published 11 years later by William McDougall (1938), Hart's fellow countryman, who had by this time come to the United States. His paper, appearing in the year of his death, was entitled "The Relations between Dissociation and Repression." He returned to some of the ideas that had been expressed in his *Outline of Abnormal Psychology* (1926), and attempted to refute some criticisms that had been made by Lundholm (1933) and Pattie (1935). McDougall felt that the basic cleavage was between Janet's doctrine of dissociation and Freud's doctrine of repression. He indicated that he had developed a balanced position, with repression as a dynamic factor that in many cases prepares the way for and leads to (or causes) dissociation. Neither Hart nor McDougall rejected dissociation.

The topic lost prominence for many years. *Psychological Abstracts* began publication in 1927, the year of Hart's presidential address. In the first 10 volumes, from 1927 through 1936, there were 20 abstracts devoted to dissociation; in the next 10 years, a total of 8 abstracts were indexed; the number dropped to 2 and 3 in the next two decades, through 1966. Book discussions did not find their way into the journals reviewed in *Psychological Abstracts*, so that this is incomplete as an account of some persisting interest, showing only lack of support through research of the kind that led to publication in the journals reviewed.

Invitations to do more research were offered during these years. Hull (1933), in his book on hypnosis, devoted a chapter to the dissociation hypothesis. After an introductory exposition of Janet's views, he proceeded to discuss in some detail the experiments of Prince (1909), Burnett (1925), and Barry, MacKinnon, and Murray (1931). He included also two experiments done in his own laboratory, those of Messerschmidt (1927–1928) and of M. B. Mitchell (1932). He concluded that "whatever else so-called hypnotic dissociation may be, it is not a functional independence between two simultaneous mental processes" (Hull, 1933, p. 185). Still, he ended his chapter with the expressed hope that "the near future will see a series of well-controlled, large-scale investigations which will completely remove the uncertainties which at present becloud this extremely important problem" (p. 191).

Sears (1936), who had done some hypnotic experimentation with Hull, wrote an important review of functional abnormalities of memory. He treated Prince's theory more completely than Hull had done. Although wedded to a stimulus–response theory, he concluded that if the proper theory could be formulated, "there is good reason for considering it as a valuable hypothesis coordinate with the repression hypothesis as an explanation for amnesias of reproduction" (Sears, 1936, p. 269).

These invitations of Hull to further experimentation, and of Sears for a theoretical reformulation, had little effect in the years immediately following.

The Revived Interest in Multiple Personality Disorder

The interest in experimental investigations of hypnotic phenomena became enhanced in the years after midcentury, and dissociation again became of interest, particularly because of increased attention to multiple personality disorder (MPD). In an important review, Greaves (1980) reported that in 150 cases he found in the literature, at least one-third had been reported in the 1970s. Cases had accumulated much more slowly in earlier years. For example, in a major review of all known cases, W. S. Taylor and Martin (1944) had uncovered only 76 cases. In a selective review of the most plausible cases, Sutcliffe and Jones (1962) accepted only 10 cases among 16 brief case histories that were well described.

Kluft (1987) indicated a further increase in cases beyond those reported by Greaves, finding some 750 between 1980 and 1985. By this time, doubts began to arise over the diagnostic criteria that led to the numerous

MPD cases, voiced by two of the authors of one of the first new cases to cause widespread attention, that of *The Three Faces of Eve* (Thigpen & Cleckley, 1957). In a later publication, they expressed the firm belief that the proliferation of later cases was based on poor diagnostic criteria (Thigpen & Cleckley, 1984). The American Psychiatric Association began its official serious interest in improved diagnosis of MPD in its *Diagnostic and Statistical Manuals* of 1980 (DSM-III) and 1987 (DSM-III-R).

Experimental Studies of Dissociation within Hypnosis

Prior to this upsurge of interest in MPD, the Stanford Laboratory of Hypnosis Research undertook some experimental studies of the much less pervasive types of dissociation found in routine hypnosis. Done without reference to MPD, these early trials proved sufficiently intriguing to invite further investigation.

One illustration of dissociation in hypnosis, repeated in demonstrations in our laboratory, was first given by Milton Erickson on a visit to Stanford. Prior to Erickson's demonstration, he asked us to provide one of our subjects known to be unusually high in hypnotic responsiveness. The demonstration proceeded as follows: The subject, already hypnotized, was asked to hold his right hand and arm up vertically from the shoulder. Then Erickson, holding the upraised hand tentatively, explained that he was lowering the arm and hand, so that the hand would rest on the subject's lap. Letting go of the hand, he touched the lap as if still holding it, indicating that the hand was now resting there. To be sure that the hallucination was working, he invited the subject to place his left hand over the right hand on his lap and hold it there. He placed his left hand over the place where his right hand was reported to be, although the observers knew that the right arm and hand were still in the upright position. This having been achieved, Erickson then pinched the hand of the upright arm and asked the subject if he felt anything. With no mention of anesthesia, the subject reported that he felt nothing, and this was explained by Erickson on the grounds that he could not feel something in the hand that was—to him—somewhere else. This became a useful demonstration of dissociation, repeatable only with highly selected subjects, yet useful in some of our later-designed experiments.

The first planned research on dissociation took the form of a doctoral dissertation written by James Stevenson in 1972, although the results (in abbreviated form) were not published until 1976. Stevenson was already familiar with an unpublished master's thesis from the University of Oregon by William A. Cass, of which only an abstract had appeared (Cass, 1941). Cass had used as the two simultaneous tasks color naming from a display of colored patches as a "conscious task" and a consecutive addition of numbers done through automatic writing as a "subconscious" task, with, of course, appropriate controls. Stevenson added simulator controls requiring "faking" of the automatic writing by subjects not responsive to hypnotic procedures.

Stevenson found important evidence denying the complete functional independence of the tasks, and some evidence supporting a "repression" or perhaps a "suppression" interpretation of the subconscious task. The interpretation arose because he was able to demonstrate that the addition task deteriorated through being kept out of awareness, compared with conscious addition, even though there was no interfering task to be performed by the subject. In other words, some cognitive effort appeared to be needed to hold the task out of awareness, and this expenditure of effort interfered with performing that task. When a conscious interfering task was added, the performance deteriorated further. The simulators, performing the two tasks without the effort to keep one out of awareness, actually showed less deterioration on both tasks. Stevenson's results supported the earlier findings of a lack of complete functional independence between the two tasks, one of which seemed to be out of awareness, and added the evidence on the cognitive cost of trying to hold an active performance out of awareness. Although his findings set limits to what might be expected through dissociation experiments, the answers were not all in.

A second experiment was performed later than Stevenson's, although the published account appeared earlier than his (Knox, Crutchfield, & Hilgard, 1975). The experiment was designed similarly to Stevenson's, except that we selected a subconscious task to permit a better analysis of the strategies used in doing two tasks at once and to show the effects of suggestions for automaticity on these tasks. As a conscious task, we chose the same color-naming task that Stevenson had used. For the arithmetic task that he had used, we substituted a key-pressing task, which called for the patterned pressing of two keys mounted in a box concealed from the subject's view. The pattern was a cycle of three pressings of the left key, followed by three pressings of the right key; this cycle was repeated throughout the single trial period of 1 minute. A voice key recorded the naming of the colors on a polygraph, and the key pressing was recorded in parallel on the same polygraph. It was thus possible to determine the time relationships between the color naming and the key pressing (when the tasks were done simultaneously), as well as the accuracy of the key pressing. Each unit of the key pressing was scored, one unit being two triplets of key pressing (correctly, 3L-3R). A unit was in error if there was an extra or an omitted press (e.g., a cycle of 3L-4R or 2L-3R).

The overall results confirmed Stevenson's findings of two interfering factors—one due to hypnotic suggestions that the key pressing was to be done subconsciously, without awareness; the other due to the interfering simultaneous tasks. The key-pressing task proved to be of roughly the same difficulty as the counting task used by Stevenson, although with 15 real subjects instead of 8, the interference between conscious and subconscious single task performance proved to be significant even with this rather easy task. The interference showed in the number of errors made rather than in the number of key pressings attempted.

The Knox et al. (1975) experiment went beyond Stevenson's because it permitted a study of the strategies employed. Six strategies were identified, all of which involved an integration between the key pressing and the color naming. The most common strategy was used successfully by 8 of the 15 subjects. Decision time is involved in color naming; hence, the subject apparently selected the name and held it in readiness to announce simultaneously with key pressing. This resulted in an order on the polygraph of L-color-LL. Then, while pressing RRR, the subject apparently registered and stored the next name to complete the cycle as before (L-color-LL). Hence two colors were named for each set of six key presses, a ratio commonly found. Among the other strategies was alternating color names with key pressings (L-color-L-color-L-color, etc.). This slowed the whole process because of the long decision time in color naming. When both tasks were conscious, a subject tended to use the preferred strategy 85% of the time, whereas when the key pressing was intended to be subconscious, the strategy was used only 39% of the time, indicating some break in the selected strategy.

Two conclusions are justified by the results of these two experiments on the dissociation of simultaneous tasks, one conscious and one subconscious. First, the subjective ignoring of the subconscious automatic tasks while a conscious task is being performed is very real to some highly hypnotizable subjects; second, the interference is increased by the effort to maintain one task as subconscious, and this effort is a function of the difficulty of the task. Mutual interferences between conscious and subconscious tasks are found; the division between the tasks depends on the strategies available for their integration.

The Unanticipated Appearance of a Hidden Observer

At the time, I was offering a course to undergraduate students on hypnosis, with emphasis upon the variety of phenomena that could be experienced by a responsive hypnotized person. In this instance, the topic was hypnotic deafness. The subject of the demonstration was a blind student of known hypnotic talent, who had volunteered to serve. His blindness was not related to the experiment, except that it eliminated any unintended visual cues, although it was important that the subject knew that hypnotic deafness would be temporary because of his normal reliance upon hearing. After the induction of hypnosis, he was given the suggestion, that, at the count of 3, he would become completely deaf to all sounds. His hearing would be restored promptly when the instructor's hand was placed upon his right shoulder.

After the slow count to 3, loud sounds made by banging together some wooden blocks close to the subject's head produced no sign of reaction. No reaction was expected because the subject had previously shown no response to the shots of a starter's pistol when hypnotically deaf. A startle response had been evident when the shots had been fired when his eyes were closed but he was not hypnotized. The students asked questions and taunted him to see whether they could get a reaction, but nothing resulted. One student in the class raised the question whether some part of him might know what was going on, for, after all, there was nothing wrong with his ears. It occurred to me to test this by a method of interrogation that I had seen some clinical hypnotists use in seeking information from a hypnotized patient. So I addressed the subject in a quiet voice:

"As you know, there are parts of our nervous system that carry on activities that occur without awareness, of which the control of the circulation of the blood, or the digestive processes, are the most familiar. However, there may be intellectual processes also of which we are unaware, such as those that find expression in night dreams. Although you are hypnotically deaf, perhaps there is some part of you that is hearing my voice and processing the information. If there is, I should like the index finger of your right hand to rise as a sign that this is the case."

To the surprise of both me and the class members, the finger rose, and the subject immediately said:

"Please restore my hearing so that you can tell me what you did. I felt my finger rise in a way that was not a spontaneous twitch, so that you must have done something to make it rise." I then placed my hand on his right shoulder, as the prearranged signal for restoring his hearing, and the following conversation took place:

"Can you hear my voice now?"

"Yes, I hear you. Now tell me what you did."

"What do you remember?"

"I remember your telling me that I would be deaf at the count of 3, and could have my hearing restored when you placed your hand on my shoulder. Then everything was quiet for a while. It was a little boring just sitting here, so I busied myself with a statistical problem that I have been working on.[1] I was still doing that when I suddenly felt my finger lift; that is what I wanted you to explain to me."

I assured the subject that he would soon be informed about everything that had transpired. At this point I dared to introduce what came to be an important innovation. As explained above, my colleagues and I had been conducting some experiments on dissociation, including automatic writing. We had found that some material not in the awareness of the hypnotized subject could be recovered through automatic writing. It seemed worth testing with this highly hypnotizable subject whether, by analogy with automatic writing, "automatic talking" might yield similar results. Hence, with the subject hypnotized but able to hear and carry on a conversation, I spoke to him as follows:

"When I place my hand on your arm like this [I demonstrated], I can be in touch with that part of you that listened to me before, while you were hypnotically deaf. But this part of you, to whom I am now talking, will not know what you are saying, or even that you are talking, until—when you are out of hypnosis—I shall say 'Now you can remember everything.' All right, now I am placing my hand on your arm."

The following conversation ensued: "Do you remember what happened when you were hypnotized and what the hypnotized part of you reported?"

"Yes." (In some instances hypnotized subjects are thought to be literal in their answers, as in this "Yes," but that is by no means universal, and in this instance the subject had already told me about the experience while hypnotized.) On further questioning he repeated much of the earlier conversation, including his surprise at the finger's lifting.

I continued, "Does this part to whom I am now talking know more about what went on?"

"Yes."

"Please tell me what went on."

"After you counted to make me deaf, you made some noises as if banging some blocks together behind my head. Members of the class asked me questions to which I did not respond. Then one of them asked if I might really be hearing, and you told me to raise my finger if I did. This part of me responded by raising my finger, so it's all clear now."

I then lifted my hand from his arm to restore his prior condition, according to what I had told him.

The next question was to the hypnotized subject in his usual hypnotic condition following induction.

"Please tell me what has happened in the last few minutes."

"You said something about placing your hand on my arm, and some part of me would talk. Did I talk?"

I told him that he would remember everything after hypnosis was terminated and then aroused him by counting backwards, a procedure with which he was familiar. He then recalled all that had happened throughout the demonstration.

This unplanned and hence unrehearsed demonstration indicated clearly that a hypnotized subject who is not aware of a sensory information (in this case, auditory) may nevertheless be registering the sensory experience in some manner and processing the information. Under appropriate circumstances, what was unknown to the subject while hypnotized can be uncovered and talked about. For convenience of reference, instead of using the expression "automatic talking" (which I had in mind in introducing the demonstration), the degree of processing of the information that was revealed led me to introduce the metaphor of a "hidden observer." The metaphor may have been unfortunate because to some it suggested a secondary personality with a life of its own—a kind of homunculus lurking in the head of the conscious person. The "hidden observer" was intended as merely a convenient label for the information source capable of a high level of cognitive functioning, not consciously experienced by the hypnotized person.

Once the existence of the hidden-observer phenomenon was demonstrated with this highly responsive hypnotic subject, it became important to find how prevalent it was and what its parameters were. This task interested others as well as those in our laboratory, and led to two camps: those who supported the original interpretation, and added to the knowledge of how it was related to other hypnotic phenomena; and those who believed it to be only another of the hypnotic phenomena whose distinctiveness should be denied.

Elucidation of the Hidden Observer's Frequency and Its Correlates

Within our laboratory, we had found the phenomenon of the hidden observer only among a small fraction of the very highly responsive hypnotic subjects. In an early study of ice water pain (the cold-pressor response) among 20 highly hypnotizable subjects, all of whom could achieve substantial pain reduction through hypnotically suggested analgesia, clear evidence of covert pain revealed through the hidden-observer procedures was significant for the group as a whole, although the mean findings depended very much on the responses of 8 subjects among the 20 who gave the most substantial evidence of having the covert pain beyond the pain reported in the usual way following hypnotically suggested analgesia (E. R. Hilgard, Morgan, & Macdonald, 1975). In another study performed later (although published earlier), the pain was that known as ischemic pain, produced by a tourniquet to the upper arm, followed by exercise of the occluded hand (Knox, Morgan, & Hilgard, 1974). In this study the eight subjects had been preselected for exhibiting the hidden-observer phenomenon in contexts other than analgesia, so that, as expected, all showed hidden observers in this study. Because the subjects had been preselected, the fact that all showed hidden observers did not contradict the less frequent appearance of hidden observers in the other study.

In a later study of hypnotically suggested hearing loss, only 4 of 16 highly responsive subjects, all of whom showed substantial hearing loss following hypnotic suggestion, gave clear evidence of covert hearing beyond that overtly reported in hypnotic deafness (Crawford, Macdonald, & Hilgard, 1979). The limited number of highly responsive subjects from whom a hidden observer can be elicited restricts the appropriate generalizations to be made regarding these phenomena. It must be recalled that the highly responsive subjects used in these experiments were already a limited sample of the general population of student subjects, so that the 1 in 4 in the deafness experiment represented something less than 5% of a general student sample. Laurence and Perry (1981) replicated the hidden-observer finding in their Montréal laboratory for hypnotically produced analgesia, finding hidden observers in only 39% of their highly responsive subjects.

A group in the same laboratory conducted additional experiments that contributed an important finding bearing upon those highly responsive subjects who report and do not report hidden observers (Nogrady, McConkey, Laurence, & Perry, 1983). Aware of some attacks by others upon the hidden observer as a possible laboratory creation (Spanos & Hewitt, 1980), Nogrady et al. (1983) were meticulous in controlling for "demand characteristics" that might produce the phenomena through pressure for compliance. By making use of the "real–simulator" design of Orne (1959, 1979a), in which if compliance cues are prominent those simulating hypnosis will respond to them, they were able to show that the cues were not operative. Then to avoid any experimenter bias in interpreting what the subject experienced, one of the experimenters, McConkey, who had done none of the hypnotizing, conducted the postsession interview. He was unaware of which of the subjects were responding as highly hypnotizable and which were merely acting "as if" highly hypnotizable, although selected as not hypnotically responsive. He made use of the Experiential Analysis Technique of Sheehan, McConkey, and Cross (1978), which he had helped develop. The technique consisted (and consists) of showing each subject some time after the session a videotape of all that took place—what was done and what was said, both by the hypnotist and by the subject. At predetermined points the videotape was stopped, and the subjects were encouraged to comment on the observed material that they found meaningful. They could also request that the tape be stopped at other points when they wished to comment. McConkey occasionally asked specific questions—for example, with regard to the hidden-observer experience, "Is this an experience you had following the instructions, or is it one you were having throughout the session?" Another member of the investigative team, unfamiliar with the subjects' hypnotizability or with the ratings made by the interviewer, rated aspects of the experience bearing on dissociation and the hidden-observer experience. This carefully designed experiment confirmed our results (E. R. Hilgard, Macdonald, Morgan, & Johnson, 1978) and those of Laurence and Perry (1981) by finding a hidden-observer response in 5 of 12 highly hypnotizable subjects, in none of 10 high-medium subjects, and in none of 10 low hypnotizables simulating hypnosis.

The study by Laurence and Perry (1981), confirmed by Nogrady et al. (1983), in addition to showing the validity of the findings, threw some light on the problem of why some "highs" showed hidden observers and others did not. In the course of hypnotic testing, these investigators included age regression, in which the subjects were to experience themselves as again children of 5 years of age. Age regression may take one of two different forms. In one form the subject becomes completely absorbed in being a child again, in a manner convincing to him or her and to an observer. In a second form, the subject feels himself or herself to be reliving the experience of a 5-year-old, but in addition there is an adult observer present. Sometimes this is reported in statements that are variants of this one: "I felt sorry for that child [myself as a child] because I was lost and frightened lest my mother would not find me, but I knew all along that she would return soon." The experience can be considered as one of duality—the subject is at once a child and an adult. In the Montréal experiments, regression was recorded before there had been an opportunity to test for a hidden observer. It turned out, however, that the presence or absence of the duality experience was almost perfectly correlated with the subsequent experience of a hidden observer.

What would be the expected relationship? Would duality be predictive of a hidden observer or absence of a hidden observer? Let us take the position that there is some conformity to expectations. When the suggestion is to become again a child of 5, there is clearly no demand that an adult observer be expected. Hence duality would not be the expected result, and hence, if the hidden observer is a result of responses by the most compliant subjects, one would expect the hidden observer to be prevalent for those without the duality experience—that is, those who complied strictly with the wording of the suggested age regression. If, on the other hand, the hidden observer is an aspect of genuinely dissociated experiences, then the duality in age regression can be taken as a mark of spontaneous dissociation and taken as a sign that a hidden observer may be more readily manifested. This was, in fact, what was found: Those who had the duality experience also manifested the hidden observer.

Care is needed in advancing plausible interpretations as though they do not require experimental justification. The possibility that some sort of amnesic process is involved in these less severe dissociations, as it is often found in reported cases of multiple personality, has led to a search for such amnesic correlates. In a subsequent paper, Perry (1983) reported new data showing that amnesia was more profound in highly hypnotizable subjects with hidden observers than in those not demonstrating hidden observers. Why should there be a greater tendency to amnesia among highs with hidden observers? A possible conjecture is that they more readily store marginal experiences behind a cloak of amnesia, ready to be recovered by the reversibility of amnesia. Then those with less access to amnesia (i.e., those without a hidden observer) fail to record and store in memory events not in focus. The events are complex, and supplementary experiments will be necessary to clarify the kinds of individual differences involved.

Although the hidden-observer experience has its bearings on how we interpret the hypnotic experience, I wish now to consdider the present situation with respect to theories of hypnosis.

Current Theories of Hypnosis

Theories of hypnosis are currently in disarray for several reasons. The basic reason for failure is that it has not been possible to find any truly distinguishing basis—psychological, physiological, or neurophysiological—by which to distinguish sharply between the established hypnotic condition (call it "trance" or any other name) and normal waking consciousness. It is an easy leap, then, to decide that there is nothing substantial about hypnotic phenomena. Consider how research on sleep and dreams has been enhanced by the discovery of rapid-eye-movement sleep, and the other stages of sleep revealed by the electroencephalogram. At the same time, it must also be kept in mind that we did not doubt the reality of sleep and dreams prior to these advances. If the study of hypnosis is at the same stage as the study of sleep and dreams before the discovery of their physiological correlates, we may ask: Why should there be such concern over the definition of what belongs to hypnosis? In other words, why should there be uncertainty about what we are studying before there is an agreed-upon bodily basis for hypnosis?

What we find is that two major orientations toward hypnosis led gradually to a conflict between those who adopt the generally accepted view of the hypnotic interaction and the experiences and behaviors associated with it, and those who adopt an opposing standpoint. The first view is that the major hypnotic phenomena have been well enough established through experimental and clinical practice over the years to provide topics for investigation that belong in the general vocabulary of psychology along with such topics as attention, emotion, learning, motivation, sensory perception, thinking, and so on. Those who adopt the accepted view, in its several forms, may or may not use the concept of "hypnotic trance" as an explanatory concept to account for what occurs. I return to what is valuable in the traditional and accepting position after looking into the alternative orientation—supported by a minority of those trying to make a science of hypnosis, but a very active and committed minority, which asserts its victories so stridently that its views are convincing to those less familiar with the many unanswered problems in research on hypnosis.

The Alternative to the Accepted View of Hypnosis

The second orientation, again in several forms, questions most of the claims of the traditionalists, through what I earlier described as a form of iconoclasm with respect to hypnosis (E. R. Hilgard, 1971a). Proponents of this orientation address their theories and experiments to debunking practically all of the ordinary beliefs about hypnosis, such as the genuineness of posthypnotic amnesia or of hypnotic hallucinations; they reflect a distaste for any interpretation that favors some distinctive identifying characteristics of hypnotic phenomena, as compared with behavioral or experiential phenomena classified under ordinary psychological topics without reference to hypnosis. This standpoint is variously described as a "nonstate" position, with variants emphasizing "role enactment," a "social-psychological" stance, or a "cognitive–behavioral" perspective.

Sutcliffe (1960) was probably the first of those interested in serious research on hypnosis to propose a dichotomy between those who had a "credulous" and those with a "skeptical" view of hypnotic phenomena. He elaborated his view by presenting experimental evidence bearing upon esthesia, hallucinations, and delusion (Sutcliffe, 1961). By sharpening this distinction, he was unfair to those who accepted the phenomena while treating them with the same skepticism that is associated with all careful scientific work. Because of the phenomena they accepted, he accused them of delusion if, for example, they achieved pain reduction without evidence that the physiological aspects were identical with those found through the use of local or general anesthetics. The logic here is faulty, for pain is the feeling that something hurts, and less pain means that it hurts less; blood flow, blood pressure changes, heart rate, or other physiological concomitants of felt pain need not be alike for insensitivities to painful stimulation to be genuine. When the pain is gone, the hurt is gone, no matter what other indicators of potentially painful stimuli are present. The hidden-observer experiments on the representation of pain bear on these issues, because sometimes pain is not felt when other methods show that some pain was registered.

The next prominent adoption of the skeptical or nonstate view was that by T. X. Barber and his associates, represented by his practice of writing the word "hypnosis" in quotation marks as though there were something phony about it. He and his collaborators wrote a series of papers expanding upon his theory in the 1960s (e.g., T. X. Barber, 1962). He early converted at least two young disciples to his views (Chaves, 1968; Spanos, 1970), and this early imprinting has persisted beyond some changes in Barber's later perspectives (S. C. Wilson & Barber, 1981). His own book, entitled *Hypnosis: A Scientific Approach* (T. X. Barber, 1969), was the culmination of this early phase of his work, although he continued for a time to elaborate it as an alternative paradigm to more conventional approaches (T. X. Barber, 1979). Chaves and Spanos, although working at widely separated universities, remained faithful, and more recently have restated their common position (with a slight change in terminology) by editing a large multiauthor book entitled *Hypnosis: The Cognitive–Behavioral Perspective* (Spanos & Chaves, 1989c). The authors, including themselves, many of their students, and a few others, all support the common perspective, so that this book, with its many chapters and 62 pages of references, is described on its dust jacket as "A Reference Guide to Current Research." To be sure, there are many references included by those with whom they disagree. Still, it must stand for some time as the most thorough guide for those who have adopted their general orientation.

It would be a mistake not to mention another pair of workers who have consistently supported a related, if not identical, position. I refer to the theory of "role taking" to explain hypnosis, with which Theodore R. Sarbin was identified for many years (Sarbin, 1950). His student, William C. Coe, joined him as a collaborating author in the book that still stands as the best exposition of their position (Sarbin & Coe, 1972). Although based primarily on the sociological concept of role enactment, it fits the position of alternative to the traditional position on hypnosis by extending characteristic role-taking behavior to what the hypnotized subject does. Some are found to have more appropriate role enactment skills and hence are "better" hypnotic subjects. As a younger partner, Coe has continued to contribute valuable experimental studies after Sarbin's retirement from his active professional career. Coe contributed two chapters to the Spanos and Chaves book (Coe, 1989a,b).

Support is given these American alternatives to traditional hypnosis by the spread of the orientation to Great Britain, prominently represented by the writings of Graham F. Wagstaff—for example, his book entitled *Hypnosis, Compliance and Belief* (Wagstaff, 1981a), in which hypnosis appears to be largely a matter of willing compliance to the implied demands by the hypnotist. The more traditional word "suggestion" does not require another word to indicate that the hypnotic subject is compliant, although in its social-psychological meaning it implies that the behavior may be involuntary. According to Wagstaff, no matter how involuntary the behavior feels to the subject, the hypnotized person is not in an altered condition; he or she is just "an ordinary person who responds to expectations and social obligations" (p. 28).

Robert A. Baker is another American convert to the general position under discussion. Although over the years he has been less involved in hypnosis research than the others mentioned, they attracted his support through their papers and books. In his book entitled *They Call It Hypnosis* (R. A. Baker, 1990), he employs the familiar metaphor of "the emperor's clothes" to signify the unreality of hypnosis. His book is throughout supportive of an extreme skepticism about hypnosis, and in a final section entitled "Recapitulation—Questions and Answers," he gives the impression to anyone more experienced with hypnosis than he that he has never witnessed a genuinely highly responsive hypnotic subject. Here are some of his answers: "Intense concentration on our internal images is what we mean by 'self-hypnosis' " (p. 289). "In fact, most of hypnosis is nothing but reassurance and distraction" (p. 289). It is easy to get such ideas about hypnosis by immersing oneself primarily in the literature of one side of the major competing viewpoints, and not listening to honest reports by hypnotized persons, in view of having accepted the belief that they are all lying in order to please the hypnotist. That is too easy a way out: Call it all "social compliance," and there are no unanswered questions about these otherwise puzzling phenomena.

There would be no point, in a brief chapter, to attempt an incisive review of the three books mentioned that have appeared in the last decade or so (R. A. Baker, 1990; Spanos & Chaves, 1989c; Wagstaff, 1981a). They are serious books, and there is much to be learned from them, but they are also polemical—written for the most part in support of a common thesis, antithetical to the more traditional view of hypnosis accepted by many whose curiosity about hypnosis is not satisfied by these authors' assurance that they have all the answers. One curious by-product of adopting the voluntary-compliance position is that the old problem of detecting those who simulate hypnosis practically disappears. If all hypnotic subjects are simulators, there is no problem!

The assertion that all hypnosis is simulation, according to the alternative view, would not be acceptable to those who support that view, because compliance, although almost synonymous with voluntary cooperation, shows individual differences (such as those that turn up in hypnotic responsiveness scales). The training methods for improving hypnotic performance, however, do indeed attempt to make all subjects more compliant by defining hypnosis in such a manner that there is nothing wrong with *trying* to do what the hypnotist suggests—that is, to *make it happen*, instead of *letting it happen*. However, a point is made (e.g., by Spanos, Robertson, Menary, & Brett, 1986) that those who have improved their hypnotic performance with the Carleton Skills Training Program have not simply become more compliant, because they can still produce changes by simulating hypnosis. The increase in visual imagery through training is said to be largely responsible for the training success, but the evidence is not wholly convincing. The large gains reported through training by Gorassini and Spanos (1986) were not readily duplicated by those in another laboratory (Gfeller, Lynn, & Pribble, 1987). In their study, 14 of the 24 initially low scorers failed to achieve a high score after training.

Although those who take this alternative view usually continue to be interested in the usual types of performance and experiences as reported by hypnotic subjects, well-established manifestations of hypnosis are occasionally rejected out of hand. Let me take as one example the complete rejection of the concept of posthypnotic amnesia by Coe (1989a). After a scholarly review of the more recent literature, the final statement is this: "Responsive hypnotic subjects can be viewed as engaging in strategic enactment to fulfill the role of good hypnotic subject as they perceive it" (p. 147). There is nothing genuine about posthypnotic amnesia! Thus we come out the same door as that by which we entered: the espousal of role theory. In the meantime, we have had to contend with such irrational attacks on posthypnotic amnesia as that it is incredible, for it is not like ordinary forgetting, since it is partially reversible (p. 111). This uses against psthypnotic amnesia the very criterion that identifies it—that it *is* a reversible forgetting! That it is easily reversible makes many of the later studies of its breaching subject to the possibility that the emphasis upon compliance used in other circumstances is applicable here. Implanting a signal for reversal also implants the possibility of breaching, and the investigator, unless extreme caution is used, may signal reversal without an explicit use of the implanted signal.

Traditional Orientations

The claims by those with alternative views on hypnosis have by no means won a complete victory over those more accepting of conventional interpretations of what happens in hypnosis. This does not mean that those who are more accepting are united in their theorietical orientations. In fact, the opposite is the case: Those with the alternative view are the more dogmatic and united in what they stand for.

Who are some representatives of the more conventional views? Many of them are rather pragmatic or eclectic; they go about their business, studying or using hypnosis without being strident in their theorizing. Still, I can list a few.

One of these is André M. Weitzenhoffer, who has been writing on hypnotism for many years, defending the position that goes back to Bernheim (Weitzenhoffer, 1978b). More recently he has written a two-volume work, *The Practice of Hypnotism,* of which the first volume is subtitled *Traditional and Semi-Traditional Techniques and Phenomenology* (Weitzenhoffer, 1989). One of his recommendations is to study some "pure cases" of unusually high hypnotic responsiveness ("somnambulists") over time, to learn what phenomena are produced in "true" hypnosis.

Another is Martin T. Orne, who has run a large and well-equipped laboratory for many years. He has produced many innovations, such as first calling attention to (and naming) "demand characteristics," so prominent among those who today are so fascinated by compliance (Orne, 1962a). As one way of bringing such demands to light he proposed the real–simulator design, in which nonhypnotizable subjects, through behaving as though they were highly responsive to hypnosis, would reveal how clearly they could infer the hypnotist's expectations (Orne, 1959, 1979a). These approaches are not indications that he is uncritical in the acceptance of hypnotic phenomena; and he would probably still defend the view expressed in an earlier paper, "The Nature of Hypnosis: Artifact and Essence," in which he relied on the reports of hypnotized persons (contrasted with simulators) to learn what the experience was like (Orne, 1959).

Then there is Erika Fromm, who also has been deeply involved in hypnosis research for many years. Her theorizing has been influenced by psychoanalysis. This has not lessened her holding to the accepted view that there is something unique about hypnosis, whether heterohypnosis as usually practiced, or self-hypnosis which she and her collaborators have studied very thoroughly (D. P. Brown, 1990; Fass & Brown, 1990; Fromm, Brown, Hurt, Oberlander, Boxer, & Pfeifer, 1981; Fromm & Kahn, 1990). Her incorporation of ego psychology from psychoanalysis has made her theory distinctive. According to Fromm, what happens in hypnosis cannot be described simply as entering a "state," for it also implies a "talent" for hypnosis. She says:

> Hypnosis is an altered state of consciousness into which people can go if they have the talent to do so: in which they experience heightened ego receptivity (equals suggestibility) *and* ego activity; attention changes; more primary process thinking, more imagery; dissociative phenomena (for instance, the observing ego versus the experiencing ego); regression in the service of the ego; [fading of] the GRO (Generalized Reality Orientation); and stronger and quicker transference phenomena. It is also an altered state of consciousness in which the repressed returns more easily. (personal communication, January 23, 1991)

One of the prominent practitioners of hypnosis, with a large number of followers, also developed an orientation that was unique. I refer to Milton H. Erickson, about whom much has been written, and whose work is now carried on with promotional zeal by the Milton H. Erickson Foundation in Phoenix, Arizona, under the directorship of Jeffrey K. Zweig. There is a related Milton Erickson Gesellschaft in Germany. One of Zweig's associates, Michael D. Yapko, director of the Milton H. Erickson Institute of San Diego, has written a useful book entitled *Trancework,* which by its very title places it in the "trance" tradition (Yapko, 1990). Although its orientation is largely Ericksonian, it is placed in a larger context by including a number of relevant comments by others (not all Erickson disciples) in 10 short boxed sections entitled "Frames of Reference," giving glimpses of the personal perspectives of others with viewpoints on hypnosis. In an appendix, three major models of hypnosis are contrasted: traditional (the generally accepted view), standardized (with routinized procedures, as in the test for hypnotic responsivity), and Ericksonian (which is characterized as "utilization," because the basic principle is to utilize whatever will work for a given patient in a given situation).

There are many other theories of hypnosis that lie, in general, within what Weitzenhoffer would describe as "semitraditional" theories (i.e., departing from the generally accepted orientation in special ways). For example, the Spiegels have propounded a theory in connection with their hypnotic scale, the Hypnotic Induction Profile. This theory of hypnosis emphasizes the role played by attention, but also takes account of individual differences in hypnotic responsiveness. How hypnotizable a person is depends upon a biological basis, represented by the eye roll sign, and an acquired set of abilities, in which the capacity to sustain attention is particularly important (H. Spiegel & Spiegel, 1978).

I could go on, but this is enough to show that the generally accepted orientation consists of a family of theories. These have in common an agreement that there exist typical hypnotic phenomena that give coherence to the field, even though a brain model is elusive.

A Pragmatic Dissociation Interpretation

Although I define myself as one who adopts the generally accepted point of view toward hypnosis as a field of inquiry on its own, and deserving of its own theories, I have never been much of an advocate of comprehensive theories that go beyond the data of observation. I suppose this derives from my continued favoring of functionalism, even though I grew up in the era of behaviorism. The general principle I followed in designing my experiments, whether on conditioned responses or hypnosis, was to raise questions that were of somewhat limited scope so that the results held promise of dependable answers. After developing an interest in establishing dissociation in a contemporary form as applicable to hypnosis, I held back against extending the theory too far. After closing the Stanford Laboratory of Hypnosis Research in 1979, I felt little like elaborating a theory in directions that I was not in a position to test.

As a consequence, I am relying rather heavily on things that I have written before, if on rereading them I find that they still seem sensible to me. I feel that way about a paper I wrote on "the domain of hypnosis" (E. R. Hilgard, 1973c), and in what follows I repeat much that appeared in that paper.

The Domain of Hypnosis[2]

We have a great deal to do in hypnotic research activities besides trying to resolve the controversy between state theories and the nonstate alternative. One way to turn aside from the endless and often fruitless debates is to look for areas of agreement. An area of possible agreement is that of the common topics we study when we engage in hypnotic research. These topics define what I like to call "the domain of hypnosis."

The General Domain

The initial focus for someone who becomes interested in hypnosis is on what happens when the hypnotist, with the consent of the subject, attempts to induce hypnosis through conventional procedures. These procedures usually include eye fixation or other immobilization suggestions of relaxation or sleep, and a fairly monotonous flow of talk from the hypnotist. When the subject has appeared to respond (or at such time as a responsive subject would have responded), the hypnotist gives suggestions for particular kinds of actions and experiences. If he or she is successful, what the subject does or experiences illustrates the kinds of behavior familiar in hypnotic lore. These behaviors have been known for a century at least, many for longer: the involuntary production of contractions and paralyses; the creation of hallucinations, both positive and negative, including absence of pain to normally painful stimuli; age regression; posthypnotic amnesia; the performance of hypnotic acts to a preestablished signal. Anyone who has witnessed such a performance knows something about the domain of hypnosis. These behaviors, especially when seen together in one session, are very seldom demonstrated in any other context.

The denotative definition of the domain of hypnosis is further enriched by the clinical successes when hypnotic procedures are used to eliminate the pain of childbirth, major burns, and cancer, or when its procedures are used in clinical psychology or psychiatry to produce relaxation, to recover memories, or to relieve anxiety. The testimony of hypnotized subjects about alterations that take place within themselves cannot be ignored.

Defining the domain is not simple, however, for there are puzzling problems of so-called "waking suggestion," in which most of the responses typical of hypnotic behavior are given without a prior induction; self-hypnosis, in which subjects do for themselves what is usually done by a hypnotist, even without any prior experience of hypnosis (Ruch, 1975); and the many related phenomena in other contexts, such as highway hypnosis, responses to a demagogue, meditation, and placebo response. Hence, one approach to the domain of hypnosis is to delimit the domain by defining its boundaries.

Delimiting the Domain of Hypnosis

It is possible to move from a general familiarity with hypnotic phenomena to a more precise delimitation of the field.

1. *The first point is that hypnotic behavior cannot be defined simply as a response to suggestion.* Liébeault and Bernheim convinced many investigators that hypnosis was primarily a matter of suggestion, and this intimate relationship has continued to be acknowledged, as, for example, in the titles of Hull's (1933) *Hypnosis and Suggestibility* and Weitzenhoffer's (1953) *Hypnotism: An Objective Study in Suggestibility*. T. X. Barber's (1965) scale is called a suggestibility scale. Shall we not then define hypnotic-like behavior as responses to suggestion? The answer is no; although hypnotic-

ike behaviors are commonly responses to suggestion, the domain of suggestion includes responses that do *not* belong within hypnosis, and the phenomena of hypnosis involve more than specific responses to suggestion.

There are three lines of evidence for excluding some kinds of responses to suggestion from the domain of hypnosis. First is the distinction made by Hull (1933) between "personal" and "impersonal" heterosuggestion, and clarified by Eysenck and Furneaux (1945) as "primary" and "secondary" suggestibility. In this classification, primary suggestibility is defined by responses to waking suggestion, such as postural sway, that predict the usual phenomena of hypnosis, and secondary suggestibility is defined as responses to waking suggestions that do not correlate with the tests classed as primary. Secondary suggestibility is represented by such tests as Binet's progressive weights, a form of test that Hull described as impersonal heterosuggestion. Later investigators have confirmed the distinction through correlational and factor-analytic studies (e.g., Stukát, 1958).

Second is the empirical demonstration that forms of social suggestibility, described by such names as conformity and gullibility, are not correlated with hypnoticlike behaviors (Burns & Hammer, 1970; Moore, 1964).

A third bit of evidence for the nonoverlap between hypnosis and all of suggestion is that response to placebo is also distinguishable from hypnotic-like responsiveness (McGlashan, Evans, & Orne, 1969).

By defining primary suggestibility as lying *within* the hypnotic domain and these other varieties of suggestibility as lying *outside* the domain, we can begin to make additional assertions about the hypnotic domain.

2. *A second point in defining the domain of hypnotic behavior is the persistence of individual differences in what has been defined as primary suggestibility.* Whenever anyone has constructed a scale to measure this kind of suggestibility or susceptibility, with or without hypnotic induction procedures, highly concordant results are obtained. A comparison between the Barber Suggestibility Scale (BSS) and the Stanford Hypnotic Susceptibility Scale, Form A (SHSS:A) shows essential similarity in outcome, regardless of some differences in detail (Ruch, Morgan, & Hilgard, 1974).

The SHSS:A was developed as a modification and extension of an earlier one by Friedlander and Sarbin (1938). These are all elementary scales, with a heavy emphasis on motor performance and without much "top"; the scales are too easy, so that the individual differences among those making the highest (top) scores are not differentiated because they all score alike. The original and the revised scale have much in common.

From other evidence, both from our laboratory and from the studies by others, we know that there is a substantial correlation (about .70) between scores on hypnotic scales when the scores are obtained with and without a prior formal induction procedure. What this means, by my criteria, is that waking suggestion of this kind belongs within the domain of hypnosis, regardless of the arguments over a state of hypnosis or over the consequences of induction. Most induction procedures use some form of waking suggestion to induce hypnosis, such as suggested eye closure or arm levitation. If there were no correlation between waking suggestion and hypnotic suggestion, these procedures would be ineffective.

Two kinds of evidence call attention to the significance of these persistent individual differences. One was a study of the hypnotizability of twins and their families, conducted in the Stanford laboratory. There is a strong suggestion that hypnotic talent may have a hereditary component, as indicated by the substantial correlations of the scores of monozygotic twins as compared with dizygotic twins or ordinary siblings. These correlations yield a heritability index (h^2) of .62, highly significant (Morgan, 1973; Morgan, Hilgard, & Davert, 1970). This finding is subject, of course, to the limitations of all twin studies.

The second line of evidence comes from the stability of hypnotic responsiveness scores over long periods of time. Fifty subjects who were tested while university undergraduates, and whose scores were available, were located through alumni records and tested at three later dates: one 10 years later after original testing, another at 15 years, and a final test 25 years after the original testing. The correlations are consistently high, despite the changes in life experience after living and working in the community after college. The results are presented in Table 3.1. The correlations compare favorably with those obtained in other studies of such measures as intelligence and personality (Piccione, Hilgard, & Zimbardo, 1989).

The relative stability of hypnotic susceptibility, without any intrusive measures to support change, does not mean that change cannot take place. The common finding is, however, that the final results correlate positively with initial baselines and the greatest improvement (when corrected for ceiling effects) is for those initially responsive. More recent reports of large

TABLE 3.1. Test–Retest Correlation Coefficients of Measured Hypnotizability (Stanford Hypnotic Susceptibility Scale, Form A) for Total Sample and by Sex

Retest	Total ($n = 50$)	Male ($n = 24$)	Female ($n = 26$)
25 years (1960–1985)	.71	.69	.73
15 years (1970–1985)	.82	.82	.81
10 years (1960–1970)	.64	.62	.67

Note. All correlations are statistically significant, $p < .01$, but no one correlation differs significantly from another, $p > .05$, two-tailed. From "On the Degree of Stability of Measured Hypnotizability over a 25-Year Period" (p. 291) by C. Piccione, E. R. Hilgard, and P. G. Zimbardo, 1989, *Journal of Personality and Social Psychology, 56,* 289–295. Copyright 1989 by the American Psychological Association. Reprinted by permission.

changes have been presented, but only when the training methods encourage a good deal of simulation of hypnosis (Gorassini & Spanos, 1986). (For comments on this study, see p. 83, above.)

The statistical evidence of stability and continuity of individual differences in responsivity to hypnosis was supported also by clinical observations made in our interviewing program, where imaginative involvements in childhood indicated a developmental aspect to hypnotizability (J. R. Hilgard, 1979b).

3. *A third point relating to the domain of hypnosis is that subjective reports illuminate the phenomenological aspects of hypnotic-like behavior and serve as correctives to objective scores.* Barber and his associates, over recent years, gave attention to subjective scores and supplemented the BSS with an inquiry regarding the reality of the experiences (T. X. Barber, 1969, p. 247). The subjective and objective scores correlated very highly, both with and without prior hypnotic induction. However, the correctives introduced by the subjective scores raised the predictive value of the BSS, when correlated with the scores on the more advanced Stanford Profile Scale of Hypnotic Susceptibility, Form 1, from a corrrelation of .58 with objectives scores to one of .70 with the subjective score correction. The increase was somewhat less with the SHSS:A, from .73 to .76 (Ruch et al., 1974).

To deny the significance of verbal reports is to lose sight of the fact that all science depends on inferences from data, and the data from overt movements as well as the data from verbal reports may lead to faulty inferences. It is as easy to falsify a muscular contraction inferred to be involuntary as it is to report verbally that it is involuntary. The movement and the words can both be interpreted as forms of social communication.

When the testimony of hypnotized subjects is taken seriously for the description of the phenomena of hypnosis, we find that variety and richness are added. It is for this reason that the domain of hypnosis includes more than responses to specific or implied suggestions.

The domain of hypnosis has been defined by showing (1) that it commonly involves suggestion, but not all kinds of suggestion; (2) that the behaviors studied reflect persistent individual differences that we are beginning to understand; and (3) that the subjective reports, correlating significantly with objective behavior, can at the same time produce correctives to reliance solely on objective performance. The testimony of subjects regarding their experiences gives the domain a coherence not completely described by responses to specific or implied suggestions.

In describing the domain of hypnosis in this way, I have indicated that it is possible to agree on the *area of inquiry*, or the *topics* under investigation, prior to an agreement on the substantive nature of any changes that take place in bodily processes, the cognitive organization within hypnosis, or the most appropriate explanatory concepts. Regardless of standpoint, it is not necessary to write "hypnosis" in quotation marks if we understand that we are talking about an area of inquiry rather than a theory or explanation.

Executive and Monitoring Functions within Hypnosis[3]

Executive Functions in Hypnosis

For many years psychologists paid little attention to central control functions, avoiding the problems of a central "will" behind acts that they felt were better understood as "habits." They introduced some ancillary functions such as "sets" or "determining tendencies" to account for sustaining one direction of activity against competing alternatives, but these were somewhat local and temporary. Of two extreme interpretations about how decisions lead to action, one interpretation may accept a powerful central control system, replacing the concept of a strong will, whereas the other may deny central control altogether, substituting instead a hierarchy of possible thoughts and actions determined by the competitive strengths of the activated subsystems (whether habits or cognitive structures). These subsystems would then fight according to their strengths for control of the final common path leading to action. Because psychologists had evaded the problems of a planning and initiating self, they tended to adopt the second of these alternatives. To the extent that human beings were thought to be controlled by external stimuli and the habits conditioned to them, it was felt that human's actions represented a compromise behavior adapted to the totality of forces upon them. However, now that planning and control functions are gaining recognition, the entire matter of central processes requires reexamination.

A central regulating mechanism characterized by both temporary and enduring aspects, limited in what it does and can do, may be accepted as a starting point. Many subsystems of habits, attitudes, prejudices, interests, and specialized abilities are available, although at any one time they may be latent; these are actuated according to the demands of the situation and the plans of the central system. This central regulatory mechanism is responsible for the facilitations and inhibitions that are required to actuate the subsystem selectively. A hierarchy of subsystems is implied, although it is a shifting hierarchy under the management of the control mechanisms. Once a subsystem has been activated, it continues with a measure of autonomy; the conscious representation of the control system may recede, leading to some degree of automatization. William James noted, as others had before him and others have done since, that as habit takes over it diminishes the conscious representation of what goes on: "A strictly voluntary act has to be guided by idea, perception, and volition throughout its whole course. In an habitual action, mere sensation is a sufficient guide, and the upper regions of brain and mind are set comparatively free"

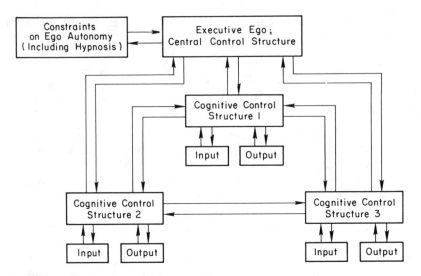

FIGURE 3.1. Subordinate cognitive control systems in a hierarchical order subject to change under a dominant executive ego or central control structure. From "A Neodissociation Interpretation of Pain Reduction in Hypnosis" (p. 405) by E. R. Hilgard, 1973, *Psychological Review, 80,* 396–411. Copyright 1973 by the American Psychological Association. Reprinted by permission.

(James, 1890, Vol. 1, pp. 115–116). The automatization of habit, setting the rest of the mind free, allows such dual actions as carrying on a conversation while engaged in habitual activity.

An earlier attempt to convey the idea of multiple subsystems under central control is presented in Figure 3.1, designed to indicate the availability of substructures in hierarchical arrangement; only three are shown (E. R. Hilgard, 1973b). Their positions in the chart suggest their hierarchical order; once activated, each has its own input and output, thus indicating a relative autonomy. At the top is an executive ego or central control structure with the planning, monitoring, and managing functions required for using the subsystems appropriately. The autonomy of the subsystems is restrained by the feedback relations among the systems, as well as by the central mechanism. The executive ego has no absolute authority, as indicated by the box representing constraints on it. These are the familiar constraints against a purely voluntary control of action and are determined by the individual history and situational influences; the constraints become particularly clear when hypnotic influences are imposed. Suggestions from the hypnotist may influence the executive functions themselves and change the hierarchical arrangement of the subsystems.

Other psychologists, whether or not they have included a central control system, have found it desirable to recognize organized subordinate cognitive structures. Once such a substructure becomes active, it has a certain degree of autonomy; a simple illustration is that of a bilingual person deciding to talk in one of his or her two languages, after which the appropriate language forms are used automatically and the other language is inhibited. Brief mention of the positions that several others have taken, without elaboration, shows that an analysis along these general lines is closely allied to other developments within general psychology. Seven of these positions follow; in only two of them does the planning function find expression.

1. The term "cognitive structure" was made familiar by Edward Tolman (1932/1949, 1948) and taken over by Kurt Lewin (1935). Such a structure may be pervasive but it is not all-embracing, and there are problems of communication between structures.

2. One of Clark Hull's central concepts was that of "habit-family hierarchy," in which a number of habits (each of which may be considered a small substructure) permit the organism to achieve its goals in a given situation, and these small substructures are organized in a preferential or hierarchical system, so that if one is blocked the next is activated (Hull, 1934).

3. Donald Hebb's conception of "cell assemblies" serves to provide a physiological substratum for cognitive structures (Hebb, 1949), and in a talk before the Canadian Psychological Association in 1974 he noted a possible coordination between his proposals and the existence of the "hidden observer" as I have described it (Hebb, 1975).

4. Sarbin's "roles" can also be considered to be cognitive substructures (e.g., Sarbin & Coe, 1972).

5. The "cognitive networks," prominent in the model proposed by Blum, Geiwitz, and Stewart (1967), serve comparable functions.

6. The "images" and "plans" of G. A. Miller, Galanter, and Pribram (1960) represent their levels of analysis that would provide for control of thought and action; these, too, may be considered to be substructures, with some hierarchy implied.

7. The "subordinate ego structures" of Gill and Brenman (1959), with a dominant ego, represent an interpretation similar to mine, at least within hypnosis. In a larger setting the various ego apparatuses of Hartmann (1939/1958), especially those in his "conflict-free ego sphere" are readily assimilated.

Repeatedly, over the past two decades, Erika Fromm has emphasized the role of the ego in hypnosis, thus continuing to propose ideas closely related to the others cited (e.g., Fromm, 1972, 1977).

Even though a central planner is lacking in several of the foregoing proposals, the idea is a congenial one and is familiar in everyday experience. Even a simple matter such as making an appointment for luncheon next week is negotiated with those involved, written down, and then acted on at a later time. This planfulness controls the possible behavior on that future date quite effectively. The many competing thoughts that occur the morning of the luncheon do not appear to be as determinative of what is going to happen in the midday as the plans that were made by some responsible part of the cognitive apparatus during the prior week. Appointments of this kind are kept with a very high probability—perhaps as high as 90% of the time—so that the planning function must be taken seriously. The event may be trivial, but its implications are not.

The support for a special executive function has come into the open from an unlikely source—the computer. Heuristic computer programs commonly have an executive program that monitors the computer's attempts to solve problems (Newell & Simon, 1972). If one direction goes on too long without reaching a solution, the executive calls a halt and a new direction is taken. This close analogy makes the idea of control a plausible one (Neisser, 1967). From another direction, control processes have been noted as important in such processes as rehearsing to hold information in short-term memory (R. C. Atkinson & Shiffrin, 1971), and since then more attention has been given to problems of control as part of the "working memory" (e.g., Bower, 1975).

The central executive functions in hypnosis are typically thought to be divided between the hypnotist and the hypnotized person. The latter retains a considerable portion of the executive functions from his or her normal state—the ability to answer questions about his or her past and plans, as well as to accept or refuse invitations to move about or to participate in specific kinds of activities. At the same time the subject turns over some of his or her executive functions to the hypnotist, so that within the hypnotic contract, the subject will do what the hypnotist suggests, experience what the hypnotist suggests, and lose control of his or her movements if this is indicated. The retained and relinquished fractions will depend upon circumstances, including the degree of hypnotic responsiveness or talent that the subject brings to hypnosis, and the depth of involvement in hypnosis as a function of what transpires between the subject and the hypnotist.

A striking illustration of what is meant by the division of the executive system into two parts is provided by what occurs in self-hypnosis. The central executive function now divides itself into two parts, representing the role of hypnotist and hypnotized. Although this appears essentially irrational, it is no more irrational than heterohypnosis, in which dissociated controls are the very essence of what happens. In fact, heterohypnosis is primarily "aided self-hypnosis" when a hypnotist is present; the person accepts the hypnotist as an aid to hypnotizing himself or herself. It has often been supposed that self-hypnosis must be a kind of response to posthypnotic suggestion of a person who has "internalized" the hypnotist. That is, once a person has been hypnotized, the hypnotist can say, "You can hypnotize yourself by counting to 10." In that way, the hypnotist has really implanted the suggestion, even though the subject engages in self-hypnosis. This is not quite correct, for with the barest of instructions a subject can proceed to hypnotize himself or herself and yield the usual responses to suggestion, *even if the subject has never had the experience of being hypnotized by another* (Ruch, 1975). Surprising as this may seem, here is an example: A hypnotizable man may suggest to himself that his arm will become stiff until he gives himself a release signal, and he will be unable to bend it, no matter how hard he tries, until he releases the suggestion (say, by counting to 5). The arm does indeed become stiff; he exerts all possible efforts to bend it without success. Then he starts to count, and at the count of 5 the arm relaxes and he can again bend it. It is as though he has created a small version of the Frankenstein monster, his own creation that then defies him by its autonomous behavior. This is the essence of the split of the executive function in hypnosis—a retained normal part that has permitted the hypnotized part to become active, with the hypnotized part then, in its own sphere, having considerable strength in conflict with the residual normal executive.

As a first step in hypnosis, the central executive function becomes sufficiently divided that the usual initiative of the executive is lost. Its planning side is inhibited, and it does not independently undertake new lines of thought or action. The hypnotized person, asked to behave normally while remaining hypnotized, finds the effort at initiative distasteful and commonly withdraws to a comfortable chair if given the opportunity. We have observed this in informal demonstrations in our laboratory. One subject, asked to show an interest in a box of small objects at the other end of the room, replied, "I don't want to but I'll do it if you insist." Interesting and convincing observations along these lines have been reported by Gill and Brenman (1959, pp. 36–37). For example, after subjects were asked how they knew they were hypnotized, if they said "I feel relaxed," they were told that they would no longer feel relaxed, but would remain in hypnosis. In this manner, one after another of the subjective signs of being hypnotized were taken away, while the subjects remained hypnotized. The final reply turned out, for several subjects, to be "I know I am in hypnosis because *I know that I will do what you tell me.*" This still defines hypnosis by suggestion, but includes *readiness to respond* to suggestions as part of the background associated with being in the state. Once initiative has been relinquished, the hypnotized person is prepared to respond to suggestions, as though the initiative resides either with the hypnotist or, in self-hypnosis, with the nonhypnotized fraction.

The type of cooperation that the hypnotized person exercises in hypnosis adds features that modify the common misconception of the subject as a passive pawn manipulated by the hypnotist. Even though the subject has turned over a large measure of his or her executive function to the hypnotist, he or she remains essentially the hypnotist's assistant in producing the phenomena. This state of affairs appears transitional between heterohypnosis and self-hypnosis. Many subjects report repeating the hypnotist's suggestions to themselves, occasionally modifying the wording to make the suggestions more acceptable. If the hypnotist requests that they select an appropriate fantasy to implement a suggestion, they cooperate by doing so; in fact, they may choose an appropriate fantasy to help out the suggestion even if not asked to do so. Spanos and his associates have shown in a series of experiments that the involuntariness of a suggestion that the arm is becoming stiff is associated with the extent to which a subject has aroused appropriate fantasies. These may include picturing the arm in a splint, or as made of wood or iron, so that it cannot bend. Spanos has named them "goal-directed fantasies" because they have the purpose of making the suggestion more convincing. They may be invoked even when the hypnotist's suggestion has made no reference to fantasy, having suggested directly, "Your arm is now becoming stiff" (Spanos, Rivers, & Ross, 1977). The subject, cooperating with the hypnotist, is exercising some initiative *within* hypnosis.

It can be argued that, except for relinquishing control over the subsystems that are specifically dissociated from control by suggestion, and the readiness for relinquishing control, the central executive functions have not been much modified in hypnosis. In superficial hypnosis, these mild dissociations can occur through waking suggestions, with little alteration of the general state of consciousness. When varied suggestions to a talented hypnotic subject have cumulative effects, as in suggestions of relaxation and detachment from the environment, the more general features of the hypnotic state begin to appear. A more massive dissociation, so far as the executive is concerned, may be the consequences of the summing up of many specific subsystems for which control has been relinquished. Such an interpretation permits hypnosis as a state to be a relative matter, the specific dissociation being identifiable, but the general state being a matter of how many specific dissociations are operative and how pervasive they are. Only when they are sufficiently pervasive is it appropriate to speak of a change of state.

Monitoring Functions in Hypnosis

The divisions in executive functions bear importantly upon the divided roles within the monitoring functions in hypnosis. Having accepted the hypnotic contract, the executive "issues an order" to the monitor to reduce the amount of critical scanning—to relinquish, as Shor (1970) has put it, the usual "reality orientation." The monitor may then repeat what occurs ("The arm is now stiff") without questioning the cause of its stiffness.

In the usual waking condition, the monitoring functions proceed in a satisfactorily integrated manner as they perceive and take account of the information that becomes available from the external world and from the body. The distortion of reality in hypnosis depends on the degree of hypnotic involvement, and much normal monitoring is retained in hypnosis. A subject who is hypnotically analgesic, or deaf, or amnesic for a list of words previously memorized, is still able to use the other senses normally and has available the usual memories. Even the behaviors that have been produced within hypnosis by way of suggestion can be described in a normal, matter-of-fact manner: "My hands are rising as if by themselves," "I see a red and white box on the table." The characteristic distortion that can be used to indicate a partial fractionation of the monitoring function is its uncritical acceptance of distorted reality as though it were undistorted, without making the usual reality tests. That is, normal persons may be subject to reality distortion, as in a size–weight illusion whereby a pound of lead feels heavier than a pound of cotton, but they are likely to be suspicious of their judgment and to test the weights on a balance. Hypnotized persons, told that one of two objects of equal weight is heavier than the other, report that that is the way they feel, but they are unconcerned about testing the reality in some other way, unless asked to do so. Examples of hypnotic distortion include hallucinations, both positive and negative, and age regression.

The exact relation between the monitoring function and the activated subsystem is not readily defined, for to the extent that the experience belongs to the subsystem in which the subject is deeply involved, the monitor may be reporting accurately. That is, the person may be reported as phenomenally a child again, on the playground of the third grade in school. All available information is not used by the activated subsystem, and the monitor does not offer a correction; hence imagination may be confused with external reality. The lack of normal criticism was called "trance logic" by Orne (1959), who used as his illustration the hallucination of a double person actually present and perceived. The hypnotic subject accepts this doubling without concern, even though he or she may at first be a little puzzled, as shown by looking back and forth between them in behavior known as a "double-take." Correspondingly, in one of the items on the Stanford Profile Scales, the hypnotized subject hallucinates a second light at the other end of a box on which a real light is present. This is not logically contradictory, as in the case of the doubled person, but it has some similar characteristics. For example, in both illustrations the subject tends to act as if the hallucinated experience is like the actual perceptual one, even when, upon questioning, he or she may often detect differences between them. The point is that the subject is typically unconcerned about exercising critical discrimination until his or her monitoring functions are again mobilized by the hypnotist.

Another way in which the fractionation of the monitoring function from the activated subsystem is shown is in the detachment of the observing part from what is happening. The monitor may express surprise that an arm cannot be bent or amusement over some fantasied reality, such as floating on a cloud. The monitoring system knows what is going on from the point of view of the hypnotized person, but some information is concealed from it. The executive system, in collaboration with the hypnotist, succeeds in giving rise to the actuated experiences. How this has been done may be concealed from the monitor or lost by the fractionation of memory. For example, if an arm is made stiff by suggestion and the subject is unable to bend it even when he or she tries, the monitor reports just that: "You said my arm would be stiff and I couldn't bend it; I have tried to bend it and I can't do it." The monitor may go further: "I fantasized having my arm in a splint, and I think that helped me to understand how stiff it was." What is lacking to the monitor is the information that some part of the person, in response to the hypnotist's suggestions and his or her own supplements, contracted both antagonistic muscle groups (one voluntarily, the other involuntarily) when the person attempted to bend the arm, so that it remained stiff, as the arm does when you "make a muscle." This would appear to have more to do with a fractionation of the executive than of the monitor, although the possibility of this resolution is not ordinarily noted by the uncritical monitor. Somewhat the same can be said about the concealments present in negative hallucinations and amnesia: The monitor can report the absence of the appropriate perceptions and the memories, without being a party to how they came about.

Except for some information denied it and the lack of criticism shown by the failure to insist on reality tests, very much of the normal monitoring function is retained in hypnosis at the ordinary levels of involvement. Less of the usual monitor is retained when the hypnotic involvement is greater, as in deep hypnosis, or when the subject becomes more deeply engrossed in an activated system that has been aroused. In such cases, the reality-oriented part of the monitor may fade out of the picture, and the unified experience seems to the subject the total reality. In these deeply involved experiences, the reports become similar to those described by ex-istentialists, in which the observer and observed merge into one. In the lighter stages of hypnotic involvement, by contrast, the central monitor may be described as an observer standing in the wings while the hypnotic events are taking place in the center of the stage. As one subject put it:

> Part of me knew I was being hypnotized; it was watching. It was like a person inside of me, looking out through my eyes but not being able to control what was happening. I thought I was still in control because I didn't do some of the suggested things. But review of the ammonia convinced me. He had made me smell it twice, and the first time there was nothing. I asked him: "Was that a trick?" When he assured me that I had smelled the same bottle twice, but hadn't smelled the ammonia the first time, I knew I was hypnotized. . . . The part that was watching always thought that *it* was in control, and that I wasn't being hypnotized, and yet I was.

The capacity for detachment from the participative events themselves has led to a distinction between the monitor and the events. At times the separation is much less than at other times. Usually there is a representation of a central monitor commenting in the detached manner of a sideline observer, reporting what is going on as the person is involved in the hypnotically experienced events. Some essential information appears to be denied the monitor, however. The subsystems do their own monitoring and uncritically accept the many reality distortions; the monitor merely describes what the subsystems experience, perhaps separating itself only enough to be surprised, pleased, or disappointed, but without reality testing of its own. This is very like a person reporting the manifest content of a dream, unaware of its latent content or how the dream was formed.

The Hidden Observer as a Fraction of the Monitoring Function

The covert experiences in hypnotic analgesia and hypnotic deafness, as studied by the hidden-observer techniques, yield additional evidence on the fractionation of the monitoring function, because some fraction of it exists behind an amnesic-like barrier. This is the part of the monitor that has been called the hidden observer and becomes accessible only through automatic writing or automatic talking.

The temptation is strong to see the hidden part as a persistent system that must have been there all along. More extremely, the hidden part may be viewed as an upsurge from a deep unconscious. Many practicing hypnotists, for example, believe that they can "talk to the unconscious" by way of the finger-signaling technique. Under the conditions of our experiments, the characterization of the hidden observer that emerges from the interviews with our subjects denies these interpretations. A summary statement of what our subjects are like would read more like this: "The hidden observer is in all respects like the normal observing part as found in waking. It is objective and well oriented to reality."

The role of the monitoring function in the several stages of the experiments indicates three divisions that occur within it:

1. There is the normal role of the monitor in waking, with its usual scanning, critical testing, and reporting of reality as it is ordinarily perceived.

2. Within hypnosis, the reality distortions reported suggest that a fraction of the monitor is involved in the ongoing experiences, is uncritical of them, and gives an overt account as though the distorted or fantasied experiences were part of the real world. A substantial part of the normal monitor is retained in the areas of behavior and experience not specifically involved in the hypnosis; it is only the hypnotic fraction that is dissociated from the normal whole.

3. The third fraction is the one concealed behind an amnesic-like barrier that can be broken by the special methods exposing the hidden observer. This turns out to be a part of the normal monitor and like it in its reality orientation.

A Final Word

A large proportion of those who are spending essentially all of their working hours engaged with hypnosis are serving the public through the practice of clinical hypnosis. Although I have chosen not to deal with the practice of clinical hypnosis in any detail in this chapter, it would obviously be a serious oversight if I said nothing about it.

It is safe to assume that most of those engaged in clinical hypnosis subscribe to a conventional acceptance of the phenomena of hypnosis. However, it would be misleading to assume that those who take the alternative view are not occasionally interested in the practice of hypnosis, even though they are uneasy about its relationship to other forms of psychotherapy. One or two illustrations may suffice to show this interest. Spanos and Chaves (1989c) devote a five-chapter section to hypnosis in applied settings. Chaves, who has been working with dental patients in the context of a school of dental medicine, has contributed important ideas with respect to the control of pain. For example, he and his collaborators have distinguished between two types of reaction to felt pain in naturalistic settings. One type manages to control pain by discovering coping strategies that minimize pain and stress. Others, however, engage in patterns of thinking that exaggerate their pains; these are characterized as "catastrophizers" (e.g., Chaves & Brown, 1987). Joyce D'Eon, in her review of hypnosis in the control of labor pain in parturition, gives a very fair summarization of the claims of both hypnosis and "prepared childbirth" methods, such as those of Read and Lamaze (D'Eon, 1969). She herself works in a center for chronic pain in Ottawa.

A problem that always arises in the study of the effectiveness of a psychotherapy is to find out what aspects of the interventions are contributing most to the outcome. Hypnosis is usually considered to be an adjunct to other forms of psychotherapy. There is one useful test of the role played by hypnosis per se: If favorable and unfavorable outcomes are correlated with measured hypnotic responsiveness, it is reasonable to assume that hypnosis is effective. If there is no correlation, it is likely that the results depend upon other aspects of the psychotherapeutic interventions.

It is true that the hypnosis is carried out by many who have little interest in the scientific aspects of hypnosis. This is an unfortunate social reality, but those who are serious in their use of hypnotic interventions should not be bracketed with those who make a mockery of hypnosis, and exploit a gullible public.

Notes

1. The blind student was preparing to take a postdoctoral course in mathematical statistics, and his professional career since then has been as a statistician in a federal agency.

2. This section is adapted and updated from "The Domain of Hypnosis, with Some Comments on Alternative Paradigms" (pp. 972–975) by E. R. Hilgard, 1973, *American Psychologist, 28,* 972–982. Copyright 1973 by the American Psychological Association. Adapted by permission.

3. This section is adapted from *Divided Consciousness: Multiple Controls in Human Thought and Action* (rev. ed., pp. 216–222) by E. R. Hilgard, 1986, New York: Wiley. Copyright 1986 by John Wiley & Sons. Adapted by permission.

CHAPTER FOUR

A Social-Psychological Approach to Hypnosis

NICHOLAS P. SPANOS
WILLIAM C. COE

In everyday life, people make the tacit assumption that those with whom they interact are wide awake, cognizing individuals whose behavior flows in meaningful and understandable fashion from their motives and from the goals they are attempting to achieve. Responsive hypnotic subjects seem to violate these tacit assumptions by appearing more asleep than awake—a demeanor creating the illusion that they are responding like automatons. These subjects behave as if they see the nonexistent scenes and hear the nonexistent voices suggested to them and, when given further suggestions, as if they feel little if any pain when exposed to noxious stimuli, and as if they no longer have volitional control over the movement of their limbs. In sum, responsive hypnotic subjects behave as if they have surrendered their volitional control to the hypnotist.

Most theories of hypnosis have been based on the assumption that the causes of hypnotic behavior differ fundamentally from the causes of "normal" everyday social behavior. According to these theories, hypnotic behavior results from an unusual psychological state (i.e., a trance) or reflects the operation of unusual cognitive processes (e.g., "trance logic," dissociation). These unusual cognitive processes are said to fully manifest themselves in only those relatively few individuals in the general population who respond highly on measures of hypnotizability.

Social-psychological theories of hypnosis reject the assumption that hypnotic behavior results from unusual mental states or processes (T. X. Barber, 1969; Sarbin & Coe, 1972; Spanos & Chaves, 1989a; Wagstaff, 1981a). Instead, these theories view hypnotic responding as fundamentally similar to other, more mundane forms of social interaction. Even the most responsive of hypnotic subjects are viewed as purposeful agents who are attuned to contextual demands and who guide their behavior in terms of their understandings of those demands and in terms of the goals they wish to achieve (Coe & Sarbin, 1977; Lynn, Rhue, & Weekes, 1989; Spanos, 1982a, 1986b; Wagstaff, 1981a). Thus, from the social-psychological perspective, hypnotic respondings are conceptualized as the enactments, constructions, or doings of sentient, motivated individuals. They are not "happenings" elicited automatically by suggestions given to "entranced" individuals.

R. W. White, Goal-Directed Action, and Altered State

The origins of all contemporary social-psychological approaches to hypnosis can be traced to the seminal work of Robert W. White (1941), the first modern investigator to reject mechanistic approaches to the understanding of hypnotic behavior. He pointed out that hypnotic behavior is purposeful, goal-directed action, and that hypnotic subjects gear their behavior in terms of their expectations concerning what the hypnotist wishes them to do. He pointed out further that the mechanistic theories of hypnosis current in his day (i.e., ideomotor responding and dissociation) could not adequately account for the complexity and goal-directed nature of hypnotic responding.

Despite White's emphasis on subjects' expectations and the importance of goal-directed strivings, he retained the notion that hypnotic responding reflects an altered state of the person. White's retention of the altered-state concept was based on two hypotheses that have been very seriously challenged by modern research: (1) that hypnotic responding transcends nonhypnotic capabilities, and (2) that hypnotic procedures lead to a "restriction in consciousness" that produces the experience of responding involuntarily, as well as to subtle changes in cognitive functioning. Research concerning these hypotheses that has been conducted since the publication of White's paper is discussed below.

The Hypothesis of Transcendence

R. W. White believed that hypnotic procedures produce enhancements in responding that transcend nonhypnotic responding. In the 1960s and 1970s, however, a large amount of research conducted primarily by T. X. Barber and his associates (T. X. Barber, 1969; T. X. Barber, Spanos, & Chaves, 1974) demonstrated that (1) nonhypnotic control subjects who were administered no special preliminaries regularly enacted the responses called for by suggestions for age regression, pain reduction, hallucination, amnesia, and so on; (2) the addition of hypnotic induction procedures produced only small increments in responsiveness to suggestion; and (3) the increments produced by hypnotic procedures could be easily matched and sometimes exceeded by the administration of nonhypnotic instructions designed to enhance subjects motivations to perform optimally (task motivation instructions). In other words, the repeated empirical demonstration that wide-awake, task-motivated subjects were as responsive to suggestion as hypnotic subjects drove home the basic ordinariness of hypnotic behavior, and thereby undercut the belief that hypnotic subjects could transcend the abilities of nonhypnotic subjects.

White's (1941) second reason for positing an altered state stemmed from his belief that the relaxation component of hypnotic induction procedures produces a "restriction in consciousness" that facilitates the experience of responding involuntarily and that leads to subtle changes in the cognitive functioning of hypnotized subjects.

Experienced Involuntariness

A good deal of research (some of which is described later) now indicates that White was correct in arguing that the responses of hypnotic subjects to suggestions are goal-directed. As White (1941) described, these enactments change to meet the changing demands of the hypnotic test situation, and they are geared to the goals that subjects are attempting to achieve and to the social impressions they are attempting to convey (for reviews, see Sarbin & Coe, 1972; Spanos, 1986c). Despite the fact that they are goal-directed, hypnotic subjects frequently describe their responses as feeling involuntary (Spanos & Barber, 1972; Spanos, Radtke, Hodgins, Stam, & Bertrand, 1983; Weitzenhoffer, 1974). For instance, when given a suggestion for arm levitation, subjects who raise their arms frequently describe the movement as something that "happened by itself."

Research has not supported White's (1941) hypothesis that the relaxation component of hypnotic induction procedures facilitates reports of involuntariness. Instead, the most important variable in this regard appears to be the wording of the communications administered to subjects. The suggestions used in hypnotic contexts are usually worded in the passive voice (e.g., "Your arm is slowly rising") and imply that the called-for responses are passive happenings that occur automatically. On the other hand, the instructions employed in most nonhypnotic contexts are actively worded (e.g., "Please raise your arm") and imply that the called-for behavior is self-generated or voluntary. A number of studies showed that *both* hypnotic and nonhypnotic subjects rated their responses to suggestions as significantly more involuntary than their responses to instructions (Spanos & Gorassini, 1984; Spanos & Katsanis, 1989). Importantly, when hypnotic and nonhypnotic subjects were given the same suggestions, they reported equivalent levels of experienced involuntariness—an observation indicating that reports of responding involuntarily are strongly related to the expectations conveyed by the passive wording of hypnotic suggestions. However, these findings provide no support for White's (1941) hypothesis that hypnotic or relaxation procedures "restrict consciousness" in a manner that facilitates attributions of nonvolition, or that such procedures induce an "altered state."

The importance of the wording of suggestions at facilitating reports of involuntariness was also illustrated by Spanos, Salas, Bertrand, and Johnston (1988–1989). In that study, subjects wrote open-ended descriptions of the movements made by an actress in a videotape. In one condition, the actress raised her arm slowly in response to a passively worded hypnotic suggestion for arm levitation; in the other condition, she slowly raised her arm while in the process of tracking and swatting a fly. Subjects who saw the hypnosis video overwhelmingly described the woman's arm movement as an occurrence (e.g., "Her arm went up") rather than as a self-generated action. On the other hand, those who saw the fly-tracking video invariably described the woman's arm movement as a self-initiated action (e.g., "She raised her arm to hit the fly"). In other words, it was the context in which subjects observed the woman that influenced them to categorize her movement as an involuntary occurrence or as a voluntary action.

On the basis of Bem's (1967) ideas concerning the process of attribution, Spanos, Salas, et al. (1988–1989) reasoned that the contextual cues that observers use to categorize the behavior of another in a particular situation are the same ones they will probably use to categorize their own behavior in that situation. Thus, subjects who lift their own arms following an hypnotic suggestion for arm levitation are likely to be influenced by cues in that situation to categorize or interpret their arm movement as an involuntary occurrence.

Despite exposure to the same contextual cues, not all subjects who respond to hypnotic suggestions rate their behavior as feeling involuntary. Some of the variability in this regard appears to be related to what subjects attend to while responding to suggestions. Those who become highly absorbed in suggestion-related imaginings (e.g., absorbed in imagining their arms pumped up with air when given an arm levitation suggestion) rate their responses as feeling more involuntary than do those who become less absorbed (Spanos & McPeake, 1974). These findings suggest that subjects tend to interpret their suggested responses as involuntary when they succeed in deflecting attention away from cues associated with the idea of voluntary arm movement, and instead attend to situational cues (e.g., suggestion wording) and imaginal cues that are consistent with an involuntariness interpretation.

Still another reason for reports of involuntariness may be compliance with experimental demands. The passive wording of suggestions, coupled with rating scales that ask subjects to circle a number that reflects how involuntary their response felt, make it clear that reports of involuntariness are a mark of a "good" hypnotic subject. Thus, at least some subjects who are motivated to present themselves as "deeply hypnotized" may exaggerate the extent to which their responses felt involuntary in order to reinforce such a self-presentation (Spanos, Burgess, Cocco, & Pinch, 1991). We shall see later that compliance appears to play an important role in hypnotic responsiveness.

Hypnotic Procedures and Subtle Cognitive Changes

R. W. White's (1941) suggestion that hypnotic procedures produced subtle changes in cognitive functioning was pursued most systematically by Orne (1959, 1979a) and his colleagues (e.g., Orne, Sheehan, & Evans, 1968). Orne (1959) emphasized that much hypnotic behavior can be adequately explained in terms of social compliance. Like social-psychological theorists, Orne (1959, 1962a) argued that highly hypnotizable subjects are motivated to please the hypnotist and to respond in terms of the social demands contained in suggestions and in other aspects of the hypnotic situation. Unlike social-psychological theorists, however, Orne (1959) also postulated that hypnotic responding involves subtle cognitive changes that do not reflect social demands, and that are not characteristic of *non*hypnotic responding.

To assess these ideas, Orne employed an experimental paradigm that compared the behavior of responsive hypnotic subjects (i.e., "reals") to the behavior of low hypnotizables who were instructed to fake hypnosis in order to fool the hypnotist (simulators). The "reals" and the simulators were exposed to the same hypnotic procedures, and the hypnotist did not know which subjects were which. Because the simulators and nonsimulators were exposed to the same hypnotic situations, Orne (1959) reasoned that these subjects were exposed to the identical social demands. According to this reasoning, any differences in the behavior of the simulators and nonsimulators had to result from the operation of variables or processes other than social demands.

Orne (1959), in fact, found subtle differences between the behavior of simulators and "reals." For example, when given a suggestion to visually hallucinate a person sitting across the room, "reals" often described their hallucinated person as transparent, whereas simulators usually reported that the hallucination was solid rather than transparent. Orne (1959) argued that this and other differences in the responding of simulators and "reals" indicated that "real" (as opposed to faked) hypnotic responding is characterized by an unusual type of cognitive activity labeled "trance logic." According to Orne (1959), trance logic responding is specific to hypnosis and cannot be explained in terms of demand characteristics.

During the 1970s and 1980s, a good deal of work was conducted on trance logic responding (for reviews, see de Groot & Gwynn, 1989; Spanos, 1986b). However, many of the behavioral differences between simulators and "reals" that Orne described as indices of trance logic could not be replicated by other researchers (e.g., Obstoj & Sheehan, 1977). Furthermore, those behavioral indices that reliably differentiated simulators from hypnotic "reals" failed to differentiate hypnotic "reals" from *non*hypnotic "reals." For example, even though high hypnotizable hypnotic "reals" exhibited transparent hallucinating to a greater extent than low hypnotizable simulators, nonhypnotic high hypnotizables who were not asked to simulate (i.e., *non*hypnotic "reals") also exhibited higher rates of transparent hallucinating than low hypnotizable simulators. In other words, so-called "trance logic" responses were not found to be hypnosis-specific, and their occurrence was more closely related to the absence of instructions to simulate than to the administration of a hypnotic induction procedure (Spanos, 1986b).

As research progressed, it also became increasingly clear that the assumption that simulators and nonsimulators are exposed to the same demand characteristics was untenable (e.g., Sheehan, 1971a). In fact, the administration of simulation instructions was found to have a very substantial influence on how subjects interpreted and responded to the later demands contained in the hypnotic session. Spanos (1986b) suggested that "real" subjects are exposed not only to demands for compliance, but also to demands for responding honestly and for reporting their experiences accurately. Thus, "reals" tend to report transparent hallucinations not because they are exhibiting "trance logic," but because they are honestly reporting that the suggested images they conjure up with their eyes open tend to be incomplete, nonvivid, and transparent. Simulators, on the other hand, are exposed only to demands for compliance, and in fact are explicitly instructed to ignore demands for honesty and to lie about their experiences. Consequently, they tend to give idealized responses and thereby describe suggested hallucinations as having the characteristics of real objects (i.e., as being vivid, complete, solid, etc.). On the basis of these ideas, Spanos, de Groot, and Gwynn (1987) showed that the reliable differences in responding between simulators and nonsimulators that Orne (1959, 1979a) attributed to "trance logic" can be more parsimoniously explained in terms of the different demands to which these subjects are exposed. In other words, differences in the behavior of simulators and nonsimulators, which Orne (1959) attributed to subtle cognitive processes unique to hypnosis, turn out to result from subtle differences in the social demands to which simulators and nonsimulators are exposed. Thus, research originally designed to highlight cognitive processes unique to hypnosis has, instead, underscored the pervasive and sometimes subtle ways that contextual variables can shape the experiences and behaviors of hypnotic subjects.

In summary, R. W. White's (1941) suggestion that hypnotic responding is expectancy-generated goal-directed action has proven highly fruitful, and forms the basis for contemporary social-psychological views. On the other other hand, White's (1941) hypothesis that hypnotic responding involves an altered state of the person has held up much less well under empirical scrutiny. Modern social-psychological theories began when investigators who adopted White's (1941) notion of hypnosis as goal-directed action dropped his corresponding notion of hypnosis as an altered state. The first of these investigators was T. R. Sarbin (1950).

Role Theory and Its Extensions

In 1950, Sarbin published the first in a highly influential series of theoretical papers that subsumed hypnotic responding under social role theory. Sarbin (1950, 1962, 1989; Sarbin & Coe, 1972; Sarbin & Juhasz, 1970) retained R. W. White's notion of hypnosis as goal-directed action and conceptualized such action in terms of the attempts of subjects to meet the social role expectations that emerge and become salient as the hypnotic situation unfolds. Unlike White, however, Sarbin (1950) explicitly rejected the notion of a hypnotic state. Instead, individual differences in hypnotic responsiveness were accounted for in terms of differences in the extent to which subjects become involved or absorbed in the hypnotic role. Although Sarbin himself conducted relatively little empirical research, his theoretical writings provided a framework for understanding hypnosis as contextually supported social action, and a viable alternative to the "hypnotic state" formulations that dominated this research area throughout the 1960s and 1970s.

Sarbin (1950) and other investigators who follow in the social-psychological tradition (T. X. Barber, 1969; Coe, 1978; Coe & Sarbin, 1977; M. J. Diamond, 1974; Kroger, 1988; Lynn, Rhue, & Weekes, 1989; Sarbin & Coe, 1972; Spanos, 1982a, 1986b; Spanos & Chaves, 1989a; Wagstaff, 1981a, 1986) begin with the view that people are continually involved in organizing sensory information into schemas or categories that can be used to guide actions. From this perspective, people use their implicit understandings to negotiate social situations. Social interaction usually proceeds smoothly because the interacting parties share similar understandings of their common situation and of the reciprocal roles they are to play within the confines of their shared definition of the situation (Coulter, 1989; Sarbini & Silver, 1982).

Interaction proceeds in terms of mutually negotiated self-presentations and reciprocal role validation. Role enactment is rule-governed and involves the tacit understandings of the actors concerning the definition of the situation and the behaviors that are considered appropriate to that definition (Goffman, 1959; Sarbini & Silver, 1982).

From a social-psychological perspective, the term "hypnosis" does not refer to a state or condition of the person. Instead, it refers to the manner in which the historically rooted conceptions of hypnotic responding that are held by the participants in the context labeled "hypnosis" express themselves in reciprocal interaction (Spanos, 1991). Hypnotic responding is viewed as context-dependent but as multidetermined. These determinants include (1) the willingness of subjects to adopt the hypnotic role; (2) their understandings of what is expected in that role; (3) the manner in which such understandings change as the situation unfolds; (4) subjects' interpretations of the ambiguous communications that constitute hypnotic test suggestions; (5) their ability and willingness to generate the imaginal experiences called for by suggestions; and (6) the way in which feedback from the hypnotist and from their own responding influences their definitions of themselves as hypnotic subjects (Sarbin & Coe, 1972; Spanos, 1982a, 1991). The remainder of this chapter examines the implications of the social-psychological view for an understanding of several phenomena that, historically, have been considered central aspects of hypnotic responding.

Hypnotizability and Special Processes

The View of Hypnotizability as a Stable Trait

At least since the early 19th century, it has been clear that people differ in their degree of responsiveness to hypnotic procedures. In the 1950s and 1960s, Weitzenhoffer and Hilgard (1959, 1962) extended the earlier work of others (e.g., Friedlander & Sarbin, 1938) in developing standardized scales for the assessment of hypnotizability. These and the similar scales developed by other investigators (T. X. Barber, 1965; Shor & Orne, 1962; Spanos, Radtke, Hodgins, Stam, & Bertrand, 1983) quickly came into common use, and it soon became apparent that hypnotizability was a relatively stable characteristic. Thus, individuals tended to obtain roughly similar scores on two administrations of the same hypnotizability test even when the two administrations were separated by long time intervals (E. R. Hilgard, 1965a; Piccione, Hilgard, & Zimbardo, 1989).

Shortly after the introduction of these scales, a number of investigators addressed the issue of whether hypnotizability could be modified through special training (see M. J. Diamond, 1974, for a review). T. X. Barber and Calverley (1964a) illustrated the influence of motivations and attitudes toward hypnosis on hypnotizability scores by demonstrating that subjects who were given negative information about hypnosis exhibited substantial decreases in hypnotizability. However, most investigators were interested in increasing rather than decreasing hypnotizability, and here the evidence was less clear-cut. Most early studies aimed at enhancing hypnotizability were premised on the assumption that hypnotic responding involves an altered state of consciousness. Consequently, the training procedures used in these studies were designed to facilitate such an altered state (e.g., repeated, individualized hypnotic inductions; electroencephalographic biofeedback; sensory isolation). Although some of these studies reported that training induced significant increments in hypnotizability, the findings were inconsistent and the increments, even when statistically significant, were usually small (Perry, 1977).

The failure of these studies to consistently obtain large gains in hypnotizability, coupled with the finding that hypnotizability scores exhibited high test–retest reliability, led to the view that hypnotizability reflects a stable-trait-like capacity that is highly resistant to modification (K. S. Bowers, 1976; E. R. Hilgard, 1977a; Perry, 1977).

Special-Process Views

Investigators who advocated a stable-capacity view of hypnotizability typically argued that hypnotic suggestions produce unusual subjective experiences and unusual changes in perception and memory that cannot be adequately explained in terms of social-psychological variables. Usually, they also qualified their statements by arguing that unusual changes in experience, perception and memory are likely to occur only in those relatively few subjects who attained high hypnotizability scores (K. S. Bowers, 1976; Orne, 1979a; E. R. Hilgard, 1977a, 1987; Kihlstrom, 1985a). We refer to investigators who adopt this line of argument as "special-process" theorists (Spanos, 1986a), and in the last 15 years they have generated a large number of studies aimed at showing that specific hypnotic phenomena (e.g., amnesia, pain reduction, and negative hallucination) require the positing of unusual cognitive processes and cannot be adequately explained in terms of contextually supported goal-directed action.

Social-psychological theorists have countered these claims in several ways. For instance, they have suggested that the stability that characterizes hypnotizability may reflect such mundane factors as stable attitudes, styles of interpretation, and skills at imagining, rather than a largely unmodifiable capacity for such unusual cognitive processes as "dissociation." Moreover, they have suggested that hypnotizability may be substantially more modifiable than early studies indicated, and that such modifiability supports a social-psychological rather than a special-process conceptualization of hypnotizability.

Social-psychological theorists have also argued that the responses of high hypnotizables to suggestions for amnesia, analgesia, and so on, are often not what they seem, and that such responses in fact reflect mundane social-cognitive processes such as compliance-induced reporting biases, alteration in attentional focus, and misattribution of experience, rather than such special processes as dissociation or trance logic. Below, we examine social-psychological approaches to the modification of hypnotizability, and to three hypnotic phenomena that special-process theorists regard as hallmarks of high hypnotizability: negative hallucination, hidden-observer responding, and hypnotic amnesia.

Stability and Change in Hypnotizability

The moderate to high test–retest correlations that characterize hypnotizability scales can be understood either as reflecting a stable capacity for unusual experiences (i.e., the special-process view) or as reflecting stability in such variables as attitudes toward hypnosis and interpretations of test demands (the social-psychological view). A number of recent studies have begun to delineate contextual variables that influence both stability and change in hypnotizability.

Defining the Situation as Hypnosis

Spanos, Gabora, Jarrett, and Gwynn (1989) administered two different hypnotizability scales to the same subjects. Administration of the two scales was separated by an interval of at least 2 weeks. For subjects in one group, both scales were defined as tests of hypnosis, and the suggestions on each scale were preceded by a hypnotic induction procedure. For subjects in the other group, only the first scale was defined as a test of hypnosis and preceded by a hypnotic induction procedure. The second scale was defined to subjects as a test of creative imagination. Nothing was said about hypnosis, and the initial hypnotic induction procedure was replaced by short instructions encouraging subjects to become actively involved in demonstrating their creativity by responding imaginatively to the suggestions.

The results showed a substantial correlation between the two scales ($r = .65$) when both were defined as tests of hypnosis. However, when one scale was defined as a test of hypnosis and the other as a test of imagination, the correlation between them was significantly lower ($r = .34$). Closer examination revealed that subjects who attained high hypnotizability scores on the first scale also tended to attain high scores on the second, regardless of whether the second scale was defined as a test of hypnosis or imagination. Subjects who obtained low hypnotizability scores on the first scale also tended to obtain low scores on the second scale when the second scale was defined as a test of hypnosis. However, when the second scale was defined as a test of imagination, subjects who attained low scores on the first scale usually attained scores in the moderate or high range on the second scale.

These findings indicate that the attitudes, motivations, and interpretations called up by the definition of the test situation strongly influence subjects' responsiveness to suggestions, as well as the extent to which such responsiveness is stable across testings. Defining the situation as hypnosis seems to facilitate responsiveness for some subjects, but it interferes with the responsiveness of others. When both testing sessions are defined in terms of hypnosis, the attitudes, expectations, motivations, and interpretations that are salient for subjects in one session are also likely to be salient in the next, and therefore lead to similar responding in the two situations. Defining a situation as "creative imagination" is likely to generate positive attitudes and motivations in most people, including those who view hypnosis in a negative light. Consequently, the subjects who responded poorly to suggestions defined as hypnosis became much more responsive to suggestions defined as assessing creativity. These findings clearly contradict the special process-view that low hypnotizables are people who simply lack the cognitive capacity to respond well to suggestions. Instead, they suggest that whether or not people respond to suggestions has a good deal to do with the attitudes and motivations they hold about the situation in which suggestions are administered.

Spanos, Gabora, et al. (1989) also conducted a second experiment, one designed to influence the motivations and expectations of subjects both high and low in hypnotizability. Subjects who had previously scored low or high on a test of hypnotizability were invited to return to the laboratory for a second nonhypnotic session. Half of the "highs" were told that they were likely to continue responding to a high degree in the second session, even though it did not involve hypnosis. They were told that hypnotizability was a skill that people expressed in nonhypnotic as well as hypnotic situations, and therefore that they should respond quite well to the nonhypnotic suggestions. The other half of the highs were informed that they were likely to do poorly on the nonhypnotic suggestions. These subjects were informed that hypnotic induction procedures were required to make people responsive to suggestions, and that without such a procedure, they were likely to be unresponsive to suggestions.

One group of "lows" was also told that hypnotizability was a capacity that expressed itself similarly in hypnotic and nonhypnotic situations. Thus, these subjects were given the expectation that they would respond as badly to the nonhypnotic suggestions as they had to the hypnotic ones. The other group of lows was told that hypnotic procedures interfered with their abilities to respond imaginatively to suggestions. Since the second session did not involve hypnotic procedures, the expectation conveyed to these subjects was that they would perform much better in the nonhypnotic session than they had in the hypnotic one.

As predicted, subjects responded in terms of the expectations conveyed to them. Highs who did not expect to do well in the nonhypnotic condition were much less responsive in that condition than highs who expected to do well. Relatedly, lows who expected to do well without hypnosis were much more responsive in the second session than lows who expected to do poorly without hypnosis.

Correlations between hypnotizability scores in the two sessions were quite high and significant for those subjects who expected to perform similarly in the two sessions. However, among subjects who expected to perform differently in the two sessions (i.e., lows who expected to do well and highs who expected to do poorly in the second session), the correlations between hypnotizability scores in the two sessions were very low and not statistically significant.

If responsiveness to suggestion reflects a stable cognitive capacity for engaging in unusual experiences, then different measures of responsiveness should correlate highly with one another. However, these findings were to the contrary and indicated that hypnotizability measures correlated with one another highly, to a low but significant degree, or not at all, depending upon how the test situation was defined.

These findings suggest that social-psychological factors such as the attitudes and interpretations held by subjects determine hypnotizability test scores to a much greater extent than special-process theorists have acknowledged. They also suggest that hypnotizability scores are probably more modifiable than many of the older studies on this topic indicated. Recall that most of these early studies attempted to change hypnotic responsiveness by training subjects with procedures designed to induce an altered state of consciousness. But if responding as a high hypnotizable does not involve such a state, then it is not particularly surprising that these training procedures failed to enhance hypnotizability.

Social-Psychological Approaches to Modifying Hypnotizability

A few early studies approached the modification of hypnotizability from a social learning perspective rather than a special-process perspective. Several of these studies obtained large gains in hypnotizability (M. J. Diamond, 1972; Kinney & Sachs, 1974; Sachs & Anderson, 1967; Springer, Sachs, & Morrow, 1977). In all of these successful studies, subjects were administered training designed to instill positive attitudes about hypnosis, and to show subjects how to interpret test suggestions.

More recently, these early studies were extended by a series of experiments that exposed low hypnotizables to a three-component social-cognitive skills training program that was designed to (1) enhance subjects' attitudes and expectations about hypnosis; (2) teach the use of imaginal strategies as an aid to experiencing responses to suggestion as involuntary; and (3) teach subjects to interpret suggestions as calling for their active participation in the enactment of the appropriate responses. Because this skills training package was developed at Carleton University (Gorassini & Spanos, 1986), it is called the Carleton Skills Training Program (CSTP).

The interpretation component of the CSTP is particularly important. It is based on the idea that many subjects fail to respond to suggestions not because they lack imaginative skills or have negative attitudes toward hypnosis, but rather because hypnotic suggestions are ambiguously worded and, therefore tend to be misinterpreted. Earlier, we have pointed out that suggestions are worded in the passive voice. Instead of telling subjects to do something, suggestions inform them that something is happening to them (e.g., "Your arm is getting heavier and heavier").

One consequence of the passive wording of suggestions is that it leads many subjects to assume that their responses will occur automatically (Spanos, 1986c). Thus, many subjects with positive attitudes, motivations, and expectations concerning hypnosis, as well as with skills at imagery, fail suggestions because the passive wording of suggestions leads them to simply wait passively for the suggested effects to "just happen" (Katsanis, Barnard, & Spanos, 1988–1989). In order to counter this passive interpretation, subjects who are exposed to the CSTP are taught that suggested responses do not happen automatically; they must be enacted. However, subjects are also informed that they can learn to experience their enacted responses as *feeling* involuntary by attending to imagery that is consistent with an involuntary response (e.g., imagining holding a heavy weight in their hand).

A number of studies (reviewed in Spanos, 1986a) from the Carleton laboratory administered the CSTP to low hypnotizable subjects and found large gains on both behavioral and subjective indices of hypnotizability. Importantly, large gains in hypnotizability with the CSTP have also been replicated in other laboratories (L. D. Bertrand, Stam, & Radtke, 1990; Gfeller, Lynn, & Pribble, 1987; Robertson, McInnis, & St. Jean, in press). Furthermore, several studies also indicate that CSTP-induced gains generalize to novel and difficult suggestions and are maintained even after long temporal intervals (Gfeller et al., 1987; Spanos, Cross, Menary, & Smith, 1988; Spanos, DuBreuil, & Gabora, 1991; Spanos, Lush, & Gwynn, 1989).

On the other hand, Bates, Miller, Cross, and Brigham (1988) failed to obtain large gains in hypnotizability using the CSTP. Importantly, Bates et al. (1988) made no attempt to develop rapport with their subjects, and simply read the CSTP script to subjects in rote-like fashion. In the Carleton laboratory, trainers are encouraged to develop high levels of rapport with subjects and to involve subjects as active participants in the training. In order to assess the role of rapport in skills training, Spanos, Flynn, and Niles (1989–1990) administered the CSTP under conditions of high rapport for one group of low hypnotizables, and under conditions of low rapport (e.g., reading instructions in a monotone, acting disinterested in the subject) for the other group. When rapport was low, Spanos, Flynn, and Niles (1989–1990) found no significant gains in hypnotizability following CSTP administration. However, when rapport was high, subjects showed very large gains on both behavioral and subjective indices of hypnotizability.

Bates et al. (1988) hypothesized that when rapport is high, subjects given the CSTP may exhibit increments in hypnotizability not because they learn to generate the experiences suggested, but instead because they fake in order to please the trainer with whom they have developed a close relationship. Spanos, Flynn, and Niles (1989–1990) tested this hypothesis in a second experiment. One group of low hypnotizables was given the CSTP under high rapport conditions, and another group of lows was given a training program that induced high rapport while informing subjects that hypnotic responses just "happened by themselves." The trainer in both groups made it clear to subjects that she expected them to show large gains in hypnotizability as a result of their training, and subjects in both groups rated themselves as liking and feeling warmly toward the trainer to the same degree. Contrary to the hypothesis of Bates et al. (1988), subjects given passive training showed no increases in hypnotizability despite their high rapport, whereas those given the CSTP plus high rapport exhibited large hypnotizability gains. These findings suggest that rapport probably achieves its effects not by simply inducing subjects to fake their responses, but instead by leading them to attend to the training information, and by motivating them to employ what they have learned when interpreting suggestions and generating the experiences called for.

Recently, the faking hypothesis of modification gain was tested by comparing three groups of subjects (Spanos, Burgess, Roncon, & Wallace-Capretta, 1991). Those in one group were subjects who scored high in hypnotizability after CSTP training, while those in a second group scored high in hypnotizability without any training. Subjects in a third group were lows instructed to simulate hypnosis. Subjects in all three groups were tested twice on a hypnotizability posttest: once while they were alone in a room (all instructions were administered via tape recording), and once while the experimenter was in the room. Unbeknownst to the subjects, a hidden camera filmed their responses while they were alone in the room. While the experimenter was in the room, subjects in all three groups exhibited high levels of response to the suggestion. Furthermore, subjects in all three groups *rated themselves* as responding to a high degree when they were alone in the room. However, the hidden camera indicated that the simulators frequently failed to respond to suggestions that they later scored themselves as passing. While supposedly responding to suggestions, these subjects were often looking around the room, flipping through their response booklet, and engaging in other behaviors indicating that they did not adopt the hypnotic role when they believed they were not being observed. The CSTP subjects, like those who attained high hypnotizability without training, responded to the suggestions in the same way when they were alone and when the experimenter was with them. These findings clearly contradict the hypothesis that hypnotizability gains induced through training are the result of faking aimed at pleasing the trainer. The trained subjects in this study continued to respond as high hynotizables when they believed that they were alone, and there was no reason to fake.

Although the above-described findings indicate that gains induced by skills training cannot be adequately understood solely in terms of faking, it is important to acknowledge that compliance with situational demands does seem to play a central role in hypnotic responding. As we discuss shortly, subjects who attain high hypnotizability scores without benefit of any training (i.e., "natural highs") frequently exaggerate and misrepresent their experiences to varying degrees in order to meet suggested demands.

Therefore, it would be surprising indeed if skill-trained subjects did not, to varying degrees, also engage in the same kinds of compliant responding.

The findings discussed thus far should not be taken to mean that social-psychological theorists reject the idea that stable cognitive abilities may play some role in hypnotic responding. For instance, even though the evidence reviewed above indicates that CSTP training produces large enhancements in hypnotizability, skill-trained subjects continue to exhibit wide individual differences in posttraining hypnotizability scores. Some of this residual variability occurs because subjects differ in their openness to the training information, and in the extent to which training actually changes their attitudes toward hypnosis. For instance, one study (Spanos, Cross, Menary, Brett, & de Groh, 1987) found that subjects who continued to hold relatively negative attitudes toward hypnosis despite CSTP training showed smaller hypnotizability gains than those who held relatively positive attitudes following training. On the other hand, two studies (Cross & Spanos, 1988–1989; Spanos, Cross, et al., 1987) found that subjects who scored relatively low on a measure of imagery vividness showed smaller hypnotizability gains following CSTP training than did those with relatively high imagery scores. These findings suggest that some subjects with positive attitudes and appropriate interpretations may nonetheless attain relatively low hypnotizability scores because they lack the imaginal abilities required to generate the subjective experiences called for by many test suggestions.

In summary, the available data support the view that hypnotizability is modifiable. Subjects show substantial changes in their responsiveness to suggestion as a function of how the test situation is defined to them, and many low hypnotizable subjects demonstrate large gains in hypnotizability when they acquire the appropriate attitudes, motivations, and interpretations of suggested demands. These findings are consistent with the view that performance on hypnotizability scales reflects subjects' attitudes, motivations, interpretations, and expectations in interaction with their imaginal propensities (M. J. Diamond, 1974, 1977; Sachs, 1971; Spanos, 1986a). In short, these findings indicate that response to hypnotizability scales can be understood as a social-psychological phenomenon.

Negative Hallucinations

The term "negative hallucination" refers to a suggestion-induced failure of perception. For example, when exposed to a loud tone following a suggestion for deafness, some highly hypnotizable subjects report that the tone sounds much quieter than it did before the suggestion, and a few report that they cannot hear the tone at all (e.g., Sutcliffe, 1960). Similar suggestion-induced perceptual failures have been reported for visual, tactile, and olfactory stimuli as well as for auditory stimuli (see Jones & Flynn, 1989, for a review). Negative-hallucination suggestions are particularly difficult, and most subjects fail these suggestions (i.e., most report having the perceptual experience despite the suggestion). Furthermore, most of the subjects who pass such suggestions also attain high hypnotizability scores (E. R. Hilgard, 1965a).

The Problem of Compliance

In most negative-hallucination experiments, the only indices of perceptual change are the subjects' reports of not perceiving. Given the inherent implausibility of negative-hallucination responding, and the strong demands for compliance contained in negative-hallucination suggestions, many investigators have been understandably critical of negative-hallucination reports (Sutcliffe, 1960, 1961). Nevertheless, on the basis of such reports alone, a number of special-process theorists have argued that negative-hallucination suggestions do, in fact, produce the experiences called for in at least some highly hypnotizable subjects (Bryant & McConkey, 1989b; E. R. Hilgard, 1977a; Zamansky & Bartis, 1985).

One strategy employed by critical investigators has been to assess objective indices of negative-hallucination responding that cannot be faked as easily as verbal reports of experience. For instance, investigators have given subjects the suggestion that they will not see the radiating background lines of the Ponzo illusion, and then assessed whether those who claim to no longer see the lines still respond to the illusion (thus indicating that the supposedly unseen lines continue to influence perception). Similarly, investigators have assessed whether those who claim to be hypnotically deaf stutter in response to delayed auditory feedback (thereby indicating that they can hear; T. X. Barber & Calverley, 1964b; R. J. Miller, Hennessy, & Leibowitz, 1973; Sutcliffe, 1961). Such experiments have consistently indicated that negative-hallucination suggestions fail to influence objective indices of perceptual change, despite their influence on subjects' verbal reports (see Jones & Flynn, 1989).[1]

The simplest account of these findings is that the demands for compliance contained in negative-hallucination suggestions induce some highly hypnotizable subjects to bias their perceptual reports in the absence of corresponding changes in perception (Wagstaff, 1981a, 1986, 1991). Direct support for this hypothesis was recently obtained by Spanos, Flynn, and Gabora (1989). These researchers postexperimentally interviewed negative hallucinators who had insisted that they saw nothing on a piece of paper (the paper contained the number 8). During the interview subjects were led to believe that only fakers report seeing nothing on the paper. They were told that deeply hypnotized people initially see what was on the paper, but that their perception gradually fades away. When asked to draw what they had initially seen on the paper, all but one subject correctly drew the number 8. In so doing, of course, they demonstrated that their earlier experimental reports of having seen nothing on the paper were inaccurate.

These findings indicate that the reports of negative hallucinators are strongly biased in terms of experimental demands. These reports can involve gross exaggerations and may sometimes involve outright fabrications. The demands for biased reports contained in negative hallucination suggestions are by no means subtle (e.g., "You will see nothing on the page; it will be completely blank"), and, at least to us, one of the most surprising aspects of this research area is the continued insistence of some special-process theorists that the unsubstantiated verbal reports of subjects can be employed as valid indicators of suggestion-induced perceptual alteration. In light of the available data, such a position seems indefensible.

Direct Assessment of Reporting Bias

Experiments like those reviewed above make it clear that reporting biases that are induced by experimental demands play an important role in hypnotic responding. Nevertheless, the extent to which demand-induced response biases influence hypnotic behavior is difficult to determine, because, to an unknown degree, suggestion-induced reports of experiential change can confound actual changes in experience with demand induced reporting biases. Several recent studies (Spanos, Burgess, Cross, & McCleod, 1992; Spanos, Burgess, & Perlini, 1992; Spanos, Perlini, Patrick, Bell, & Gwynn, 1990) have addressed this issue by using a paradigm that provides a direct index of demand-induced reporting bias that is independent of actual experiential change. For instance, in several experiments subjects heard a loud tone on a 30-second baseline trial. Ten seconds after termination of the tone, subjects rated its loudness on a 21-point scale. They were then given a hypnotic suggestion for deafness and a second presentation of the same tone. Ten seconds after the second presentation of the tone, subjects again rated its loudness. The hypnotic suggestion was then canceled, and subjects were presented with the same tone a third time. However, in the 10 seconds that followed termination of the third presentation, but before rating the tone's loudness, subjects in one condition were given an instruction designed to induce compliance. These subjects were told that they had probably slipped back into hypnosis and therefore had heard the tone less loudly than they otherwise would have. Following this demand instruction, subjects rated the loudness of the tone as presented the third time. Control subjects rated the loudness of the tone without the intervening demand instruction.

It is important to keep in mind that both the subjects administered the demand instruction and the control subjects were treated identically up until the termination of the trial 3 tone. Consequently, any differences in reported loudness between the groups for the trial 3 tone could not reflect actual differences in the loudness with which subjects in the two groups heard that tone. Instead, a reduction in reported loudness for the demand instruction group could only reflect a reporting bias.

Studies using this paradigm (Spanos, Burgess, Cross, & McCleod, 1992; Spanos, Burgess, & Perlini, 1992) found that control subjects reported that the tone was equally loud on trials 1 and 3, and less loud on trial 2 (hypnotic deafness) than on trials 1 and 3. On the other hand, the demand instruction subjects reported that the tone was less loud on trial 2 (hypnotic deafness) and on trial 3 (reporting bias) than on trial 1. Furthermore, on trial 3 these subjects reported the tone as less loud than did control subjects. These findings indicate that hypnotic subjects bias their perceptual reports in terms of experimental demands, independently of any changes in perceptual experience.

Among subjects in the demand instruction condition, extent of reporting bias can be assessed by subtracting trial 3 (reporting bias) loudness ratings from trial 1 (baseline) ratings. In these two studies (Spanos, Burgess, & Perlini, 1992; Spanos, Burgess, Cross, & McCleod, 1992), the loudness reduction reported on trial 3 (reporting bias) was almost as large as the loudness reduction reported on trial 2 (hypnotic deafness). Moreover, the correlation between loudness reduction of trials 2 (hypnotic deafness) and 3 (reporting bias) was quite high, and the correlation between hypnotic deafness ratings and hypnotizability did not differ in magnitude from the correlation between trial 3 reporting bias and hypnotizability. In other words, subjects who reported high levels of hypnotic deafness tended to be the same people who compliantly biased their reports in the absence of any perceptual change. Furthermore, hypnotic high hypnotizables biased their reports of perceptual change to a greater extent than did hypnotic low hypnotizables.

Spanos, Burgess, Cross, and McCleod (1992) extended these findings in a two-part experiment that assessed hypnotic blindness as well as hypnotic deafness. In the first session, it was suggested to hypnotic subjects that they would be unable to see a word that was clearly printed on a page. After the suggestion, subjects rated the extent to which they had used strategies in an attempt to distort visual perception (e.g., unfocusing the eyes, creating an image to "cover" the target word). All subjects reported using one or more strategies to distort visual perception, but there was no relationship between the extent of such strategy use and subjects' reports of blindness. In the second session, subjects were tested in the deafness/reporting bias paradigm described above. The extent to which subjects biased their loudness reports following the demand instruction correlated significantly with their degree of reported blindness as well as with their degree of reported deafness. Once again, subjects who were willing to bias their auditory reports in terms of situational demands, and independently of any real perceptual change, tended to be the same people who reported perceptual change when given suggestions for hypnotic deafness and hypnotic blindness. Probably the subjects in this study did use various strategies in an attempt to induce perceptual distortion following the blindness suggestion. However, the extent to which any resultant perceptual alterations were defined by subjects as "blindness" was un-related to strategy usage. Instead, reports of blindness were related to subjects' self-presentational concerns and to their motivations to bias their perceptual reports in terms of compliance demands.

Taken together, the results of the studies reviewed above suggest that the tendency to bias responses in terms of suggested demands is a central component in hypnotic responding. Hypnotic subjects who are unable to generate the experiences called for by suggestions to the degree that they believe is required sometimes exaggerate their experiences to meet ex-perimental demands. Such exaggeration is by no means uncommon, and occurs more strongly in high than in low hypnotizable subjects. Because pressures toward compliance are strong, and the perceptual changes called for by negative-hallucination suggestions are improbable, the verbal re-ports of perceptual change proffered by hypnotic subjects should not be taken at face value. On the contrary, it now seems clear that the kinds of reports taken by special-process theorists as indices of unusual suggestion-induced perceptual change tell us little about perception, but much about how social pressures in experimental settings induce subjects to exaggerate in order to maintain their self-presentations as "deeply hypnotized."[2]

The Hidden-Observer Phenomenon

As indicated above, it is commonly found that suggestion-induced reports of perceptual change are not accompanied by corresponding changes on objective indices of perceptual functioning, and these findings have been used to support the hypothesis that the verbal reports of hypnotic subjects are strongly influenced by reporting biases. An alternative hypothesis for these findings, which has been promulgated by some special-process theorists, holds that highly hypnotizable hypnotic subjects may process perceptual information on two levels simultaneously (E. R. Hilgard, 1977a, 1991; Zamansky & Bartis, 1985). According to this hypothesis, negative hallucinators process stimulus information unconsciously, which accounts for why they exhibit evidence of perceiving on objective indices. Despite such unconscious processing, however, these subjects supposedly do not consciously experience the stimulus information. The findings most often cited in support of this hypothesis were generated in a series of so-called "hidden-observer" experiments conducted by Hilgard and others (see Hilgard, 1991, for a review). Most of these experiments employed only highly hypnotizable subjects and used noxious events as perceptual stimuli.

In a typical hidden observer experiment, subjects were exposed to pain on a baseline trial (e.g., 60 seconds of limb immersion in ice water), and at set intervals reported their level of pain intensity. Next, subjects were given a hypnotic induction procedure and informed that they pos-sessed a hidden part that remained aware of their experience even after suggestions for pain reduction. Later, during hypnotic analgesia testing, subjects were instructed to give overt (verbal) reports that indicated the intensity of pain felt by their "conscious, hypnotized part," and hidden reports (numerical ratings tapped out in a pretaught code) that purportedly reflected the degree of pain felt by their "hidden part." Typically, the high hypnotizables exposed to these procedures exhibited hypnotic analgesia by reporting low levels of overt pain. However, many of these subjects also reported (via the pretaught code) high levels of hidden pain.

According to E. R. Hilgard (1979a, 1991), reports of hidden pain do not result from suggestions or other experimental demands. Instead, Hilgard (1979a) argued that hypnotically analgesic subjects simultaneously experience high levels of hidden pain and low levels of overt pain, regardless of whether they have been administered hidden-observer instructions. Supposedly, however, the hidden pain remains dissociated from consciousness by an "amnesic barrier" unless and until the experimenter obtains hidden reports. In other words, it is Hilgard's (1979a) contention that explicit hidden-observer instructions do *not* provide subjects with the idea that they have a hidden part or with the idea that hidden-pain reports should be higher than overt-pain reports. Supposedly, these instructions simply provide a structured setting that allows pre-existing hidden pain to come to light more easily.

A social-psychological alternative to E. R. Hilgard's (1991) dissociation hypothesis suggests that reports of experiencing a hidden part and ratings of hidden pain reflect the construals that subjects develop from the instructions used in hidden-observer experiments (Coe & Sarbin, 1977; Spanos & Hewitt, 1980). According to this hypothesis, motivated subjects are led by the content of hidden-observer instructions to construe themselves as possessing hidden parts that feel pain differently. These subjects then behave in a manner consistent with these construals when giving their ratings of overt and hidden pain.

Two experiments (Spanos, Gwynn, & Stam, 1983; Spanos & Hewitt, 1980) obtained support for the social-psychological hypothesis by varying the content of hidden-observer instructions and demonstrating that hidden-observer reports were closely tied to the expectations conveyed by these instructions. For example, Spanos, Gwynn, and Stam (1983) found that high hypnotizables rated hidden and overt pain as being of equal magnitude unless they were given explicit instructions informing them that one type of pain was supposed to be more intense than the other. These findings contradict E. R. Hilgard's (1979a) hypothesis that hidden-observer instructions simply access a pre-existing cognitive subsystem that "holds" high levels of hidden pain. In addition, Spanos, Gwynn, and Stam (1983; see also Spanos & Hewitt, 1980) also found that instructions implying that hidden pain was *less* intense than overt pain (the opposite of the pattern predicted by E. R. Hilgard, 1979a) led subjects to report hidden pain as less intense than overt pain. In short, the subjects in these experiments did not behave as though they possessed high levels of hidden pain that they were invariably made aware of when the experimenter communicated with their "hidden part." On the contrary, these subjects reported no difference between hidden and overt pain, higher hidden than overt pain, or lower hidden than overt pain, depending upon the content of their experimental instructions. These findings support the hypothesis that the hidden-observer phenomenon is a social construction shaped by the demands of the instructions to which subjects are exposed, rather than an intrinsic and unsuggested aspect of hypnotic responding.

Zamansky and Bartis (1985) acknowledged that hidden-observer responding is influenced by experimental demands, but contended that they obtained such responding even when minimizing experimental demands. Zamansky and Bartis (1985) gave high hypnotizables the suggestion that when they opened their eyes, they would not see anything on a piece of paper that clearly had a number written on it. After removal of the paper, subjects who insisted that they saw nothing on the paper were informed that a hidden part of their minds remained aware of everything they had experienced during the suggestion period, and that the experimenter could talk with their "hidden part." While giving their "hidden-observer reports," all of these negative hallucinators named the number on the paper that they had supposedly been unable to see consciously.

Like E. R. Hilgard (1979a), Zamansky and Bartis (1985) argued that negative hallucinators really do possess hidden parts that remain aware of stimulus information. They further assumed that the information obtained from these hidden parts is accurate and uninfluenced by experimental demands. In contrast, a social-psychological account suggests that the subjects in that experiment initially saw the number, but in conformance with the demands of the suggestion, denied having done so. Following the hidden-observer instruction, which made it clear that accurate reporting was now expected, subjects then reported the number.

Spanos, Flynn, and Gwynn (1988) tested these ideas by replicating the Zamansky and Bartis (1985) study. In this case, the number on the paper was an 18. Half of the negative hallucinators were informed that their hidden part would report what had been on the paper. The other half were told that their hidden part experienced everything in reverse. The implication, of course, was that the hidden part saw the number 81. Since hidden-observer instructions were given only after the stimulus paper was no longer visible, subjects could report an 81 only by knowing that the stimulus number had been an 18 and by following demands to reverse the 18 and report 81. Contrary to Zamansky and Bartis's (1985) assertion that hidden reports are always accurate, subjects given the modified hidden-observer information always reported an 81, while those given the standard hidden-observer instructions always reported an 18. Clearly, subjects in the reversal condition were misrepresenting what they had actually seen on the paper in order to follow the demands of the hidden-observer instruction.

In summary, the hidden-observer reports proffered by subjects in the Zamansky and Bartis (1985) paradigm, like the hidden-observer reports proffered in E. R. Hilgard's (1979a) paradigm, are strongly influenced by instructional demands. The available evidence fails to support the hypothesis that hidden-observer reports reflect the activity of an unsuggested unconscious cognitive subsystem that holds perceptual information out of conscious awareness. The evidence suggests instead that such reports reflect subjects' use of unfolding contextual information to guide their hypnotic enactments in terms of their beliefs concerning what is expected of them in the experimental situation.

Hypnotic Amnesia

Since the late 18th century, the purported inability of hypnotic subjects to recall the events of the hypnotic session after its termination (i.e., "hypnotic amnesia") has been considered a hallmark of the highly responsive hypnotic subject (Sarbin, 1962). Throughout the 19th and early 20th centuries, hypnotic amnesia was thought to often occur spontaneously. However, the available data now indicate that in experimental settings, hypnotic amnesia results from implicit or explicit suggestions to forget (T. X. Barber, 1969). Typically, hypnotic amnesia is operationalized as a temporary and reversible failure to recall or to recognize some or all of the target material specified in the suggestion (Coe, 1978, 1989a). Standardized hypnotizability scales include an explicit suggestion for amnesia that asks subjects to forget the test suggestions they were administered earlier in the session. However, amnesia suggestions can cover any material (e.g., a previously learned word list, one's own name, the number 4).

Hypnotic amnesia has been intensively studied in the last 20 years, and a number of findings are now well established (for a review, see Coe, 1989a). For instance, studies indicate that nonhypnotic subjects given amnesia suggestions often recall as poorly as hypnotic subjects (T. X. Barber & Calverley, 1966; Spanos, Radtke-Bodorik, & Stam, 1980); that high hypnotizables exhibit more amnesia than low hypnotizables (F. J. Evans & Kihlstrom, 1973; Spanos, Radtke-Bodorik, & Stam, 1980); and that lows exposed to skills training can be taught to exhibit as much or even more amnesia than corresponding highs (Spanos, de Groh, & de Groot, 1987).

A good deal of research has been devoted to determining whether hypnotically amnesic subjects exhibit disorganized recall. The research findings in this area are complex and sometimes contradictory (see Spanos, 1986b, for a review). Special-process theorists initially claimed that disorganized recall indexed an inability on the part of subjects to use organizational strategies to aid recall (F. J. Evans & Kihlstrom, 1973). The available research data fail to support this hypothesis, and a good deal of evidence indicates that disorganization in recall, when it does occur, reflects the operation of attention diversion strategies sometimes used by subjects in their attempts to generate forgetting (Spanos, 1986b).

A number of other studies have attempted to validate hypnotic amnesia by testing for it with indirect memory assessment procedures that are not under subjects' voluntary control (e.g., proactive and retroactive interference procedures). These studies have uniformly yielded negative results (Coe, Basden, Basden, & Graham, 1976; Dillon & Spanos, 1983; Graham & Patton, 1968). In other words, when hypnotically induced "forgetting" is assessed by indirect means, there is no evidence that any forgetting has actually occurred.

Theories of hypnotic amnesia, like theories of negative hallucination, can be distinguished on the basis of the amount of credibility that investigators are willing to give to subjects' verbal reports. When given amnesia suggestions, many highly hypnotizable subjects fail to recall the targeted material. Some of these subjects fail to recall even when given several opportunities to remember and when encouraged to be honest and try their best. Nevertheless, after a prearranged cue that "cancels" their amnesia, these subjects easily remember the "forgotten" material. Many of these subjects report afterwards that they were unable to recall during the suggestion period, despite trying their best (Coe & Yashinski, 1985; Howard & Coe, 1980; Spanos & D'Eon, 1980).

Special-process theorists have typically taken the reports of hypnotically amnesic subjects at face value. Consequently, they have developed theories assuming that hypnotically amnesic subjects have actually lost control over their normally voluntary memory processes. From their perspective, hypnotic amnesia involves (1) an inability to access retrieval cues, or (2) the development of an "amnesic barrier" between certain memories, or (3) a dissociation between cognitive subsystems (F. J. Evans & Kihlstrom, 1973; E. R. Hilgard, 1977a; Kihlstrom, 1978; Kihlstrom, Evans, Orne, & Orne, 1980).

Social-psychological theorists do not assume that hypnotically amnesic subjects have lost control over remembering, but rather that hypnotic amnesia reflects an output inhibition phenomenon (Coe, 1978, 1989a; Spanos, 1986b; Wagstaff, 1981a). In other words, these investigators hypothesize that amnesic subjects retain control over their ability to retrieve target information, and guide their recall (and failures to recall) in terms of the unfolding social demands of the amnesia test situation.

The social-psychological position acknowledges that, depending on the requirements of particular amnesia suggestions, subjects may carry out various cognitive strategies in an attempt to define themselves as having forgotten. For instance, when instructed to forget all of the words on a previously learned list, many subjects engage in attention diversion in order to define themselves as not remembering the list (Spanos & Radtke, 1982). When instructed to forget a subset of items (e.g., only the animal words on a multicategory list), many subjects selectively rehearse the to-be-remembered items as a strategy for avoiding the retrieval of the to-be-forgotten items (L. D. Bertrand & Spanos, 1984–1985). When challenged to remember, it is difficult for subjects both to use such strategies and simultaneously to recall the to-be-forgotten items. Such temporary self-induced difficulties in recall may help subjects to define themselves as being amnesic. Nevertheless, such self-induced recall difficulties do not imply an inability to recall, because subjects retain the ability to employ or not to employ the disruptive strategies as a function of the changing demands contained in the amnesia situation.

In short, the central theoretical issue dividing special-process and social-psychological theories of amnesia may be stated as follows: Do hypnotically amnesic subjects lose control over memory processes and thereby become unable to recall target material, or do they retain control over memory processes while behaving as if they are unable to recall? This question has been addressed most directly through a series of amnesia-breaching studies.

Can Hypnotic Amnesia Be Breached?

Kihlstrom et al. (1980) gave hypnotic subjects an amnesia suggestion and then asked them on two successive trials to try to recall the target material. Between these two trials, experimental subjects were administered various instructions designed to break down (i.e., to breach) their amnesia. For example, subjects in one condition were instructed to be honest on the second trial; those in a different condition were urged to try their best to recall on the second trial; and control subjects were administered no intervening instructions between the two trials. Following the second recall trial, amnesia was canceled, and subjects in all conditions were given a third and final recall attempt. Subjects in *all* conditions recalled more on the second trial than on the first, and still more after cancellation of amnesia than on trial 2. Importantly, subjects in the breaching instruction conditions did not recall more on the second trial than did controls.

These results were interpreted as strong evidence against a social-psychological conceptualization of hypnotic amnesia (Kihlstrom, 1978). According to Kihlstrom (1978), the instructions to breach used in that study constituted strong demands for enhanced recall. Since subjects given these instructions failed to recall any more on trial 2 than controls did, they must have been unable to follow the demands for enhanced recall. In other words, despite their best efforts, these subjects were unable (as opposed to unwilling) to exhibit any greater recall on trial 2.

In order to explain why subjects in all treatments (including the controls) recalled more on trial 2 than on trial 1, Kihlstrom et al. (1980) suggested that the "amnesic barrier" that separates the dissociated memories from consciousness tends to "wear down" with time. As a result, previously forgotten material tends to leak into awareness with the passage of time.

The Strength of Demands

Coe (1978) pointed out that the failure of Kihlstrom et al. (1980) to obtain breaching of amnesia may have occurred because the breaching instructions employed in that study were simply too weak. In a series of studies, Coe and his associates (Coe & Yashinski, 1985; Howard & Coe, 1980; Schuyler & Coe, 1981; Coe & Sluis, 1989) assessed this hypothesis by varying the strength of the demands to breach. For example, before a second recall trial, amnesic subjects in one condition might simply be instructed to report honestly everything they could remember; those in another might be attached to a "lie detector" and informed that their physiological responses indicated that they were not being completely truthful. In general, the results indicated that many of the breaching manipulations employed in these studies produced a good deal more breaching than the instructions used by Kihlstrom et al. (1980).

Although subjects in Coe's studies exhibited significant amounts of breaching, they did not breach completely. At least some of the subjects in all of these breaching conditions failed to recall at least some words on trial 2 that they recalled later after cancellation of the amnesia suggestion. Moreover, subjects who rated themselves after the first amnesia trial as being *not* in control of memory ("involuntaries") were less likely to breach than subjects who rated themselves as in control ("voluntaries").

The finding that involuntaries were less likely to breach than voluntaries is, of course, consistent with the view that the involuntaries were unable to recall because they had lost control over memory processes. Recently, however, Coe and Sluis (1989) exposed both highly hypnotizable voluntaries and involuntaries to a strong, composite breaching manipulation. First subjects were given honesty instructions; second, they received bogus "lie detector" feedback; and, third, they were shown a videotaped playback of their own hypnotic session. When exposed to these strong demands for increased recall, both the involuntaries and the voluntaries exhibited substantial breaching. These findings indicate that most amnesic subjects, including those who claim that they have lost control over memory, breach amnesia when exposed to sufficiently strong social pressure to recall.

Even in the Coe and Sluis (1989) study, a few subjects failed to breach amnesia completely (i.e., recalled items after cancellation of the suggestion that they had not recalled on the breaching trials). In order to account for such findings, Spanos, Radtke, and Bertrand (1984) suggested that highly hypnotizable subjects are often intent on presenting themselves as deeply hypnotized during the test session. For this reason, they tend to ignore or reinterpret instructions that, if followed, would compromise their hypnotic self-presentations. Presenting as deeply hypnotized means, among other things, being highly responsive to test suggestions. The complete reversal of hypnotic amnesia following exposure to breaching manipulations would not only violate the role requirements for presenting as deeply hypnotized; it would also call into question the legitimacy of subjects' failures to recall on earlier trials. For example, recalling all of the target items after being instructed to "be completely honest" or to "try harder this time" would imply that the subjects had not been completely honest or tried hard when failing to recall these items on previous trials. In short, amnesic subjects have a vested interest in not recalling, despite exhortations to the contrary. For this reason, many of them fail to breach unless they can be fooled into believing (e.g., via a lie detection manipulation) that the experimenter can accurately determine the validity of their responses. And even some of these subjects may choose to "bluster through" rather than to acknowledge that they have been deceitful.

The Congruence of Role Demands

If hypnotically amnesic subjects actually lose control over memory, then they should be unable to reverse amnesia even if they wish to do so. However, if they actually retain control over memory, it should be possible to induce them to breach amnesia completely by constructing a situation that convinces them that the recall of target items (rather than continued nonrecall) is congruent with their role as deeply hypnotized.

To test these ideas, Spanos, Radtke, and Bertrand (1984) used eight very highly hypnotizable hypnotic subjects who had described their responses to suggestions as involuntary in previous testing, and who had failed repeatedly to breach amnesia despite exhortations to report honestly. A modification of E. R. Hilgard's (1977a) hidden-observer paradigm was used: These subjects were informed that during hypnosis, hidden parts of their minds remained aware of things that they could no longer consciously remember. Specifically, these subjects were told that one hidden part remained aware of everything that occurred in the left hemisphere of the brain, while a different hidden part remained aware of everything that occurred in the right hemisphere. Subjects learned a list of abstract and concrete words. Half were told that abstract words were stored in the left hemisphere and concrete words in the right; the remaining half were given the *opposite* information about storage location. Following an amnesia suggestion to forget the words, all subjects failed to recall most of them (i.e., exhibited very high levels of amnesia). However, before canceling the amnesia suggestion, the experimenter "contacted" each subject's right and left "hidden part" in succession. When informed that contact had been made with their "left hidden part," all subjects correctly recalled all of their "left-hemisphere words" but none of their "right-hemisphere words." These subjects exhibited the opposite pattern of recall when informed that contact had been made with their "right hidden part." In other words, amnesia was breached easily and completely in every one of these highly hypnotizable hypnotic subjects when breaching supported rather than challenged a self-presentation as deeply hypnotized.

A related study by Silva and Kirsch (1987) also obtained very high levels of breaching in highly hypnotizable hypnotic subjects. In this case, amnesic subjects were informed that they would be put into a very deep hypnotic state. Half were told that they would be able to remember even less while in this deep state (i.e., that recall would be reduced), and the remainder were told that they would remember more in the deep state (i.e., that recall would be enhanced). Subjects in the two treatments exhibited equivalent amounts of amnesia on their initial recall trial. However, following the "deep state" manipulation, 8 of the 10 subjects in the recall-enhanced condition exhibited a complete breaching of amnesia, while 8 of the 10 in the reduced-recall condition remained completely amnesic. Thus, to an overwhelming degree, subjects behaved in terms of the expectations conveyed to them when these expectations did not conflict with a self-presentation as deeply hypnotized.

In summary, experimental findings indicate that hypnotic amnesia can be breached by a wide variety of social-psychological manipulations. Findings like those of Spanos, Radtke, and Bertrand (1984) and Silva and Kirsch (1987), which demonstrated complete or almost complete breaching as a function of changes in subjects' expectations concerning what is consistent with the hypnotic role, are clearly inconsistent with special-process accounts. Such studies demonstrate that amnesic subjects, regardless of what they may sometimes say, retain control over memory and guide their recall (and failures to recall) in terms of the changing demands of the amnesia test situation. In short, hypnotic amnesia, rather than being an event that "happens" to passive subjects, is a "doing"—a pattern of interpersonal responding that is geared to the expectations conveyed in the hypnotic situation, and that is designed to communicate a self-presentation as having lost control of one's memory.

Conclusion

A social-psychological perspective is premised on the notion that the suggested phenomena most closely tied to the concept of hypnosis are historically rooted social actions that are fundamentally similar to other, more mundane forms of social behavior. According to this view, traditional conceptualizations of hypnosis as a "trance state" that is induced by certain rituals (hypnotic induction procedures), and that in turn produces unusual behavior, is misleading. Instead, hypnotic induction procedures are viewed as historical artifacts that arose from misguided 19th-century attempts to conceptualize the behavioral phenomena that became associated with hypnosis as somehow related to sleep. In fact, from a social-psychological perspective, hypnotic behaviors are themselves social artifacts (Radtke, 1989; Spanos, 1991). Rather than reflecting the essential characteristics of an invariant "trance state," these behaviors constitute rule-governed, context-dependent social actions that are rooted in the shared conceptions of hypnosis held by subjects and hypnotists in particular historical circumstances.

A social-psychological conceptualization acknowledges that hypnotic responding may involve faking. In other words, hypnotic subjects who are unable to generate the experiences that they believe are required by suggestions sometimes exaggerate and misdescribe the experiences that they do have (e.g., reporting deafness when they actually hear) or enact behaviors implying an experience that they do not have (e.g., raising an arm to an arm lightness suggestion even though it does not feel light). On the other hand, a social-psychological conceptualization does not view faking as a sole or adequate account of hypnotic responding. On the contrary, one of the most interesting aspects of hypnotic responding is that subjects, to varying degrees, appear to convince themselves temporarily that their arms are rising involuntarily, that a nonexistent cat is sitting in their laps, that they can no longer remember well-learned material, and so on. A good deal of research and theorizing from the social-psychological tradition has focused on delineating the variables that underlie subjects' acceptance of such counterfactual beliefs (Sarbin & Coe, 1972; Spanos, 1986c; Spanos, Menary, Gabora, DuBreuil, & Dewherst, 1991). From a social-psychological perspective, then, the goal of research is not the isolation of some subtle will-of-the-wisp hypnotic essence, but instead the integration of hypnotic responding into a more general theory of social action.

Notes

1. A number of investigators have investigated the effects of suggestions for negative hallucinations on evoked responses (ERs; Amadeo & Yanovski, 1975; Andreassi, Balinsky, Gallichio, De Simone, & Mellers, 1976; A. F. Barabasz & Lonsdale, 1983; Beck & Barolin, 1965; Beck, Dustman, & Beier, 1966; Halliday & Mason, 1964b; Shagass & Schwartz, 1964; D. Spiegel, Cutcomb, Ren, & Pribram, 1985). In most of these studies, negative-hallucination suggestions failed to influence the ERs of even highly hypnotizable subjects. Although some studies have reported decreases in the amplitude of ERs with suggestion (e.g., D. Spiegel et al., 1985), others have reported increases in amplitude (A. F. Barabasz & Lonsdale, 1983). The area is complicated further by a lack of consensus concerning the inferences about psychological functioning that can validly be drawn from late-

component ER amplitude changes. In short, the findings from these studies do little to challenge the hypothesis that the reports of perceptual change proffered by negative hallucinators strongly influenced by reporting biases.

2. The findings of the reporting bias studies described above can be interpreted in terms of at least two hypotheses (Spanos, 1991). Both hypotheses are based on the notion that subjects who responded to the demand instruction were invested in the role of being "good subjects," and motivated to guide their behavior in terms of the demands associated with that role. The first hypothesis suggests that subjects who exhibited a reporting bias were simply lying about the degree of loudness that they experienced. According to this hypothesis, subjects were aware that they were reporting the tone as less loud than they actually heard it on trial 3. The second hypothesis suggests that the demand instruction led subjects to reinterpret the trial 3 tone as being less loud than they initially believed it to be. This hypothesis does not imply that subjects were lying. Instead, it suggests that the compliance instruction initiated a process of motivated reinterpretation that led subjects to change the way that they classified the loudness of the trial 3 tone.

Deception and reinterpretation are not mutually exclusive explanations; in fact, both processes may occur in the same subject. For instance, some subjects may initially lie and report the tone as less loud than they actually believed it to be. However, as they reflect on the situation, at least some of these subjects may convince themselves that "maybe it wasn't as loud as I first thought" (Spanos, 1991).

CHAPTER FIVE

An Ego-Psychological Theory of Hypnosis

ERIKA FROMM

This chapter presents an ego-psychological theory of hypnosis. It is a cognitive theory based to a great extent on a number of concepts developed in classical and neoclassical psychoanalysis.

Antecedents

Altered States of Consciousness

Hypnosis is an altered state of consciousness (ASC), a state different from the waking state. Until about 1885, psychology acknowledged two mental states only: the waking state and the state of sleep. The waking state was defined as the state in which we operate with consciousness. Sleep was considered to be a no-consciousness state and therefore not worth exploring.

Then, at the turn of the century, Freud (1900/1953) made his great discovery: the unconscious. He identified three mental states: the "conscious" (that which at a given moment is in full waking awareness), the "preconscious" (that which is not in full awareness but can be brought into consciousness by simply turning one's attention to it), and the unconscious (those mental contents—memories, fantasies, thoughts, and affects—that resist being brought into consciousness). He conceived of dreams as a special state of consciousness of great significance—namely, as "the royal road to the unconscious activities of the mind" (Freud, 1900/1953, Vol. 5, p. 608).

I contend that dreams are not the only royal road to the unconscious. Hypnosis is another. And so are most other ASCs.

William James did the first research on ASCs in 1902. He wrote that our normal waking consciousness

> is but one special type of consciousness, whilst all about it, parted from it by the flimsiest of screens, there lie potential forms of consciousness entirely different. We may go through life without suspecting their existence; but apply the requisite stimulus, and at a touch they are all there in all their completeness, definite types of mentality . . . discontinuous with ordinary consciousness. (James, 1902/1935, p. 298)

An ASC is a cognitive–perceptual state different from the waking state. It has its own felt reality. One of its characteristics is involuntarism or nonconscious involvement (Shor, 1962, 1979). An ASC is a state in which the barrier between Freud's unconscious and the conscious becomes more permeable, and in which the individual can make contact with the contents of the unconscious much more easily than in the waking state. The hypnotically altered state of consciousness can be recognized subjectively by the individual as being different from the waking state. However, subjectively very vivid altered states do not necessarily translate into overt behavior that is measurable or observable by an outside observer (Fromm, 1979; Shor, 1979).

The Psychoanalytic Concept of the Ego

Psychoanalysis has existed for over a century now. It was started by Freud as the libido theory, a theory of the unconscious and the instincts. Other psychoanalytic theories were added later—namely, ego psychology, object relations theory, and the theory of the self. Freud himself (1923/1961) originated ego psychology. Object relations theory began in England in the late 1940s (Fairbairn, 1946/1952) and in the United States in the 1950s (Jacobson, 1954). And the theory of the self originated in the United States in the 1960s (Kohut, 1966, 1971). These four theoretical strands form the broad braid that currently constitutes psychoanalysis.

My theory of hypnosis rests on concepts stemming from the ego-psychological strand of psychoanalysis. The "ego" is a conglomeration of functions: perception, cognition, defenses, decision making, judgment, memory, attention, imagery, sensations, and affect. The ego organizes and structures all of the above in conscious and in unconscious awareness, in relationship to the outside world as well as to the individual's inner world.[1]

In 1953, Rapaport (1953/1967) initiated a (psychoanalytic) theory of ego activity and ego passivity. The ego is active or autonomous, he said, when a person is free to make choices and decisions; it is passive when the ego lacks autonomy and is overwhelmed by instinctual drives or by demands coming from the environment. We (Stolar & Fromm, 1974) extended Rapaport's theory later to include the ego's reaction to demands coming from the superego.

Rapaport showed that there are two forms of ego activity and two forms of ego passivity. Decision making and coping with challenges can be sovereign, smooth, and masterful, or they can be protective and defensive. In masterful coping, a person actively meets the demands coming from the instincts or from reality and handles them creatively or at least smoothly, at his or her own leisure and pace. In protective coping, the individual also makes a decision—the decision to defend the self against demands coming from the instincts, the outside world. But the action is not free, sovereign, and smooth. Defenses represent mastery of a lower order—namely, choosing to do what feels the least uncomfortable under the circumstances. But still a (usually unconscious) decision is actively being made by the ego. Rapaport differentiated ego activity and ego passivity from active and passive behavior. Each can occur without the other. For instance, the person who sits motionless in a chair and thinks is ego-active but physically inactive; the serial killer who feels *driven* to murder people is ego-passive but physically very active.

These are the antecedents to my ego-psychological theory of hypnosis. Next, I describe my own theory and its place in the context of other theories.

Theoretical Concepts and Principles

In the early 1880s, Freud became familiar with hypnosis through attending the lectures of Charcot at La Salpêtrière in Paris; after his return to Vienna, working with Breuer (Breuer & Freud, 1893–1895/1955), he used authoritarian hypnosis. He demanded from his patients that they go deep down into their unconscious and bring up with them memories not available in the waking state. Frequently, in the hypnotic state, they would remember incestuous experiences; however, when brought up to the waking state, they would deny ever having had such experiences as well as having talked about them in trance. Freud therefore came to believe that hypnosis circumvents the ego, and for this and other reasons gave it up.

I contend that hypnosis does not circumvent the ego. Quite the contrary: The hypnotic subject or patient can hear, see (if his or her eyes are open), and smell, and can produce imagery, thoughts, and even defenses. All of these are ego functions. In the following, I discuss ego-psychological concepts and principles that I feel explain important aspects of hypnosis. Put together as a whole, they form my theory of hypnosis.

Dissociation of the Observing Ego from the Experiencing Ego

My psychoanalytic model of conscious, preconscious, and unconscious *awareness* (Fromm, 1965b, 1977, 1979) in trance is a vertical one in which, as in psychoanalytic theory, the unconscious, the preconscious, and the conscious are viewed as mental states ranged in ascending order. E. R. Hilgard, in his research on the "hidden observer" (1977a, 1979; see also Chapter 3, this volume), speaks of divided consciousness as consisting of several subsystems of cognitive control structures, some of which can be dissociated in hypnosis from central cognitive control. Hilgard's model of hypnotic consciousness is a horizontal one in which all subsystems are on the same level. His theory of hypnosis is a neodissociation theory. In my own theory (Fromm, 1965a, 1976), I interpret the dissociation process that takes place so easily in the hypnotic state as a dissociation of the experiencing ego from the observing ego.

Hypnosis as a Regression in the Service of the Ego

Letting go of some of one's usual activities and controls, and going backward a step on the developmental ladder in order to be able to take two steps forward, is called a "regression in the service of the ego" (Kris, 1934/1952) or an "adaptive regression" (Hartmann, 1939/1958) in the psychoanalytic literature. For instance, instead of running around with a fever and continuing to work, a person with light pneumonia curls up in bed like a child, looks for hours at lightweight TV programs, and lets himself or herself be taken care of by others. This helps the person to get well and become independent again more quickly. Taking a nap or a vacation, in order then to return to work with greater vigor and joy, is another example of regression in the service of the ego or of adaptive regression. Regressions in the service of the ego are nonpathological and healthy.

Gill and Brenman (1959), and my collaborators and I (Fromm, 1977, 1978–1979, 1979; Fromm & Gardner, 1979; Fromm & Hurt, 1980), have theorized that hypnosis is an adaptive regression or a regression in the service of the ego. Hypnotic relaxation is thought to cause an ego-modulated relaxation of defensive barriers, with a return to earlier, less realistic, primary-process thinking. It is also temporary (i.e., limited to the time of a relatively deep hypnotic trance).

Ego Activity, Ego Passivity, and Ego Receptivity

The issue of ego activity is tied to the concepts of choice, free will, and mastery; that of ego passivity is tied to feeling overwhelmed and failing to cope.

I define "ego activity" with regard to the hypnotic state as a volitional mental activity during trance. It can be a decision by the subject *not* to go along with what the hypnotist is suggesting, or to go along with it because the subject *wants* to do it (Fromm, 1972). In self-hypnosis (SH), it can be the act of giving oneself a self-suggestion or of deciding to break off the trance (Fromm, Brown, Hurt, Oberlander, Boxer, & Pfeifer, 1981; Fromm, Lombard, Skinner, & Kahn, 1987–1988; Fromm & Kahn, 1990).

"Ego passivity" is a state in which the person feels overwhelmed or helpless and is unable to handle the situation. Except perhaps in highly masochistic people, this is always accompanied by unpleasant affect. The ego-dystonic demand may come from the instincts, from the external world, or from the superego (Stolar & Fromm, 1974). The person goes along with the demand—as, for instance, the drug addict or the individual who runs amok does—even though he or she does not want to, or because the person feels overwhelmed and experiences that he or she *has* to submit. In hypnosis, ego passivity may occur when an authoritarian hypnotist forces a patient into doing, feeling, or experiencing things that the patient definitely does not want to experience (Fromm, 1972).

In 1971 Deikman, a psychoanalyst interested in meditation, added to Rapaport's scheme the exciting concept of "ego receptivity." In ego receptivity voluntarism, critical judgment, and deliberate control of internal emotional experiences are temporarily relinquished, and the subject allows unconscious and preconscious material to emerge freely. I have applied this concept to the field of hypnosis, and found that in hypnosis ego receptivity occurs when the "generalized reality orientation" (GRO) has faded into the background of awareness. Then there exists a greater openness to the experiencing of stimuli that arise from within or stem from just *one* outside source, the hypnotist, on whom the subject's attention is concentrated and to whom the subject has a special relationship. Active, goal-directed thinking and strict adherence to reality orientation are temporarily relinquished, and the subject or patient can "just let go." The hypnotist's suggestions, as well as the subject's own unconscious and preconscious material, float effortlessly into awareness (Fromm, 1976, 1977, 1979).

With regard to SH, I hypothesized that ego receptivity would be an important variable. When the ego is receptive, defenses are supposed to be relaxed, allowing into consciousness the emergence of fluid thoughts, associations, and images—phenomena that in the waking state usually are below the level of conscious awareness. In heterohypnosis, ego receptivity is encountered primarily as suggestibility (i.e., increased openness to stimuli coming from the hypnotist) (Fromm, 1979). Ego receptivity to stimuli arising from within, of course, appears in heterohypnosis as well, and has highly beneficial consequences for hypnotherapy and hypnoanalysis. It aids in speeding up the processes of uncovering and reintegration.

Ego receptivity in hypnosis is basically the same as what P. G. Bowers (1978, 1982–1983) has called "effortless experiencing." She has found this to be an important aspect of heterohypnosis and creativity.

Primary-Process and Secondary-Process Imagery

Imagery is thinking in pictorial forms. It has been well researched with regard to hypnosis by J. R. Hilgard (1965, 1979a,b). Primary process (Freud, 1900/1953) is the mental functioning typical of early childhood—

that is, before reality orientation and the ability to delay immediate gratification have developed. In primary process, the form of thinking is nonverbal imagery. Functioning is still fluid and undifferentiated, and several ideas are often represented by a single image, or a word that contains a double entendre. Primary-process thinking, to a great extent, is nonsequential and does not follow the rules of logic.

Secondary-process thinking occurs in words and in sentences—in language rather than in imagery, pictures, and symbols. It results from the impact of reality; is reality-oriented and goal-directed; and operates by logically ordered practical, or abstract concepts. It is the dominant, every-day cognitive mode of the adult. When primary process occurs spontaneously in the healthy adult, it represents an input from the drives or from the unconscious ego, both of which can creatively enrich waking logic and ordinary modes of thought.

Primary-process thinking is not given up when secondary-process thinking has developed. Even in the adult waking state, our thoughts are hardly ever devoid of some minor form of imagery; and even in the deepest stages of trance or in the state of nocturnal dreaming, some elements of realism and logic can be found.

Primary and secondary processes range themselves along a continuum (Fromm, 1978–1979), and no sharp line of distinction separates one from the other. Figure 5.1 illustrates this continuum. The primary-process end is drive-dominated, characterized by vivid, healthy imagery, or be hallucinations; the secondary-process end is characterized by step-by-step logic and reasoning and by full reality orientation. Healthy primary processes are particularly characteristic of the inspirational phase of the creative act and of intuitive thought. Examples of pathological primary processes are schizophrenic hallucinations and psychotic thinking. In the psychotic, primary process overwhelms and drowns out secondary-process logic and reality orientation.

Either primary-process or secondary-process energy can be invested in imagery. For instance, when one plans to drive from Los Angeles to San Francisco and pictures in one's mind the beautiful highway by the ocean along which one will drive, one uses reality-oriented, secondary-process type of imagery. It can be produced voluntarily (but not equally vividly by all people). Primary-process imagery usually arises spontaneously from within. It has fantastic and nonrealistic qualities. But both primary- and secondary-process imagery and thinking are products of the ego, because only the ego can perceive, think, and produce imagery. Voluntarily produced fantasy represents an ego-active process. Imagery that arises spontaneously from within—as, for example, in dreams—is an ego-receptive process.

On the continuum from primary process to secondary process, the "waking entranced" state is relatively close to the secondary-process pole of mental functioning. The state of absorption or fascination, depending on the content or nature of the thing one is fascinated with or entranced by, is

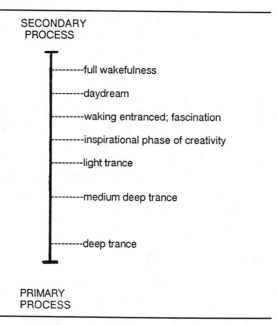

SECONDARY
PROCESS

--------full wakefulness

--------daydream

--------waking entranced; fascination

--------inspirational phase of creativity

--------light trance

--------medium deep trance

--------deep trance

PRIMARY
PROCESS

FIGURE 5.1. Primary and secondary process in waking and hypnotic states. From "Primary and Secondary Process in Waking and in Altered States of Consciousness" (p. 118) by E. Fromm, 1978–1979, *Journal of Altered States of Consciousness, 4,* 115–128. Copyright 1979 by Baywood Publishing Co., Inc. Reprinted by permission.

located somewhat farther from secondary process. For instance, if the content in trance is primary-process imagery with which the subject is fascinated, it would probably require at least a medium depth of hypnosis and contain more primary process than the ordinary book-reading fantasy.

Attention, Absorption, and the Generalized Reality Orientation

Three other concepts that play a role in my theory of hypnosis are attention, absorption, and the GRO (Shor, 1959/1969). Attention and absorption are concepts that stem from cognitive psychology, but I feel they can also be considered to represent ego functions. I have not yet been able to conceive of the GRO as an ego function—given the fact that for the person in hypnosis the GRO usually fades into the background of awareness. Absorption and the fading of the GRO have long been recognized as important characteristics of hypnosis. The former has been researched by Tellegen and Atkinson (1974) and Tellegen (1981), the latter by Shor (1959/1969).

With regard to attention, I differentiate between "concentrative" or "focused" attention on the one hand, and "expansive" or "free-floating" attention on the other (Fromm, 1977, 1979). In expansive attention the subject "lets go," and a wide variety of thoughts, feelings, memories, and images are picked up consecutively and momentarily in the attentional field.

Although attention and absorption are not concepts first described in the psychoanalytic literature, I have looked at them from a psychoanalytic point of view of my own and conceive of both of them as ego functions, in the same way in which perception and cognition are ego functions. Attention is a cognitive function, and cognition is a function of the ego. Absorption is a result of both concentrated attention and ego receptivity. It denotes the extent to which a subject's concentrated attention has been gripped at a given moment by an outside event or by an ongoing inner experience. The content of *hypnotic* experiences involving absorption is usually—though not necessarily—imagery.

Structural and Content Categories

In the studies done in my laboratory we have come to differentiate between Structural and Content variables that separate SH and heterohypnosis from the waking state. Structural variables are those that essentially characterize the nature of the state. They are Absorption/Fascination, concentrative and expansive Attention, Ego Activity and Ego Receptivity, the disruption of the GRO, and Trance Depth. Content categories comprise the phenomena of increased Imagery Production (Lombard, Kahn, & Fromm, 1990; Fromm & Kahn, 1990), memories (particularly hypermnesia), strong affect, enjoyable or conflictful thoughts, hypnotic dreams, working on personal problems, and self-suggestions of sensory and motor phenomena (Fromm et al., 1981; Fromm, 1988).

Structural Differences between Hypnosis and the Waking State

Although there certainly is a felt difference between the waking state and ASCs (among them hypnosis), it is doubtful whether there is a real hiatus between them. E. R. Hilgard (1977a) found that hypnotizability is distributed along a bimodal curve, with only very deeply hypnotized subjects attaining the full ASC. Waking and ASCs can shade into each other. For example, let us take the waking state that I have called "waking entranced" (Fromm, 1977, 1978–1979). It is a state in which the individual is awake, watching a particular event or detail in the outside world with fascinated attention. The person may focus on such an event—for instance, the busy life of ants in an anthill, or a piece of music he or she is hearing (Shor, 1970)—with such intense attention and concentration that great parts of the rest of reality fade into the background of awareness. The person is awake, so entranced by what he or she is doing or thinking as to be unaware of anything else going on. The "waking entranced" person is awake, but does not make as clear a distinction between reality and fantasy as people do in the normal waking state. Thus, particularly in this second type of entrancedly being awake, one can question whether the person is not already in an ASC (of SH).

Awareness versus Consciousness

When it comes to hypnosis and other ASCs, I have felt the need to differentiate between consciousness and awareness (Fromm, 1965b). The inner reality is as real to the deeply hypnotized person as objective reality is to the waking human being. Is the hypnotized person "conscious" of this inner reality in the state of trance, or is he or she "aware" of it? Frequently, material that in the waking state has been unconscious comes up in the state of trance, because in hypnosis a person makes closer contact with the unconscious. But can one say that in this state the person is *conscious of the unconscious?* That would be a contradiction in terms. I therefore have introduced the differentiation between "awareness" and "consciousness" (Fromm, 1965b), and have compared awareness to a flashlight that can be directed at the conscious, the preconscious, or the unconscious (see Figure 5.2). In the waking state it is directed at consciousness. In the hypnotic state, with the fading of the GRO, the light of awareness moves from consciousness—perhaps over preconsciousness—to shining onto parts of the unconscious.

Shaping My Theory of Hypnosis

I have developed my theory of hypnosis by applying to the understanding of the phenomena of hypnosis the above-described psychoanalytic concepts, as well as the three others stemming from cognitive psychology. At times I made theoretical formulations first and followed them up with experimentation that would prove or disprove the theory I had made. At other times the experimental findings came first and led me to add to, modify, or discard parts of the theory I was building.

Pertinent Research Evidence

Adaptive Regression and Primary-Process Imagery

Gill and Brenman's (1959) theory that hypnosis is a regression in the service of the ego had become a cornerstone of our thinking, but it had never been tested experimentally. In the late 1960s I found an opportunity

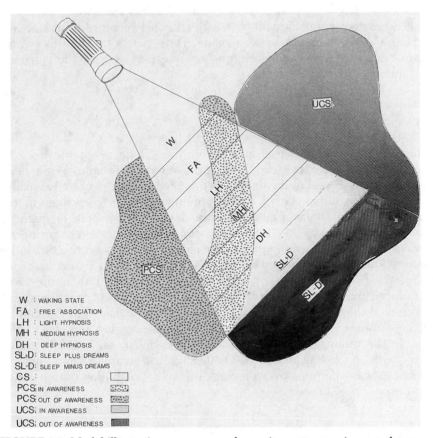

FIGURE 5.2. Model illustrating awareness of conscious, preconscious, and unconscious process in waking states, in hypnotic states, and during sleep. From "Awareness versus Consciousness" (p. 712) by E. Fromm, 1965, *Psychological Reports, 16,* 711–712. Copyright 1965 by *Psychological Reports.* Reprinted by permission.

to do this. Holt and his collaborators (Holt, 1963, 1969) at that time developed a Rorschach scoring method that measures three dimensions of perceptual–cognitive functions and their implications for regression in the service of the ego: (1) degree and kind of primary-process manifestations and defenses; (2) their fluctuations; and (3) content and structure of thought processes.

Regression in the service of the ego has been defined as a "partial temporary lowering of the level of psychic functioning . . . [in which the ego permits] relatively free play to the primary process thinking in order to accomplish its adaptive tasks" (Silverman, 1965, p. 232). Rather than to repress or otherwise to defend against it, the ego makes constructive use of the primary process. In the healthy individual, as I have described earlier, adaptive regression consists of a short-term going backwards for one step on the developmental ladder in order to take two steps forward. It often results in a creative act. In contrast, psychotic regression is a pathological process, a long-term breakdown of reality testing and secondary-process thinking; it is not adaptive. With the Holt method, one can score the increase in primary process and the ego-modulated relaxation of control and defense on the Rorschach, as well as the healthiness or pathology of the content of the responses. So I decided to use this method to test whether hypnosis indeed is a regression in the service of the ego.

We gave the Rorschach (Rorschach, 1954) to 32 subjects, in the waking state as well as in the hypnotic state. It was administered in counterbalanced order with a 4-week interval between the two administrations. The subjects were selected from a relatively normal student population who demonstrated good or excellent hypnotizability. Each subject went through both conditions with the same examiner and served as his or her own control. The Rorschach protocols were scored blindly by three psychologists according to both the Holt (1963) and the Klopfer (Klopfer & Kelley, 1942) methods. Discrepancies in scoring were then discussed until consensus was reached. Design, methodology, and the statistical analysis of the results have been fully reported in two publications (Fromm, Oberlander, & Gruenewald, 1970; Gruenewald, Fromm, & Oberlander, 1979). Our results showed that in hypnosis there was a significant increase ($p <$ .01) of primary-process mentation. However, contrary to expectation, a concomitant increase in defense and coping functions was not uniformly present. Hypnosis had no significant effect on subjects' scores on Holt's Adaptive Regression Scale. Only the well-adjusted subjects engaged in predominantly flexible and far-ranging ego activity in the hypnosis condition, with a preponderance of higher-level coping mechanisms. Male subjects with strong ego controls (the somewhat more rigid subjects) tended to become more constricted and to produce more maladaptive defenses in the hypnotic than in the waking state. Instead of comfortably accepting hypnosis and "letting go," they defended themselves against what they must have feared was a potentially disorganizing influence of hypnosis by clinging to realistic features and to more rigid intellectual functioning. They, too, produced significantly more primary process in the hypnotic state than in the waking state. But in them, the expected increase in healthy defense effectiveness during trance did not occur.

Levin and Harrison (1976) have replicated and extended our study. In the waking as well as in the hypnotic state, they asked their subjects to make up a story for a Thematic Apperception Test card and used a Rorschach card to induce dreams. They arrived at the same results as we did: Their data showed a significant increase in primary process in hypnosis, but their subjects did not universally demonstrate the hypothesized increase of controls and defenses under hypnosis that is supposed to make it possible to adaptively utilize the regression from mostly secondary-process to more primary-process thinking.

Levin and Harrison themselves speculated that their failure to obtain a full confirmation of the adaptive regression hypothesis may have resulted from the fact that many of their subjects "were only lightly hypnotized and no subjects were deeply hypnotized during the duration of the hypnosis procedures" (1976, p. 413).

From their statistical analyses, they concluded that the two facets characteristic of regression in the service of the ego (i.e., increases both in primary process and in healthy controls and defenses) are two relatively independent factors, and that the presence of just one of them—namely, increase in primary process—suffices to indicate adaptive regression.

I must confess I find it difficult to relinquish the idea that hypnosis is a regression in the service of the ego. On the other hand, I find it equally difficult to accept the thought that increase in primary process alone is all that is needed to demonstrate adaptive regression. To me it is the *combination,* the dynamic balance of the two factors, that constitutes regression in the service of the ego. Gill and Brenman (1959) felt that hypnosis for healthy as well as for emotionally disturbed people is a regression in the service of the ego. And notwithstanding our own and Levin and Harrison's research results—which do not seem to prove this—I still find myself clinging to the hypothesis that hypnosis *is* an adaptive regression. I hope that some day other researchers will pick up where my research group and Levin and Harrison left off. New indices of primary-process mentation and creativity have yet to be applied to the question of adaptive regression in hypnosis (Dudek, 1980; Martindale, Covello, & West, 1986).

In hindsight, it occurs to me that perhaps our subjects too, even though they were somewhat more deeply hypnotizable than Levin and Harrison's, could not maintain a deep enough trance during the hypnotic session. They had to open their eyes, and had to keep them open for at least an hour, during the administration of the Rorschach and the Holt inquiry. It is very likely that during this long, open-eyed period their trance lightened so much that it simply was not deep enough to produce a regression in the service of the ego. Our data were collected in the 1960s, and the Tart Self-Report Scales of Hypnotic Depth (North Carolina Scales) were not published until later (Tart, 1970b). Thus, unfortunately, we could not repeatedly test our subjects for depth of trance during the Rorschach experiment. I would advise future researchers who want to test the adaptive regression hypothesis to employ a method that does not require eye opening during the hypnotic experiment. Perhaps then these future researchers will be able to show that, indeed, hypnosis is a regression in the service of the ego in which *both* facets are demonstrably present in healthy, flexible personalities. As long as this cannot be shown, I am reluctant to say that hypnosis per se is a regression in the service of the ego, though I clinically really feel it is. The exceptions, perhaps, are psychotics and relatively normal but quite rigid individuals. When not expertly handled in hypnosis, psychotics can go into a *pathological* regression. And highly defended rigid persons, we later found, do not allow themselves to go into a deep enough SH state to experience the regression in the service of the ego (Fromm & Kahn, 1990).

The Modes of the Ego

Other pertinent research evidence for various facets of my ego-psychological theory of hypnosis stems from a research project on SH in which my students and I were engaged over many years (Fromm et al., 1981; Fromm & Kahn, 1990).

In this longitudinal study of SH, 33 subjects selected for high (heterohypnotic) hypnotizability were asked to practice SH for an hour per day for 4 weeks. Only highly hypnotizable subjects were selected to participate in the study—that is, those who attained a score of 9 or above out of a possible score of 12 points on the Harvard Group Scale of Hypnotic Susceptibility, Form A (Shor & Orne, 1962) and on the Stanford Hypnotic Susceptibility Scale, Form C (Weitzenhoffer & Hilgard, 1962). Prior to participating in the month-long experiment, all potential subjects were given the Minnesota Multiphasic Personality Inventory (Dahlstrom, Welsh, & Dahlstrom, 1972) and the Rorschach as screening tests, so that we could exclude individuals with psychopathology from the sample. Subjects practiced SH alone, in a small, quite stimulus-free room of my laboratory, for 1 hour daily. No hypnotist was present or watched them. The subjects had been instructed beforehand to make daily journal entries immediately after each session, describing their SH experiences. At the end of the 4 weeks, their diaries were collected, and only then were they given three large questionnaires (Fromm et al., 1981) containing questions about their SH experiences. Thus, what they wrote in their diaries about the phenomena they experienced in SH was not influenced or distorted by the questions we asked, based on our own hypotheses. The questionnaires and the diaries were analyzed separately and carefully. They form our data base.

One of the studies based on our analyses of the SH diaries was a study on the modes of the ego (Fromm et al., 1987–1988; Fromm & Kahn, 1990). We had postulated that three modes of the ego would be among the variables involved in SH: Ego activity, Ego Passivity, and Ego Receptivity. And we had also wondered whether something like Ego Inactivity, a suspended state in which nothing at all happens, does at times exist in SH. We had hypothesized that people in hypnotist-absent SH would naturally open themselves up to stimuli that arise spontaneously from within—in other words, that they would demonstrate a high degree of Ego Receptivity in hypnosis. We also expected that subjects in SH would show Ego Activity in giving themselves self-suggestions. In our healthy population, we did not expect to find much Ego Passivity—that is, a feeling of being overwhelmed by affect, imagery, or thoughts, or an inability to take one-self out of the SH trance when feeling overwhelmed.

We hypothesized (1) that both Ego Activity and Ego Receptivity would be present in SH, with Ego Receptivity being more frequent than Ego Activity; (2) that Ego Receptivity would be positively related to hypnotic susceptibility, Trance Depth, and Absorption; and (3) that Ego Receptivity would be related to personality characteristics associated with openness to internal self-initiated experiences, whereas ego activity would be related to personality characteristics associated with independent initiative and the need to structure internal experiences for oneself in SH instead of just letting them happen.

Roughly 900 diary reports, one for each daily SH session of each subject, were scrutinized and scored on a 5-point scale for the presence or absence of the four ego modes. The modes were mutually exclusive and exhaustive, but *not* independent. If one mode was given a score of 2 (or between 25% and 50% of the total trance experience per day), the scores of the three other modes on that day, when added, could not total more than 50% of the trance experience. Reliability for identification of ego modes from 81% to 90% was achieved by two independent raters.

The results (see Table 5.1) showed indeed that Ego Activity and Ego Receptivity were both present in SH. However, the hypothesis that Ego Receptivity in SH would predominate over Ego Activity was not sup-ported. Upon closer scrutiny, we found out that this was a result of the fact that we (intentionally) had not instructed our subjects in the techniques of deepening and maintaining the SH state or in what the phenomena of SH might be, because we did not want to contaminate the results by our

TABLE 5.1. Four Modes of Ego Functioning in Self-Hypnosis ($n = 30$)

	Mean	SD
Ego Activity	2.4427	0.8043
Ego Receptivity	1.6747	0.9644
Ego Inactivity	0.5360	0.5405
Ego Passivity[a]	—	—

Note. From "The Modes of the Ego in Self-Hypnosis" (p. 340) by E. Fromm, L. Lombard, S. H. Skinner, and S. Kahn, 1987–1988, *Imagination, Cognition and Personality, 7,* 335–349. Copyright 1988 by Baywood Publishing Co., Inc. Reprinted by permission.

[a]The incidence of Ego Passivity was so infrequent across subjects that it was virtually nonexistent.

hypotheses. Perhaps because of their lack of information (and also because we wanted them to report their experiences in diaries), the subjects needed to direct and organize their SH sessions to a greater degree than we had foreseen—that is, to use more Ego Activity. In a few instances, subjects defended themselves against too much affect by *deciding* to change the content of their imagery to a more neutral topic or even to terminate a particular trance session. That is, they employed Ego Activity as a defense, to protect themselves against being overwhelmed by affect.

Ego Activity in the form of self-suggestion, decision making, and problem solving provides a scaffolding for the ego-receptive, effortless SH experiencing. In three of our subjects (all very rigid personalities), there was so much Ego Activity and so little Ego Receptivity that they really were not able to go into SH experiences of any depth. Rather than just providing structure for SH, Ego Activity in these cases overshadowed Ego Receptivity. And thus the phenomena of SH became constricted (Fromm et al., 1987–1988).

Ego Passivity (feeling overwhelmed) was indeed as rare as we had expected it to be in our normal population. It occurred in only one or two instances. And although we expected that many subjects for extended periods would report Ego Inactivity ("nothing happened"), only a very few subjects ever reported that. Perhaps our volunteer subjects were all too interested in discovering the phenomena of SH to let Ego Inactivity happen. Or perhaps when there is no stimulation from the outside, the ego needs to provide stimulation for itself—as we do in dreams—in order to keep ego structures from withering (Holt, 1965).

Statistically, our findings showed a strong link between Ego Receptivity and phenomena indicative of a powerful SH experience. Trance Depth, Absorption/Fascination, Imagery (vivid realistic as well as primary-process imagery), and hypnotic susceptibility were all strongly related to Ego Receptivity (Fromm et al., 1987–1988). These results indicate, as hypothesized, that Ego Receptivity is at the very heart of SH—perhaps even more central than it is to heterohypnosis. The high correlation between Ego Receptivity on the one hand and Imagery and Absorption/Fascination on the other shows that in SH the ego opens itself up and becomes receptive to stimuli coming from within. We hope that future research will show whether or not there is any correlation between Ego Activity on the one hand and Imagery and Absorption on the other.

Imagery

Results of the statistical analyses of the diaries in our SH studies also showed that Ego Receptivity and Vivid Imagery are the most important aspects of SH. The presence of vivid imagery was a dramatic common denominator in the SH diaries of all but the above-mentioned three rigid subjects (Lombard et al., 1990). It, too, may be considered to be a marker of the SH state itself: The more imagery (particularly the more primary-process imagery), the deeper the trance. Indeed, one of the studies done by our research group has shown that Imagery in SH correlates positively with Trance Depth (Kahn, Fromm, Lombard, & Sossi, 1989). As noted earlier, the imagery was either reality-oriented or fantastic primary-process imagery. Ego Receptivity, we found, is an essential precondition for the occurrence of primary-process imagery.

Attention

In our SH questionnaire study (Fromm et al., 1981), we found that SH is characterized by more concentrated *as well as* by more expansive Attention than is the waking state, and by more frequent vacillation between expansive and concentrated Attention. In trance, particularly in SH trance, there are fast fluctuations between concentrated and expansive Attention. These are characteristics of the SH state.

When we tried to score the diaries, too, for attention modes, we found that expansive Attention was *invariably* tied to Ego Receptivity, and focused Attention to Ego Activity. When a subject is in an ego-receptive state, his or her Attention is expansive and free-floating. However, at times of Ego Activity—for instance, when one gives oneself a suggestion—Attention is focused.

Structural and Content Factors

Structural factors are state-related factors, variables that relate to the differences between hypnosis and the waking state. In our research (Fromm et al., 1981), we found two factors that are common denominators of SH and heterohypnosis, and two that differentiate between them. Absorption and relinquishing of the GRO are important common features of heterohypnosis *and* of SH. They set the stage for all (deep) hypnotic experiences and are essential characteristics differentiating hypnotic states from the waking state. Together they form the sine qua non, the axis on which SH as well as heterohypnotic experiences rest (Fromm et al., 1981). If they are absent, neither deep heterohypnotic nor deep SH phenomena occur. In addition, there are two structural factors that differentiate SH from heterohypnosis: expansive, free-floating Attention and Ego Receptivity. A good deal of expansive Attention and Ego Receptivity to stimuli arising from within characterize SH. In contrast, concentrative, steadily focused Attention and receptivity to stimuli coming from a single outside source (the hypnotist) typify much of what happens in heterohypnosis.

The content categories we established on the basis of the analyses of the questionnaires (Fromm et al., 1981) were these: imagery, personal memories, dreams (usually induced by self-suggestion) working on problems, strong affect, sensory and motor phenomena induced by self-suggestions, and self-suggested age regression (which rarely worked). In the content analysis of the diaries, which was done 5 to 7 years later than that of the questionnaires (Fromm et al., 1981) and independently of it, the very same content categories were found. This serves to validate my theory, particularly as much the same occurred with regard to the structural components. It should be noted, however, that Absorption was not found to be as powerful a factor in the analysis of the diaries as it was in the analysis of the questionnaires.

Conclusions

Hypnosis is an ASC in which the ego functions in a manner that is different from the way in which it functions in the waking state. People in hypnosis retain the capacity to observe, to reflect, to think, and even to guide the experience if they wish to do so. All of these capacities are ego functions. The deeply hypnotized subject may vividly "see" a person who is actually not there, or may hallucinate away objects that are actually present. Whereas thinking in the waking state is mainly reality-oriented and proceeds along secondary-process lines, hypnosis is a state in which the balance shifts toward the primary-process pole of the primary–secondary process continuum. A hypnotized person has greater ego receptivity than the person in the waking state; that is, most hypnotized people relax some of their vigilance and defenses and allow stimuli from the inside (their own unconscious thoughts and feelings) to drift into awareness. The material that emerges is often a significant emotional experience for the subject or patient, because the hypnotic state is characterized by greater intensity of affect than the waking state, and by a tendency to experience imagery as real.

Freud abandoned hypnosis because he thought, as did his daughter, Anna Freud (A. Freud, 1926/1948), that hypnosis circumvents the ego. This statement, however, I feel I have proven to be wrong. Many of the essential characteristics of hypnosis are ego functions: ego receptivity and ego activity, primary- and secondary-process thinking, concentrated and expansive attention, imagery, absorption, hypermnesia, and heightened affect. The state-dependent capacity to move back and forth from unconscious to conscious experience, from secondary-process to primary-process thinking, from experiencing to observing ego, from ego activity to ego receptivity, and from concentrated to expansive attention (not discussed in this chapter) facilitates problem solving and coping, which also, of course, are ego functions. It is this mobility—this ability to vacillate so easily within each of the above-named bipolar parameters of the ego—and the increase in such ego functions as imagery and available memory that create the major advantage of hypnotherapy over waking-state therapy.

Our clearest and most important set of findings established a strong relationship between our SH variable of Ego Receptivity and other phenomena that signify a powerful SH experience. Absorption, Trance Depth, and Vivid Imagery were all strongly linked to Ego Receptivity. Thus, as we had hypothesized, Ego Receptivity is one of the most essential aspects of SH. It represents what commonly has been called "suggestibility," as well as the ability and inner freedom to allow unconscious fantasies, memories, thoughts, and affects to rise into awareness during the state of trance.

Hypnosis is a wondrous, "many-splendored thing." My theory, I believe, explains its essential structure and content. However, it does not cover a few other facets of hypnosis and hypnotherapy—for instance, the transference relationship. Such phenomena can only be understood with the help of either psychoanalytic libido theory, object relations theory, or self theory. Just as I believe that psychoanalysis is not only that which the libido theory *or* ego psychology says it is, but that it must be understood as a fabric woven out of four theoretical strands of different colors (libido theory, ego psychology, object relations theory, and self theory), so do I believe that hypnosis has many facets, which can best be understood from the viewpoint of one or more of these four psychoanalytic theories, and by intertwining them with concepts taken from cognitive psychology. We can and must strive for a unified theory of hypnosis. But the total multihued tapestry that will emerge must be one that is woven from solid, well-selected fibers of interesting, compatible colors.

Note

1. Note that the way in which the word "ego" has been used in popular parlance since the 1960s is quite different from the psychoanalytic concept of the ego, which is the concept I have described on page 132. Laypeople may talk about a person's having a "big ego" or needing to enhance his or her ego. This popular usage of the word "ego" in the sense of self-respect is closer to what in the psychoanalytic theory of the self would be called "narcissism."

CHAPTER SIX

Hypnosis, Psychopathology, and Psychological Regression

MICHAEL R. NASH

Questions about the relationship between what we now think of as hypnosis and psychopathology actually predate the full scientific definition and elaboration of either term. Before the fields of psychiatry, psychology, or even neurology had been articulated, Mesmer was faced with some of the same puzzling observations I examine in this chapter: The attempt at cure produces a condition that somehow seems connected to the disease process itself. Mesmer's aim was in part to secure for science what was once priestly healing. The aim of this chapter is to critically examine in what sense there is—and in what sense there is not—a shared process underlying hypnosis and psychopathology.

Definitions

Since, unlike Mesmer, we do have the benefit of over 150 years of scientific work on the issues at hand, it seems prudent to define the three components of our objective in as precise a way as possible, taking advantage of what the scientific community has learned about hypnosis, psychopathology, and mental processes.

First, "hypnosis" is a social interaction in which one person, the subject, responds to suggestions offered by another person, the hypnotist, for experiences involving alterations in phenomenal awareness, memory, and action (adapted from Kihlstrom, 1987a, p. 1449).

Second, although the term "psychopathology" can and often does refer to every conceivable mental disorder, including organically based dementias and intoxication/withdrawal syndromes, the working definition for this chapter is as follows: A psychopathological condition is a disturbance in experience, emotion, behavior, soma, and relationships arising from mental or psychological problems (adapted from Cameron & Rychlak, 1980, p. 2).

Finally, a "shared underlying process" is a biological, psychological, or social mode of functioning that characterizes and explains some essential feature of two conditions (in the present case, hypnosis and psychopathology).

Hypnosis and Psychopathology: Clinical Observations and Research Findings

Before we can meaningfully explore how clinical theorists have struggled with the relationship between hypnosis and psychopathology, we must understand what moved them to do so. The answer is straightforward. Four fundamental observations concerning hypnosis and psychopathology have been noted by researchers and clinicians from Puységur, Braid, Charcot, and Bernheim to Freud, Pavlov, E. R. Hilgard, and Fromm:

1. Both hypnosis and psychopathology can involve dramatic and deviant shifts in behavior or experience in the absence of obvious impairment in relevant biological structure (e.g., tumor, central nervous system lesions, chemical imbalance).

2. Certain symptoms of psychopathology can emerge during hypnosis with seemingly normal subjects.

3. Hypnosis can be effective as a treatment for some forms of psychopathology.

4. The description given by patients of some pathological states often resembles the report of normal subjects describing their experience during hypnosis.

Together, these four observations pose an intriguing possibility, one that was not lost on the earliest investigators of abnormal psychology (e.g., Charcot, Janet, Prince, Freud, and Sidis)—that by understanding hypnosis we may better understand psychopathology. Below, I elaborate on these four core observations, citing relevant research.

Deviant Function with No Obvious Organic Basis

The lay and professional communities alike have noted the dramatic and unusual behaviors elicited during hypnosis and seen in pathological conditions. As a first component of this observation, there is little disagreement that both hypnosis and psychopathology broadly yield peculiar behaviors and experience. But this impression must be tempered by the general consensus of researchers that hypnosis does not enable subjects to transcend waking volitional capacities (Kihlstrom, 1985a). Motivated, nonhypnotized subjects can simulate the behavior of genuinely hypnotized subjects quite accurately (Orne, 1979a); similarly, reasonably bright, motivated subjects can accurately fake various forms of psychopathology with little or no prior detailed information concerning criterion responses or nature of patient diagnosis (Rogers, 1988). It appears that the ways in which hypnotized subjects and psychiatric patients deviate from the norm are fairly predictable. Social expectations, demand characteristics, and cultural preconceptions of hypnosis and psychopathology undoubtedly affect how these phenomena are expressed (Sarbin & Coe, 1979). Whether there is some other process linking the two is a focus of this chapter.

The second component of this observation is that whatever unusual behaviors are manifested during hypnosis or during a psychopathological condition, they are not attributable to some obvious structural aberration of the central nervous system. It was just this notion that compelled Charcot and others to propose that an underlying, more subtle "nerve weakness" linked hypnosis and hysteria, and that the ability to experience hypnosis was essentially a symptom of hysteria. But contemporary research with hypnosis has as yet found no reliable biological marker for either the hypnotic condition or hypnotic susceptibility (Galbraith, London, Leibovitz, Cooper, & Hart, 1970; Dumas, 1980; F. J. Evans, 1979). The research on biological markers in psychopathology is far more complex. With the advent of very sophisticated twin studies and of more sensitive computerized methods for probing brain anatomy, it appears that some forms of psychopathology may involve brain pathology (Nasrallah & Coffman, 1985; Coffman, Mefferd, & Golden, 1981; Mathew & Partain, 1985; Free & Oei, 1989; Kendler, 1983; Kendler & Robinette, 1983). But the findings for specific reliable biological markers in even the most debilitating and chronic forms of psychopathology are still mixed. It seems probable that for many forms of pathology, as well as for hypnosis, psychosocial and biological aspects interact to produce a pattern or mode of responding. The original observation that hypnosis and many forms of psychopathology do not involve gross anatomical aberrations is reasonably secure.

Phenotypic Similarity between Suggested Hypnotic Phenomena and Symptoms of Psychopathology

When otherwise nonsymptomatic subjects are hypnotized, they can elicit a host of behavioral and experiential phenomena characteristic of psychopathology. Hypnotic alterations in perception and sensation (hallucinations, time sense distortion, anesthesia, deafness, blindness, anosmia), cognition (amnesia, obsessions, false beliefs, hypermnesia, agnosia, aphasia, depersonalization, derealization), emotion (rage, lability, depression, anxiety), and behavior (compulsions, automatic writing, impulsivity, paralysis) are quite common, even in the relatively neutral context of the experimental laboratory. Functional disorders of psychogenic origin (psychogenic amnesia, hysterical blindness, anesthesia) and their hypnotic counterparts are alike in that they generally do not conform to patterns of organic illness that might otherwise explain the shift in function or experience (Grosz & Zimmerman, 1965; Theodor & Mandelcorn, 1973; Blum, Porter, & Geiwitz, 1978; M. R. Nash, Lynn, Stanley, & Carlson, 1987; Loomis, Harvey, & Hobart, 1936; Pattie, 1935). But beyond the impressionistic observations beginning at the turn of the century, few studies have carried out a fine-grained analysis of whether psychogenic symptoms (e.g., hysterical blindness) and their hypnotically produced counterparts (e.g., hypnotically induced blindness) are really similar in other ways. That is, in addition to not looking like an organic disturbance, do they share cognitive or affective properties? What findings are extant generally support the notion that, at least in the case of conversion reactions, hypnotically induced functional aberrations are behaviorally and cognitively similar to their hysterical counterparts, and dissimilar to organically based disease (Malmo, Boag, & Raginsky, 1954; Sackheim, Nordlie, & Gur, 1979).

Hypnosis as an Effective Treatment in Certain Disorders

Probably the strongest argument for a shared underlying process linking hypnosis and psychopathology has been the long and well-documented record of hypnosis as an agent of cure for many types of mental disorders over two centuries of clinical practice. The claims have sometimes been exaggerated, but there remains a solid and respectable research literature that supports the clinical efficacy of hypnosis (Wadden & Anderton, 1982; Beutler, 1979; Deabler, Fidel, Dillenkoffer, & Elder, 1973; Friedman & Taub, 1978; Scagnelli-Jobsis, 1982; DePiano & Salzberg, 1979). It seems reasonable that if an intervention can alter or even cure debilitating symptoms, then it probably affects whatever process underlies the symptoms. Though reasonable, the logic of this argument is not without flaw. Certainly there are ameliorative interventions that may have only obscure and very limited relevance to the essential features of the disease process (e.g., aspirin for headaches). Still, the clinical efficacy of hypnosis is highly suggestive, especially as it relates to the disease process underlying the disorders traditionally treated by hypnosis—dissociative, posttraumatic stress, psychophysiological, and other neurotic-level disorders of a circumscribed nature.

Subjective Experience of Hypnosis and Some Pathological Conditions

For some types of pathology, there is a striking similarity between patients' description of their subjective experience and reports of subjective experience given by normal hypnotic subjects. If we examine some items from a standard inventory of subjective experience of hypnosis (Field's Scale of Hypnotic Depth; Field, 1965), it becomes clear that unsuggested shifts in experience occur during hypnosis—shifts that in another context could easily be mistaken for signs of psychotic, dissociative, anxiety, posttraumatic stress, or impulse control disorders, or for drug-related phenomena: "Time stood still," "I felt dazed," "Everything happened automatically," "Sometimes I did not know where I was," "Things seemed unreal," "Parts of my body moved without my conscious assistance," "I felt uninhibited." Breuer and Freud (1893–1895/1955), Janet (1919/1925), Frankel (1974), and H. Spiegel and Spiegel (1978), among others, noted these similarities and hypothesized that various pathological states (pathological anxiety, conversions, stupors, ruminations, and gross dissociations) were actually examples of spontaneously occurring self-hypnosis episodes.

Taken together, these four observations are as difficult to ignore now as they were 100 years ago at La Salpêtrière. The similarities between hypnosis and certain forms of psychopathology, along with the clinical efficacy of hypnosis, seem to be valid and highly suggestive of shared processes. There are two further considerations central to any meaningful evaluation of shared underlying processes in hypnosis and psychopathology. First, it seems unlikely that there is *just one* mental process determining the nature of hypnotic response. Contemporary theorists (Spanos & Barber, 1974; Orne, 1959; K. S. Bowers, 1973a; H. Spiegel & Spiegel, 1978) view hypnotic response as multiply determined by contextual, social, psychological, and, for some, biological factors (the relative weight attributed to each factor depends upon the theorist). Certainly the same can be said for experimental psychopathology as theorists wrestle with such ambitiously integrative terminology as the "psychosociobiological model" to explain the enormous range of abnormal human behavior and experience. Thus, the possibility that hypnosis and all forms of psychopathology can both be fully explained by one single mental process gone askew seems quite remote. Both phenomena are far too complex. It seems more likely that hypnosis and psychopathology overlap across only one or two shared processes, and that the remainder of their variance is determined by factors that may be unique to each.

This leads us to the second important consideration in the determination of shared processes. We not only must examine similarities between hypnosis and psychopathology, but must consider differences as well—for they can be just as instructive. Among these differences, two figure prominently. First, hypnotic phenomena are far more transient than psychiatric symptoms: hypnotic alterations in perception, mood, behavior, and experience are quickly and easily reversed. Second, manifestations of psychopathology are more often accompanied by some form of dysphoria than is the case with hypnosis; hypnosis is usually experienced by the subject as either unremarkable or pleasant (Coe & Ryken, 1979).

Proposed Shared Processes Underlying Hypnosis and Psychopathology

Many explanations for our four key observations have been offered by clinical theorists in the 200 years since Mesmer began his work in earnest. Most early attempts used metaphors borrowed from scientific developments current at the time. It is certainly no coincidence that mesmerism was understood to act upon the patient via an invisible fluid or force (Mesmer, 1779/1948). Other invisible forces (e.g., electricity, magnetism, oxygen, gravity) had recently been proposed by the elite of science to explain a host of natural phenomena. For Mesmer, then, the underlying shared substrate of mesmeric trance and physical disease was electromagnetic and biological in nature. Disease was a disharmony in a fluid; mesmerism affected corrective shifts in this ethereal fluid via an initial exaggeration of the fluidic imbalance, followed by a restorative convulsive "crisis." Although this formulation may seem quite obtuse, an enduring and respectable tradition developed that construed hypnosis and psychopathology as manifestations of essentially similar irregularities in a physical substrate. Thus for Puységur (1784–1785), hypnosis was a variant of sleepwalking; for Pavlov (1923), the common process was cortical inhibition; for Charcot (1882), hypnosis was a symptom of a neurological disease, hysteria.

Early Formulations

Though the emphasis on a physiological substrate common to both hypnosis and psychopathology faded, it still persists in somewhat muted form today (H. Spiegel & Spiegel, 1978; E. L. Rossi, 1986). But beginning with the work of Faria (1819/1906), A. J. F. Bertrand (1823), Braid (1843/1960), and Bernheim (1886), hypnosis and to some extent psychopathology came to be construed as products of psychological processes. Two of these theories are of particular importance because they bear most directly on contemporary formulations.

First, Janet (1919/1925) understood most psychopathology and all genuine hypnosis to be manifestations of a common process, dissociation; under special circumstances, certain ideas, motives, sensations, and memories operate outside of conscious awareness. These fixed ideas can function quite automatically via amnesic barriers separating clusters of perceptual–cognitive activity from one another. Janet's ideas lost currency for several reasons most thoroughly reviewed by Ellenberger (1970). Experiments failed to support the idea that dissociated tasks could be so completely separated that they would not, and could not, interfere with one another (R. W. White & Shevach, 1942). Furthermore, in the first quarter of the 20th century, the mushrooming of interest in psychoanalysis obscured Janet's important work.

Second, Freud was acutely interested in hypnosis and its relationship to psychopathology, especially hysteria. In an early work coauthored with an older colleague, Josef Breuer (Breuer & Freud, 1893–1895/1955), Freud theorized that symptoms of hysteria were actually manifestations of self-induced "hypnoidal states" brought about by the threatened eruption of early traumatic memories into awareness and the subsequent conversion (expression) of these memories in the somatic or functional sphere. In this very early Freudian formulation, the underlying process shared by hypnosis and hysteria was a "splitting off" of certain mental contents from the mainstream of awareness. Therapy then was curative to the extent that the therapist could exploit the ability of hypnosis to isolate and focus on the somatically expressed yet profoundly repressed affect-laden memories. Hypnotherapy sessions with these patients were often very dramatic, with violent explosions of emotion when the original memories surfaced; these were then followed by symptom relief. There are certainly echoes of Mesmer's disharmony hypothesis in Breuer and Freud's early abreactive therapies. Later, Freud came to view both hypnosis and psychopathology from a more developmental perspective, with psychopathology and hypnosis representing a return to earlier modes of psychological functioning and relating (Freud, 1915/1957). I elaborate on this hypothesis in the final section of the present chapter.

Two Promising Current Theoretical Formulations

Before presenting a view of hypnosis and psychopathology from a contemporary psychoanalytic perspective, I wish to summarize two exceedingly important and well-researched current models of hypnosis that bear directly on the question of shared processes.

A Role Theory View

Operating from a social-psychological or contextualist paradigm, some contemporary theorists contend that both psychopathology and hypnosis are examples of counterexpectational conduct reflecting learned, interpersonal strategies designed to communicate dissatisfaction or to obtain social reinforcement (Sarbin & Coe, 1979; Spanos & Gottlieb, 1979; Chodoff, 1974; Spanos & Chaves, 1989c). These theorists acknowledge that there are behavioral similarities between hypnosis and psychopathology, but they claim that there is no need to posit an underlying shared mental process. They would explain the four key observations concerning hypnosis and psychopathology as products of role enactments leading to self-deception on the part of the subject or patient. Hypnosis and psychopathology look alike because they have evolved from the same 19th-century world view based on the same ideological constructs. Counterexpectational behavior presented in a medical clinic (e.g., glove anesthesia) came to be attributed to some internal, diseased mental process. Counterexpectational behavior presented in the context of hypnosis (e.g., hypnotic glove anesthesia) came to be attributed to similar internal biological or psychological aberrations (Sarbin & Coe, 1979). From this point of view, there is no need to posit an internal mechanism of any kind to explain either psychopathology or hypnosis; they are both manifestations of the individual's participation in a particular role. Any resemblance between the two is a function of similarities in expectations concerning the role as communicated by the mental health professions to the individual and society. In a word, these similarities are artifactual.

Despite its "bold and perhaps strident" claim that "psychopathology has been, and continues to be an exercise in futility" (Sarbin & Coe, 1979, pp. 523–524), the paradigm is not really an anathema to other points of view. Clearly, context, role enactment, and strategic social factors influence the nature of psychopathology (Chodoff, 1974; Szasz, 1967; Smith-Rosenberg, 1972). Just as clearly, they influence hypnotic response (Spanos & Chaves, 1989c). Most theorists acknowledge the importance of contextual factors in determining behavior of subjects and patients, but they also emphasize interpersonal and cognitive factors (Orne, 1977; Sheehan, 1977; Kihlstrom, 1984).

Whether or not one fully embraces the role theory view, its message to investigators in the area is a clear and chilling one indeed. Sarbin and Coe (1979, p. 506) accurately note that "the history of attempts to understand the phenomena associated with the terms hypnosis and psychopathology points to a graveyard of abandoned beliefs" (e.g., animal magnetism, somnambulism, Charcot's neuropathology, monomania, vapors). These terms stumbled into their graves in large part because of the unrecognized contribution of contextual factors. Any contemporary formulations that posit a mental process linking hypnosis and psychopathology must be grounded in empirical work that considers and controls for the influence of role and demand.

Hypnosis as a Division of Consciousness

It is beyond the scope of this chapter to review the research relevant to the formulation of hypnosis as a relaxation of the monitoring or executive functions in the overall cognitive structure (see E. R. Hilgard, Chapter 3, this volume). The impact of Hilgard's neodissociation theory has been immense as psychology struggles to bring the study of consciousness back into the mainstream scientific inquiry. The revitalization of the concept of dissociation spawned more vigorous experimental and clinical interest in the related phenomena of absorption, imaginative involvement, fantasy proneness and dissociative disorders (J. R. Hilgard, 1979b; Tellegen & Atkinson, 1974; Lynn & Rhue, 1986; Bliss, 1984a). Not surprisingly, given the wealth of research suggesting that dissociation is a core feature of hypnosis, clinicians have begun to examine whether some forms of psychopathology might share a common dissociative pathway with hypnosis.

The logic of much of this research is as follows: There are types of psychopathology characterized by intense absorption, amnesias, fantasy proneness, automatism, depersonalization, or cognitive inconsistencies. Since these same phenomena figure so prominently in hypnosis, a propensity for spontaneous self-hypnosis may then underlie these disorders. If true, then patients suffering from these disorders should test as more hypnotizable than control individuals. The findings on this approach are quite mixed, but some interesting possibilities have emerged.

Frankel (1974) observed that the descriptions of panic states given by phobic patients are strikingly similar to the self-reports of hypnotic subjects—ego-alien experiences, depersonalization, derealization, absorption, and distorted perceptions. He reasoned (not unlike Breuer & Freud, 1893–1895/1955) that the experience of panic may be a variant of spontaneous self-hypnosis ("hypnogenic phobias"). Thus low hypnotizables would be unlikely to develop this type of pathology, but high hypnotizables would be likely to do so. It then follows that phobic patients suffering panic attacks would, as a group, score higher than nonphobic controls on measures of hypnotizability. Of six studies examining this hypothesis, four supported Frankel's position (Foenander, Burrows, Gerschman, & Horne, 1980; Frankel & Orne, 1976; S. F. Kelly, 1984; John, Hollander, & Perry, 1983) and two did not (Frischholz, Spiegel, Spiegel, Balma, & Markell, 1982; Owens, Bliss, Koester, & Jeppsen, 1989). There have been problems in this literature with measurement of hypnotizability, control groups, experimenter awareness of group assignments, and assessment of phobic pathology (Owens et al., 1989). Until these methodological difficulties are resolved, no definitive inference can be made linking panic and hypnosis.

Approaching this problem from a slightly different angle, Herbert and David Spiegel (1978) posited that an ability to focus attention and maintain concentration is a core physiologically based feature of hypnotic capacity. Because schizophrenics are, as a group, more easily distractible and cognitively impaired, they should obtain lower hypnotizability scores than nonschizophrenic controls. Here again, the findings have been mixed. Of 11 empirical studies, 6 found schizophrenics to be less hypnotizable than controls (H. Spiegel & Spiegel, 1978; Frischholz, Spiegel, Spiegel, Lipman, & Bark, 1988; Lavoie & Elie, 1985; D. Spiegel, Detrick, & Frischholz, 1982; T. X. Barber, Karacan, & Calverley, 1964; Ham, Spanos, & Barber, 1976), and 5 found schizophrenics to be as hypnotizable as, or more hypnotizable than, controls (E. L. Baker & Copeland, 1978; Kramer, 1966; Gordon, 1973; Kramer & Brennan, 1964; Vingoe & Kramer, 1966). Frischholz (1985a) has noted a peculiarity in this research: Schizophrenics earn consistently lower hypnotizability scores on one scale (the Hypnotic Induction Profile; H. Spiegel & Spiegel, 1978), but not on another set of scales (the Stanford scales; Weitzenhoffer & Hilgard, 1959, 1962). Again, without more comprehensive studies using careful controls and broad dependent measures, it is difficult to resolve this question, which is both interesting and clinically relevant.

Happily, there does seem to be some convergence of findings on dissociative disorders and hypnotizability. A group of dissociation theorists (Frischholz, 1985b; Kluft, 1984, 1987; F. W. Putnam, 1985; D. Spiegel, Hunt, & Donnershine, 1988) contends that early trauma leads to repeated overuse of dissociation until it becomes the child's primary psychological defense, manifesting itself in dramatic alterations in the experience of self and the world—experiences similar to those of hypnosis. In turn, this ability to separate from awareness certain experiences, motives, and emotions could reasonably be expected to enable the patient to score quite high on hypnotizability tests. Very high hypnotizability is indeed a feature of multiple personality disorder, and perhaps of dissociative disorders (Bliss, 1984a; Frischholz, 1985b). The research in this area is not extensive, but the findings are consonant with clinical observation. The dynamics of hypnosis and dissociative psychopathology may share an underlying process involving a division in consciousness.

If psychopathology were, broadly speaking, a manifestation of spontaneous hypnotic-like processing, then we, like Charcot, would expect to see more pathology among high hypnotizables and practically no pathology among low hypnotizables (a positive correlation). But this is decidedly not the case. Overall hypnotizability does not appear to be related to general level of psychopathology or any broad-band type of pathology, such as neuroticism, psychoticism, or acquiescence (Deckert & West, 1963a; for reviews see T. X. Barber, 1964, E. R. Hilgard, 1965). There is no patterned systematic covariance between hypnotizability and psychological health.

If we confine ourselves to one rather rare type of pathology, dissociative disorder, then we find some suggestive evidence that there is a common underlying dissociative process between hypnosis and this one form of psychopathology. However, if we persist in a more broad-based definition of psychopathology and seek to find common ground between it and hypnosis, we must explain two sets of data: first, the four key observations mentioned earlier; second, the findings that there is no relationship between measures of gross pathology or personality style and hypnotizability. What follows is just such a formulation, framed in terms of contemporary psychoanalytic theory.

Psychological Regression as a Shared Underlying Process in Hypnosis and Psychopathology

Relatively early in his career, Freud identified two types of psychological regression—"temporal" and "topographic"—which he invoked to explain a host of special mental conditions (e.g., dreaming, psychopathology, hypnosis, and certain clinical phenomena evidenced during analysis). Though Freud was elegantly concise in drawing the distinction between these two types of regression (Freud, 1917/1957), the difference became quite muddled again even during his lifetime (S. W. Jackson, 1969; Tuttman, 1982). If we are to consider how psychological regression may underlie both psychopathology and hypnosis, then we must re-examine Freud's important distinction between temporal and topographic regression.

Temporal Regression

Patterning his concept of temporal regression on work in developmental morphology, Freud posited that psychic development proceeds from less complex forms to more advanced, organized forms. But Freud maintained that these old forms remain intact and accessible. Under certain circumstances, these early stages "again become the mode of expression of the forces in the mind" (Freud, 1915/1957, p. 285), and "the essence of mental disease lies in a return to earlier states of affective life and of functioning" (p. 286). Freud explicitly defined hypnosis as a temporal regression—a return to an infantile mode of functioning (Freud, 1921/1955). Many contemporary psychoanalytic theorists and cognitive-developmental psychologists have embraced the idea that old developmental stages remain imperishable and that psychopathology is most essentially a temporal regression to one or more of these previously abandoned modes of relating to self and others (Balint, 1968; Bion, 1977; Kohut, 1971; Langer, 1970; Stolorow & Lachmann, 1980; Werner, 1948). The notion that temporal regression is possible and that psychopathology is a lawful undoing of development is exceedingly appealing to clinicians and theorists who struggle to make sense of the seemingly random disorganization arising from pathology. A formulation based on temporal regression defines a certain continuity between presumed etiological factors in childhood and the adult symptoms themselves. It charts a course for treatment involving a therapeutic regression to the developmental stage in question, and a gradual resumption of development from that point. Similarly, hypnosis theorists have invoked Freud's concept of temporal regression to explain aberrant changes in the cognition, perception, and behavior of hypnotic subjects (Erickson & Kubie, 1941; Ferenczi, 1909/1980; Kubie & Margolin, 1944; Weitzenhoffer, 1957).

But there is serious doubt among many developmental and clinical theorists as to whether temporal regression is even a possibility. They argue that the psychic structure of a child is unalterably changed during the course of development; as a consequence, old stages or infantile modes of functioning are simply not "there" to be retrieved (Gill, cited in Tuttman, 1982; Peterfreund, 1978; Piaget, 1973; Rubinfine, 1981; Spitz, 1965; Westin, 1989). Indeed, a growing research literature fails to support the

notion that adult psychopathology is similar to, or even properly analogous to, normal phases in child development (Harter, 1977, 1983, 1986;
Harter & Buddin, 1987; Donaldson & Westerman, 1986; Flavell, 1985;
Westin, 1989). Furthermore, an exhaustive review of over 100 years of
hypnosis research on temporal regression failed to find any special correspondence between the behavior and experience of hypnotized adults and
that of actual children (M. R. Nash, 1987). Because there are such serious
doubts about whether a temporal regression underlies either psychopathology or hypnosis, it is certainly a poor candidate for a shared
process. However, the theoretical and research literatures are much less
clouded on Freud's other type of regression—topographic.

Topographic Regression

Freud's concept of topographic regression (Freud, 1917/1957) was based on
his understanding of the reflex arc in neurology and physiology. In this
theory, too, regression is a backward movement, but in space rather than
time. It is a reverse movement along a path "from the region of thought-
structures to that of sensory perceptions" (Freud, 1905/1960, p. 162); "in
this process thoughts are transformed into images" (Freud, 1917/1957, p.
227)—a backward course that results in a transformation of thoughts into
visual imagery (Freud, 1933/1964). Freud noted that the regressive shift
from thought to imagery carries with it a shift in form, from secondary
process to primary process (Freud, 1916–1917/1963, 1917/1957). Indeed, a
rich literature suggests that imagery and primary process are linked, and
that these manifestations of topographic regression can be operationalized
and reliably measured in the consulting room and the laboratory (Atwood,
1971; Bogen, 1973; N. F. Dixon, 1981; Erdelyi, 1985; Galin, 1974; Marcel,
1983; Paivio, 1971; G. E. Schwartz, Davidson, & Maer, 1975; Sperling,
1960).

   Thus, a cornerstone of psychoanalytic thinking is the notion that
psychopathology involves a regressive shift away from secondary-process
thinking toward primary-process thinking—a form of cognition characterized by symbolization, displacement, condensation, nonlogical forms of
reasoning, and relative equivalence of memory and current experience
(Rapaport, 1950; Suler, 1980; Dudek, 1980). As Freud saw it, primary-
process thinking is not restricted to pathological conditions alone; rather, it
serves as a constant backdrop to all our waking and sleeping hours. It is in
wit, slips of the tongue, art, inebriated states, dreaming, and hypnosis that
we encounter primary process in everyday life (Freud, 1916–1917/1963).
Although Freud's formulation of pathological states as involving this type
of regressive shift came to be widely accepted, rigorous empirical examination awaited refinement of projective and behavioral measures that could
operationalize the construct of regression or primary process (notably Holt

& Havel, 1960; Martindale, 1975). The research literature is clear on two points. First, the regressive shift from secondary to primary process is not temporal, but topographic: Primary-process thinking in adults does not resemble the "normal" thinking of small children or infants (Dudek, 1980; Holt, 1967; Suler, 1980). Second, various forms of psychopathology do involve a prominence of primary-process thinking, including thought disorder, alcohol intoxication, marijuana intoxication, paranoid schizophrenia, childhood anxiety, neurophysiological disorder, hemispheric asymmetry, borderline personality disorder, process schizophrenia, and sociopathy (Harrow, 1976; Zimet & Fine, 1965; Gustafson & Kallmen, 1989; Salwen, Reznikoff, & Schwartz, 1989; A. N. West & Martindale, 1988; Kleinman & Russ, 1988; Ducat, 1985; Martindale, Covello, & West, 1986; F. Schwartz & Lazar, 1984; A. N. West, Martindale, Hines, & Roth, 1983). Thus, topographic regression of this sort does seem to underlie many forms of psychopathology. The question then becomes this: What evidence is there that the same, or a similar, process underlies hypnosis?

Topographic Regression and Hypnosis

It is the premise of this chapter that the similarity between hypnosis and many forms of psychopathology is that they involve an underlying shift in mental processing that can be characterized as a topographic regression. Though the physiological and/or psychological mechanisms leading to this shift may vary, a similar pattern of responding emerges in hypnosis and many forms of psychopathology: a disruption of ego and sensorimotor functioning, and a relative prominence of primary-process mentation. It is further posited that an essential difference between psychopathology and hypnosis is that in the latter, the topographic regression is transient, contained, and reversible, perhaps enabling the subject to utilize primary-process material in the service of adaptation ("regression in service of the ego"; Hartmann, 1939/1958; Kris, 1934/1952; Schafer, 1958). Thus, among the general population, a capacity to experience hypnosis fully is no more related to manifest psychopathology than is a capacity to dream a great deal, or an ability to be creative, or a capacity for quick wit. These expressions of a topographic regression are contained; psychopathology is not (Dudek, 1980; Suler, 1980).

If hypnosis does involve a topographic regression, then hypnotic response, when compared to normal waking response, should be characterized by (1) changes in thought processes in the direction of symbolic, primary-process mentation (Gill, 1972; Gill & Brenman, 1959); (2) increased availability of affect marked by vivid and intense outbursts of feeling (Gill & Brenman, 1959); (3) fluctuations in how the body is experienced (Gill & Brenman, 1959); and (4) displacement and condensation in the relationship with the hypnotist. As to whether the regression in hypnosis is reversible and contained, it is easily demonstrated that the effects of hypnosis are reversible. But it is another matter to claim that hypnosis is an *adaptive* regression. If this is so, then (5) we should find evidence that hypnosis enables subjects to respond in a more flexible or effective fashion. I briefly examine the relevant research on these five points.

Changes in Thought Processes

In seven studies, projective tests were administered while or just after the subjects were hypnotized. Some studies compared these protocols to those of a baseline control group; others compared them to within-subject baselines. If hypnosis does involve a shift in mental functioning from secondary-process to more primary-process thinking, then the hypnosis protocols should contain more imagistic, nonlogical, and other primary-process characteristics. Many of these studies used Holt and Havel's (1960) measure of primary process on the Rorschach.

Easily the most comprehensive study examining changes in thought processes during hypnosis was carried out at the University of Chicago (Fromm, Oberlander, & Gruenewald, 1970; Gruenwald, Fromm, & Oberlander, 1972; Oberlander, Gruenwald, & Fromm, 1970). Thirty-two subjects were administered the Rorschach in counterbalanced order—once when hypnotized, once when not hypnotized. Although the Rorschach protocols were scored according to two systems (Holt's and Klopfer's), the relevant dependent measure for our consideration was Holt's measure of primary-process mentation. Within-subject analysis revealed that across all orders and all experimenters, more primary-process material was evident in the hypnosis condition. Though an outstanding example of the careful application of the within-subject design, this programmatic research could not fully eliminate an explanation of the results based on demand expectations.

Two studies that did control for demand characteristics found similar results. Wiseman and Reyher (1973) examined whether subjects who reported hypnotically induced dreams in response to Rorschach cards would evince more primary-process material on Holt's Rorschach measure than either nonhypnotized or simulating subjects; their results confirmed that this was indeed the case. Hammer, Walker, and Diment (1978) found more primary-process thinking in the response of hypnotized subjects to a spoken poem. The response of two nonhypnotized control groups consisting of highly hypnotizable subjects indicated that primary-process thinking during hypnosis was not simply an effect of hypnotizability or demand characteristics.

Four studies examined projective test responding, perception, and dream activity in light of primary-process activity. J. V. West, Baugh, and Baugh (1963) reported more primary process during hypnosis on both Rorschach and Draw-A-Person tests when they were administered, with and without hypnosis, to 10 randomly selected male volunteers. A much more rigorously designed investigation (Levin & Harrison, 1976) administered two projective tasks (a Rorschach-card-induced dream and a Thematic Apperception Test story). In the hypnotized condition, as opposed to the nonhypnotized condition, there was increased incidence of primary-process material. In a clever study reported by Barrett (1979), the hypnotic dreams, daydreams, and nocturnal dreams of medium to high hypnotizable subjects were examined over a 6-week period. Hypnotic dreams differed from daydreams and were more similar to nocturnal dreams in terms of emotional themes and cognitive distortions. This finding provides some additional evidence of a link between hypnosis and a shift to more primary-process mentation. Finally, a series of studies examining the eidetic-like imagery of hypnotized and nonhypnotized subjects suggested that hypnosis may facilitate imaginal processing of information, with a shift from a sequential, verbal, and logical mode during the nonhypnotized condition to a more visual, "holistic" style during hypnosis (N. S. Walker, Garrett, & Wallace, 1976; Crawford, Wallace, Nomura, & Slater, 1986; B. Wallace, 1978).

There is a reasonable amount of evidence suggesting that there may be a change in thought processing during hypnosis in the direction of symbolic and primary mentation. It is important to note, however, that few of these studies attempted to control for demand characteristics. It is conceivable that Sarbin's contextualist position may account for these findings in terms of role play. However, the two studies that did address demand characteristics still found evidence for a shift in mental processing that was not so easily explained by role enactment.

Increased Availability of Affect

In a series of studies, my colleagues and I found that hypnotically age-regressed subjects were no more childlike than simulating controls, but they had freer access to more intense emotions. In these studies (M. R. Nash, Johnson, & Tipton, 1979; M. R. Nash, Lynn, Stanley, Frauman, & Rhue, 1985; M. R. Nash, Drake, Wiley, Khalsa, & Lynn, 1986), hypnotized and simulating subjects were given suggestions to regress to the age of 3 and asked to imagine themselves in various home situations. The experimental procedures assessed how subjects related to their transitional objects (e.g., teddy bears, blankets). The hypnotically age-regressed subjects were significantly more spontaneous, specific, and emotionally intense in relation to their transitional objects than the simulating controls. Initially, we suggested that under some circumstances there might be a partial reinstatement of interpersonally relevant affective processes during hypnotic age regression. But our follow-up study (Nash et al., 1986) defined some limitations on the nature of the presumed regression. To determine whether the transitional object reported by each hypnotically age-regressed subject was the same that the subject had had as a child, we independently interviewed the mothers of both the hypnotized and control subjects used in the earlier study. Despite their dramatic emotional reactions to transitional objects, hypnotized subjects were significantly less able than nonhypnotized controls to identify their specific childhood transitional objects correctly (23% accuracy for hypnotized subjects, compared to 70% accuracy for controls). Furthermore, all recollections obtained during hypnosis were incorporated into posthypnotic recollections, regardless of accuracy. We therefore concluded that hypnotic age regression may enhance access to important emotional material (a topographic regression), but may not necessarily involve an accurate reliving of a specific event.

A cautionary note was sounded by Bryant and McConkey (1989c) in a study comparing hypnotically induced emotions and physical sensations with those produced by simulating subjects. In this very carefully controlled study, the authors found that *both* hypnotic and simulating subjects described and enacted suggested emotions with remarkable accuracy. There were no differences between hypnotized and simulating subjects on the evoked emotional intensity or accuracy. As Bryant and McConkey point out, "This similarity does not indicate that the performance of [hypnotized subjects] was due to demand characteristics, but it does not allow us to rule out that possibility" (p. 315).

Taken together, findings from these two laboratories seem to suggest that when suitably personalized and subtle procedures are used to elicit and measure emotional response, hypnotized subjects may evince more intense affect. However, emotions are easily faked, and any examination of affective response during hypnosis must control thoroughly for the effects of role expectations.

Fluctuations in Body Experience

The ego is considered first and foremost a body ego (Freud, 1923/1961). If hypnosis involves a topographic regression, one would expect unusual fluctuations in how the body is experienced during hypnosis. There are no systematic, empirical investigations of such changes during hypnosis; however, there is a rich clinical literature, as well as some suggestive evidence from studies on spontaneous "side effects" of hypnosis. Gill and Brenman (1959) cited occurrences of hypnotized subjects spontaneously reporting feelings of shrinking, swelling, or loss of equilibrium. Freundlich and Fisher (1974) found that depersonalization and body distortions were pronounced during hypnosis, and that the extent of distortion was positively correlated with hypnotic susceptibility. In studies of common unsuggested sequelae to hypnosis, distortions in body awareness were found even during routine experimental administration of standard hypnotic scales (Crawford, Hilgard, & Macdonald, 1982). More distortions were reported by highly hypnotizable subjects, and more negative transient experiences of a general nature were reported following individual (as opposed to group) administration. Four cases of apparently spontaneous depersonalization following termination of hypnosis have been reported (Haber, Nitkin, & Shenker, 1979; J. R. Hilgard, Hilgard, & Newman, 1961; Starker, 1974b; Wineberg & Straker, 1973). Although no definitive study of regressive body experience has been undertaken, future researchers may wish to assess body experience as an index of topographic regression.

Displacement and Condensation in the Relationship with the Hypnotist

Many theorists in addition to Freud have regarded hypnosis as a regressed relationship (Ferenczi, 1909/1980; Gill & Brenman, 1959; Gruenewald, 1982; Kubie & Margolin, 1944). But this regression was almost universally viewed as temporal in nature. That is, theorists observed the compliance of hypnotic subjects to the "will" of the hypnotist, likened it to the presumed blind obedience of a small child, and inferred that hypnosis must be a temporal regression to an infantile mode of relating to a parent. Although any involved parent of a 2-year-old will immediately question just how compliant a small child really is, the notion of hypnosis as essentially a transference phenomenon (in the temporal sense) was embraced by the psychoanalytic community. Forgotten was the fact that transference is an example of displacement and condensation—the quintessential features of primary-process thinking and therefore of topographic regression.

Two nonanalytic investigators have offered particularly thoughtful and measurable working definitions of transference during hypnosis; both, interestingly enough, have emphasized the topographically regressive features of hypnosis. Shor (1979) defined "archaic involvement" with the hypnotist as "the extent to which there occurred a temporary displacement or 'transference' onto the . . . hypnotist of core personality emotive attitudes . . . most typically in regard to parents" (p. 133). Sheehan (Sheehan & Dolby, 1979) suggested that "when transference is operable, the subject can be assumed to respond beyond the role demands of the hypnotic test situation as they are normally defined and to interact with the hypnotist in an especially motivated and personally meaningful way" (p. 573). Although these definitions place a different emphasis on past versus contemporary components of a relationship, they have generated some interesting empirical work on transference and hypnosis.

Bitter (1974/1975) defined transference as the semantic similarity between the hypnotist and the more similar parent (as measured by semantic differentials). He administered a semantic differential measure concerning the experimenter to 86 females both before and after hypnosis. When the results were compared with those of the same measure administered to 34 nonhypnotized control subjects at the beginning and end of the study, they indicated that perceived similarity between hypnotist and either parent did not facilitate hypnotic response. Nor did the hypnotic procedure itself enhance perceived similarity between the hypnotist and either parent. Transference, at least as measured by semantic differentials, did not appear to be an important feature of hypnosis in this study.

In a carefully designed double-blind study, Frauman, Lynn, Hardaway, and Molteni (1984) examined subliminal activation of symbiotic fantasies as a way to help subjects experience more fully the archaic/ positive aspects of the hypnotic relationship. Before hypnosis, the experimental group received subliminally presented symbiotic stimulation ("Mommy and I are one"); a control group received a neutral message ("People are walking"). Comparisons of subsequent hypnotic performance revealed that the experimental treatment did indeed result in increased ratings of rapport with the hypnotist. Subjects in the "Mommy" group were also marginally more responsive to hypnosis than were controls, indicating the importance of relationship factors in hypnosis.

A few years ago, a colleague and I attempted to operationalize Shor's construct of archaic involvement by adapting 20 of his phenomenological descriptions of the subject's experience of the hypnotist (M. R. Nash & Spinler, 1989). Each of these items was transformed into a self-rated Likert-type scale, yielding a 20-item scale to be administered following hypnosis. Preliminary findings indicated a significant positive correlation between hypnotizability and posttreatment scores on this measure ($r = .52$). Factor analysis suggested three clusters of variables relevant to archaic involvement and hypnotic response: (1) perceived power of the hypnotist, (2) positive emotional bond to the hypnotist, and (3) fear of negative appraisal. All three factors correlated significantly with hypnotic susceptibility.

Sheehan (1971b, 1980; Sheehan & Dolby, 1979) examined the extent to which good hypnotic subjects evidence an especially motivated interaction with the hypnotist, along with increased involvement in the experience of suggested events. Using appropriate imagination, task motivation, and simulating control groups, Sheehan found that hypnotic subjects characteristically participated more personally in hypnotic dream experiences than did control subjects. Hypnotized subjects more often reported dreams (manifest content) in which they perceived the hypnotist in a positive light and spontaneously expressed feeling protected, cared for, and supported. This special commitment superseded demand characteristics and was sensitive to manipulations for reducing rapport. Sheehan interpreted these findings less in terms of analytic theory and more in terms of a special "motivated cognitive commitment" to the hypnotist and the hypnotic task. Either way, Sheehan's research suggests the importance of relationship factors in hypnosis and offers new ways to investigate an often elusive phenomenon.

Facilitation of Adaptive Responding

If hypnosis is an adaptive regression (Kris, 1934/1952), as claimed by many contemporary psychoanalytic theorists (Fromm & Gardner, 1979; Gill & Brenman, 1959), then we should find evidence that hypnosis enables subjects to respond in a more flexible and effective fashion. That is, in the presence of evidence for a topographic regression, there should also be evidence of enhanced creative problem solving. Three studies mentioned earlier examined the extent of primary-process thinking and defense effectiveness during hypnosis (Wiseman & Reyher, 1973; Levin & Harrison, 1976; Fromm et al. 1970). The three studies used Holt's composite measure of regression in service of the ego derived from the Rorschach as the primary dependent measure (Holt & Havel, 1960). The findings across all three studies were quite similar: The component of the Holt score sensitive to primary-process material was indeed elevated during hypnosis, as noted earlier, but there was no evidence of any significant change on the component measuring effectiveness of defense. In general, the subjects' defense effectiveness scores were more closely associated with general psychological adjustment than with whether they were hypnotized or not. Some well-adjusted subjects did reveal enhanced adaptive functioning in the hypnosis condition, but poorly adjusted subjects seemed to rely even more on maladaptive styles of coping during hypnosis. To date, there is no empirical evidence supporting the contention that hypnosis per se enables subjects to respond more adaptively.

The research on the five points discussed above may be summarized as follows. Investigators have uncovered evidence for topographic regression during hypnosis by comparing hypnotic to nonhypnotic response on standardized measures of regression. These investigators do not claim a return of childhood functioning, but assert that some aspects of hypnotic response seem to reflect a form of mentation characteristic of (but not limited to) certain types of psychopathology. It does appear that when compared to control conditions, hypnosis is more likely to elicit more imagistic, primary-process material; a greater extent of unusual body sensation; and more displacement of core attitudes about important others onto the hypnotist. Whether hypnosis enables subjects to display more spontaneous and intense affect is at this point still underresearched. It must be cautioned that all hypotheses relevant to a topographic regression must still be viewed as tentative, pending carefully designed research addressing the extent to which demand characteristics may account for this altered pattern of responding. In contrast, the idea that hypnosis is a form of *adaptive* regression, though an intuitively appealing one, is not supported by the literature despite several attempts. It is important to note here that all studies examining adaptiveness have used the same dependent measure derived from the Rorschach (Holt & Havel, 1960). Other measures of adaptive regression sampling different domains of experience may be more sensitive to the presumed ego-enhancing potential of hypnosis.

If the concept of topographic regression does describe some essential shared feature of hypnosis and psychopathology, then it must be noted (with Gill & Brenman, 1959) that in hypnosis this regression does not encompass the entire "I-ness" of the subject, but operates only in a subsystem of the ego. Here the role enactment formulation (Sarbin & Coe, 1979; see also Spanos & Coe, Chapter 4, this volume) and the present psychoanalytic formulation of hypnosis dovetail quite nicely. Whether on the theatrical stage or in our everyday lives, we attend and respond to social cues to enact certain roles. With or without forethought, we can become inattentive to competing cues and role demands that might distract us from the drama in which we find ourselves most immediately embedded. But these cues are nonetheless processed (after all, an actor will leave the stage if the fire alarm is sounded). From a psychoanalytic perspective, it would seem that even during the most compellingly absorbing hypnotic experience there is a portion of the ego that does not engage—that does not participate in the regression. If hypnosis *were* a topographic regression across the entire ego, then it would indeed be quite indistinguishable from a psychotic state or a dream, with little or no chance for the subject to initiate, focus, change, or participate. Across the social-psychological, psychoanalytic, and neodissociation literatures, it is clear that hypnotic subjects do respond to cues that are incompatible with their immediate hypnotic enactment.

Conclusions

Perhaps Freud's most fundamental discovery was to note the similarity in how information is processed during pathological states and dreaming. If we ignore for the moment his unfortunate propensity to weave temporality into almost every aspect of his metapsychology, we are left with the more hearty and empirically sound inferences surrounding his concept of topographic regression. Dreaming and pathological states do share an underlying process. But this does not mean that dreaming and psychopathology are identical, or that people who dream a great deal are at special risk for development of pathology, or even that the functional similarities of the two phenomena are products of the same physiological or psychological pathway. Rather, embedded in all the differences between a pathological state and dreaming is a similarity—a relative shift from thought to image, from logic to nonlogic, from control to expression, from time to timelessness.

My general contention is that hypnosis is of this same ilk. That is, along with psychopathology, dreaming, parapraxes, and some forms of humor, hypnosis involves a topographic regression, albeit in a subsystem of the ego. It is not that psychopathology is really a form of spontaneous hypnosis, nor that hypnotizable people are more vulnerable to psychopathology, nor that the neurological or psychological pathways leading to a topographic regression in hypnosis are the same as those in all forms of psychopathology. However, there is a phenotypic similarity between hypnosis and psychopathology—a similarity that has impressed and challenged clinical theorists and researchers since the very inception of experimental psychopathology. It is my contention that this similarity reflects the operation of a shared form of mentation best characterized as a product of topographic regression.

PART THREE

SURVEYS OF
BROAD AREAS

CHAPTER SEVEN

Research Designs and Considerations

ARREED F. BARABASZ
MARIANNE BARABASZ

The investigation of hypnotic phenomena presents several intriguing and complex research design challenges. If strong inference is to be achieved and scientific progress is to continue, we must recognize, accept, and address these demanding issues. The endeavor is both fascinating and rewarding. The creativity and rigorous controls required ensure that there is seldom a dull moment in hypnosis research. Such demands make the investigation of hypnotic phenomena one of the best avenues for teaching research methodology, because of its applicability to the solution of a breadth of behavioral science research problems. On the basis of our experience, involvement in hypnosis research can become so intriguing that graduate and postdoctoral students who begin study with a focus on practice alone may complete their degrees as true scientist/practitioners with an enduring interest in scientific inquiry. Jack Hilgard (E. R. Hilgard, 1990) mused, "When I run a subject in a hypnosis experiment I learn something new every time. I found this to be different from other studies in psychology, where running a subject just meant getting a number."

This chapter attempts to emphasize specific design considerations that provide both stringency and sensitivity for clinical case studies, quasi-experimental studies, and controlled experimental research. The primary emphasis is on progressive hypothesis testing, because this route is most likely to lead to the kind of strong inference essential to scientific progress (Platt, 1964). The process necessarily involves recognition of the contributions of both coarse qualitative and fine quantitative data. The value of integrating quantitative and qualitative data is new to many areas of behavioral science (Polkinghorne, 1991), but not to hypnosis research, which has a long history of gleaning inference from a combination of both approaches. For example, conclusions about the validity of a theory may be drawn from a combination of numerical experimental test data and postexperimental clinical interview information (A. F. Barabasz, 1990c; A. F. Barabasz & Barabasz, 1992; Sheehan & McConkey, 1982). Hypnosis investigators can also take pride in the knowledge that our enterprise is not characterized by the study of "hypotheses" about correlational relationships masquerading as tests of experimental effects, or by grossly inappropriate practices such as the use of correlational techniques to assess relationships between multiplicative composites and independent variables (M. G. Evans, 1991). These problems have been confined to those operating in the ex post facto realm of nonexperimental or nonclinical designs.

The major goal of the present chapter is to help researchers and clinicians design experiments and evaluate work that has been published. Procedures are detailed, as are some pitfalls, biases, artifacts, and bases of controversy. The chapter discusses (1) clinical and experimental approaches; (2) design sensitivity; (3) subject factors; (4) institutional review and risks to subjects; (5) effects of experimental-context demand characteristics; and (6) M. T. Orne's real–simulator design.

Clinical and Experimental Approaches

Hypnosis research almost certainly owes its early development to the clinical method. As part of the therapy session, the clinician would first observe certain reactions during the waking condition. Then changes would be noted following the hypnotic induction and direct or indirect suggestions. Alterations in the client's responses were attributed to the power of the hypnotic state, as they often are today.

Clinical Case Study Research

Clinical case study research can be an important first step in furthering our knowledge. If a specific hypnotic intervention appears to work with one or a few patients, perhaps it will work with others. The keys to useful clinical case study research are careful observation and description. We have seen hundreds of case interventions by psychologists and psychiatrists that had the potential of contributing new theoretical or applied knowledge to the field. Unfortunately, the failure to address certain minimal requirements meant that these "proto-studies" were never articulated in writing or were unsuitable for publication. Researchers who sometimes scoff at clinical research might consider that (1) theories in the physical sciences, such as in astronomy, have been built entirely on observations; and (2) major theories in psychology, such as psychoanalysis, may be based entirely on systematic case study research.

Because psychologists in practice can solve major problems, creatively develop new techniques, and stringently test existing procedures, their lack of research productivity is a "social and professional tragedy" (Barlow, Hayes, & Nelson, 1984, p. 18). In addition to being directly relevant to patients' needs, such work would push back the frontiers of psychological science. The scientist/practitioner model directly addresses this dilemma by providing a true integration of both research and practice. The Ph.D. program accreditation criteria of the American Psychological Association, for example, now emphasize the importance of licensure in psychology for core teaching faculty, and an active, ongoing program of experimental and clinical research. These role models should go a long way in improving the present situation in the near future.

Many practicing psychologists, psychiatrists, and dentists have not had the benefit of such crucial role models. However, their doctoral training has included the development of the key skills essential to clinical research. The essential elements of clinical research are quite straightforward. The lack of one or more of these essentials makes many potentially valuable contributions unpublishable.

Fromm (1981) has stated, "The purpose of a clinical manuscript must be to communicate to other clinicians new hypotheses, observations, and findings which expand the professional horizon; or to present in detail new or modified techniques. It is important to state in clear cut, concrete form what was actually done so that others can replicate, test, or apply the procedure to their own patients" (p. 6). To be useful to others in practice and to contribute to science, clinical case studies must usually include (1) a literature survey; (2) a clinical diagnosis; (3) hypnotizability testing data; (4) the patients' history, including previous treatment and the referral source; (5) details of the hypnotic induction procedures used, including specific suggestions given; and (6) follow-up data on treatment outcomes, including unsuccessful as well as successfully treated cases. There is no need to provide details of all cases treated. Three to five representative cases, including a representation of case failures, seems ideal in the present clinical literature.

A recent case study of trichotillomania (chronic hair pulling resulting in alopecia) demonstrated how these criteria can be met (M. Barabasz, 1987). First, the literature survey highlighted 17 studies reporting attempts to cure trichotillomania. In these predominantly behavior-therapy-based treatments, a common thread of compliance problems was identified as a probable cause or contributing factor to treatment failure and relapse. The long history of documented successes in using hypnosis in the treatment of habit disorders, without the complexity of the behavioral interventions, was cited. The entire literature survey, which included the few hypnosis case reports available from the literature, was summarized in a table showing the type of clinical research design used, the number of subjects employed, and treatment outcome for each study. Next, subjects' diagnoses (M. Barabasz, 1987) were given on the basis of _Diagnostic and Statistical Manual of Mental Disorders_, third edition (DSM-III) criteria. Relevant medical tests (Steck, 1979; Wright, Schaffer, & Solomons, 1979) germane to the trichotillomania diagnosis were cited. Subsequently, procedural details were given, and the effort to employ identical treatment procedures for all client cases was emphasized. For example, clients' first sessions emphasized (1) establishing the onset, duration, present condition, and history, including a review of the referral sources' data; (2) discussion of hypnosis; (3) introduction to the hypnotic experience; (4) administration of the Stanford Hypnotic Clinical Scale (SHCS; Morgan & Hilgard, 1975); and (5) specifics of the hypnotic induction procedure used, including the exact wording of suggestions.

Cases were then described, with demographic data and specific histories disguised to protect the identity of clients. Previous treatment information was provided, including success–failure (quantitative) data and clients' perceptions (qualitative data). Intervention procedures were elucidated with adequate detail for replication. The frequency and massing of treatment sessions was indicated. Treatment outcome data were shown for posttreatment and 1-month, 4-month, 6-month, and 12-month follow-ups for each of the client cases. Finally, the discussion section of the paper emphasized the major finding of the study, which was the strong relationship between the SHCS scores and successful treatment outcomes. The need for additional research in controlled settings was explained, and questions still to be answered were formulated. Limitations of the study were discussed, and recommendations for improvements in further clinical trials were made. Questions were raised about accepting certain specific kinds of referrals that might have contributed to a negative outcome in the single failure among the five cases discussed.

The importance of obtaining hypnotizability data on the basis of standardized scales with accepted psychometric properties cannot be overemphasized. Indeed, little can be said about the specificity of hypnosis in treatment unless a relationship between hypnotizability and treatment outcome can be demonstrated (F. J. Evans, 1983; Frankel, 1982). Of course, the relationship between hypnotizability scale scores and treatment outcomes is probabilistic in nature rather than absolute (E. R. Hilgard, 1979c, 1987). However, obtaining such data is of critical importance if we are to further our understanding about operative variables in clinical hypnosis, in contrast to mere assumptions about hypnotic effectiveness. For example, the relationship between SHCS (Morgan & Hilgard, 1975) scores and treatment outcomes has been established in many smoking cessation studies. Although not universal, the findings are so strong in some studies as to suggest that subjects of extremely low susceptibility would be very unlikely to reduce or terminate smoking following a hypnotic procedure (A. F. Barabasz, Baer, Sheehan, & Barabasz, 1986; Baer, Carey, & Meminger, 1986; Holroyd, 1986, 1991; H. Spiegel, 1990; H. Spiegel & Spiegel,

1978). A similar treatment outcome relationship has been demonstrated in a study of the reduction of habitual overeating for weight control (M. Barabasz & Spiegel, 1989) and in the clinical and experimental reduction of pain (A. F. Barabasz & Barabasz, 1989; E. R. Hilgard & Hilgard, 1975; E. R. Hilgard, 1979c).

Hypnotizability data obtained in clinical settings can also be useful in helping to establish a diagnosis, such as in the cases of dissociative experiences and high hypnotizability scores shown by bulimics (M. Barabasz, 1991). The use of standardized scales to test hypnotizability with patients can also provide other benefits directly relevant to clinical needs. For example, we have found hypnotic susceptibility test data to be of particular assistance in identifying specific hypnotic interventions for both chronic and acute pain patients. The absolute score is helpful in indicating a patient's hypnotic capacity, but this may not be as important as identifying specific hypnotic talents, such as the capacity for age regression. A patient who is not able to attenuate pain on the basis of suggestions for anesthesia may be able to employ his or her age regression talents in self-hypnosis for periods of pain relief. Such relief may help decrease depression and reduce dependency on chemical analgesic drugs (A. F. Barabasz & Barabasz, 1989).

Experimental Research Designs

This brief discussion is not intended as a substitute for the many volumes that have been written on experimental research designs. Instead, it highlights some within- and between-groups design considerations that are of particular relevance to the study of hypnotic phenomena.

Within-subjects designs use subjects as their own controls in much the same way as clinical case study trials are conducted. For example, subjects may be asked to perform a specific task under some sort of placebo or control condition and then to repeat the task following a hypnotic induction. Between-groups designs use at least two independent samples of subjects. For example, the experimenter may use a hypnotic procedure with one sample and a nonhypnotic procedure with another sample. A between-groups, within-subjects split-plot design might involve pre- and posthypnosis measures within subjects, and a comparison between two or more independent groups. E. R. Hilgard and Tart (1966) demonstrated that between-groups-only designs and the between-groups component of split-plot designs may be insensitive to important differences resulting from the hypnotic intervention. The concern for researchers is that the between-groups approach may fail to show a true effect even when one exists (a type II or beta error).

E. R. Hilgard and Tart (1966) articulated the rationale in favor of within subjects designs to minimize the risk of a type II error. First, it was suggested that subjects who are high in hypnotizability can enter hypnosis spontaneously without a prior hypnotic induction. This hypothesis was recently confirmed (A. F. Barabasz, 1990b,c). High hypnotizables were exposed to 45 minutes of flotation restricted environmental stimulation (REST), in which subjects float supine on a solution of Epsom salts and tap water at skin temperature in a tank that resembles an enclosed bathtub. The REST environment is sound-attenuating and light-free. The results of the study showed significantly reduced cold-pressor pain scores following a simple suggestion without a prior hypnotic induction. We (A. F. Barabasz & Barabasz, 1992) further tested the E. R. Hilgard and Tart (1966) hypothesis by administering eight items from the Stanford Hypnotic Susceptibility Scale, Form C (SHSS:C) and the SHCS during flotation REST. This study also showed that hypnosis could be induced without a formal induction procedure. Significant differences were found between high- and low-susceptibility subjects in the mean number of items passed, but there was no significant difference between the scores for subjects receiving REST only and subjects receiving REST with a formal hypnotic induction. These studies indicate that the use of the within-subjects research design may be of critical importance if effects of hypnosis are to be detected. The changes from waking to hypnosis for high hypnotizables under the same suggestion conditions can easily be minimal or nonexistent.

High within-group variability of responses to behavioral criteria for high hypnotizables (A. F. Barabasz, 1990a,b) also greatly reduces the probability of identifying significant differences between means produced by alternative group treatments. The variability problem may be further increased by high hypnotizables' capacity to enter self-hypnosis and their tendency to do so contrary to the experimenters' intentions. In addition to the quantitative findings discussed above, we (A. F. Barabasz & Barabasz, 1992) conducted an independent postexperimental inquiry and found that 5 high hypnotizables out of 14 admitted using self-hypnosis during the experiment. Because of the occurrence of spontaneous hypnosis or the practice of self-hypnosis by high hypnotizables under noninduction conditions, production of statistical significance in group comparisons is left to those few subjects who make dramatic gains between waking and hypnosis conditions. As E. R. Hilgard and Tart (1966) noted, overall between-groups comparisons that fail to account for waking–hypnosis responsiveness correlations will understate the changes that take place for some subjects as a result of hypnosis.

E. R. Hilgard, Weitzenhoffer, Landes, and Moore (1961) identified a high degree of response variability to hypnotic suggestions between subjects. The distributions are flat or bimodal with extreme scores at either end of the scale. Between-groups designs may thus be inappropriate because differences in responses between groups of subjects in hypnosis and nonhypnosis conditions can easily be obscured by such variability. Alternatively, random assignment of subjects to hypnosis or nonhypnosis groups can erroneously produce statistical significance (a type I or alpha error) simply through the chance appearance of disproportionate numbers of extremely high or extremely low hypnotizable responders in either group (E. R. Hilgard & Tart, 1966). A few subjects showing large changes in the predicted direction may move the mean enough for significance, while the majority of subjects show no effect.

Between-groups designs using subjects randomly assigned to waking or hypnotic conditions can also be confounded by the substantial number of low hypnotizable subjects in normal populations. E. R. Hilgard (1965a) noted that insufficiently hypnotizable subjects can account for as much as two-thirds of a volunteer general sample. The presence of such subjects will dilute potential effects, because subjects incapable of hypnotic responding would be unlikely to contribute to real differences between waking and hypnosis conditions. The presence of these low susceptibles would contribute to low means and high variability relative to average scores in waking and hypnosis conditions, thereby reducing the probability of significant differences between the compared groups (A. F. Barabasz, 1976; A. F. Barabasz & McGeorge, 1978; E. R. Hilgard & Tart, 1966).

The number of subjects required when using a random-assignment between-groups design is necessarily large if significant differences are to be detected. Running large numbers of subjects is effortful, costly, and time-consuming. The statistically significant differences produced may be brought into question because the percentage of variance accounted for by a particular variable can be trivial, especially in terms of potential clinical applications (Hays, 1963, pp. 329–333). Canonical methodology where random assignment to alternative treatment groups and large numbers of subjects are the norm may be most appropriate for many experiments in psychology, but its use in hypnosis research can bias results in unpredictable directions.

Within-subjects designs have been criticized because differences apparently attributable to hypnosis may be confounded by differences in baseline responses. Low hypnotizables may show better baseline scores than high hypnotizables, so that the performance gains attributed to hypnosis for the highs are artificially enhanced because of the lower pre-hypnosis starting point. Zamansky, Scharf, and Brightbill (1964) believed that these differences may result from the restriction or "holding back" of prehypnotic performance to please the hypnotist by later performance. Another explanation suggests that low hypnotizables may be more compulsive than high hypnotizables and may try harder in the baseline testing (E. R. Hilgard, 1979c). Assumptions about baseline differences are tenuous at best, because prehypnosis baseline differences between highs and lows are far from reliable. E. R. Hilgard, Morgan, and Prytulak (1968) found no significant differences between tranceable and untranceable subjects in normal waking reactions to cold-pressor pain. This important finding suggests that the holding back or compulsiveness criticisms of within-subjects designs are not valid unless baseline differences are shown to exist in a specific experiment. As long as baseline differences are nonsignificant, the within-subjects design appears to be the design of choice when investigators are attempting to evaluate waking versus hypnosis effects, because the limitations of the between-groups design make it more likely to fail to show a true effect when one actually exists.

Design Sensitivity

Because the investigator is focused on establishing support for his or her hypothesis, a statistical power analysis (Cohen, 1977, 1988) of the planned study can sometimes be advantageous. Power analysis is intended to indicate how many subjects are needed to give a hypothesis predicting a true effect a fair chance of being supported as correct.

To determine the minimum number of subjects, the investigator makes the assumption that the true-effect hypothesis can be supported by data gleaned from either within-subjects or between-groups comparisons. Then the minimum value by which the experimental condition data must differ from the control condition data must be established. Let us assume, for example, that an investigator is attempting to test the effects of hypnosis versus a placebo on experimental pain relief. The investigator decides that the hypnotic procedure will be deemed clinically useful only if hypnosis can reduce reported pain scores by an average of 50% for the group below that produced by the placebo. The 50% value is determined on the basis of a pilot study that generates the same kind of data (e.g., cold-pressor pain scores) as the proposed major test-of-effects study to estimate both the parameter of interest and the variability. Next, the hoped-for difference between the mean placebo score (the control mean) is divided by the standard deviation. Kraemer and Thieman (1987) refer to the result of this calculation as the "critical effect size." They suggest that substantial quantitative pilot study data should be obtained before commencement of the major study. A meta-analysis of related issues may also be valuable, although it is seldom undertaken.

Once the critical effect size has been determined, the power of the statistical test of significance should be realistically specified. Choosing a power of .95–.99 might seem attractive, because statistical significance could be shown with near-certainty if the hypothesis is correct. The number of subjects required would be enormous, however and the result, although statistically significant, might be of little clinical relevance. In our opinion, values of .60–.80 appear to be quite appropriate for hypnosis research, as is the case for research on psychotherapy outcomes and psychopharmacological studies. Finally, the acceptable probability level (alpha) should be decided upon for rejection of a null hypothesis. This is typically .05 or .01, but alphas as high as .10, as suggested by Orne and Scheibe (1964), may be appropriate for certain kinds of data. Once critical effect size, power, and alpha have been determined, the number of subjects for the major experiment can be readily determined by reference to tables provided by Kraemer and Thiemann (1987). Alternatively, statistical power analysis can be conducted by computer simulation and calculation of power. Borenstein and Cohen (1988) developed a program that runs on personal computers. It is intended to allow the investigator to create tables and graphs showing how statistical power would be affected by alterations in a study's design. Another useful option includes the capacity to run Monte Carlo simulations to demonstrate alternative effects of statistical power in research planning.

A general understanding of what is involved in statistical power analysis can be far-reaching. Power analysis can help avoid potentially irrevocable investigation planning errors. The investigator will have an estimate of how many subjects to run and will know what kind of data to collect for the major hypothesis-testing study. The process discourages post hoc analyses, which might most charitably be viewed as fishing expeditions involving a variety of statistical tests as hooks (Kraemer & Thieman, 1987, p. 96), or other ex post facto approaches, which represent little more than trolling for significance.

Despite the contribution of statistical power analysis to experimental planning, scientist/practitioners should not ignore data collection opportunities offering only small numbers of subjects. Power calculations become particularly inaccurate for the sample cell sizes available in most clinical settings. Failing to collect data because of the discouragingly large numbers of subjects predicted to be necessary by a power analysis might also result in failure to make an important breakthrough. For example, despite a total n of 20 and cell sizes of only 5 volunteers per group, statistically significant reductions of both experimental and clinical pain were demonstrated for chronic pain patients (A. F. Barabasz & Barabasz, 1989). The study also appeared to produce effects that were of immediate clinical significance. High hypnotizable subjects significantly reduced their dependence on addictive pain medications. Power analysis might have easily discouraged conduct of the investigation, because the computation is notoriously inaccurate with cell sizes of less than 10 subjects. In our study, dramatic and lasting clinical effects were produced with half that number.

Subject Factors

Subject Types

The findings of laboratory settings using primarily college student populations are of little value unless the results can be generalized to a wide range of different settings, populations, and clinical situations. Questions have been raised as to whether or not college student research populations provide valid inference. Riecken (1962) suggested that some apparent treatment effects might best be interpreted in terms of the power relationship between the experimenter in control and the subject's perception of his or her best interests. Rosenberg (1969) speculated that some apparent treatment effects might be the result of pretest sensitization or a subject's apprehension about evaluation. Masling (1966) raised concerns about noncooperative subjects, while Orne (1962a) observed apparent cooperative behavior. All of these conclusions were based on either speculation or observations of a very few subjects.

Weber and Cook (1972) identified four types of alternative subject roles. Each involves arousal of motivation to adopt a role and perception of cues that guide behavior to make it congruent with the aroused motivation: (1) The "good subject" attempts to provide responses that, in his or her view, confirm the experimental hypothesis; (2) the "faithful subject" tries to follow experimental instructions scrupulously; (3) the "negativistic subject" gives responses that are of little use to the experimenter (demonstrating Masling's [1966] "screw you" effect); and (4) the "apprehensive subject" responds in a manner suggesting fears that the performance will be used to evaluate his or her abilities or adjustment. Crowne and Marlowe (1964) suggested that apprehensive subjects attempt to provide responses that they perceive as socially desirable.

Given a sociopsychological context consistent with experimental instructions that emphasize possible danger to subjects, apprehensive subjects can be created. Orne and Scheibe's (1964) findings suggest that these subjects can generate responses to experimental interventions that are independent of the potency of such interventions. Alternatively, we (M. Barabasz, Barabasz, & O'Neill, 1991) found that the potency of an anxiety-arousing experimental atmosphere may be minimal, so that only nonsignificant effects are produced, if the general sociopsychological context is not consistent with anxiety arousal specific to the experimental demands.

Weber and Cook (1972) demonstrated that valid inferences about causality can be drawn from subjects adopting the "faithful subject" role, as long as care is taken to camouflage hypotheses. However, adoption of the "apprehensive subject" role can threaten valid inferences. These findings emphasize the importance of employing subject instructional packages that are not anxiety-arousing in nature. Once such antianxiety instructional procedures are employed—including, for example, opportunities to view and to experience experimental settings before the day in which the experiment is to take place—apprehension can be entirely eliminated in most cases. Eliminating unnecessarily anxiety-producing aspects of instructions, informed consent forms, and props seems to be an effective way of controlling apprehension in even the most demanding experiments (A. F. Barabasz, 1982; A. F. Barabasz & Barabasz, 1989). As Suedfeld (1980, p. 71) noted in regard to REST research, investigators came to realize that the panic button was ancillary and that experiments could be conducted without it; this has enabled them to eliminate the effects of such props and to find out with as little contamination as possible what is produced by experimental procedures.

Consistent with Fromm (1975a,b), Fromm, Brown, Hurt, Oberlander, Boxer, and Pfeifer (1981), Fromm and Kahn (1990), and a review of our own work (A. F. Barabasz & Barabasz, 1990) in 50 experiments involving over 1,000 subjects, we believe it is now appropriate to name a fifth type of subject—the "scientist subject." Scientist subjects seem to join with the experimenter in maintaining multiple hypotheses and having an honest interest in seeing whether an intervention works. When treated in the context of a partnership with the experimenter, these subjects are interested in seeking the truth rather than trying to identify the hypothesis with the goal of providing supportive responses. Scientist subjects' data resemble that of faithful subjects' data, but the former subjects go beyond a scrupulous or robotic following of experimental instructions by volunteering information that they believe may improve the conduct of the experiment. In a demonstration of trance logic (Orne, 1959), for example, scientist subjects readily volunteer details as to the completeness or incompleteness of the suggested hallucination in an effort to facilitate further scientific inquiry. The data provided by "scientist subjects" seems ideally valid. Hypnosis researchers can help maximize the probability of working with scientist subjects by developing rapport that emphasizes a partnership between investigator and subject. Careful attention to the informed consent procedure and subject recruitment process can help develop subjects who recognize that they can further the cause of science by providing accurate data. A subject who knows in advance of experimental participation that his or her reactions and advice will be sought at some point seems particularly likely to adopt the scientist subject approach.

Subject Self-Selection

Subject self-selection to treatments, a characteristic of quasi-experimental and many clinical designs, reduces the generalizability of the findings because personality variables can be expected to be involved in subjects' choices of alternative treatments. We (A. F. Barabasz et al., 1986) completed a 3-year follow-up of hypnosis and REST therapy for smoking, and concluded that apparent differential effects of alternative treatment procedures might have been accounted for by self-selection factors rather than the treatments themselves. Clinic policy allowed subject self-selection to group or individual treatment, freedom of choice as to hypnotist experience level, and the addition of REST therapy as an adjunct to hypnosis.

An analogous problem can occur even in a true experimental design study. Human subject protections permit a subject to withdraw from a study at any time. Differential deselection from treatment conditions can potentially alter the results of the study. In a recent study of abstract figure inversion perception following relaxation or flotation REST, a significantly higher dropout rate was found for the relaxation condition (M. F. Miller & Barabasz, 1990). In situations where subjects become aware of the nature of alternative experimental conditions, and a certain condition is perceived as "more interesting" than others, subject deselection can become problematic. One way to control for skewed subject deselection among treatment groups is to provide the "interesting treatment" to all subjects. Subjects assigned to conditions perceived to be less interesting are less likely to deselect themselves from the study any more frequently than subjects assigned to other treatments, as long as they are assured eventual participation in the more interesting treatment. After participation in the condition deemed less interesting, and collection of data, these subjects are then involved in the treatment of interest as promised. Assignment to treatment conditions should be counterbalanced and a statistical analysis conducted to determine whether or not order of treatment has any systematic effect on the results. It is interesting to note that F. J. Evans (1963) found that differences between hypnosis and the waking state persisted, regardless of which condition came first.

Subject self-selection according to the invitation to participate has also been raised as a threat to experimental validity. Several studies have shown a significant positive relationship between electroencephalographic (EEG) alpha density (the amount of time a person produces alpha during a particular recording period) and hypnotizability, whereas others have failed to support such a significant positive correlation (these studies are reviewed in A. F. Barabasz, 1980a). On the basis of a review of the literature, Dumas (1977) concluded that the only consistent covariate of EEG alpha–hypnotizability correlations was the method by which subjects were selected. In experiments where the sample consisted of non-naive volunteers, there was a significant correlation, while investigations employing invited subjects or subjects unaware of the experimental focus found no such correlation. Although Dumas's conclusions were later found to be inconsistent with some of the reported data (A. F. Barabasz, 1983), no experimental study testing the hypothesis had been conducted to that date.

To test Dumas's (1977) hypothesis that EEG alpha density would not be significantly correlated with hypnotizability in a sample of subjects unaware of the experimental focus, EEG data were collected in an experimental context completely isolated from hypnotizability. Data were collected in the context of a study of the effects of Antarctic isolation. All measures were administered at Scott Base, Antarctica, before and after wintering-over isolation. Eight channels of EEG and skin conductance response (SCR) data were collected in the context of an olfactory experiment (A. F. Barabasz & Gregson, 1979). Independently of the EEG and

SCR data collection context, a modified hypnotizability scale was administered. In order to provide the basis for a stringent test of Dumas's hypothesis, the naiveté of subjects was maintained by administration of the test of hypnotic susceptibility without hypnosis induction. Contrary to the findings of Dumas (1977), a significant relationship was found between hypnotizability and EEG alpha density, and this was increased by a mathematical correction procedure for subject arousability using the SCRs (A. F. Barabasz, 1980a). These results, combined with a re-evaluation of the earlier studies (A. F. Barabasz, 1983), demonstrate that EEG alpha–hypnotizability correlations are not simple covariates of subject self-selection.

Despite the failure to support the potency of subject self-selection postulated by Dumas, researchers should not ignore other potential effects of this moderator variable. Lynn (1990) reported that mean scores on the Harvard Group Hypnotic Susceptibility Scale (HGSHS:A; Shor & Orne, 1962) were significantly higher for subjects tested at the beginning of a university academic quarter than for those tested near the end of the same academic quarter. Lynn's (1990) findings are consistent with our own data and those of Crawford (1992). Similarly, E. R. Hilgard (1979c) found significantly higher HGSHS:A scores for university subjects who volunteered early in the academic year than for subjects who were asked to volunteer for further (later) experiments with a small stipend for participation. This result supports the conclusions of the earliest reported study addressing this question. Boucher and Hilgard (1962) reported that subjects volunteering at large from the university community tended to have mean hypnotizability scores higher than those of subjects who volunteered "because of class requirements."

Institutional Review and Risks to Subjects

The usual prerequisite step to undertaking research with human subjects is to obtain the approval of one's institutional review board (IRB). IRBs serve a gate-keeping function (Ceci, Peters, & Plotkin, 1985) that can have a substantial influence on research procedures. In the United States, the Department of Health and Human Services (DHHS) stipulates IRB approval of a research proposal prior to release of funds. Any institution that receives DHHS funds is also required to include an institutional general assurance (IGA). Under the principle of "pre-emption," the IRB cannot contradict or lessen the impact of federal statutes. The IGA commits the institution to protect human subjects through fully informed consent, the option to deny participation (or terminate participation without penalty), freedom from coercion, minimization of risk, and ethical review. Review of nonfunded research is considered evidence of an institutional willingness to afford human subjects protection. Ninety-one percent of national IRBs use the same procedures to review both funded and nonfunded research proposals (Ceci et al., 1985).

Conclusions drawn by an IRB regarding a research proposal can have major effects on research design, the conduct of the experiment, and the inferences that may be drawn from the findings. We (M. F. Miller, Barabasz, & Barabasz, 1991) investigated the effects of active/alert and relaxation hypnotic inductions on cold-pressor pain. The study used Orne's (1979a) real–simulator subject design, in which a group of subjects established to be essentially nonhypnotizable is asked to simulate hypnosis. An IRB consultant advised that simulators were to be instructed to provide real rather than simulated pain reports in response to the cold-pressor procedure. It was felt that the experimenter administering the pain measure would not be able to protect subjects adequately if the subjects were instructed to simulate throughout the experiment and give pain ratings equivalent to what they thought real hypnotized subjects would provide. In the present case, the study was conducted without a negative influence on the power of the design, because high hypnotizable subjects could be given the identical real pain report instructions. The requirement of a change from simulation to veridical reporting for the final minute of data collection in this study was, however, quite a departure from the traditional manner in which simulator subjects are employed. (Orne's real–simulator design is discussed later in this chapter.)

Risks to subjects in hypnosis research should be addressed in IRB proposals by reference to the specific samples under consideration. In order to avoid unwarranted precautions, which may have negative consequences for implementation of the research design, it is important that proposals produced for IRBs acknowledge that there have been occasional reports of disastrous consequences of hypnotherapy (see E. R. Hilgard, 1965a, p. 52) in cases of severely ill patients with long histories of illness who were treated by incompetent therapists.

A competent psychological evaluation of a potential patient is essential before the use of hypnosis for symptom removal is considered. In particular, this use of hypnosis with patients on the verge of an acute psychotic episode is ill advised, because hypnosis may threaten defense mechanisms. Early reports indicated that some patients treated for symptom removal with hypnosis developed much more severe symptoms following treatment. H. Rosen (1960) reported that a male patient treated with hypnosis to relieve phantom limb pain later developed schizoaffective psychosis; he also noted that a female treated for smoking developed overeating, which was then replaced by alcoholism. H. Rosen and Bartemeier (1961) reported that a male treated for numbness in one arm developed schizophrenic psychosis, while Teitel (1961) found that lower back symptoms were replaced with paranoid psychosis. In contrast to these early findings, data obtained from over 600 patients treated in a hypnosis and psychosomatic medicine unit in a large metropolitan general hospital (A. F. Barabasz & Sheehan, 1983) revealed negative sequelae of hypnosis in only a single case, and these were successfully ameliorated in 3 hours of counseling over a 2-week period. Although no control data were available for comparison, it appeared that the routine clinic practice of obtaining psychological evaluations and mental status prior to hypnosis was successful in precluding the kinds of negative consequences reported in the early studies.

Unfortunately, the rare problems occurring in clinical situations have been misgeneralized to the kinds of normal subject populations typically used in hypnosis research. In contrast to the potential problems following hypnosis with psychiatric patients, particularly those treated for psychosomatic symptoms, the incidence of hypnotic sequelae with university student populations presents a much less worrisome picture. Even the much-maligned university sophomore has shown at least 1 year of successful adjustment to academia (Zubek, 1969, p. 295). Despite the fact that the Department of Health, Education and Welfare listed hypnosis as an "at-risk" procedure in the late 1970s (Coe & Ryken, 1979), there are very few data to support the notion that the use of hypnosis with university student populations is any more problematic than many of the normal activities students are subjected to in their daily lives.

Student volunteer subjects who respond to induction procedures in hypnosis testing experience a number of unique phenomena. Therefore, it is not surprising to find reports of some transient experiences after exposure to hypnosis testing sessions. J. R. Hilgard, Hilgard, and Newman (1961) interviewed 220 college student subjects after administration of the Stanford Hypnotic Susceptibility Scale, Form A (SHSS:A; Weitzenhoffer & Hilgard, 1959). A positive relationship was found between unpleasant childhood experiences with anesthesia and negative aftereffects of hypnosis; however, most sequelae were "minor and fleeting." Only 17 subjects reported sequelae, and only 5 of these (2.3%) reported effects that lasted as long as a few hours. J. R. Hilgard et al. (1961) concluded that hypnosis is generally harmless in a student population.

Faw, Sellers, and Wilcox (1968) compared the aftereffects of three group hypnosis sessions on 102 subjects with the aftereffects of discussion groups over the same period of time (but no actual hypnosis) on 105 subjects. Subjects in the hypnosis group who were judged prepsychotic on the Minnesota Multiphasic Personality Inventory improved more on neurotic and behavior problem scales than did the nonhypnotized controls. At posttest, the no-hypnosis control subject group produced one psychotic and a higher incidence of difficulties with insomnia or nervous tension than the hypnotized-subject group. J. R. Hilgard (1974b) compared sequelae of the HGSHS:A (Shor & Orne, 1962) with those of the more demanding and more cognitively oriented SHSS:C (Weitzenhoffer & Hilgard, 1962). In contrast to the findings obtained with the HGSHS:A (and with the findings of the earlier studies using scales of similar item content), 31% of subjects reported transient experiences that lasted from 5 minutes to several hours after administration of the SHSS:C. Fifteen percent of subjects reported such experiences lasting more than 1 hour. Coe and Ryken (1979) further explored this finding, employing 209 introductory psychology students as subjects. The aftereffects of the SHSS:C were compared with the aftereffects of participating in a verbal learning experiment, taking a college exam, attending a college class, and college life in general. Coe and Ryken's results indicated that hypnosis was no more bothersome than any of the comparison activities.

Crawford, Hilgard, and Macdonald (1982) explored possible differences in the occurrence and type of transient experiences following the HGSHS:A and the SHSS:C with 172 undergraduate introductory psychology student volunteers. On 2 days, sessions were conducted according to procedures common to the appropriate conduct of research involving hypnosis. The procedures emphasized establishing good rapport through development of a positive, trusting relationship between hypnotist and subject. A short lecture about hypnosis, aimed at dispelling its myths, was also presented. Subjects were encouraged to present their queries during a question-and-answer period. The HGSHS:A was then administered. Subjects were individually instructed as to how to use an open-ended scale to estimate hypnotic depth, before administration of the SHSS:C. Reports were obtained following the induction, after it was determined that the age regression item had been successfully completed and after posthypnotic amnesia had been lifted. Only 5% of the 172 subjects reported minor, transient posthypnotic experiences after the HGSHS:A; however, 29% reported these reactions following the SHSS:C. Only one case involving cognitive distortion or confusion was found after the SHSS:C. Subjects scoring significantly higher on the cognitively oriented SHSS:C were those who reported feeling drowsy. A special termination procedure involving exercise and conversation had no significant effect on report of transient experiences. The transient experiences found were not viewed as constituting a risk to subjects. Any slight discomforts and uneasiness reported by subjects were easily dealt with by a well-trained psychologist/hypnotist. Crawford et al. concluded that it is important to define the end of the hypnotic experience clearly and to ensure that the subjects are no longer in hypnosis before leaving. No suggestions should be made about potential difficulties. However, it was emphasized that it should be made easy for subjects to come back if they feel troubled in any way, but to indicate subtly that this is not expected.

The most recent thorough examination of hypnotic sequelae (Strauss, 1990) also found little if any risk to subjects. The Strauss study confirmed the importance of screening prior to hypnosis. One subject reported paranoid ideas about hypnosis prior to the time that he would have been scheduled to experience hypnosis. The point was made that had only a posthypnotic interview been conducted, the paranoid ideation might have been attributed to the hypnotic experience. Another subject had a transient experience involving discomfort of an arm, but this problem was quickly self-correcting.

Experimental Context: The Demand Characteristics Issue

Concerns about experimental-context demand characteristics may be traced to Campbell's (1957) explication of internal and external experimental validity. However, there can be little argument that Martin T. Orne has contributed the greatest richness to our knowledge about these variables crucial to our design, execution, and interpretation of experiments (F. J. Evans, Kihlstrom, & Orne, 1973; F. J. Evans & Orne, 1965; Orne, 1959, 1961, 1962a,b,c, 1965, 1966, 1969, 1970, 1971a,b). This important contribution, developed in the hypnosis laboratory, has influenced human experimental research in many fields of psychology and in the wider arena of the behavioral sciences in general. If strong inference is to occur and findings are to be generalizable, it is essential that scientists studying human behavior recognize that observed responses occur in a social context and that a subject's responsivity will reflect that social context, as well as, (let us hope) the effects of the experimental procedure per se. Indeed, research subjects are not stupid.

In the papers cited above, Orne elaborated upon unwitting cues and their impact on every piece of research involving humans as subjects. The effects of such unwitting cues must "always" (Orne, 1981) represent an alternative hypothesis to be considered. An experiment in behavioral science may be viewed as two completely distinct experiments: the one that has been designed by the experimenter to test his or her hypothesis, and, quite separately, the experiment that the subject conceptualizes on the basis of the experiment's demand characteristics (Orne, 1969). Orne (1969, p. 145) defined "demand characteristics" as the "sum total of all cues available to the subject before the experiment (the experimental context), the instructions during the experiment, the covert communications during the experiment, and the nature of the procedure itself that communicate the experimental purposes and the desired behavior." Experimenters' recognition of the role of demand characteristics is crucial, because the generalizability of the study's findings, beyond the immediate experimental context, will be largely dependent upon the parity between the experiment as conceptualized by the investigator and the experiment as conceptualized by the subject. Operator variables in successful hypnotherapy (Lazar & Dempster, 1984), which can greatly influence the outcome of therapy (A. F. Barabasz et al., 1986), can also be conceptualized within the domain of demand characteristics. Unlike particles in a physics experiment, both subjects and clients are thinking, conscious human beings.

Human beings respond not only to specific experimental stimuli, but also to their perception of the stimuli in the total context of the experimental or clinical milieu.

How powerful are these extraexperimental cues? Orne and Evans (1965) demonstrated that research subjects would be quite willing to carry out high-risk activities, including, for example, picking up a poisonous snake, removing a penny from nitric acid with their bare hands, or throwing acid in the face of the experimenter. Contrary to appearances, the subjects complied because of their conceptualization that precautions for safety were somehow in place.

Failure to be attuned to the potential effects of demand characteristics can lead to misleading experimental results. In a clever demonstration of this point, K. S. Bowers (1966) cited a study of visual and auditory hypnotic hallucinations by T. X. Barber and Calverley (1964e), in which no significant differences were found in the ratings of hypnotic and "task-motivated" subjects. Barber and Calverley (1964e) erroneously concluded that both groups "imagined but did not actually see and did not actually hear that which had been suggested" (p. 19). Bowers identified the experimental demand characteristics confound in this study by noting that the person who administered the original hypnotic and task-motivational instructions was the very same person who collected the subjects' testimony ratings as to the reality of hallucinations. Consistent with Levitt and Brady (1964), Bowers noted that subjects in the Barber and Calverley experiment might have easily inferred that they were supposed to report hallucinations, regardless of whether or not hallucinations were actually experienced. As in the Barber and Calverley (1964e) study, Bowers's subjects were not selected for hypnotizability. Twenty subjects were randomly assigned to the Barber and Calverley task-motivated condition, while the remaining 20 subjects were assigned to an "honesty" condition. The situational demand characteristics of the task-motivational group produced significantly higher hallucination rating reports than the honesty group, thus demonstrating the demand characteristics confound in the Barber and Calverley study.

Instructional Demand Effects

Instructional demand characteristics can produce dramatic effects regardless of the objectivity of the dependent measure. A. F. Barabasz and Lonsdale (1983) demonstrated an increase in the P300 amplitude responses component of the EEG cortical event-related potential during a test of hypnotically induced anosmia. Contrary to this finding, D. Spiegel, Cutcomb, Ren, and Pribram (1985) found a decrease in P300 amplitude after instructing high hypnotizables that an imaginary cardboard box blocked their view of a stimulus generator. Both studies were conducted with scrupulous attention to methodological controls. The differences in findings of the two studies were reconciled (D. Spiegel & Barabasz, 1988) on the basis of differences in the hypnotic instructions given. The Barabasz and Lonsdale study employed language drawn from item 9 of the SHSS:C, which was directed at complete negation of a stimulus ("You will not smell anything at all"), whereas the Spiegel et al. study had subjects focus on a competing obstructive hallucination. The anosmia subjects in the Barabasz and Lonsdale study were surprised when they smelled anything at all, leading to the enhancement of P300 response, whereas subjects in the Spiegel et al. visual study were so absorbed in the hallucinated obstruction that perception of the stimulus was reduced. The differences in instructional demand characteristics created alternative findings.

One way to deal with the potential effects of instructional demand characteristics is to deliberately vary demands between control and experimental groups. A. F. Barabasz (1982) studied the effects of 6 hours of laboratory REST on hypnotizability. Control subjects were given instructional demands that intentionally favored an increase in hypnotizability, while no such demands were placed on experimental subjects. Consistent with the findings of Suedfeld, Landon, Epstein, and Pargament (1971), control subjects' subjective self-reports were indicative of increases in hypnotizability (as might be expected from the instructional demand characteristics), but these expectancies did not influence performance on the objective dependent measures of the study.

Studies using factor analysis are particularly susceptible to instructional demand characteristics. Significant factor-loading swings can occur in response to relatively minor instructional variations. The results of a study may be equivocal if instructional demand characteristics are ignored (Sheehan & McConkey, 1982, pp. 68–69).

Conclusions about the effects of context are difficult to draw, because contextual cues exist correlatively with the experimental intervention. Investigators are always on very shaky ground indeed when they attempt to draw causal inferences from correlative observations. Council, Kirsch, and Hafner (1986) attempted to examine the effects of context on correlations between absorption (Tellegen & Atkinson, 1974) and hypnotizability. Tellegen and Atkinson's (1974) Absorption Scale is a 34-item true–false test that is intended to measure the predisposition to be highly involved or absorbed in imaginative or sensory experiences. Similar to the kinds of observations Dumas (1977) made about subject self-selection and EEG alpha–hypnotizability correlations (discussed above in "Subject Factors"), Council et al. observed that the numerous studies showing a significant correlation between measured hypnotizability and Absorption Scale scores were conducted in the context of a hypnosis experiment. Council et al. (1986) administered the Absorption Scale to 64 subjects in the context of a hypnosis experiment and to another 64 subjects in a context unrelated to hypnosis. They found absorption to be significantly correlated with hypnotic responsivity and expectancy, but only when it was assessed in the hypnotic context. Findings based on their path analysis supported the notion that inductions alter expectancies for hypnotic suggestions and that altered expectancies determine subsequent hypnotic behavior. Analogous to the Dumas (1977) study, the Council et al. (1986) study appeared to demonstrate that absorption–hypnotizability correlations are covariates of experimental context. A significant correlation occurs when absorption is measured in a hypnosis experiment but no such correlation can be found outside of that context.

Contrary to the findings of Council et al. (1986), A. F. Barabasz and Tellegen (1992) obtained a statistically significant correlation between hypnotizability and Absorption Scale scores in a context unrelated to hypnosis. The Absorption Scale and the SHCS (Morgan & Hilgard, 1975) were administered to patients seeking treatment at an outpatient "Psychosomatic Unit" of a large metropolitan general hospital without expectations for hypnosis, and to patients appearing at the identical physical setting and location under the name "Hypnosis and Psychosomatic Unit" with the expectation for hypnotic treatment. Data obtained in the context unrelated to hypnosis generated statistically significant correlations between absorption and hypnotizability, similar to the data obtained in the context of expectancy for hypnosis. As in the earlier re-evaluation of the Dumas (1977) data (A. F. Barabasz, 1983), it appears that absorption–hypnotizability correlations cannot be conceptualized as simple covariates of context. It appears that contextual effects, although not robust, are indeed complex. It is difficult if not impossible to draw conclusions about the extent of such effects, because context exists at a merely correlative level with data collection. The experiment in the eye of the researcher may not be as broad as the experiment in the eye of the subject.

General and Immediate Context Effects

We (M. Barabasz et al., 1991) demonstrated that immediate contextual experimental demand characteristics may not have a significant effect when they are contrary to an overall or general social context. Early laboratory research on the effects of "sensory deprivation" involved unnecessarily high stress (M. Barabasz & Barabasz, 1987; Suedfeld, 1980). These early studies were conducted in the context of an era of newspaper headlines about brainwashing, which very likely contributed to the creation of many apprehensive subjects (see "Subject factors," above). This sociopsychological context was replete with reports of negative reactions, including spatial disorientation, fugue states, inability to concentrate, visual–motor impairment, and visual–auditory hallucinations (reviewed by Zubek, 1969). It was then, amidst this anxiety about sensory deprivation, that Orne and Scheibe (1964) conducted their landmark study highlighting the effects of experimental demand characteristics.

Orne and Scheibe (1964) hypothesized that "sensory deprivation" effects could be produced simply by manipulating situational variables and experimental demand cues in a normal rather than a sensorially deprived environment. Experimental subjects were exposed to anxiety-laden pre-experimental conditions congruent with the sociopsychological context of the 1960s (i.e., fear-inducing reports of sensory deprivation). The same normal stimulation physical characteristics—a fully lighted room with a desk, chair, and no soundproofing—were provided for the control group subjects, who were actually told that they were serving as controls. The controls were intentionally led by these instructions to expect nothing to happen. As expected, experimental subjects showed significantly greater "sensory deprivation" effects than controls on certain objective tests and in interviews, despite the fact that neither group was actually exposed to "sensory deprivation." This clever demonstration raised behavioral scientists' awareness about the potentially far-reaching effects of experimental demand characteristics. The study has been frequently cited by journal reviewers, despite the fact that it was confounded in almost the same fashion as the T. X. Barber and Calverley (1964e) study discussed earlier; the same investigators who administered the instructional and situational demand cues were the ones who obtained the dependent measures. It is not surprising that subjects who were told they were serving as "controls" provided data consistent with what might be expected from such subjects.

We (M. Barabasz et al., 1991) attempted to replicate the classic Orne and Scheibe (1964) study to see whether their findings still held true. Replicating the procedure of Orne and Scheibe as exactly as possible, the experimental condition employed cues to increase subjects' expectancy for "deprivation effects," including an aura of great seriousness, a tray containing drugs and medical instruments labeled "Emergency Tray," and the presence of a red button labeled "Emergency Alarm." Experimental subjects were encouraged to report "any visual imagery, fantasies, special or unusual feelings, difficulties in concentration, hallucinations, feelings of disorientation," indicating that such experiences are "not unusual under the conditions" to which the subjects were subjected (Orne & Scheibe, 1964, p. 5).

The control subjects were informed that they were part of a control group for a sensory deprivation experiment. The anxiety-producing props were deleted, and subjects were told that it was necessary to place them in the same chamber for the same period of time as experimental subjects, so that the effects of the more restrictive sensory deprivation conditions could be differentiated from the effects of simply being left alone in a room for a period of time (Orne & Scheibe, 1964). Despite every effort to replicate the procedures of Orne and Scheibe as faithfully as possible, and our expectations for replication of findings, no significant differences were found between experimental and control groups on either objective or interview data. The findings of the study were further elucidated by the addition of an independent postexperimental inquiry employing a clinician not involved in any other aspect of data collection. The inquiry revealed subjects' awareness of modern human subject safeguards and awareness of the supposed beneficial effects of REST via newspaper and magazine articles, which were not part of the general context of the original Orne and Scheibe study. Our (M. Barabasz et al., 1991) investigation demonstrated that highly loaded experimental demand characteristics and immediate situational contextual cues may not be powerful enough to contradict the demands of the general sociopsychological context, which now recognizes REST as beneficial (A. F. Barabasz, Barabasz, Dyer, & Rather, 1992; M. Barabasz, Barabasz, & Dyer, 1990; McAleney, Barabasz, & Barabasz, 1990; Suedfeld, 1990; Wagaman, Barabasz, & Barabasz, 1991).

M. T. Orne's Real–Simulator Design

Humans are active and thinking beings; research is flawed if the design assumes them to be motivationless or neutral. Unlike the physical sciences, research involving human subjects cannot be conducted in a vacuum. Humans bring their own life experiences, expectancies, and attitudes to the experiment. M. T. Orne (1959) recognized the active participation of subjects in the socially defined experimental interaction and concluded that they were "eager to please" in their effort to "contribute to science" (p. 278). Orne's "eager-to-please subject" represents one of five subject types discussed earlier in this chapter, the "good subject" (A. F. Barabasz & Barabasz, 1990; Weber & Cook, 1972). All five subject types may artifactually respond to experimental treatments and contexts. Orne's rigidly scientific real–simulator design is intended to address this problem directly, by providing a methodology for obtaining the effects or essence of the consequences of hypnosis for highly hypnotizable subjects in observable behavioral terms, unconfounded by subject artifacts that are results of the experimental context. There is probably no more powerful design available to the serious researcher who wishes to evaluate clinical judgments or critically test apparent experimental findings attributed to hypnotic interventions.

There are several prerequisites to the proper conduct of Orne's real–simulator design. First, it is essential to differentiate subjects who are highly susceptible to hypnosis from those who are insusceptible. Great care must be taken in establishing both subject groups. It is not sufficient to administer a single measure of hypnotizability. The HGSHS:A (Shor & Orne, 1962) or the SHSS:A (Weitzenhoffer & Hilgard, 1959) can serve as an initial coarse means of grading of subjects, but even top scores on these instruments are not good enough (E. R. Hilgard, 1987). Next, subjects should be provided with further orientation to hypnosis, including opportunities to observe and participate in various hypnotic inductions, ideally with alternative hypnotists. Finally, a stringent test of hypnotic capacity should be administered, such as the SHSS:C (Weitzenhoffer & Hilgard, 1962). Specific subject responses to scale items should be considered, because the scales are not just artificial measuring devices; they should be regarded as depositories of information about hypnotic responding (E. R. Hilgard, 1987). The total score achieved by a subject can provide only part of the selection criteria required by the experiment. For example, it would be ridiculous to conduct an experiment on hypnotically induced deafness if the high hypnotizable real subjects in the study were not universally demonstrated to have this capability.

The real–simulator design cannot be implemented successfully without clearly defined high and low hypnotizable subject groups. It is vital that the assumption can be made that subjects in the low hypnotizable group will not become hypnotized, and that subjects in the high hypnotizable group are in fact capable of deep levels of hypnosis. This is probably the most painstaking part of the procedure. Studies claiming to identify dozens of high and low susceptible subjects from initial samples of fewer than 100 should be evaluated with considerable suspicion, because there can be little doubt that both groups will be contaminated with several subjects who are only moderately hypnotizable. In a study using the real–simulator design, A. F. Barabasz and Lonsdale (1983) tested the effects of hypnosis on EEG P300 olfactory-evoked potentials. The SHSS:C was administered to 93 student volunteers. Subjects' plateau susceptibility was established by repeated hypnosis for the 19 subjects scoring below 3 or above 9 on the SHSS:C. These sessions reduced the number of subjects meeting high or low hypnotizability criteria. After plateauing, the SHSS:C was readministered. High susceptible subjects ($n = 4$) scored 10 or higher (all had passed the anosmia item), and low susceptible subjects ($n = 5$) scored 0 or 1 in the final SHSS:C session before beginning the experiment. Fewer than 10% of the subjects in the initial sample met the exacting criteria of the real–simulator design.

Low hypnotizable or nonsusceptible subjects comprise the simulator group because of their preselection for insusceptibility to hypnosis. These unique subjects are critically important to the experiment because they are able to stay out of hypnosis. They can role-play hypnotic performance for the experimenter involved in data collection, who must remain blind with respect to subjects' membership in the high or low susceptible group. Before commencing the actual experiment, another researcher instructs the low susceptible subjects to simulate hypnosis. The simulators are told to behave just as they believe an excellent hypnotic subject would behave; they are also asked not to reveal that they are unaffected by hypnosis, either during hypnosis or after administration of instructions for awakening. Simulator subjects are further motivated by the instruction that the experimenter will stop the experiment if it is determined that they are simulating, but that intelligent subjects have previously been successful at fooling experimenters (Orne, Sheehan, & Evans, 1968). The objectives of the procedure are still further enhanced by the finding that simulator subjects are more highly suspicious of the experiment than hypnotized subjects, thus further differentiating this population from the highly hypnotizable group. This characteristic, combined with the selection process and role to be played by the simulators, identifies simulators as unique. They should not be regarded as a normal control group. Sheehan and Perry (1976, p. 187) noted that hypnosis researchers have sometimes confused normal control groups with simulators, and that this mistake has led to considerable misunderstanding about the adequacy of this research design model.

Once the simulation instructions have been administered, each subject is sent directly to another experimenter, who administers the hypnotic procedure under study. High and low hypnotizable subjects are exposed to the same hypnotic procedures because of the experimenter's blindness with respect to group membership. Of course, the simulator subjects are aware of the existence of the high hypnotizable subject group, but the highs are not told about the simulators. Orne (1971b) explained that the two groups differ sharply in both their task and the mental set they bring to it; however, both simulator and real subjects must be drawn from the same general population. Contrary to Raikov (1982, 1990), who used trained actors to simulate hypnosis, Orne's design requires that simulators have no special training or special set that they bring with them to the experiment. The simulation task itself is intended to be independent of the hypnotic induction. Simulators simply respond to available cues.

A study by Orne et al. (1968) provides a classic example of how the real–simulator design can be used to provide the same kind of strong inference, unconfounded by artifact, that has characterized major breakthroughs in the biological sciences. The study investigated posthypnotic behavior outside the experimental setting, to provide a critical test of the state-oriented theoretical account of hypnotic behavior versus the role-playing view of the nature of hypnosis. High and low hypnotizable groups were carefully differentiated on the basis of HGSHS:A and SHSS:C testing from a large pool of volunteers. The highly hypnotizable real subjects participated in a 48-hour experiment, which they were told would involve many personality tests. During the first day, the subjects were given the suggestion, under hypnosis, that for the next 48 hours they would touch their foreheads each time they heard the word "experiment." The experimenter, unaware of subjects' group membership, tested the suggestion in the experimental setting. However, the critical test came shortly thereafter in the waiting room. The secretary/receptionist mentioned the word "experiment" innocuously as part of schedule checking for subjects as they were leaving the office on the first day, and then again as they arrived on the following day. The low hypnotizable subjects served as a quasi-control group. They were instructed to simulate hypnosis, to facilitate evaluation of whether the experimenter may have unwittingly cued subjects to respond to the posthypnotic suggestion outside of the experimental setting. The results of the study demonstrated that both real and simulator subjects responded to the suggestion in the laboratory, but that only the real hypnotic subjects responded consistently away from the experimental setting. Not one simulator subject showed a comparable posthypnotic response outside of the experimental setting. The role-playing explanation of hypnosis was therefore not supported: The real hypnotizable subjects not only responded when they thought they should, but their responses, to a significant level, existed independently of the context in which they originated.

The real–simulator design is enormously valuable in providing an artifact-free modality to evaluate whether or not the experimenter may have unwittingly cued subjects differentially because of their level of hypnotizability. In the only EEG study to employ Orne's simulator design, A. F. Barabasz and Lonsdale (1983), as noted earlier, tested evoked potential responses to item 9 from the SHSS:C (which instructs subjects to become anosmic to all odors). All subjects were treated in an equivalent manner, because the design prevented the experimenter from becoming aware of subjects' hypnotic susceptibility level. A strong-odor, weak-odor, or no-odor condition was administered by computer control to each subject in random sequence under hypnosis and waking conditions. The three alternative odor conditions provided an extension of the usual simulator design because, in this study, the experimental situation was double-blind. Neither the simulator subjects nor the experimenter knew what treatment conditions were administered. The standard simulator design is single-blind, in the sense that subjects know quite precisely which treatment they are receiving.

The simulator design has also been successfully varied in studies involving testing of the effects of hypnosis on cold-pressor pain. A. F. Barabasz (1990b) exposed 10 high and 10 low hypnotizable simulator subjects to three experimental conditions consisting of (1) flotation REST without a hypnotic induction, (2) a hypnotic induction outside of the REST lab, and (3) a no-hypnotic-induction condition. Cold-pressor pain data were obtained by standardized methodology after administration of a dissociative suggestion. Human subject considerations demanded that the subjects in both groups provide accurate pain reports. This variation was contrary to the standard real–simulator design, which would have required simulator subjects to continue simulating their pain reports. Since the pain reports were obtained within the last minute of the study, and verbal interaction on the part of the experimenter at that point was limited to the word "report" to obtain pain data at 5-second intervals, the variation did not create bias with respect to treatment of subjects. The study benefited from the feature that direct comparisons could be made between high and low subjects in each of the three within-subjects experimental conditions on the basis of true pain report scores obtained in the experiment, rather than having to rely on postexperimental descriptions of pain (as would have been the case with traditional real–simulator methodology). An independent postexperimental inquiry—also a key characteristic of Orne's real–simulator design—showed that both highs and lows viewed REST as relaxing, but that only the highs added vivid imaginative descriptions of their experiences that were consistent with E. R. Hilgard's (1977a) neodissociation theory of hypnosis. Only the highs demonstrated significantly lowered pain scores in the hypnosis condition. Both highs and lows demonstrated significantly lower pain scores in flotation REST, but pain reduction was significantly greater for highs than for lows.

The use of veridical pain scores was again found to be useful in a study testing the effects of active/alert and relaxation hypnotic inductions on cold-pressor pain (M. F. Miller et al., 1991). Relaxation and active/alert hypnotic inductions were contrasted with or without a specific suggestion for cold-pressor pain analgesia. A total of 304 volunteers were tested for hypnotizability; highly hypnotizable real subjects and low susceptible simulator subjects were plateaued for responsiveness. Testing on the SHSS:C resulted in high susceptible ($n = 38$) and low susceptible ($n = 27$) groups. Cold-pressor pain data were obtained after counterbalanced exposure to a traditional relaxation hypnotic induction or an active/alert induction involving riding of a bicycle ergometer. The highly hypnotizable real subjects demonstrated significantly lower pain scores than the lows. Pain reports did not significantly differentiate between the active/alert or traditional relaxation hypnotic induction conditions. Highs given a specific analgesic suggestion showed significantly lower pain scores than highs exposed only to hypnosis. Again, the experimenter's behavior during the last minute of the experiment, in which pain scores were obtained, did not influence interactions with subjects. The findings demonstrated that relaxation is not necessary for hypnotic analgesia. A postexperimental inquiry provided qualitative data supporting E. R. Hilgard's (1977a) neodissociation theory.

The power of Orne's real–simulator design to produce strong inferences suffers from a few limitations. It is cumbersome to use because several researchers must work together to meet the exacting procedural constraints of the model. E. R. Hilgard (1987) has found that simulators tend to overplay their parts. Sheehan and Perry (1976, p. 183) criticized Orne's stress on establishing the veridicality or essence of hypnosis on the basis of the subjective experience of the subjects. Other than subjects' testimonies, obtained in the postexperimental inquiry, the model gives no real basis upon how to achieve this goal. The model itself is strictly behavioral in nature and provides no confirmable quantitative methodology to assess the subjects' reported experiences of imagined events. Specific strategies to test the honesty of postexperimental inquiry reports are lacking. The greatest strength of the real–simulating model lies in its ability to analyze largely artifact-free responses of highly hypnotizable subjects.

However, nondifferential responses between reals and simulators cannot be assumed to be due to situational artifacts. Sheehan and Perry (1976, p. 196) explained that such similarity in responding suggests only that the real hypnotizable subjects may be reacting to procedural artifacts. Apparent differences between the reals and the simulators may be the effects not of hypnosis, but of simulation. The design does not address artifacts associated with subject selection variables or confounding of hypnosis with relaxation. There is also the problem of confounding hypnotizability with group assignment (all reals are highs; all simulators are lows). Group differences may be attributable to trait, not state. The need for subsequent research using alternative methodologies is not precluded. The A. F. Barabasz and Lonsdale (1983) study focused on independent EEG criteria to evaluate the responses of real and simulator subjects exposed to various odor conditions. Had the experiment been conducted using subjects' self-reports as to whether or not they responded to hypnotically induced anosmia, or had both reals and simulators responded similarly, true hypnotic performance on the part of the reals could not have been excluded as an explanation. Artifacts may have produced simulators' reports of anosmic responding that were identical to the reports of the reals, but the reals may also have been genuinely unable to smell any of the odors! The EEG criteria used in the study provided an outcome of testing hypnotic performance, whereas the real–simulator model played a secondary role in the experiment; it served to help minimize the probability of introducing procedural biases.

Final Remarks

The most clever research design cannot compensate for failure to take a comprehensive approach in planning an investigation. Such rigor may impede the flow of studies, but the final result may serve to propel hypnosis research to new levels of strong inference.

Design sensitivity is a primary consideration. The alternative approaches to statistical power analysis discussed in this chapter may help the researcher to determine how many subjects must be run to give the hypothesis of interest a fair chance of being supported. However, power analysis should be viewed as only one guiding consideration. The approach is inaccurate for the small sample sizes available in clinical settings, so investigators are cautioned not to be discouraged from making potential inquiries on this basis alone.

Research subjects vary. The five distinctly different types of subjects discussed can greatly influence the results of an investigation. The ideal "scientist subject" can be cultivated in both clinical and experimental laboratory settings by forming an investigator–subject partnership aimed at producing the most accurate data. Generalizability of the results obtained in laboratory settings using college student populations must be addressed in studies aimed at clinical utility. The data on subject self-selection and volunteering behavior should be considered at both the planning stage and the interpretation-of-results stage. Procedures that provide opportunities for all subjects to participate in the treatment of interest can minimize, if not eliminate, one major source of self-selection confounds.

IRB recommendations and safeguards for risks to subjects can influence a study's procedure, design, and inferences to be drawn. Rare problems occurring in clinical settings have been misgeneralized to research with college students, where risks have been demonstrated to be minimal. Consideration of risks to subjects should always be addressed by reference to the specific sample under consideration. The use of well-trained hypnotist/researchers, and emphasis on a clearly defined end to the hypnotic experience (without suggestions about potential difficulties), both help to minimize the potential for problems.

Unwitting cues of the experimental context must always represent an alternative hypothesis to be considered. Conclusions about effects of context are difficult to draw, because contextual cues exist at a merely correlative level with the intervention of interest. Attempts to replicate classic studies of context effects have yielded mixed results. The effects of experimental demand cues and situational variables appear to be most likely to produce significant effects when such cues are consistent with the general sociopsychological context. Since experimental demand cues cannot be eliminated, researchers should consider their deliberate manipulation to help determine whether their effects confound a particular investigation.

Within-groups and real–simulator research designs seem to be particularly powerful approaches to some of the problems facing hypnosis researchers. Despite some unique limitations, the real–simulator design is particularly appropriate for studies attempting to focus on the veridicality of hypnosis as free from artifact as possible. The real–simulator design is also adaptable to studies such as those involving pain reports, where the simulation must be incomplete. Clinical research, based on observations of patients' responses following the hypnotic induction, served as the original basis for systematic experimental hypnosis research. Clinical studies that include the key elements required for publishability continue to fill lacunae, to generate curiosity, and to produce testable hypotheses.

Acknowledgments

We thank Helen Crawford, Peter Suedfeld, and Dennis Warner for their comments on a preliminary draft of this chapter. Research conducted by ourselves and cited herein was supported in part by the New Zealand Antarctic Research Program; the Department of Psychology, University of Canterbury–New Zealand; the National Science Foundation; the National Aeronautics and Space Administration; and Harvard University.

CHAPTER EIGHT

Hypnosis as a Methodology in Psychological Research

JEAN HOLROYD

The history of hypnosis as a research method is intertwined with the investigation of hypnosis itself. The hypnosis method has generally been used to create special effects (e.g., to induce emotion, amnesia, or relaxation), although it is increasingly being used as an approach that is complementary to other experimental psychology methods. Scientists who understand how hypnosis can be used to explore other content areas in experimental psychology and neuroscience are in a position to investigate a wider range of human phenomena. Given the historical contributions of hypnosis as a research method dating to the earliest years of experimental psychology (e.g., Bernheim, 1886/1887; Hull, 1933), it is shocking to learn that hypnosis is not on a recent list of "must know" words for psychology students (Boneau, 1990)!

In exploring how a researcher might use hypnosis, it becomes important to distinguish between a number of closely related experimental manipulations: neutral hypnosis, hypnotic suggestion, and waking suggestion. For example, amnesia was taken to be an effect of (neutral) hypnosis per se in earlier times, whereas it is now attributed to hypnotic suggestion (E. R. Hilgard, 1977b) or to strategic enactment (Spanos, 1986b). Moreover, hypnosis, suggestion, and motivation effects are often confounded, so that what may appear to be an effect of hypnosis may be an effect of waking suggestion or of motivational instructions. The principal question of the present chapter is this: If there are predictable changes associated with hypnosis, how might they be exploited by psychologists, sociologists, and physiologists in their respective areas of research?

In previous discussions of this nature, use of the hypnotic method was predicated upon general impressions of how behavior might be influenced by hypnosis. At various times, hypnosis has been said to increase suggestibility, perceived involuntariness, vividness of imagery, fantasy, imagination, dissociation, mind–body interaction, lateralization of brain function, access to memories, amnesia, absorption, sense of relaxation, confidence, strategic social enactment, and role enactment or "as if" behavior; to cause changes in attention, awareness, the stream of consciousness, sense of time, and the hypnotic relationship; to make information processing less sequential and chronological; and to decrease intention or desire to make and carry out plans, sense of executive identity, reality awareness, and reality testing (P. G. Bowers & Bowers, 1979; D. P. Brown & Fromm, 1986; Frumkin, Ripley, & Cox, 1978; E. R. Hilgard, 1977b; Holroyd, 1985–1986; MacLeod-Morgan & Lack, 1982; Sarbin & Coe, 1972; Sheehan & McConkey, 1982; Shor, 1962; Spanos, 1982b; Spanos, Radtke, & Dubreuil, 1982). A careful consideration of research developments in the last decade should lead us to qualify this list, and permits us to be more specific about how the changes inherent in hypnosis can benefit the research endeavor.

The present chapter also considers hypnotizability as a person variable, because experimental results often depend upon subjects' responsiveness. In fact, for some investigations it may be more important to have subjects who are preselected for hypnotizability than to do a hypnotic induction procedure. The distinction among experimental effects attributable to a personality trait (i.e., hypnotizability), those attributable to hypnosis context (i.e., an induction), and those attributable to the interaction between the two is particularly important in using hypnosis as a research strategy. Effects of the interaction have been shown to be very important in the psychology of personality (Tellegen, 1981), attention (Pekala & Kumar, 1987–1988), learning (Crawford, Allen, & Kiefner, 1983), cognition (Coe, Basden, Basden, Fikes, Gargano, & Webb, 1989), and physiology (Gruzelier, Brow, Perry, Rhonder, & Thomas, 1984).

This survey of representative contemporary literature is intended to demonstrate how hypnotic inductions (and waking suggestions) may be used as experimental manipulations. This chapter is concerned with how hypnosis can be used to study behavior, physiology, and cognition. For convenience, the chapter is organized according to four types of effects one could expect hypnosis to provide: changes in suggestibility, imagery, mind–body relationship, and cognition.

Suggestibility

People tend to be more responsive to suggestions following a hypnotic induction than in normal conditions and to describe their behavior as nonvoluntary—a combination known as the "classic suggestion effect" (Weitzenhoffer, 1980). Expectations and commitment to the experience account for much of the increased response to hypnotic suggestions (Spanos, 1986c). The tendency for at least some people to be more responsive to suggestion following a hypnotic induction has been used to explore a number of traditional subject domains in experimental psychology, such as sensation and perception, attitude change, learning, and social processes. Increasing the power of suggestions by using a hypnotic induction is useful when it is expected that a particular communication should affect subjects' behavior, cognitions, or physiology. However, even waking suggestion is a potent experimental manipulation, and simply putting subjects into a "hypnosis group" is a potent form of suggestion.

Four contemporary investigations illustrate how hypnosis has been used for its suggestibility-enhancing characteristic to investigate a range of behavioral and attitudinal phenomena. In this approach, hypnotic suggestion is used to modify the behavioral or attitudinal characteristics of subjects. These investigations also provide an opportunity to discuss some of the experimental controls needed for drawing unambiguous conclusions when using hypnosis is used as a research method.

A. F. Barabasz (1980b) used hypnotic suggestion to influence vigilance performance in a radar target detection task. Navy volunteers were randomly assigned to four groups: hypnosis with a suggestion to augment vigilance; hypnosis with a suggestion to decrease vigilance; hypnosis with no vigilance suggestion; and a usual-activities control group. Suggestions to improve vigilance reduced errors, whereas other experimental manipulations increased errors, compared to those of controls. Hypnotizability correlated significantly with reductions in error scores ($r = .68$) for the suggested-improvement group. Thus vigilance performance was strongly influenced by hypnotic suggestion, especially for hypnotically responsive people. Other control groups would have provided additional information. If there had been a waking-suggestion control group, we would know whether the experimental effect was a result of *hypnotically* increased suggestibility rather than waking suggestion, and if there had been a task motivation group, we would know whether the effect was a result of suggestion or simply of trying harder. Since each group's hypnotized performance was compared to the group's own waking baseline performance rather than to the performance of a simulator group (Orne, 1979a), it is possible that the results were a function of changes the subjects expected to obtain from hypnotic suggestions. Nonetheless, the hypnosis experimental manipulation did modify the behavioral attributes of subjects differentially.

Hypnosis also can be used to increase the frequency of a particular behavior under investigation. M. A. Kelly, McKinty, and Carr (1988) gave both hypnotized and waking subjects one session of suggestions about flossing their teeth. After 8 months the gingival health of the experimental group had improved, whereas that of the control group had deteriorated. We would understand more about this behavior change if hypnotizability had been measured. The increase in flossing could have resulted from expectations and motivation based on being in a hypnosis condition, or from an interaction between personality and hypnosis condition. The importance of measuring hypnotizability is illustrated even better by the next example, in which hypnosis was used to modify the attitudes of research subjects.

Malott, Bourg, and Crawford (1989) investigated college students' responses to a taped message advocating a pregraduation comprehensive examination. Low and high hypnotizable subjects in hypnosis or waking conditions listened to the recording and then wrote down the thoughts that they had had while listening. Subjects in the hypnosis condition agreed more with the message than did waking-suggestion subjects (a hypnosis context effect). Also, highs agreed more with the message than lows (an individual-difference effect). However, none of the interaction effects were significant. That is, subjects who were in the hypnosis condition *and* were highly hypnotizable were not persuaded more than the other three groups. When one is using hypnosis as a method of investigation, one can obtain effects that are not necessarily results of increased suggestibility following an induction.

Even when it appears that suggestibility accounts for positive results following a hypnotic induction (the interaction effect), other factors may be more important. Van Denberg and Kurtz (1989) examined whether a suggestion that was relegated to the unconscious by virtue of hypnotically suggested amnesia would be more potent than a suggestion that remained in conscious memory (Erickson & Erickson, 1944; Sheehan & Orne, 1968). They evaluated the proposition by giving women positive suggestions for changes in attitudes toward their bodies under different conditions. The women were divided into five groups: high hypnotizables with and without amnesia suggestions; low hypnotizables simulating hypnosis with and without amnesia; and high hypnotizables who remembered the positive suggestions despite suggested amnesia. High hypnotizables who were amnesic for the positive suggestions reported the most positive self-image changes, whereas high hypnotizables for whom the amnesia suggestion broke down reported the fewest changes. Hence, those expected to be most suggestible (highs in hypnosis) became least suggestible if they experienced spontaneous breeching of amnesia. The results are concordant with self-efficacy theory (Bandura, 1982), suggesting that feelings of self-efficacy promoted by passing hypnosis items mediate a positive response to later suggestions. The results also indicate that subjects who are unable to respond positively to a suggestion may become less responsive to other suggestions that are part of the experimental manipulation.

The foregoing investigations used hypnosis for its behavior- or attitude-enhancing effects. They were well designed compared to most in the literature; yet, although suggestion effects were demonstrated, we usually cannot rule out the possibility that an experimental effect might have been attributable to personality or to the mystique implicit in a hypnotic induction. An effect also might have been observable with waking suggestions. This underscores that in any research employing hypnosis, it is important to measure hypnotizability; to use contrasting conditions in order to account for hypnosis versus waking suggestion or heightened motivation; and to allow for the possibility of interactions between personality trait and hypnotic condition.

If we accept that hypnotic inductions lead to increased suggestibility (E. R. Hilgard & Tart, 1966; Weitzenhoffer & Sjoberg, 1961) or increased role enactment (Sarbin, 1950, 1989), then the greatest experimental effects can be expected from high hypnotizable subjects in a hypnosis condition. Not everyone shows increases in suggestibility following a hypnotic induction, however (E. R. Hilgard & Tart, 1966). Success with suggestions may depend upon the nature and extent of subjects' previous experiences with the type of phenomenon being suggested (for examples, see P. G. Bowers, Laurence, & Hart, 1988; Raynaud, Michaux, Bleirad, Capderou, Bordachar, & Durand, 1984; Spanos, Stenstrom, & Johnston, 1988). Success and failure with suggestions may increase or decrease the power of other suggestions that are intended to be experimental manipulations (Van Denberg & Kurtz, 1989). Furthermore, many experimental effects attributed to hypnotic suggestion are obtainable with unhypnotized (but highly hypnotizable) subjects or with specially motivated subjects. Finally, when hypnosis is being used for its suggestion effect, it may be advisable to have subjects rate the extent to which their behavior during hypnosis was experienced as nonvolitional. P. G. Bowers et al. (1988) found that people rated only about a third of the suggestions they passed as happening nonvoluntarily rather than being enacted, while another 48% were rated as partly nonvoluntary.

Given the exquisite sensitivity of high hypnotizables to expectancy manipulations (Kirsch & Council, 1989), the enlightened researcher will also be alert to the possibility of waking-suggestion effects on such subjects for *any* communications in the research situation, including instructions, admonitions, and screening procedures.

Imagery

Hypnosis purportedly enhances imagery, and for that reason hypnosis has been used in research where imagery is an important part of a psychological process. For example, imagery has been considered important in therapy (J. R. Hilgard & LeBaron, 1984; Reyher & Smeltzer, 1968; M. R. Nash, 1988; Sheikh & Jordan, 1983), creativity, and problem solving (Adams, 1974; Barrios & Singer, 1981–1982; Dave, 1979; Ernest, 1977; S. Sanders, 1976, 1978). Recent research suggests that hypnosis does not necessarily enhance imagery vividness,[1] and yet the more complex relationship between hypnosis and imagery that is emerging is creating even more opportunities for research.

It has become apparent that much of the presumed experimental effect of hypnosis on imagery is a function of the superior imaging ability of high hypnotizables, with or without hypnosis.[2] The consensus is that highs generally report rich and vivid imagery, but that lows vary and may report good or poor imagery. The researcher wishing to use hypnosis as a methodology should realize that vivid imagery is generally necessary for hypnosis (see reviews by de Groh, 1989; Spanos & Flynn, 1989b) and for improving hypnotizability (Cross & Spanos, 1988-1989). However, this does not mean that the imagery reports of highs have been described as any more vivid than those of lows in a simple eyes-closed condition (Pekala & Bieber, 1989–1990; Pekala & Kumar, 1989).[3]

It has been said that the imaging abilities of high hypnotizables may reflect fundamental differences in cognitive style, particularly in the early stages of imagery-mediated information processing. Thus highs have shown differences from lows in gestalt closure, visual illusion reversals, afterimage perseveration, and rapid visual perception even in the absence of hypnosis (Acosta & Crawford, 1985; Priebe & Wallace, 1986; Saccuzzo, Safran, Anderson, & McNeill, 1982; B. Wallace, 1988, 1990a; B. Wallace & Patterson, 1984; see also Crawford, 1981). Nadon, Laurence, and Perry (1987) suggested that preference for the use of imagery in cognitive activities, not stronger imagery per se, is the salient characteristic of highs. Kearns and Zamansky (1984) suggested that highs simply have more ability to expand imaginatively upon verbal input, but the results of research testing this proposition are mixed (t'Hoen, 1978; Kearns & Zamansky, 1984; Sweeney, Lynn, & Bellezza, 1986).

Given the evidence for different imagery-mediated cognitive abilities in high and low hypnotizable subjects, it has proved fruitful to investigate imagery-related cognitive processing using highs and lows, in and out of hypnosis. Hypnotized highs performed better than a nonhypnotized control group composed of both highs and lows on speed of visual information processing (Friedman, Taub, Sturr, & Monty, 1987). Highs in hypnosis performed better than in a waking condition, and better than lows in either a waking or a hypnosis condition (the interaction effect) on a number of imagery-mediated information-processing tasks: perception of stereograms (Crawford, Wallace, Nomura, & Slater, 1986); visual signal detection (R. P. Atkinson, 1990); and visual memory discrimination (Crawford & Allen, 1983). Theories of cognitive processing will need to account for these interaction effects.

In contrast, several studies have found that highs exhibit more perceptual interference than lows, *especially* in hypnosis or in what amounts to a low-signal condition (M. Dixon, Brunet, & Laurence, 1990; Blatt, Dixon, & Laurence, 1990; Sheehan, Donovan, & MacLeod, 1988). For example, highs may exhibit more automatic processing of an iconic (image-dominated) memory in tasks where automaticity interferes with performance, as in the Stroop phenomenon.[4] Research on the retention of high-

and low-imagery paired-associate words in and out of hypnosis has produced mixed results (Crawford, Allen, & Kiefner, 1983; Sweeney et al., 1986). Friedman, Taub, Sturr, and Monty (1990) proposed that differences between highs and lows may not be observed with complex cognitive tasks, but may be found in more basic perceptual processes.

Hypnosis offers an opportunity to alter parameters of cognitive and physiological functioning *temporarily,* for a dynamic approach to classical psychological problems implicating imagery processes.[5] High hypnotic responsivity may lead to superior performance in the earliest stage of visual information processing (Friedman et al., 1987), especially when the information is literal or untransformed (Crawford, Wallace, et al., 1986). Hypnosis then may enhance holistic processing, perhaps through greater right-hemisphere involvement (e.g., Crawford & Allen, 1983; Crawford, Nomura, & Slater, 1983; Gruzelier et al., 1984; see also Crawford & Gruzelier, Chapter 9, this volume). It should be noted that hypnosis-related changes resulted in poorer inhibition of competing visual stimuli in the Stroop test, but facilitated visual signal detection, perception of stereograms, speed of visual information processing, and visual memory discrimination.

As the above-cited studies suggest, exploiting hypnosis-related changes in imagery processing enriches research in cognitive psychology (e.g., lateralization of brain function and information processing) and in perception (e.g., signal detection, synesthesia, the Stroop effect, and illusions). The associated changes in imagery processing are more complex than simply changes in vividness, which heretofore was the principal attribute of interest. In effect, the opportunity for using hypnosis as a research method has broadened as our understanding of the relationship between hypnosis and imagery has deepened.

The role of imagery when hypnosis is used for the manipulation of physiological states is another important area of research. For example, remission of warts following hypnosis has been attributed to more intense sensory imagery, such as tingling (Spanos, Williams, & Gwynn, 1990). This leads us into a discussion of hypnosis as a research method in the area of psychosomatic and psychoneuroimmunological phenomena.

Mind–Body Relationship

Across centuries and cultures, we find a belief that the mind can cure illness, and psychoneuroimmunology has given some credence to the concept of mental healing (Ader, Felton, & Cohen, 1990; Geiser, 1989; Solomon & Amkraut, 1981). Hypnosis has been used to evaluate whether the belief in mental healing is warranted, and more broadly to explore how mind can influence matter. Hypnosis and suggestion have demonstrated remarkable clinical effects (see reviews by T. X. Barber, 1984; DePiano &

Salzberg, 1979; E. R. Hilgard & Hilgard, 1983; Mott, 1979; Paul, 1963; Perry, Gelfand, & Marcovitch, 1979). Unfortunately, clinical investigations have usually not been designed in ways permitting unambiguous conclusions about the manner in which mind has influenced body. Often it is not clear whether the outcome was a result of hypnosis, relaxation, education, emotional support, or expectancy (Paul, 1969; Stam, McGrath, Brooke, & Cosier, 1986; Swirsky-Sacchetti & Margolis, 1986).

A few investigators have found that the physiological effects of hypnotic suggestions are more powerful than those of relaxation (Gruzelier & Brow, 1985; Pagano, Akots, & Wall, 1988) and are not simply the result of subject expectancy (Spanos, Williams, & Gwynn, 1990). Hence, hypnosis may be the method of choice if an investigator wishes to maximize physiological responses in order to study mind–body phenomena. Physiological responses to hypnotic suggestions may be regarded as a variant of the "classic suggestion effect," especially since most suggestions for physiological changes cannot be enacted voluntarily. The causal relationships are not yet clear, but a few theorists have tentatively proposed mechanisms (e.g., Kissin, 1986; E. L. Rossi & Cheek, 1988; Wagner & Khanna, 1986).

Clinical improvement attributable to hypnosis probably results from an interaction among a number of cascading psychophysiological events. Research on a viral disease, the common wart (recently reviewed by R. F. Q. Johnson, 1989), provides a model for how hypnosis may be useful as a research methodology to investigate relevant physiological processes. Hypnosis has been used both to establish the fact that people can mentally banish their own warts, and to explore how those beneficial results may come about. Warts have offered a good treatment model, because afflicted populations are readily available and results are more easily evaluated than for many pathological conditions. Furthermore, researchers have used hypnosis to investigate mental control of physiological mechanisms that may relate to mentally shrinking or obliterating warts (blood flow, coagulation, and immunology).

Two remarkable studies have documented warts' being removed selectively from one part of the body by means of hypnotic suggestions (Noll, 1988; Sinclair-Gieben & Chalmers, 1959).[6] These case studies indicate that the hypnotized person can target physiological changes associated with healing to specific locations of the body; the person does not just create system-wide changes, as would be expected with relaxation. The drama of these two cases is reinforced by a large-scale study that controlled for placebo-induced expectancy and waking suggestion (Spanos, Williams, & Gwynn, 1990). Subjects in three treatment groups received either hypnosis, a topical medication (salicylic acid), or a topical placebo medication. Only the hypnosis subjects lost significantly more warts than subjects in a no-treatment control group. Success was associated with more vivid suggested imagery (e.g., sensations of tingling), though not with higher hypnotizability. Since imagery often implicates a specific corporeal location, targeting physiological changes to one area of the body may depend on hypnotic imagery.

The actual death of warts may result from the combined effects of hypnotically restricted blood supply and hypnotically improved immunity (Ullman, 1959; Birkett, 1982). Hypnosis has in fact been used to demonstrate how the mind can affect blood supply, blood-clotting mechanisms, and the immune response. Interaction among these three factors not only could account for warts disappearing, but also could explain localized effects.

Blood Supply and Clotting

There are case reports of hypnotic suggestion preventing people from bleeding to death (Bishay, Stevens, & Lee, 1984; Fredericks, 1967). Dentists who use hypnosis have claimed that it helps stem blood loss (e.g., Newman, 1971), and there is supportive evidence from a controlled intervention (Chaves, 1980, cited in T. X. Barber, 1984). Paul (1963) concluded after reviewing the literature that vasoconstriction and dilation could be influenced by both hypnosis and waking suggestion. In fact, people can voluntarily warm one hand while cooling the other by means of hypnosis (Bishay & Lee, 1984; Maslach, Marshall, & Zimbardo, 1972; Roberts, Kewman, & Macdonald, 1973). In one person with Raynaud's disease (attacks of poor circulation in the hands), a fourfold increase in finger blood volume was produced within 45 seconds following a hypnotic suggestion (Conn & Mott, 1984). Thus, in addition to a targeted physiological response, hypnosis can create a rapid physiological response.

Researchers may wish to use waking suggestion rather than hypnosis to study how thinking about physiological changes brings them about. Subjects receiving waking suggestions for wart removal did as well as those receiving hypnotic suggestions (Spanos, Stenstrom, & Johnston, 1988). Bennett, Benson, and Kuiken (1986) used waking suggestion with spinal surgery patients to control blood loss. The waking-suggestion subjects were told, "the blood will move away from your back, beginning now and continuing through your operation." The suggestion subjects lost approximately half as much blood as the control and relaxation groups. As the authors noted, it is not clear whether suggestions altered vasoconstriction or the clotting mechanism.

Hypnosis has been used as a method to investigate mental control over blood clotting in severe hemophilia (Swirsky-Sacchetti & Margolis, 1986). A hypnosis treatment group used less clotting factor concentrate compared to baseline levels, while the waiting-list group used more. There was a significant correlation ($p = .56$) between self-hypnosis practice and change scores, although treatment effect and hypnotizability were uncorrelated. Since the treatment group received a multimodal intervention (education in stress management, deep relaxation, and hypnosis; tape-assisted self-hypnosis training), we cannot be sure that hypnosis per se reduced blood loss. In research like this, contrasting hypnosis and suggestion with other treatments such as relaxation would offer more opportunity for understanding the mechanisms of change.

Immunology

The proposition that the mind may positively influence the body's defense systems has been investigated through the use of hypnosis with viral disease (warts), allergens, and burns, as well as through a few experiments in which hypnotic suggestion was used to manipulate the immune system directly. Black, Humphrey, and Niven (1963) showed that the Mantoux reaction to tuberculin could be inhibited by direct suggestion under hypnosis in highly hypnotizable Mantoux-positive subjects. Zachariae, Bjerring, and Arendt-Nielsen (1989) had highly hypnotizable subjects increase the Mantoux reaction in one arm and decrease it in the other arm, using guided imagery, extensive hypnotic suggestions, and daily audiotaped hypnotic suggestions. Three days later the difference between arms in erythema area was 35% and in palpated induration was 84%; control subjects exhibited no such differences. The same highly hypnotizable subjects were able to inhibit the immediate response to histamine skin prick by 41% compared to their own baseline levels, whereas control subjects exhibited no significant difference. Neither Black et al. (1963) nor Zachariae et al. (1989) attempted to determine whether waking suggestion would be just as effective as hypnotic suggestion.

Other investigations suggest that hypnosis may be useful for exploring "learned" psychosomatic associations and the limiting conditions for mental cures. At least two careful attempts to replicate the Black et al. (1963) experiment have not met with success (Beahrs, Harris, & Hilgard, 1970; Locke, Ransil, Covino, Toczydlowski, Lohse, Dvorak, Arndt, & Frankel, 1987). Locke et al. (1987) speculated that since Black et al.'s work involved people with histories of psychosomatic disorders, it might be necessary to use that type of subject. In a similar vein, Spanos and Chaves (1989b) noted that hypnotic treatment of warts is more effective with severe cases than with light cases. They speculated that successful wart removal may relate to more pathogens in the body. However, it is also possible that the pathological condition of warts is associated with thinking about (imaging?) affected areas more intensively, which may contribute to better mind–body communication. Raynaud et al. (1984) noted that even among highly hypnotizable subjects, only some were able to lower core body temperature while raising skin temperature. E. L. Rossi (1989) has suggested that physiological responsivity may be more important than hypnotic responsivity for mind to influence body.

For the most part, research in psychoneuroimmunology has focused on a stress model and breakdown in normal protective functions (Ader et al., 1990). Hypnosis offers a method for experimentally improving healing processes, not just interfering with them. For example, hypnosis has resulted in enhancement of immune system components: beta-endorphin-like immunoreactive material in the blood of arthritic pain patients (Domangue, Margolis, Lieberman, & Kaji, 1985); B cells, white blood cells, and (not significantly) lymphocyte count for young highly hypnotizable volunteers (Hall, 1982–1983; Hall, Longos, & Dixon, 1981); and salivary immunoglobulin A in children (Olness, Culbert, & Uden, 1989). A clinical investigation showed that women with terminal cancer who attended group therapy and learned self-hypnosis for pain reduction lived almost twice as long as a control group (D. Spiegel, Bloom, Kraemer, & Gottheil, 1989; see Stam, 1989, for a critical review of the scant literature on hypnosis used as an immunological treatment for cancer). Attempts to increase immunological response with other kinds of psychological methods have also been successful (Futterman, 1990), so it remains to be seen whether hypnosis and suggestion will continue to be the most potent methods for effecting such changes.

It may be that the attractiveness of hypnosis for experimental investigation of the mind–body connection has to do with a well- established complementary relationship between clinical reports and laboratory research. There is a vast body of clinical literature to which controlled laboratory studies can be related. For example, hypnosis has been shown to be clinically effective in limiting the pathological response to burns, thereby preventing tissue damage (Ewin, 1986a,b; reviewed by Patterson, Questad, & Boltwood, 1987). In a now-classic study, Chapman, Goodell, and Wolff (1959) demonstrated that hypnotic suggestions could augment or diminish the histamine-mediated inflammatory response to burns created with a standarized heat stimulus. (Histamine dilates blood vessels, reduces blood pressure, stimulates gastric secretions, and causes uterine contractions.)

Another use of hypnosis methodology in this area is found in the literature on gastrointestinal changes. Whorwell, Prior, and Faragher (1984) showed that hypnotherapy was more beneficial than psychotherapy plus placebos for patients with severe irritable bowel syndrome. Outcome measures included abdominal pain, bowel habits, abdominal distension, and sense of well-being. (Since hypnotizability was not measured, we lack information about whether people who were responsive to hypnosis benefited more.) In an experimental analogue, Klein and Spiegel (1989) examined stimulation and inhibition of gastric acid secretion in highly hypnotizable subjects. When suggestions were given to imagine eating delicious meals, acid output rose 89%. When hypnotic suggestions to relax and not think about hunger were given, there was a 39% reduction in basal acid output and an 11% reduction in pentagastrin-stimulated peak acid output compared to the nonhypnosis condition. Klein and Spiegel (1989) provide an example of how hypnosis may be used as a safe and simple method for studying the central nervous system (CNS) mechanisms in digestive processes. The research also illustrates how hypnosis may be used both to increase and to reduce a physiological response to mental or physical stimulation.

An unexplored application for hypnosis in clinical research would be to use it to create a very powerful placebo control group. Would a new medication for irritable bowel syndrome outperform hypnosis or a placebo plus hypnosis in responsive individuals? Given the strong effects associated with the personality variable of hypnotizability, would a hypnotizability measure improve the prediction of who will benefit from medication?[7]

The role of hypnotizability continues to be an important issue when hypnosis is used as an experimental method for psychosomatic phenomena. When attempting to create an effect for subsequent study, the researcher probably should consider using subjects selected for hypnotizability and, where appropriate, subjects who have had experience with the physiological phenomena of interest. When unselected subjects are used, a measure of hypnotizability can provide information about possible mechanisms of action; for example, Collison (1975) found that asthmatics' response to hypnotherapy related to hypnotizability.

When the hypnosis methodology is used for psychosomatic phenomena, it may not be important whether the hypnosis intervention is actually called "hypnosis." In a controlled study, Kohen (1985) found that children with asthma who learned relaxation/mental imagery (self-hypnosis) benefited significantly more at a 1-year follow-up than did children in the waking suggestion, attention placebo, or pure control groups. (It should be noted that this study would seem to suggest that hypnotic suggestion, not waking suggestion, is the critical contributor to benefits for asthmatics.)

Pain

The vast literature on hypnotic pain control is a foundation for using hypnosis to study pain itself, although most pain–hypnosis investigations have been designed to increase our understanding of hypnosis rather than our understanding of pain. To the degree that hypnotic pain control entails mechanisms of action different from those involved in medication, acupuncture, biofeedback, relaxation training, or electrical stimulation, it offers a new perspective and different information. For example, hypnotic analgesia is rapidly reversible, offering a model to contrast with more long-acting analgesic procedures such as medication.

Hypnotic suggestion frequently reduces pain to a significant degree (E. R. Hilgard & Hilgard, 1983; J. R. Hilgard & LeBaron, 1982; D. Spiegel &

Bloom, 1983; Zeltzer, Fanurik, & LeBaron, 1989; Zeltzer & LeBaron, 1982). For experimental pain in one study it was more effective than a placebo, and at least as effective as morphine and acupuncture (J. A. Stern, Brown, Ulett, & Sletten, 1977); it was more effective than acupuncture for highs but not lows in another study (Knox, Gekoski, Shum, & McLaughlin, 1981). A third study found that it was more effective than waking suggestion, relaxation, and even a guided-imagery hypnotic induction that lacked specific analgesia suggestions (Van Gorp, Meyer, & Dunbar, 1985). However, Houle, McGrath, Moran, and Garrett (1988) found relaxation and hypnosis-induced analgesia to be equally effective for electrical tooth pulp stimulation; and a number of investigators have reported that for clinical pain hypnosis is no more effective than a variety of other psychological interventions (E. Katz, Kellerman, & Ellenberg, 1987; Spinhoven, 1988; Spinhoven & Linssen, 1989; Stam, McGrath, & Brooke, 1984). A review by Spanos (1986b) indicated that waking suggestion and a variety of other strategies may result in as much pain reduction as hypnosis. At the very least, these studies indicate that investigations of pain experience and behavior could include waking suggestion as well as hypnotic suggestion, although as Stam (1989) indicates, equivalence of outcome does not indicate equivalence of mechanism.

Among other things, the pain–hypnosis research suggests that many investigations of psychological pain control that do not use hypnosis or suggestion would nevertheless benefit from measuring hypnotizability. Amount of pain reduction produced by psychological procedures has correlated with hypnotizability whether or not there was a hypnotic induction (Reeves, Redd, Storm, & Minagawa, 1983; Spanos, Kennedy, & Gwynn, 1984; Spinhoven, 1988; Stam et al., 1986; Tenenbaum, Kurtz, & Bienias, 1990).[8]

Pain research using hypnosis has contributed to distinctions between the effects of suggestion, distraction, compliance, expectancy, and cognitive strategies (Farthing et al., 1983; M. E. Miller & Bowers, 1986; Stam et al., 1986; Stam & Spanos, 1980; but see Spanos, Perlini, & Robertson, 1989). It has fostered the distinction between a general relaxation effect benefiting all subjects and a specific effect of dissociation that is observed with highly hypnotizable subjects (E. R. Hilgard, 1974, 1975).[9] It has also sharpened a distinction between sensory and affective components of pain (Price & Barber, 1987). Hypnotic analgesia suggestions have been found to reduce pain intensity but not unpleasantness, and hypnotic relaxation suggestions have been determined to reduce unpleasantness but not intensity of pain (Malone et al., 1989). These distinctions arise in part because hypnosis represents a mix of pain-relevant psychological processes different from that in other psychological approaches, such as biofeedback and relaxation. The difference in processes is a basis for expecting unique contributions to our understanding of pain and pain control when hypnosis is used as a research method.

There is some indication that hypnotic analgesia may entail CNS inhibitory processes. Karlin, Morgan, and Goldstein (1980) found that contralateral occipital–temporal electroencephalographic (EEG) activation, which was correlated with reported pain ($r = .56$) during cold pressor stimulation of the arm, was not seen in highs given hypnotic analgesia suggestions. (The usual activation pattern was seen in moderates.) Chen, Dworkin, and Bloomquist (1981) observed reduction in overall cortical activation during hypnosis for surgery, with a shift away from left-hemisphere dominance. It is interesting that hypnotic analgesia, unlike acupuncture, does not appear to be mediated by CNS opiate processes (J. Barber & Mayer, 1977; Goldstein & Hilgard, 1975). By inference, hypnosis is probably associated with neurophysiological events different from those involved in acupuncture, and perhaps from those involved in other pain control techniques such as biofeedback. Potentially, hypnosis could be useful as a method to investigate CNS changes associated with mental control of pain.

Central Nervous System Effects

CNS effects associated with hypnosis and hypnotizability are emerging as the neurosciences develop new assessment procedures. Earlier efforts to identify CNS indicators of a hypnotic state or condition essentially failed (Sarbin & Slagle, 1979). Now Gruzelier and his colleagues claim to have demonstrated electrophysiolgical evidence of an altered state associated with hypnosis (Gruzelier & Brow, 1985; Gruzelier et al., 1984; Gruzelier, Allison, & Conway, 1988; Gruzelier, 1988; Gruzelier, Thomas, Conway, Liddiard, Jutai, McCormack, Golds, Perry, Rhonder, & Brow, 1987). The current literature suggests that hypnosis may be useful as a nonintrusive method to study shifts in cerebral activity patterns accompanying shifts in psychological activity.

As in other research areas, it is necessary to distinguish the CNS conditions associated with a hypnotizable personality from those associated with a hypnotic induction. High hypnotizables are generally less aroused, as evidenced by greater prevalence of alpha EEG, less fast EEG activity (40 Hz), and lower tonic skin conductance (A. F. Barabasz, 1983; Gruzelier & Brow, 1985; De Pascalis, Marucci, Penna, & Pessa, 1987; De Pascalis & Penna, 1990; De Pascalis, Silveri, & Palumbo, 1988). Moreover, highs may show waking EEG laterality patterns different from those of lows during emotion or task performance (De Pascalis & Palumbo, 1986; De Pascalis et al., 1987). Greater CNS asymmetry for highs is reflected in galvanic skin response (GSR) and manual object-sorting time (Gruzelier & Brow, 1985; Gruzelier et al., 1984).

In addition to baseline differences, high hypnotizables show changes in CNS functioning as they enter hypnosis. Alpha density is higher (reviewed by De Pascalis & Penna, 1990), although there is no change in total

EEG spectrum power (Edmonston & Moscovitz, 1990). The GSR habituates faster and there is lower skin conductance, suggesting less sympathetic nervous system activity (Gruzelier et al., 1987; Gruzelier, 1988). The differences between highs and lows during hypnosis are particularly evident while subjects are engaging in hemisphere-relevant tasks. EEG lateralization ratios during these tasks generally shift for highs more than for lows (De Pascalis & Penna, 1990; LaBriola & Karlin, 1984; Mészáros, Bányai, & Greguss, 1985). GSR lateral dominance shifts from left hand to right hand, and manual object-sorting time lateral preference also shifts (Gruzelier & Brow, 1985; Gruzelier et al., 1984).

Although hypnosis has been described as a right-hemisphere function (MacLeod-Morgan & Lack, 1982; reviewed by Edmonston & Moscovitz, 1990), the relative increase in right-hemisphere activity may be due to a reduction in left-hemisphere influence (Edmonston & Moscovitz, 1990; Gruzelier & Brow, 1985; Zaidel, Clarke, & Suyenobu, 1990; Zeig, 1978; Chen et al., 1981). Gott, Hughes, and Whipple (1984) reported an interesting case of a woman who could shift voluntarily between two states of consciousness that were reflected in EEG lateralization measures. The rapidly accumulating evidence of cortical changes during hypnosis suggests that hypnosis may be used to study functional cerebral dominance in a variety of standard laboratory tasks.

Functional cerebral dominance is often studied with laboratory perception tasks such as dichotic listening, in which subjects respond to discrepant auditory material stimulating each ear. The shifts in functional lateral dominance associated with hypnosis make it a logical method to be used along with the dichotic listening paradigm. To date, experiments employing hypnosis have yielded interesting albeit conflicting results, with gender, handedness, and hypnotizability interacting to determine right-ear or left-ear preference (Frumkin et al., 1978; Pagano et al., 1988; Spellacy & Wilkinson, 1987; Zaidel et al., 1990). In fact, Spellacy and Wilkinson (1987) have suggested that much of the atypical ear preference shown in dichotic listening experiments that do not employ hypnosis may reflect the variability of high hypnotizables in different states of consciousness! As I have observed regarding the literature on psychological control of pain, measures of hypnotizability may prove useful even if the experiment itself does not use hypnosis.

Functional independence and interdependence of the cerebral hemispheres are of current interest in cognitive neuroscience (Zaidel et al., 1990). The functional role of the hemispheres has often been studied with more intrusive methods—for example, collosectomy (Gazzaniga, 1970) and altering the brain state with alcohol (Sterman, 1990). The CNS research suggests that hypnosis offers a nonintrusive method for examining the human potential for voluntary shifts in cerebral lateralized activity.

Finally, there is some evidence that highly hypnotizable people may have the potential for exquisite cortical inhibition. If so, hypnosis may offer a way to correlate behavioral data that are suggestive of psychological inhibition with neurological data. Evidence of cortical inhibition accompanying psychological inhibition during hypnotic suggestion is scattered but suggestive. Late components of the cortical evoked potential appear to be inhibited when hypnotized subjects are told not to perceive stimuli in a negative hallucination (Blum & Nash, 1981; J. Nash, 1983; D. Spiegel, Cutcomb, Ren, & Pribram, 1985; D. Spiegel & Barabasz, 1988; D. Spiegel, Bierre, & Rootenberg, 1989; Zakrzewski & Szelenberger, 1981). As mentioned previously, contralateral cortical activation, which is observed when a person is experiencing pain in one arm, was diminished when highly hypnotizable people were given hypnotic analgesia suggestions (Karlin et al., 1980). Some time ago, Blum and Barbour (1979) suggested that hypnotic inhibitory processes such as negative hallucinations constitute an extreme case of selective inattention. Cortical changes associated with waking suggestion for selective inattention have not been investigated extensively. However, Hogan, MacDonald, and Olness (1984) found that children could increase interwave latencies in *brainstem* auditory evoked responses following waking suggestion. With the current rapid developments in electrophysiological measurement and brain imaging, the investigation of neurophysiological and psychological inhibitory processes with hypnosis should be a rich area.

Cognition

Psychology's increased attention to cognition in recent years has opened opportunities for hypnosis as a method of investigation, because many hypnotic effects can be understood as changes in cognitive processes (e.g., attention, awareness, memory, etc.). Hypnosis may be used to extend the range of cognitive phenomena and processes studied. Although it seems as if every cognitive change obtainable with hypnosis can be observed in at least some subjects under waking conditions, hypnosis increases the number of subjects in whom the process can be observed. As an example, more subjects report amnesia following hypnotic suggestions than in a non-hypnotized control condition (Williamsen, Johnson, & Eriksen, 1965). Critical reviews indicate that experimental conditions, subject expectancy, and role enactment (Spanos, 1986b,c), as well as person differences (Kihlstrom, 1985b; Kirsch & Council, Chapter 10, this volume), account for some of the cognitive changes associated with hypnosis.

Many of the cognitive changes associated with hypnosis have to do with attention, memory, awareness, and rationality (Pekala & Kumar, 1987–1988; Kumar & Pekala, 1988). High hypnotizable subjects differed from low hypnotizable subjects in the waking state (eyes closed) in their self-reports regarding body image, time sense, meaning, and state of awareness, and such differences were magnified following a hypnotic induction. Hypnosis was associated with a greater increase in altered perception and state of awareness, and a greater decrease in rationality, volitional control, and memory, for high and medium subjects than for low subjects. Whereas highs reported a more absorbed attentional focus and experiencing more unusual meanings during hypnosis, lows reported being less absorbed (or more distracted) and having less unusual meanings during the induction.

Thus research on attention, memory, rationality, and awareness may benefit by including hypnosis conditions. Lawful relationships regarding cognitive processes observed in the waking brain state may not generalize to the hypnotized brain state, and a fuller understanding would probably emerge from data collected in hypnosis as well as in waking conditions. (As an analogy, social scientists have learned not to generalize psychological principles on the basis of data obtained solely with white male college students.) Experimental results obtained when hypnosis is or is not introduced as part of the experiment call for superordinate principles. The following sections on attention, learning and memory, and awareness illustrate how hypnosis may be used to broaden the scope of investigation and understanding in cognitive psychology.

Attention

Past reviews have suggested that hypnosis is a useful research methodology because attention can be hypnotically narrowed (Holroyd, 1985–1986; Levitt & Chapman, 1979), but that is an oversimplification. Hypnosis affects various kinds of attention differently, and the use of hypnosis as a research method for studying attention should take these variations into account. Furthermore, attention differs for highs and lows both in hypnosis and in waking conditions (Pekala & Kumar, 1987–1988). Highs reported less attentional flexibility, control, and vigilance, and more attentional perspicacity, absorption, inward focus, and "out-of-the-body" attentional locus, than lows in the waking state. In fact, hypnosis was associated with increased absorption for highs but decreased absorption (compared to the waking condition) for lows (Kumar & Pekala, 1988).

Depending on the attentional task under investigation, hypnotized subjects may excel or do poorly. When highs were absorbed in a hypnotic induction, they were *less* adept at signal detection than lows (Smyth & Lowy, 1983). Attention to time is impaired. They tend to underestimate time by about 40%, although a few hypnotized subjects significantly overestimate time (K. S. Bowers & Brenneman, 1979; Zimbardo, Marshall, & Maslach, 1971).[10]

In contrast, there is extensive evidence that high hypnotizable subjects excel in tasks involving divided attention, passive receptive attention, or inhibition of competing stimuli, even in the waking state. This finding points to the need to account for or control hypnotizability as a source of variance in research on these aspects of attention. Highs fare better than lows on divided-attention tasks in which stimuli compete for a (limited) cortical processor (Zamansky & Bartis, 1984; Sigman, Phillips, & Clifford, 1985; but see Stava & Jaffa, 1988). Some highs with a posthypnotic suggestion to respond only to target stimuli actually did as well on a divided-attention task as on a task with a single attentional focus (K. S. Bowers & Brenneman, 1981).

Not only can highs engage in two cognitive processes at once with less performance degradation than lows, but they also perform better than lows when incompatible suggestions are given simultaneously (Bartis & Zamansky, 1990; Zamansky & Clark, 1986). With respect to inhibition of competing stimuli, Sheehan et al. (1988) found that highs given instructions to ignore competing stimuli in hypnosis could significantly improve their performance on an attentional task (the Stroop test) over waking-state performance, whereas lows improved only slightly. A series of investigations of attention, employing forward and backward masking designs, yielded both positive and nil relationships to hypnotizability (summarized by Friedman & Taub, 1986).

To summarize the research relevant to attention experiments, it appears that hypnosis is particularly useful for increasing an absorbed attention quality, which may in some cases impair task performance. The absorption can be countervailed by suggestions for focusing attention, as A. F. Barabasz (1980b) showed with naval radar operators. On the other hand, subjects high in hypnotic responsivity should perform very well on tasks involving divided attention, inhibited attention, or passive attention. Hypnosis can be used as a research method either to preselect subjects with certain attentional predispositions, or to modify parameters of attentional processing such as divided attention, when one is investigating cognition.

Learning and Memory

Hypnosis does not appear to help learning (Stager & Lundy, 1985) and may actually interfere with it (Sweeney et al., 1986; but see Crawford, Allen, & Kiefner, 1983). At the present time, applications of hypnosis in learning research are limited, and there is little in the contemporary literature to indicate how hypnosis might contribute to our understanding of how people learn.

The evidence for memory improvement with hypnosis (hypermnesia) is also mixed, but positive findings on hypnotic hypermnesia for meaningful material suggest possible research directions. Studies that reported memory facilitation without increase in errors all used live events or films and long retention intervals (Geiselman & Machlovitz, 1987). Whereas recall of meaningful material may be improved, recall of nonsense material is not (Relinger, 1984). In fact, Dywan (1988) concluded that in a repeated-recall situation, hypnotized subjects sometimes provide new correct information but almost invariably increase their errors.

There is some evidence that being hypnotized may actually interfere with reasoning and memory. Kumar and Pekala (1988) found a negative correlation between hypnotizability and self-reported rationality (–.41) as well as memory (–.41) *during neutral hypnosis* (i.e., improved recall was not suggested). The paradox of subjects' reporting poorer memory, given the reputation of hypnosis for producing hypermnesia, relates to an "emptying out" of consciousness experienced by most high hypnotizable subjects in neutral hypnosis (R. J. Pekala, personal communication, January 3, 1991). One obvious contribution for hypnosis as a research method would be to explore the degree to which "emptying out" would be conducive to long-term recall of meaningful or life event materials.

The ability of highly hypnotizable subjects to remember a greater amount of meaningful material when hypnotized has been used by several investigators exploring cognitive processes. One example is provided in research on depth of cognitive processing (Cermak & Craik, 1979). Meaningful material is said to be processed at deep rather than shallow levels. High hypnotizable subjects perform better than lows when remembering deep-process material in hypnosis, though there is no difference for shallow-process material (McKelvie & Pullara, 1988; Shields & Knox, 1986). If recalling meaningful material is enhanced by hypnosis, then investigations of recall for meaningful material could use hypnotized subjects across experimental conditions. This approach might be particularly fruitful in research investigating memory for life events.

Because of known hypermnesia effects for meaningful material, Geiselman, Fisher, MacKinnon, and Holland (1985) used hypnosis as a very potent control condition for their innovative technique to enhance memory for meaningful events. They confirmed that a hypnosis interview for recalling a violent crime scene yielded more correct information (without increasing errors) than did a standard police interview. However, their "cognitive interview" based on techniques derived from memory theory did as well as hypnosis. Geiselman et al.'s work is an interesting example of using hypnosis as a contrast or control method in general experimental psychology without necessarily using it to discover new relationships.

Awareness

To be unaware and yet aware is a long-standing problem for psychological investigation, not just hypnosis research. Investigations of subliminal perception, implicit memory, and automatized perceptual–cognitive or motor skills involve special problems, shared with investigations of hypnotic amnesia, analgesia, and other hypnotic sensory loss. Kihlstrom (1987a) has postulated a tripartite division of the cognitive unconscious: Truly unconscious mental processes are thought to operate on knowledge structures that may be either preconscious or subconscious. Hypnosis seems promising as a method for studying nonconscious mental processes.

Following hypnotic suggestion people report that they are remarkably unaware (e.g., of pain, sound, and memories), and yet at some other level they demonstrate awareness. For example, subjects who reported being unable to see or smell certain stimuli when given a negative hallucination suggestion were able to remember the (unperceived) stimuli after the suggestion was canceled (Zamansky & Bartis, 1985). High hypnotizables with suggested deafness performed as well as lows on a test for words presented to their "deaf" ears (Spanos, Jones, & Malfara, 1982). In fact, hypnotically deaf subjects chose words that sounded like the (unperceived) target words at a rate much *lower* than chance, as if avoiding the appearance of hearing (M. R. Nash, Lynn, Stanley, & Carlson, 1987). Similarly, hypnotically blind subjects performed as if they registered visual cues, although their description of awareness differed from that of simulators (Bryant & McConkey, 1989c).

Advances in research on unawareness have established hypnosis as perhaps the pre-eminent method for investigating different levels of consciousness. Hypnosis is nonintrusive and does not rely on finding patients with pathological conditions of unawareness. A number of hypnosis procedures are useful, but two that involve special inquiry methods have proven particularly fruitful.

Inquiring about a "hidden observer" during hypnotic analgesia may yield reports of pain of which the subject is unaware (E. R. Hilgard, 1974, 1979a). Inquiring about experience during age regression may yield reports of subjects' observing themselves as children rather than feeling like children—a "duality" of experience (Orne, 1951; Perry & Walsh, 1978). Both the hidden observer and age regression duality imply parallel processing of experience, with the sense of self accompanying only one aspect. There appears to be an association between the two phenomena (Laurence & Perry, 1981).[11] Age regression duality and the hidden observer also seem to be linked to the capacity to experience hypnotic amnesia (Nadon, D'Eon, McConkey, Laurence, & Perry, 1988; Nogrady, McConkey, Laurence, & Perry, 1983). All three phenomena are reflected in the distinction between experiential and behavioral memory that may be teased out by interviewing hypnotically amnesic subjects (McConkey & Sheehan, 1981). McConkey, Sheehan, and Cross (1980) noticed that hypnotically amnesic subjects watching their hypnotic performance on videotape often commented that they were able to recall the physical events on the videotape, but were not able to recall the experiences. (See also F. J. Evans & Kihlstrom, 1973.)

Duality experiences or the changed sense of self may occur outside hypnosis and apparently without suggestion, as in out-of-body experiences (Twemlow, Gabbard, & Jones, 1982). People who reported a hidden observer during pain experiments frequently indicated that duality was something they experienced in everyday life (Nogrady et al., 1983). Alterations in body image, meaning, and awareness are described by highs more often than by lows in the waking state, but these differences in self-experience increase during hypnosis (Kumar & Pekala, 1988). Hence, duality experiences of everyday life and the associated experiences of the self can be investigated readily using hypnotic suggestion.

In the last decade, most of the research on suggested unawareness has used a hypnotic amnesia paradigm, but (as with hypnotic pain control research) investigators have been primarily involved in establishing the characteristics of hypnotic amnesia rather than using hypnosis as a method to study forgetting. Because the "forgotten" information of hypnotic amnesia remains in the cognitive system and is immediately available when subjects are given a release signal, hypnosis is useful to psychologists interested in studying flexible forgetting. Suggested amnesia does not appear to be the same phenomenon as repression, despite surface similarities (Kunzendorf & Benoit, 1985–1986; Stam, Radtke-Bodorik, & Spanos, 1980), so hypnotic amnesia probably is not an adequate model for investigating repression.[12]

Suggested amnesia is a fairly robust phenomenon. Although highs are more likely than lows to experience amnesia (Kihlstrom, 1978, 1983), lows may become hypnotically amnesic when taught how to direct their attention away from the learned material (Spanos & de Groh, 1984, cited in Spanos, 1986c). Although amnesia dissipates with repeated trials (L. D. Bertrand, Spanos, & Parkinson, 1983), it does not seem to be simply pretending to forget (Kihlstrom, 1982, 1983). Amnesia is resistant to breaching (Coe & Yashinski, 1985; Kihlstrom, Evans, Orne, & Orne, 1980), particularly for people who experience the amnesia as nonvoluntary or effortless (Howard & Coe, 1980). However, amnesia *can* be breached with virtually all subjects through increasing social pressure (Coe & Sluis, 1989) or manipulating expectancies (Silva & Kirsch, 1987; Spanos, Radtke, & Bertrand, 1984).[13] The ability to turn memory on and off without the amnesia's dissipating (Dubreuil, Spanos, & Bertrand, 1982–1983; Spanos, Tkachyk, Bertrand, & Weekes, 1984) is what makes hypnotic amnesia useful for investigating memory processes.

Three recent investigations illustrate how hypnosis as a research method has contributed to our understanding of flexible forgetting. Geiselman, MacKinnon, Fishman, Jaenicke, Larner, Schoenberg, and Swartz (1983) compared directed forgetting to hypnotic amnesia. ("Directed forgetting" is what is required of short-order cooks, who, once having filled an order, should forget it and proceed to the next order.) Geiselman et al. concluded that the mechanisms for directed forgetting and hypnotic amnesia were closely related, and that retrieval inhibition and inhibition release were implicated in both. (See also Kihlstrom, 1983.)

However, Coe et al. (1989), concluded that the memory processes in hypnotic amnesia and directed forgetting were *not* the same, and also that lows and highs responded differently in the two contexts. (Highs did not show the usual directed-forgetting response in the hypnosis condition.) Significantly, and as emphasized in this chapter, they suggested that theories of cognitive psychology may need to include interactions between person variables and experimental conditions for an adequate understanding of some cognitive phenomena. Hypnotizability may be as important as more traditional subject variables, such as gender and age, in investigations of certain cognitive phenomena.

In the third experiment, Huesmann, Gruder, and Dorst (1987) proposed output inhibition in order to explain how amnesic subjects solved problems or gave word associations as if they were actually aware of the "forgotten" information. Their research illustrates how the dissociation between experiential memory and functional memory can be explored with the hypnotic method.

Coe (1989b), who as a social psychologist has emphasized context, expectancy, and so forth in explaining hypnotic phenomena, moved toward hypnosis state theorists in writing that "The to-be-forgotten material is retrieved into working memory, *but perhaps not awareness,* where it is searched for tags. Output is then suppressed for material with forbidden recall tags, although the material is still available for generativity uses" (p. 147; emphasis added). Coe's analysis would also apply to the data from hypnotic blindness and deafness, where it can be demonstrated that subjects operate on the basis of available information, despite extensive sensory "blocks."

Conclusion

In 1979 Levitt and Chapman listed six possible advantages for hypnosis as a research method, noting that the advantages were based on "allegedly unique properties" of hypnosis, most of which had not at that time been verified by research. The supposed advantages were that artificial states (e.g., emotions) can be created or terminated quickly, and intensified or diminished; suggestion can create amnesia for the research experience; different suggested conditions can be examined with the same subjects in within-subjects designs; subjects' attention can be narrowed; subjects are less self-conscious about what is done to them; and subjects experience less postexperimental disturbance if they have been subjected to stress. The principal disadvantages had to do with sampling bias, because many subjects are not responsive to hypnosis, and because hypnotizability is associated with a number of personality characteristics that might influence experimental results.

Research in the intervening years has vitiated most of the statements regarding advantages, turned the disadvantages into advantages, and provided new understanding of how hypnosis can enable us to answer important questions in traditional areas of interest. First, let us critically consider the six supposed advantages to the hypnosis method. Suggested effects (e.g., deafness) are complex and not necessarily the same as the condition that is being emulated. The "effects" can often be created by special motivational instructions or use of alternative strategies (e.g., imagery, relaxation); perhaps, therefore, hypnosis has no special advantage as an experimental manipulation. In addition to the effect investigators are attempting to create (e.g., fear, joy), they may also be contributing to significant changes in cognitive functioning that may influence experimental results in unknown ways. As for amnesia for the research experience, what is "forgotten" is not necessarily forgotten and may influence behavior in the experiment and afterward.

Instead of supporting the use of within-subjects designs for studying differences between conditions, hypnosis research has illustrated the vulnerability of such designs to subject expectancy. Furthermore, the attentional changes promoted by hypnosis have been found to be increases in passive receptive attention, divided attention, and absorption in inner experience, rather than increases in the focusing of attention. As for less self-consciousness of subjects and diminution of possible carryover effects following stress induction procedures, the dearth of relevant research leaves that proposition open for examination.

Levitt and Chapman (1979) mentioned that in addition to using hypnosis as a research strategy because of its methodological advantages, investigators may use it because it is complementary to other experimental approaches. The intervening years have indicated that indeed hypnosis does offer new information when introduced into traditional content areas. For example, in cognitive psychology it has reintroduced the importance of studying experiential aspects of cognition (e.g., "*I* think," "*I* remember"), or self-reference (Kihlstrom, 1987b). It also offers promise of data important to understanding the mind–body interface, a contribution to the neurosciences as well as to psychology.

What was viewed as a problem of sampling bias—the fact that hypnotizability is associated with a number of personality variables—may become an advantage for investigators who understand the implications of hypnosis responsivity. Social psychologists have underscored the active participation of subjects engaging in a hypnosis experience. Sheehan and McConkey (1982) noted that subjects sometimes make a large effort to respond within a framework of suggestion, so as to prevent reality from interfering with their performance. Tellegen (1981) describes subjects scoring high and low on the Absorption Scale as having experiential and instrumental "sets," respectively, and the same could be said for subjects who are high and low in hypnotizability. If for some reason the experimenter wishes subjects who have an experiential set—who will, at both conscious and unconscious levels, endeavor to experience effects desired by the experimenter—he or she should select people who are responsive on hypnotizability scales. One of the best examples is in the area of psychosomatic phenomena, where investigation of mental control over physiological processes is improved by choosing subjects with an experiential set—those who are able and willing to experience physiological changes.

Hypnosis as a research method will continue to benefit from contributions of radically different theoretical views of hypnotic phenomena. Social-cognitive psychologists have contributed significantly toward unifying the fields of hypnosis research and general experimental psychology. At the same time, advances in neurophysiology and psychosomatic medicine employing hypnosis indicate that there is a role for hypnosis as a research strategy, solely because of its altered-state characteristics. If theoretical physics can reconcile both wave and particle theories of light, it is conceivable that psychology can accommodate both behavioral and state theories of hypnosis.

Notes

1. The evidence for imagery enhancement in hypnosis is mixed. When a between-groups design is used, differences in imagery vividness between waking and hypnosis conditions tend to disappear (see review by Spanos, 1986c). Self-reports may be influenced by a prior belief that hypnosis increases imagery over the waking state (but see A. M. Rossi, Sturrock, & Solomon, 1963, for contrary evidence). Improved imagery was reported by Crawford and Allen (1983), A. M. Rossi et al. (1963), and Spanos, Bridgeman, Stam, Gwynn, and Saad (1982–1983); Coe, St. Jean, and Burger (1980) reported mixed results; Starker (1974a) did not find improved imagery. Spanos (1986c) cites negative evidence in T. X. Barber and Wilson (1977) and three other studies that investigated hallucinations, not enhanced imagery (Ham & Spanos, 1974; Spanos, Ham, & Barber, 1973; Spanos, Mullens, & Rivers, 1979).

2. For reviews, see Sheehan (1979a) and Sweeney, Lynn, and Belleza (1986). A positive relationship between hypnotizability and imaging ability was reported by P. G. Bowers and Bowers (1979), Coe et al. (1980), Crawford (1982a), Crawford and Allen (1983), Farthing, Venturino, and Brown (1983), and K. White, Sheehan, and Ashton (1977). Authors who did not observe such an association include Crawford, Wallace, Nomura, and Slater (1986), A. M. Rossi et al. (1963), and Van Dyne and Stava (1981). Kahn, Fromm, Lombard, and Sossi (1989) found a relationship between imagery in self-hypnosis and depth of trance. The correlation between hypnotizability and imagery ability may be an artifact associated with imagery inductions (de Groh, 1989; Friedland, 1976), or may reflect the fact that both variables are related to a third variable, absorption (P. G. Bowers, 1978, 1979;

Kearns & Zamansky, 1984; Roche & McConkey, 1990). Dywan (1988) located a group of high hypnotizables who had low imagery ability.

3. In neutral hypnosis (no imagery suggestions), the majority of highs experienced *no* thoughts or images, while a minority had very vivid imagery (Kumar & Pekala, 1988; Pekala, 1991).

4. The Stroop effect occurs when subjects are asked to identify colors but the color stimulus is printed in ink of an incompatible color (e.g., the word "green" printed in red ink). Instead of naming the color as instructed ("red"), highs are more likely than lows to respond "green."

5. Hypnotically altered imagery processes reach an apogee in the experience of hypnotically suggested hallucinations. However, other processes—notably inhibitory processes—appear to be involved (S. Sanders, 1967/1969; D. Spiegel, Bierre, & Rootenberg, 1989; D. Spiegel, Cutcomb, Ren, & Pribram, 1985). Hallucinations are discussed briefly in the section on "Cognition."

6. A number of investigations have failed to replicate Sinclair-Gieben and Chalmers (1959); see review by Spanos, Stenstrom, and Johnston (1988).

7. Although McGlashan, Evans, and Orne (1969) found that placebo response was not related to hypnotizability in an investigation of experimental pain, the relationship of suggestion, suggestibility, and placebo has not been investigated thoroughly.

8. The association of hypnotizability with degree of analgesia following an induction may be a function of induction characteristics (J. Barber, 1977, 1980; Fricton & Roth, 1985), or it may reflect the fact that analgesia suggestions emphasize imagery strategies (Spanos, McNeil, Gwynn, & Stam, 1984). Feelings of self-efficacy generated by hypnotic responsivity testing also may give highly responsive subjects a sense that they can accomplish great feats of self-control (Bandura, 1982; Spanos, Hodgins, Stam, & Gwynn, 1984). Spanos (1986b) concluded following his review that the analgesia–hypnotizability correlation is context-dependent; that is, it is only evident if testing for hypnotizability occurs in the context of a hypnotic pain control experiment.

9. Spanos and his colleagues regard the concept of dissociation as unnecessary (Chaves, 1989; Spanos, 1986b, 1989).

10. Time underestimation may be a function of task absorption in the hypnosis activities (K. S. Bowers, 1979) or of the cognitive demands associated with hypnosis (St. Jean & Robertson, 1986). Time underestimation seems to be correlated with hypnotizability (K. S. Bowers, 1979; S. W. Brown, 1984). The amount of underestimation was unrelated to hypnotizability or absorption in other investigations (K. S. Bowers & Brenneman, 1979; St. Jean, MacLeod, Coe, & Howard, 1982; St. Jean & Robertson, 1986).

11. Duality experiences also may be akin to the out-of-the-body experience that can be promoted with hypnotic suggestion (M. R. Nash, Lynn, & Stanley, 1984). The dual track of awareness has been attributed to dissociation (E. R. Hilgard, 1977b), or to social relationship variables such as expectancy, compliance, role taking, and honest admissions of partly failed suggestions (Coe, 1989b; de Groot & Gwynn, 1989; Spanos, de Groot, Tiller, Weekes, & Bertrand, 1985; Spanos & Hewitt, 1980; Spanos, 1989). Zamansky and Bartis (1984) forged a conceptual link between the hypothetical construct of dissociation and the previously mentioned

divided-attention capabilities of high hypnotizables. Hypnosis could be used to determine whether people skilled at divided-attention tasks are more likely to report duality experiences in hypnosis.

12. Hypnotic amnesia has been attributed to dissociation (E. R. Hilgard, 1977b), disrupted search (F. J. Evans & Kihlstrom, 1973; Kihlstrom & Evans, 1979b), distracted attention (Spanos, 1986b), strategic enactment (Spanos, 1986b), and output inhibition (Huesmann, Gruder, & Dorst, 1987). Disruption in the retrieval process has been noted by a number of authors (Ham, Radtke, & Spanos, 1981, cited by Coe, 1989b; Kihlstrom, Brenneman, Pistole, & Shor, 1985; Kihlstrom & Wilson, 1984; Radtke-Bodorik, Planas, & Spanos, 1980; Spanos, Stam, D'Eon, Pawlak, & Radtke-Bodorik, 1980; St. Jean & Coe, 1981; for reviews see Coe, 1989b; Radtke & Spanos, 1981; Spanos, 1986b). Explanations for memory disorganization during hypnotic amnesia include disrupted retrieval as opposed to acquisition or storage functions (F. J. Evans & Kihlstrom, 1973; Kihlstrom & Evans, 1979b; St. Jean & Coe, 1981; Pettinati, Evans, Orne, & Orne, 1981; but see Spanos & D'Eon, 1980); dissociation between episodic and semantic memory (Kihlstrom, 1980); disruption in contextual relationship among memory items (Kihlstrom & Wilson, 1984; L. Wilson & Kihlstrom, 1986); strategic enactment, or the tendency for subjects to maintain behavior confirming that they are deeply hypnotized (Coe, 1989b; Spanos, Radtke, & Bertrand, 1984); response strategies such as inattention (Spanos, 1986b); experimental demands (Spanos, Gwynn, Della Malva, & Bertrand, 1988); and compliance (Wagstaff, 1981a,b).

13. Manipulation effects have also been summarized by Spanos (1986b), and by Coe (1989b); see Spanos, Stam, D'Eon, Pawlak, and Radtke-Bodorik (1980) for contrary evidence of the manipulation effect.

CHAPTER NINE

A Midstream View of the Neuropsychophysiology of Hypnosis: Recent Research and Future Directions

HELEN J. CRAWFORD
JOHN H. GRUZELIER

We are in the midst of the "decade of the brain," a stimulating period in psychophysiology in which new, sophisticated techniques and theories are being applied to the investigation of the underlying neurophysiological processes of cognitive functioning. New technologies, such as computerized electroencephalographic (EEG) frequency analysis, EEG topographic brain mapping, positron emission tomography (PET), regional cerebral blood flow (rCBF), single photon emission computed tomography (SPECT), and nuclear magnetic resonance imaging, allow more direct evaluation of the function of the brain. Within this evolving context, this chapter is presented as a working paper in midstream—an examination of very exciting and challenging research that investigates the neuropsychophysiology of hypnosis.

This chapter contains a critical analysis of the following questions: Are there neuropsychophysiological differences between low and high hypnotizable individuals in nonhypnotic (waking) or hypnosis conditions? And are there any systematic changes in such neuropsychophysiological processes during hypnotic rest or during specific hypnotic phenomena that differ from those obtained in nonhypnotic conditions? Furthermore, are these moderated by hypnotic susceptibility level?

Emphasis is placed upon studies of neuropsychological tests and neurophysiological functioning. These include electrocortical activity (both computerized EEG and evoked potentials [EPs]), rCBF, electrodermal reactivity, dichotic listening, divided visual fields, haptic tactile processing, and neuropsychological cognitive tests. No attempt is made to address the claim that specific hypnotic suggestions can modulate certain physiological functions (such as respiration and cardiovascular activity). Readers are referred to earlier reviews on these topics (T. X. Barber, 1961; Chertok, 1969; Crasilneck & Hall, 1959; Gorton, 1962; Levitt & Brady, 1963; E. L. Rossi, 1986; Sarbin, 1956; Sarbin & Slagle, 1979; L. J. West, 1960).

As part of this critical analysis, we discuss a number of conceptual as well as methodological problems that need to be addressed in future research. Often forgotten in the early research was the issue of the moderating effects of hypnotic susceptibility level. If low, medium, and high hypnotizable individuals do not differ from one another in hypnosis, it is impossible to argue for effects being due to hypnosis per se, rather than relaxation or some other variable. Thus, the importance of the moderating effects of hypnotic susceptibility level is a recurring issue.

A difficulty of this review, particularly with older studies, is the inability to compare results adequately across laboratories and even across studies within the same laboratories because of methodological differences, variations in screening procedures, failure to consider the hypnotic level of subjects, differences in analytic techniques applied to similar physiological data, and so on. Averaging effects is no answer. Whenever studies are poorly designed, use poor methodology, and/or apply incorrect or weak statistical techniques to the collected data, they cannot be compared with equal weight to well-designed and well-executed experiments.

Overview of Our Neuropsychophysiological Working Model of Hypnosis

Hypnosis is a state of altered attention that may be focused or diffuse, depending on instruction (e.g., E. R. Hilgard, 1965a, 1977a, 1986; Sheehan, Donovan, & MacLeod, 1988). As a hypnotically responsive individual enters and becomes deeply absorbed in the hypnotic experience, there is a shift in consciousness—typically, a shift away from more analytical and sequential modes of processing toward more imaginal and holistic processing (e.g., Crawford, 1982b, 1989, 1990a, 1991b; Crawford & Allen, 1983; Crawford, Nomura, & Slater, 1983; Crawford, Wallace, Nomura, & Slater, 1986). A decrease or cessation in generalized reality testing (Shor, 1959, 1970), and an increase in dissociative experiences during hypnosis, occur as a result of such attentional and cognitive strategy shifts. Fromm (1987) has noted that the "most important structural components of the hypnotic process are imagery and fantasy, absorption, dissociation, and various ego modes and attention postures" (p. 216).

Numerous studies have demonstrated that those individuals who have the ability to refocus their attention and shift cognitive strategies when given a hypnotic induction are generally also capable of vivid imagery, holistic thinking, extremely focused and sustained attention, and absorption in imaginative activities during nonhypnotic conditions (e.g., Crawford, 1981, 1982a,b, 1989). Furthermore, Crawford (1991b; Crawford, Brown, & Moon, 1991; Atkinson & Crawford, in press), B. Wallace (e.g., B. Wallace, 1986; B. Wallace & Garrett, 1973; B. Wallace & Patterson, 1984), and others have shown that high hypnotizable individuals are capable not only of extremely focused attending to task-relevant stimuli, but also of disattending to task-irrelevant environmental stimuli. These highly responsive individuals also demonstrate greater abilities than less responsive persons in shifting from one strategy to another and from one alternate state of awareness to another—an ability we have referred to as "cognitive flexibility" (e.g., Crawford, 1989, 1990a; Crawford & Allen, 1983).

Recent research shows an evolution toward a more complex and theoretically sound, neuropsychophysiological model of hypnosis. This model replaces earlier, more general models (e.g., Gur & Gur, 1974; Graham, 1977), which proposed overall right-hemisphere involvement during hypnosis and a relationship between being "right-brained" and being highly responsive to hypnosis. There is clearly no evidence that individuals rely on only one hemisphere for thinking or activate only one hemisphere during cognitive tasks (e.g., Hellige, 1990). Recent research demonstrates that most cognitive activity may be broken down into componential stages, which then correlate with activation of different parts of the brain (e.g., Kosslyn, 1987; Posner & Petersen, 1990; Posner, Petersen, Fox, & Raichle, 1988).

Because there are substantial cognitive differences between those individuals who are highly responsive and unresponsive to hypnotic inductions and suggestions, it is likely to follow that differential brain activation patterns between and within hemispheres, both anterior and posterior (e.g., Pribram, 1991; Pribram & McGuinness, in press), should be found in nonhypnotic as well as hypnotic conditions. Shifts in cognitive functioning during hypnosis and specific hypnotic suggestions should be accompanied by shifts in patterns of brain activation. In fact, growing evidence supports our view that high hypnotizable individuals show greater hemispheric specificity than do low hypnotizable individuals under both hypnosis and nonhypnosis conditions (e.g., Crawford, 1989; MacLeod-Morgan, 1979, 1982; MacLeod-Morgan & Lack, 1982; Mészáros, Crawford, Szabó, Nagy-Kovács, & Révész, 1989; Sabourin, Cutcomb, Crawford, & Pribram, 1990), and that hypnotically responsive individuals may show greater shifts in brain activation patterns during hypnosis. Specifically, prior to and at the beginning of an induction of hypnotic relaxation, the high hypnotizable individual's attention is more fully engaged by focused attentional inductions; thus, there may be evidence of greater frontal left-hemispheric activation in susceptible than in unsusceptible subjects, as shown in studies of bilateral electrodermal orienting responses to tones (Gruzelier &

Brow, 1985). As the highly responsive individual enters into hypnosis, there is an alteration in cognitive strategies, which is exhibited in an inhibition of left-hemispheric involvement and a shift in hemispheric balance toward greater right-hemispheric involvement (Gruzelier, Brow, Perry, Rhonder, & Thomas, 1984; Gruzelier, 1988, 1990). These shifts differentially involve the anterior and posterior regions of the brain (Crawford, 1989; Mészáros et al., 1989). In addition, tasks (e.g., math or imaginal problems) and hypnotic suggestions (e.g., age regression or hypnotic analgesia) that call upon differing cognitive processes should evidence different brain activation patterns.

In summary, what this evidence demonstrates to us is that there are differences between low and high hypnotically susceptible individuals in the nonhypnotic state, and that systematic changes in brain functional organization occur with hypnosis, in keeping with a neuropsychophysiological interpretation of hypnotic induction procedures. We return to this model in the final section of the chapter with a synthesis of supporting evidence.

In the subsequent sections, each research modality is reviewed with reference to the following issues: Do high and low hypnotically susceptible individuals differ in a nonhypnotic state, both in resting and task conditions? And does hypnosis alter neuropsychophysiological processes differentially for high and low susceptible individuals?

Electrophysiological Activity during Hypnosis

Many attempts, often futile, have been made to identify possible electrocortical correlates of hypnosis (for reviews of earlier literature, see Crasilneck & Hall, 1959; Perlini & Spanos, 1991; Sabourin, 1982; Sabourin et al., 1990; Sarbin & Slagle, 1979). With the advent of quantified electrophysiological techniques (computer-based acquisition, storage, and analysis of EEG or stimulus-bound evoked responses, either in the time domain or converted to the frequency domain) and two-dimensional topographic maps, new questions have been investigated. These studies have resulted in some suggestive evidence that there may be electrocortical differences (1) between low and high hypnotizable individuals in waking and hypnosis, and (2) between nonhypnotic and hypnotic conditions as moderated by hypnotic susceptibility level.

Early research was polarized around the issue of different frequency bandwidths, whereas regional topography has been a more recent development. Initially, major historical and theoretical interest led investigators to examine whether the EEG during hypnosis was comparable to the EEG recorded during sleep. Investigators accordingly focused on slow-wave activity such as theta and alpha. As reviewed by F. J. Evans

(1979), it became quite clear that hypnosis did not share any important EEG properties with sleep.

To give structure to a complex literature, we first consider hypnosis and hypnotic susceptibility with regard to EEG activity subdivided by hertz (Hz) bandwidth before considering newer issues such as hemisphere differences and within-hemisphere specificity, and fast-frequency (40-Hz) cognitive EEG correlates. Second, we consider hypnotic analgesia studies that have examined EEG, EPs, rCBF, and cardiovascular measures as dependent measures. Finally, we examine work on EEG recorded from electrodes implanted in deep brain structures.

EEG Differences between Low, Medium, and High Hypnotizables

Alpha Frequency Differences

Alpha density (the amount of time alpha is present above a minimum amplitude criterion) and power (integrated or mean amplitude), which do not necessarily correlate strongly with each other, have been evaluated. Alpha waves occur at a frequency of 8 to 12 or 13 Hz, with amplitudes varying from 20 to 60 microvolts. Because early research found enhanced alpha production associated with relaxation and with other alternate states of awareness, such as those produced by biofeedback or meditation, some researchers hypothesized a relationship between alpha production and hypnotizability.

Early studies often reported that high hypnotizable subjects produced a higher density of bipolar occipital alpha waves than low hypnotizable subjects (e.g., Bakan & Svorad, 1969; A. F. Barabasz, 1980a, 1982; Engstrom, London, & Hart, 1970a,b; London, Hart, & Leibovitz, 1968; Morgan, Macdonald, & Hilgard, 1974; Morgan, McDonald, & Macdonald, 1971; Nowlis & Rhead, 1968; Ulett, Akpinar, & Itil, 1972a,b), although others found no such relationships (e.g., Cooper & London, 1976; R. A. Dumas, 1977; Edmonston & Grotevant, 1975; F. J. Evans, 1979; Mészáros & Bányai, 1978).

Correlations between alpha amplitude and hypnotic susceptibility have been reported in eyes-closed, but not eyes-open, resting conditions (Morgan, Macdonald, & Hilgard,, 1974; MacLeod-Morgan, 1979; De Pascalis & Palumbo, 1986) and in an eyes-closed condition when performing tasks (De Pascalis & Palumbo, 1986). De Pascalis, Silveri, and Palumbo (1988) found significant correlations between hypnotizability and mean integrated alpha amplitude (not spectral power), but not alpha density scores, at occipito-parietal bipolar locations during verbal and visual tasks. Mészáros, Crawford, and their colleagues (Crawford, 1989; Crawford, Mészáros, & Szabó, 1989; Mészáros et al., 1989) found no correlations between hypnotizability and alpha mean spectral power at F3-C3, F4-C4, P3-O1, and P4-O2 derivations. Sabourin et al. (1990) found no differences in mean alpha power between subjects very low and very high in hypnotizability at frontal (F3, F4), central (C3, C4), and occipital (O1, O2) unipolar derivations during eyes-open and eyes-closed resting conditions in waking and hypnosis, nor during hypnotic suggestions with eyes closed. Studies of self-induced happy, sad, and neutral emotional states (Crawford, Clarke, Kitner-Triolo, & Olesko, 1989; Crawford, Kitner-Triolo, Clarke, & Brown, 1988) and rest versus pain (Crawford, 1990a,b, 1991b), using unipolar recordings at F3, F4, T3, T4, P3, P4, O1, and O2, found no relationships between alpha mean power in either low-frequency (8- to 10.5-Hz) or high-frequency (10.5- to 13-Hz) bands and hypnotizability with or without hypnosis.

When evaluated further, the earlier-reported alpha–hypnotizability relationships were found sometimes to hold only for low and not high hypnotizable subjects (F. J. Evans, 1979; for a review, see Perlini & Spanos, 1991). The reported alpha–hypnotizability relationships were found to be unstable over repeated measurement occasions (e.g., Paskewitz, 1977). Given that eyes-closed alpha density was found to be highly unreliable across 3 days (Lynch, Paskewitz, & Orne, 1974), other factors, such as drowsiness or adjustment to the experimental setting, may greatly influence alpha production.

Reported alpha–hypnotizability correlations were thought to be results of situational or methodological factors (F. J. Evans, 1979) or of subject selection biases (R. A. Dumas, 1977), rather than of hypnosis per se. However, A. F. Barabasz (1983) showed that the correlations are "not simple covariates of subject self-selection," as his article title put it. De Pascalis et al. (1988) point out that differences in choice of alpha density or alpha amplitude may influence the outcome of results. In the above-discussed studies by Sabourin, Crawford, Mészáros, and their colleagues, subjects had become well acquainted with the experimenters and the laboratory facilities prior to the study, and thus they may have experienced less situational anxiety. Yet Orne and Paskewitz (1974) did not observe that apprehension or heightened arousal always led to reduced alpha activity. Thus, we must be cautious in our conclusions, but aware of the great importance of addressing and overcoming potential experimental confounds.

Finally, the choice of alpha band ranges (e.g., 7–12 Hz or 8–13 Hz) may have influenced findings in unknown ways. Recent studies suggest that the alpha band, traditionally a range of 8 to 12 Hz, may be functionally multidimensional (Andresen, Stemmler, Thom, & Irrgang, 1984; Coppola, 1986; Herrmann, 1982). Topographic analysis of EEG activity reveals two alpha bands; a 7- to 10-Hz band that displays a parietal maximum and a 10- to 13-Hz band that displays an occipital maximum (Coppola, 1986).

Although both types of alpha can be found within a person's EEG, "the individual's EEG spectrum peak will be exclusively of a slow parietal or fast occipital alpha type" (Coppola & Chassy, 1986, p. 41). As reported earlier, Crawford and her associates found no alpha–hypnotizability relationships in either low or high alpha bands. That the traditional alpha band of 8–12 Hz is apparently multidimensional and may be associated differentially with fluctuations in alertness must be taken into consideration in future research.

Laterality effects in the alpha band are considered in a later section.

Theta Frequency Differences

Perhaps the most consistent finding is that theta power (3–7 Hz) is sometimes strongly and positively related to hypnotic susceptibility. These effects seem to be topographically widespread, including occipital (Apkinar, Ulett, & Itil, 1971; Crawford, 1990a,b, 1991a,b; Galbraith, London, Leibovitz, Cooper, & Hart, 1970; Sabourin et al., 1990; Ulett et al., 1972a,b), parietal (Crawford, 1990a,b, 1991a,b; Tebecis, Provins, Farnbach, & Pentony, 1975), temporal (Crawford, 1990a,b, 1991a,b), central (Sabourin et al., 1990), and frontal (Crawford, 1990a,b, 1991a,b; Sabourin et al., 1990) locations. In fact, when hemispheres have been considered, enhanced theta power differences between low and high hypnotizable subjects have been found in both hemispheres (Crawford, 1990a,b, 1991a; Sabourin et al., 1990).

Aside from susceptibility-related differences in resting nonhypnotic baseline, the hypnosis condition itself is also associated with the production of theta. Sabourin et al. (1990) found that high hypnotizable individuals generated substantially more mean theta power than did low hypnotizable individuals in unipolar occipital, central, and frontal locations in both hemispheres (see Figure 9.1). In addition, both groups showed a substantial increase in mean theta power after hypnotic induction and during hypnotic suggestions, although the high hypnotizable subjects continued to have significantly more mean theta power than did the low hypnotizable subjects.

There have been negative studies. MacLeod-Morgan (1979) found that high hypnotizable subjects generated more theta in an eyes-open, but not eyes-closed, condition in bipolar occipito-parietal deviations of both hemispheres. No low (4- to 5.9-Hz) or high (6- to 7.9-Hz) theta power differences at bipolar anterior (F3-C3, F4-C4) and posterior (P3-O2, P4-O4) locations between stringently screened low and high hypnotizable subjects were found during eyes-closed rest, imagery of taking a walk, or doing mental arithmetic in nonhypnotic waking; however, during hypnosis highs generated more theta during the math and imagined-walk tasks (Crawford, 1989; Crawford, Mészáros, & Szabó, 1989; Mészáros et al.,

FRONTAL: LEFT

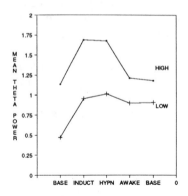

FRONTAL: RIGHT

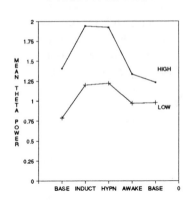

CENTRAL: LEFT

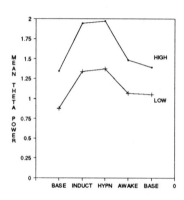

CENTRAL: RIGHT

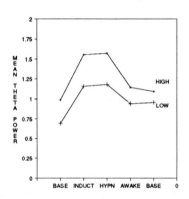

OCCIPITAL: LEFT

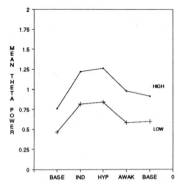

OCCIPITAL: RIGHT

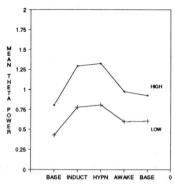

FIGURE 9.1. Theta mean power at frontal (F3, F4), central (C3, C4), and occipital (O1, O2) locations for low and high hypnotizable subjects across eyes-closed conditions of initial waking baseline, hypnotic induction after eye closure, hypnosis

1989). De Pascalis and Imperiali (1984) found no significant hypnotizability–theta relationships in temporal or parietal locations.

One factor that may lead to a reconciliation of the discrepant studies concerns the relative contribution of low and high theta. Like Galbraith, Cooper, and London (1970), who found 5- to 6-Hz theta in occipital locations to be most correlated with hypnotizability in eyes-closed resting, Crawford (1990a,b, 1991a) found that high hypnotizables generated significantly greater power than low hypnotizables in the high theta (5.5- to 7.5-Hz) but not the low theta (3.5- to 5.5-Hz) range in frontal, temporal, parietal, and occipital locations in both hemispheres. (Laterality differences in hypnotic pain and analgesia conditions are discussed further in a subsequent section on pain correlates.) When these studies are compared with previous ones in the literature, discrepancies in results may be attributed to the range of theta band examined, differing locations of electrode derivations, unipolar versus bipolar recording, differing tasks performed, and type of subjects. Nevertheless, a majority of studies have found theta production to be a characteristic of hypnotic susceptibility.

What is the behavioral significance of theta? Increments in theta (3- to 7-Hz range) EEG activity have been associated with sleep and drowsiness, as well as with problem solving, perceptual processing, cognitive tasks, and the production of imagery (for review, see Vogel & Broverman, 1964; Schacter, 1977). Increased theta in the midline frontal region (Fz), particularly that around 6 Hz, is associated with attentive performance of cognitive tasks (e.g., Lang, Lang, Kornhuber, Diekmann, & Kornhuber, 1988; Mizuki, Tanaka, Isozaki, Nishijima, & Inanaga, 1980; Nakagawa, 1988; Yamamoto & Matsuoka, 1990). Presence of theta power at Fz correlates positively with increased performance and decreases as performance declines (e.g., Nakagawa, 1988; Yamamoto & Matsuoka, 1990). This midline frontal area is directly above the anterior cingulate, which has many fibers connecting the fronto-limbic-hippocampal system of attention. Thus, the enhanced theta may be generated by this system (see below).

Increases in theta similar to those in hypnosis have been associated with restricted environmental stimulation (REST), autogenic training, and meditation. A. F. Barabasz (1990d) reported that immediately after flotation REST, high but not low hypnotizable subjects generated more theta power. During autogenic training, there was an increase of theta as individuals practiced focusing their attention (Dierks, Mauer, & Zacker, 1989; Jacobs & Lubar, 1989). Increased theta power during quiescent

---

baseline, awakening, and final waking baseline. Adapted from "EEG Correlates of Hypnotic Susceptibility and Hypnotic Trance: Spectral Analysis and Coherence" (p. 132) by M. E. Sabourin, S. D. Cutcomb, H. J. Crawford, and K. H. Pribram, 1990, *International Journal of Psychophysiology, 10,* 125–142. Copyright 1990 by Elsevier Science Publishers. Adapted by permission.

meditative states has been reported, often more so in experienced than in naive meditators (Banquet, 1973; Corby, Roth, Zarcone, & Kopell, 1978; Delmonte, 1984; Elson, Hauri, & Cunis, 1977; Fenwick, 1987; Hebert & Lehmann, 1979; Kasamatsu & Hirai, 1969; Saletu, 1987; Taneli & Krahne, 1987; T. Wallace, Benson, & Wilson, 1977). Increases in theta power have been found typically in frontal rather than occipital or parieto-temporal regions during meditation.

Vogel, Broverman, and Klaiber (1968) differentiated between "Class I" and "Class II" theta. "Class I inhibition" is associated with general inactivity or drowsiness, whereas "Class II inhibition" is associated with cognitive activity and represents "a selective inactivation of particular responses so that a continuing excitatory state becomes directed or patterned" (Vogel et al., 1968, p. 172). A large body of animal research (e.g., Isaacson, 1982) demonstrates that when an animal is exploring its environment or focusing attention on learning tasks, there is enhanced firing of theta generators (increased theta bursts) in the hippocampal region, a phylogenetically ancient cortex. With electrodes implanted in the hippocampus, Arnolds, Lopes Da Silva, Aitink, Kamp, and Boeijinga (1980) demonstrated increased theta when a patient was attending to tasks. R. Miller (1989) suggests that the hippocampus, through a cortico-hippocampal relay, transmits information by theta wave modulation and Hebbian synaptic modification so that there is selective disattention. In studies of primates learning to respond to go/no-go task conditions, Crowne, Konow, Drake, and Pribram (1972) found increased hippocampal theta generated during no-go conditions. Pribram (1991) notes that "it is as if these systems were processing 'don't look there' rather than 'look here' " (p. 224).

Given the research described above, Crawford (1990a,b, 1991b) has argued that high-amplitude, regular theta may be reflective of a disattentional process—the acknowledgment of irrelevant stimuli, with a decision not to attend to such stimuli in the environment. Thus, the greater mean theta power found in high hypnotizable individuals may reflect their

> greater efficiency in processing relevant environmental stimuli—the process of disattending and ignoring stimuli requires first the recognition of it and then the decision not to look there. This disattending ability is correlated with greater theta power, a reflection of the fronto-limbic system of attention. (Crawford, 1991b)

If so, the enhanced "Class II inhibition" theta is correlated with the high hypnotizable individuals' greater focused attentional and disattentional skills (e.g., Crawford et al., 1991; Tellegen & Atkinson, 1974). That theta increases during hypnosis in low and high hypnotizable subjects (e.g., Sabourin et al., 1990) may be indicative of the enhanced focused attention and cognitive effort of the condition.

Beta and Higher-Frequency Differences

Until recently, little interest centered on fast-frequency activity in hypnosis, in view of hypothesized relationships between hypnosis and reduced levels of arousal, and because of potential muscle activity confounds in fast-frequency activity. De Pascalis and Imperiali (1984) found no relationships between beta and hypnotizability at temporal and parietal derivations, bipolarly referenced to central vertex (Cz), in eyes-open and eyes-closed waking rest. Apkinar et al. (1971) and Ulett et al. (1972a,b) reported regression analysis of 0.5- to 70-Hz spectral power bands and demonstrated that high hypnotizable subjects had greater beta EEG activity at the right occipital (O2) derivation in a resting, nonhypnotic condition.

Recently, Sabourin et al. (1990) reported hemispheric asymmetry in the beta band (13–28 Hz) for high hypnotizable individuals, supportive of the hypothesis previously discussed of these individuals' often showing greater hemispheric asymmetries in certain EEG frequency bands. In eyes-open resting conditions, during both nonhypnotic and hypnotic conditions, high hypnotizable individuals showed significantly more mean beta power in the left hemisphere across frontal (F3), central (C3), and occipital (O1) unipolar derivations than did low hypnotizables. The low and high groups did not differ significantly in mean beta power in the right hemisphere.

Differences in 40-Hz Power

A high-frequency, low-amplitude EEG signal centered at 40 Hz within a narrow band (36–44 Hz) has been found to be a covariate of focused arousal (a component of cognitive activity) that is separate from tonic or phasic arousal and uncorrelated with other beta and alpha frequency bands (e.g., Sheer, 1970, 1976, 1984, 1989; Spydell, Ford, & Sheer, 1979; Spydell & Sheer, 1982). This "cognitive 40-Hz event-related potential (ERP)" is loosely coupled with complex stimuli and problem solving. It is distinct from a "sensory 40-Hz ERP" that is closely coupled with sensory stimuli, and is associated with " 'a selective facilitory process, believed to result from activity in the rostral brain-stem reticular formation that produces a circumscribed state of cortical excitability' (Sheer, 1975)" (Loring & Sheer, 1984, p. 34). When peak counts above a preset threshold are used, the number of 40-Hz peaks recorded from the parieto-occipito-temporal cortex junction is asymmetrically distributed over the brain area maximally engaged in cognitive activity: left hemisphere more than right with a verbal task, and right hemisphere more than left with a visuospatial task (Loring & Sheer, 1984; Spydell et al., 1979; Spydell & Sheer, 1982). In a visual search task, left-hemisphere 40-Hz activity was highly correlated with percentage of errors until the task was automated and errors eliminated, when there was a greater right-hemisphere 40-Hz ERP (R. C. Rogers, 1984). To address concerns that 40-Hz oscillations may be the results of muscle artifact, great methodological care is taken to record 70-Hz electromyographic (EMG) activity simultaneously and to eliminate from analysis 40-Hz EEG segments that have such 70-Hz EMG activity present. Thus, the resulting 40-Hz EEG is distinct from and not influenced by EMG activity (for a review, see Sheer, 1989).

If a positive relationship is assumed between hypnotizability and focused-attention skills, it would be predicted that high hypnotizable subjects would show more 40-Hz activity than low hypnotizable subjects. Apkinar et al. (1971) reported more 40- to 50-Hz activity during rest and reaction time tasks during a nonhypnotic condition in high than in low subjects. De Pascalis and his colleagues examined the density (seconds per minute rather than number of oscillations) of cognitive 40-Hz ERPs of low and high subjects, mainly women, in several studies in a nonhypnotic condition (De Pascalis, Marucci, Penna, & Pessa, 1987) or in hypnotic and nonhypnotic conditions (De Pascalis, Marucci, & Penna, 1989; De Pascalis & Penna, 1990). During nonhypnotic rest after listening to music, high hypnotizable subjects produced significantly lower 40-Hz EEG density in both hemispheres as compared with low hypnotizable subjects. Music as a nonhypnotic control condition may introduce an as yet uninvestigated potential confound, since greater absorption in music may be related to hypnotic susceptibility.

Of further interest is the consistent finding that high hypnotizables showed greater 40-Hz density hemispheric specificity than low hypnotizables when induced emotional states were compared to rest conditions in both nonhypnotic (De Pascalis et al., 1987) and hypnotic (De Pascalis et al. 1989) conditions. The low hypnotizables showed no significant shifts in 40-Hz density from rest to induced positive and negative emotions. The high hypnotizables showed bilateral hemispheric 40-Hz density increases during the recollection of positive emotions, and a reduction of density in the left hemisphere and an increase in the right during negative emotions.

Evoked Potential Differences

The disposition for more sustained attention and deeper attentional involvement is related positively to hypnotizability (e.g., Crawford et al., 1991; Roche & McConkey, 1990; Tellegen & Atkinson, 1974). Such attentional involvement may also be reflected neurophysiologically in hypnotizability-related differences of either the amplitude or latency of certain wave components of averaged EP responses.

Based upon the hypothesis that hypnotically susceptible individuals are augmenters and will show significantly greater vertex visual evoked responses (VERs) than low susceptibles, Dragutinovich and Sheehan

(1986) presented five intensities of light to 40 subjects (assessed on the Harvard Group Scale of Hypnotic Susceptibility [HGSHS]) and asked them to count mentally the number of flashes. Subjects relatively high in susceptibility had significantly greater VER amplitudes summated across the five stimulus intensities at P200 than did low hypnotizable subjects. There were no differences at P100. High hypnotizables had significantly shorter P200s than did low hynotizable subjects. These results suggest that a greater attentive involvement among the susceptible subjects when instructed to attend to environmental stimuli resulted in larger amplitudes and shorter latencies of the more cognitively oriented P200.

In a study of selective attention during a dichotic listening task, Corby, Crawford, Hink, Capell, and Roth (1980) measured auditory evoked responses (AERs) to frequent and infrequent tones during counterbalanced nonhypnotic and hypnotic conditions. Twelve subjects very low in hypnotic susceptibility (Stanford Hypnotic Susceptibility Scale, Form C [SHSS:C] scores of 0–2) and 12 subjects very high in susceptibility (SHSS:C scores of 11–12) were asked to attend to either the left or right ear and to push a button when a higher-frequency tone was detected in that ear while tones were presented to both ears. Analyses were limited to frequent tones. There were no significant group or condition effects on selective attention as measured by N1 amplitude (150–250 msec, negative peak). The later P2 amplitude (150–250 msec, positive peak) was significantly smaller for the high hypnotizables, implying that the N1 negative enhancement with selective attention was prolonged. There was a highly significant interaction (Figure 9.2) showing that high hypnotizables increased N1 latency with attention, particularly when tones were presented on the left side (and thus processed by the right hemisphere). If we postulate that highs have greater hemispheric specialization, the latency increases in highs may reflect increased right-hemisphere difficulty in processing the analytical, left-hemisphere tone task.

On a separate occasion, these same subjects participated in an auditory augmenting–reducing task. Tones of 50-, 60-, 70-, and 80-dB intensity were presented while subjects read or counted in a nonhypnotic condition. Since there were no amplitude differences between low and high hypnotizable subjects, we can conclude that they were augmenting equally in response to the stimuli when asked to disattend them. As the intensity of the tones increased (Figure 9.3), the low hypnotizables decreased their N1 latencies while the high hypnotizables increased their N1 latencies. Thus, the highs appeared to process distracting stimuli more slowly than did the lows, as the intensity of the distracting stimuli increased during conditions when they were instructed to ignore the tones and be involved in a task. Both hypnotizability and the Tellegen Absorption Scale (Tellegen & Atkinson, 1974) score correlated significantly (.44 and .58, respectively) with the latency slope measurements. Thus, both low and high hypnotizable subjects diverted equal amounts of attention to the distracting stimuli, as

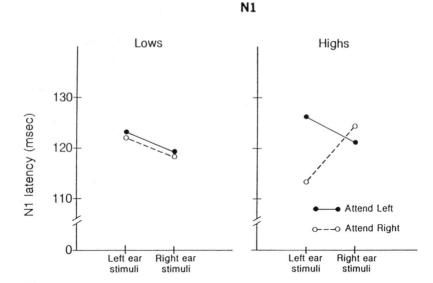

FIGURE 9.2. N1 latency means in the auditory evoked response during a dichotic tone task, when low and high hypnotizable subjects were asked to attend to the left or the right ear while stimuli were presented to either ear. Adapted from *EEG Correlates of Hypnosis and Hypnotic Susceptibility* by J. C. Corby, H. J. Crawford, R. Hink, B. S. Capell, and W. T. Roth, 1980, October, paper presented at the annual meeting of the Society for Clinical and Experimental Hypnosis, Chicago. Adapted by permission of the authors.

measured by the amplitude measures, but the highs had delayed attentional processing relative to the lows.

Lateralization and Regional Specificity: Changes Accompanying Hypnosis

A commonly espoused hypothesis popular since the 1970s is that hypnosis involves right-hemispheric generalized activation. Researchers using laterality ratios have reported shifts toward greater right-hemisphere relative to left-hemisphere involvement during hypnosis for bipolar derivations of occipito-parietal alpha (MacLeod-Morgan, 1982), occipito-temporal total power (Karlin, Cohen, & Goldstein, 1982; LaBriola, Karlin, & Goldstein, 1987), and fronto-occipital alpha and beta (Bányai, Mészáros, & Csokay, 1985; Mészáros, Bányai, & Greguss, 1985). LaBriola et al. (1987) reported greater overall total amplitude in the right hemisphere at occipito-vertex bipolar derivations, whereas two other studies (Mészáros & Bányai, 1978; Morgan, Macdonald, & Hilgard, 1974) did not. It should be noted

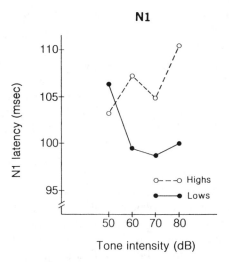

FIGURE 9.3. N1 latency means in the auditory evoked response during an auditory augmenting–reducing task in which subjects were given tones of differing intensity during reading and counting tasks. The significant interaction shows that lows demonstrated the typical decrease in N1 latencies as the tone intensities increased, whereas the highs showed increased N1 latencies. Adapted from *EEG Correlates of Hypnosis and Hypnotic Susceptibility* by J. C. Corby, H. J. Crawford, R. Hink, B. S. Capell, and W. T. Roth, 1980, October, paper presented at the annual meeting of the Society for Clinical and Experimental Hypnosis, Chicago. Adapted by permission of the authors.

that laterality ratios have been criticized because investigators cannot gauge the relative contribution of left- and right-hemisphere activity (e.g., Beaumont, Young, & McManus, 1984). Using mean power with hemisphere as a factor in their analyses, Crawford, Mészáros, and their associates (Crawford, 1989; Crawford, Mészáros, & Szabó, 1989; Mészáros, et al., 1989) reported enhancements in alpha and beta power in the right parietooccipital derivation during hypnosis in resting baseline as well as in math and imaginal tasks, in high but not low hypnotizable subjects. During visual discrimination tasks, similar enhancements in alpha and beta power in the bipolarly recorded right parieto-occipital region (Mészáros et al., 1989) and the unipolarly recorded right parieto-temporal region (Mészáros & Révész, 1990) have been found. Lubar, Gordon, Harrist, Nash, Mann, and Lacy (1991) examined EEG recorded at fronto-temporal and occipito-parietal locations before and during hypnotic tasks; complex interaction effects suggested potential effects from hypnotic level and condition, but were not broken down adequately for complete evaluation.

Furthermore, evidence also suggests a difference between low and high hypnotizable individuals in their characteristic patterns of hemispheric activation as measured by EEG frequency bands outside the hypnotic conditions. During baseline, high hypnotizable subjects show significantly greater EEG hemispheric specificity at several bipolar recording sites in the alpha band, or total power, which is greatly influenced by alpha power: Their EEGs are more activated in the left hemisphere relative to the right during analytic tasks, whereas they are more activated in the right hemisphere relative to the left during holistic, visuospatial tasks (e.g., De Pascalis et al., 1988; Karlin et al., 1982; MacLeod-Morgan & Lack, 1982; Mészáros & Bányai, 1978). Mészáros, Crawford, and their associates (Crawford, 1989; Crawford, Mészáros, & Szabó, 1989; Mészáros et al., 1989) found differential bipolar fronto-central and parieto-occipital asymmetries in the low and high alpha bands during waking and hypnosis in low and high hypnotizables during rest and during imaginal and arithmetic tasks. Specifically, in the anterior region highs showed more left-hemisphere dominance than lows, whereas in the posterior region highs were more right-hemisphere-dominant. In a study of EEG correlates of induced happy and sad emotional states, Crawford and her associates (Crawford, Clarke, et al., 1989; Crawford et al., 1988) found, regardless of nonhypnotic or hypnotic conditions, that high hypnotizables showed substantially more right-hemisphere power in low and high alpha hertz bands during the two emotional states (even greater for happiness than sadness), whereas low hypnotizables were fairly equilibrated in alpha power between the two hemispheres.

Nevertheless, when unipolar recordings were used, no hemispheric shifts during hypnosis were found at frontal, central, and occipital derivations during rest and hypnotic suggestions (Sabourin et al., 1990) or during sad and happy emotional states (Crawford, Clarke, et al., 1989; Crawford et al., 1988). These studies used subjects who were stringently screened as to hypnotic susceptibility level, and employed quite sophisticated recording methods. The fact that shifts were not observed in unipolar recordings but were observed in bipolar recordings brings up interesting methodological and theoretical issues that need to be resolved through further research. In the first comparison of bipolar and unipolar recordings in similar brain regions, R. J. Davidson, Chapman, Chapman, and Henriques (1990) demonstrated differential hemispheric asymmetries with the two recording techniques in theta, alpha, and beta power during cognitive task performance by the same subjects.

Several researchers (Karlin et al., 1980, 1982; Edmonston & Moscovitz, 1990) have preferred examining the total spectral power in comparisons of left- and right-hemisphere activity, but we feel that such general analyses do not indicate which power bands contribute to power shifts within and across derivations. Karlin et al. (1982) demonstrated greater hemispheric specificity in high than low hypnotizables for total power (1.3–30 Hz) at O1, O2, T3, and T4 referenced to Cz, similar to that discussed above for alpha band density and power, and a shift toward greater right-hemisphere activation for highs than for lows during hypnosis. Edmonston and Moscovitz (1990) found no differences between waking and hypnosis for total density (band unspecified) at bipolar O1–C3 and O2–C4 in highs only. Although these authors claim that their study calls "into question the right hemisphere activation interpretation of lateralized brain function during hypnosis" (p. 70), their study examined density rather than power, examined only one region of the brain, and used subjects screened only on the less cognitively oriented HGSHS (Shor & Orne, 1962). Density measures are time-dependent and often unrelated to amplitude-related power measures; the latter are now the preferred measures of electrocortical activity accompanying cognitive processing.

The cognitive 40-Hz ERP band associated with focused attention (e.g., Sheer, 1989), discussed in a previous section, disclosed laterality effects in hypnosis. De Pascalis and Penna (1990) found 40-Hz EEG density to shift toward greater right-hemisphere dominance during the course of a hypnotic induction in high hypnotizable women. Left- and right-hemisphere density decreased in the low hypnotizable women. During the SHSS:C (Weitzenhoffer & Hilgard, 1962) mosquito, anosmia, and voice hallucination suggestions, highs showed a greater left-hemisphere 40-Hz density, whereas during taste and negative hallucinations the two hemispheres were more balanced. Lows exhibited a greater density increase in the left hemisphere during the taste, anosmia, and negative hallucinations, and hemispheric equivalence during the mosquito and voice hallucinations. During rest lows had more 40-Hz density than highs, whereas during imaginative responses highs had a greater 40-Hz density than lows. This suggests that the highs may have been more focused in their attention during the imaginative suggestions. In a study of the recall of positive and negative emotional events in hypnosis, De Pascalis et al. (1989) found that highs showed an increase of 40-Hz density in both hemispheres during positive emotion states, and an increase only in right-hemisphere 40-Hz density during negative emotions. Lows showed no shifts in 40-Hz density during negative and positive emotional states in comparison to rest. These data were similar to those obtained in a nonhypnotic condition (De Pascalis et al., 1987).

Topographic mapping of EEG during nonhypnosis and hypnosis conditions, both at rest and during cognitive performance conditions with validated neuropsychological tests, has recently been initiated by Gruzelier and his associates. Gruzelier, Hancock, and Maggs (1991) compared the data from six high and six low hypnotizable individuals, stringently screened, on a 28-electrode array in a counterbalanced baseline–hypnosis design. Task conditions involved memorizing words (left hemisphere) or unfamiliar faces (right hemisphere), and a spatial test (right hemisphere). During hypnosis highs were distinguished from lows by more slow-wave activity (delta, theta, and alpha), which had a generalized right-hemispheric distribution both during the verbal task and while subjects were resting after the induction. During baseline the right hemisphere again differentiated the groups, but this time while resting at the beginning of the study and during the right-hemisphere tasks; highs had more alpha than lows. These EEG mapping results support earlier evidence (e.g., Sabourin et al., 1990) of more slow-wave activity in highs in nonhypnotic baseline and control conditions as well as in hypnosis, but here the findings were validated through an extensive electrode array. The relative imbalance in hemispheric activity without hypnosis supports a left-hemisphere bias in highs, at least in some conditions. With hypnosis, although it was the right hemisphere that distinguished the groups, the nature of the effect indicates that it is not a straightforward increase in right-hemispheric activation that distinguishes highs from lows; rather, highs evince more slow-wave activity in the right hemisphere, which is in line with the discussion above of the cognitive significance of "Class II" theta. Further research is needed to elucidate this hypothesis.

Neuropsychologically, highs maintained in hypnosis their nonhypnotic baseline memory for faces but showed a decline in word memory, whereas lows showed a decline in face memory and an increase in word memory after a hypnotic induction instruction (Gruzelier, Hancock, & Maggs, in press; see Figure 9.4). That highs showed a decrease in left-hemisphere verbal performance is supportive of earlier psychophysiological and neuropsychological work by Gruzelier and colleagues (Gruzelier et al., 1984). In several studies, Crawford and her colleagues demonstrated that highs, but not lows, showed increased performance during hypnosis on visual memory (Crawford & Allen, 1983), spatial memory (Crawford, Nomura, & Slater, 1983), eidetic-like imagery, and figural memory (Crawford, Wallace, et al., 1986) tasks. In addition, mainly highs reported increased use of holistic strategies during hypnosis, which correlated with enhanced visual memory performance (Crawford & Allen, 1983; Crawford, Nomura, & Slater, 1983). The neuropsychological results of Gruzelier et al. (1991, in press) and earlier work by Crawford and her colleagues are consistent with our model of lateral imbalances and the dynamics of hypnotic susceptibility. Neuropsychological studies of hypnotic and nonhypnotic conditions are discussed further in a later section.

Hypnotically Modified or Eliminated Perception of Pain

An evaluation of the effects of hypnotically suggested analgesia to painful stimuli is so far confounded by there being little consensus regarding the involvement of the cerebral cortex in pain processing (e.g., Willis, 1985). Using magnetic resonance imaging and PET in humans, Talbot, Marrett, Evans, Meyer, Bushnell, and Duncan (1991) demonstrated that painful heat applied to one arm caused significant activation of three cortical structures: the contralateral anterior cingulate, secondary somatosensory,

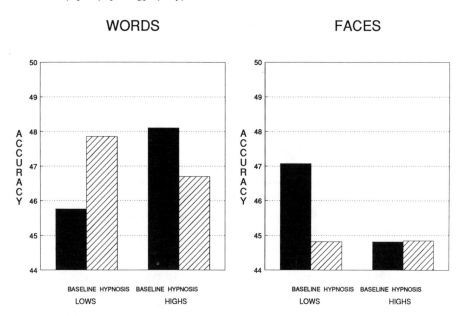

FIGURE 9.4. Mean performance on the words and faces tasks of the Warrington Recognition Memory Test during nonhypnotic baseline (solid bars) and hypnosis (hatched bars) for low and high hypnotizable subjects. Adapted from "Susceptibility-Related Changes in Recognition Memory for Words versus Faces after Instructions of Hypnosis" by J. H. Gruzelier, J. Hancock, and R. Maggs, in press, *International Journal of Psychophysiology.* Copyright by Elsevier Science Publishers. Adapted by permission.

and primary somatosensory cortices. By contrast, nonpainful, vibrotactile stimuli predominantly activated only the primary somatosensory cortex in the posterior region. This research implicates two separate attentional systems in the perception of pain: the far frontal anterior region, which is thought to regulate comfort–discomfort and emotional responses to pain, and the posterior parietal region, which is associated with sensory, time, and space aspects of pain (for a relevant review, see Crawford, 1991b; Pribram, 1991).

The frontal cortex, with its many fibers connecting to the thalamic and limbic systems, has been implicated in pain processing in other studies. Noxious electrical stimuli resulted in an increase in cerebral blood flow to the frontal lobes (e.g., Lassen, Ingvar, & Skinhoj, 1978). Prefrontal lobotomized patients report thresholds to pain similar to those of normal individuals, but there is often a dramatic decrease in the reported intensity or duress, as if the pain no longer bothers them (e.g., Hardy, Wolff, & Goodell, 1952; K. H. Pribram, personal communication, 1991). High hypnotizable individuals who learn to modify perceptions of pain often act similarly to prefrontal lobotomized patients: Pain may be still present, but little or no perception of distress is present (Crawford, 1991a; for a review, see E. R. Hilgard & Hilgard, 1975, 1983). The high hypnotizable individual who can eliminate totally the perception of both sensory and emotionally distressful pain, thus producing anesthesia as well as analgesia, should show dramatic involvement of the frontal region as well as parts of the limbic system (e.g., Crawford, 1990a,b, 1991a). We propose that in the case of hypnosis frontal inhibition is a dynamic process and is easily reversed through instruction.

The relationship between hypnotizability and reduced pain perception following suggested analgesia is about .50 (for a review, see E. R. Hilgard & Hilgard, 1975, 1983). A paradox has been noted (e.g., E. R. Hilgard & Hilgard, 1975, 1983): High hypnotizable individuals can completely eliminate the perception of pain while physiological reactivity is still evidenced. In general, cardiovascular responses are not inhibited (E. R. Hilgard & Hilgard, 1975, 1983; Olesko, Arany, & Crawford, 1989; Crawford, 1991a). For instance, although anticipated increases in blood pressure occurred with cold-pressor pain, no changes in systolic and diastolic blood pressure or in heart rate occurred as a function of hypnotic level or suggested analgesia during hypnosis in groups of low and high hypnotizable subjects (Olesko et al., 1989).

The question has arisen whether hypnotic analgesia is mediated by some endogenous opiate-like system or stress-induced analgesia mechanisms. Naloxone, a specific narcotic antagonist, is effective in reversing analgesia with opiates. Although a single-case study of repeated reversals of hypnotic analgesia by naloxone has been reported (Stephenson, 1978), controlled studies do not support its reversing hypnotic analgesia (J. Barber & Mayer, 1977; Goldstein & Hilgard, 1975; D. Spiegel & Albert, 1983). Frid and Singer (1980) found that the reversal effect of naloxone on hypnotic analgesia was enhanced by a stressful experimental condition. Using direct measurements of plasma beta-endorphin concentrations as indices of endogenous opiate activity, three studies (Domangue, Margolis, Lieberman, & Kaji, 1985; Guerra, Guantieri, & Tagliaro, 1985; Olness, Wain, & Lorenz, 1980) failed to find significant changes associated with hypnotic analgesia. De Benedittis, Panerai, and Villamira (1989) reported that beta-endorphin concentrations during waking baseline were positively related to pain endurance but not hypnotizability. Once again, hypnotic analgesia was not seen to be mediated by opiate systems.

Changes in cortical activity of rCBF metabolism, as measured by the 133-xenon method, have been reported during pain and hypnotic analgesia (Crawford, 1989; Crawford, Skolnick, Benson, Gur, & Gur, 1985; Crawford, Gur, Skolnick, Gur, & Benson, 1986). As reviewed in the section on blood flow metabolism studies of hypnosis, they found that low hypnotizable men had essentially the same rCBF metabolism patterns across all measured regions of the brain in both waking and hypnosis conditions, regardless of whether or not ischemic pain was applied to the arms. High hypnotizable men showed dramatic increases in rCBF (particularly in the temporal region), equally in both hemispheres, during pain and suggested analgesia hypnosis conditions but not a waking condition.

Research on pain perception with hypnotically suggested analgesia has also utilized cortical EP measures. Recordings of somatosensory EPs suggest that early components of the EP correlate with the sensory magnitude of somatosensory stimuli, whereas the later components reflect more the sensory-discriminative and exogenous aspects of conscious pain perception. It is the later components that are correlated with subjective pain magnitude estimates more than with objective stimulus parameters (for a review, see Stowell, 1984). Although early EP studies of hypnotic analgesia were plagued with methodological flaws, there is some evidence (Clynes, Kohn, & Lifshitz, 1964; Galbraith, Cooper, & London, 1972; Guerrero-Figueroa & Heath, 1964; Hernandez-Peon & Donoso, 1959; N. J. Wilson, 1968) that the amplitude of the EP is diminished in response to hypnotic suggestion and that the stimulus is attenuated in high hypnotizable individuals, although other studies (Amadeo & Yanovski, 1975; Andreassi, Balinsky, Gallichio, De Simone, & Mellers, 1976; Beck & Barolin, 1965; Beck, Dustman, & Beier, 1966; Halliday & Mason, 1964a; Serafetinides, 1968; Zakrzewski & Szelenberger, 1981) found no changes. A review of the psychophysiology of hypnotic hallucinations may be found in D. Spiegel and Barabasz (1987).

Mészáros et al. (1985) reported decreases in the amplitude of P200 somatosensory EPs to short electrical impulses to the median nerve when subjects experienced hypnotic analgesia. D. Spiegel, Bierre, and Rootenberg (1989) compared somatosensory EP responses to stimuli "just below the threshold of discomfort" at unipolar derivations (F3, F4, Cz, P3, P4, O1, and O2) in 10 high hypnotizable and 10 low hypnotizable subjects in four counterbalanced conditions: normal attention (attend and press button), passive attention (attend but do not press button), hypnotic attention (attend and press button), and hypnotic obstructive hallucination (suggested local anesthetic—press button if any stimuli felt). Interestingly, highs had lower P100 amplitudes, regardless of condition. In addition, in comparison to normal attention, highs showed a decrease of 45% in P100 amplitude in the hypnotic obstructive hallucination condition at all seven recording derivations. Lower P300 amplitudes were also demonstrated by the highs during the hypnotic obstructive hallucination condition, in comparison to normal attention at the right frontal (F4) and parietal (P3) derivations and at both left and right occipital (O1, O2) derivations. During hypnotic attention, highs showed a 35% increase in mean P100 amplitude. Thus, during hypnotic analgesia to mildly uncomfortable stimuli, there appears to be an alteration in signal detection (P100) as well as less cognitive awareness of the incoming stimuli (P300). D. Spiegel, Bierre, and

Rootenberg (1989) failed to train the highs to eliminate the perception of pain completely. Research using similar methodologies but with more stringently screened and trained subjects, as well as stronger painful stimulation, may elucidate these exciting results further.

In a study of hemispheric differences, D. Spiegel, Cutcomb, Ren, and Pribram (1985) found that when asked to experience a visual obstructive hallucination, high but not low hypnotizable subjects showed significant suppression of the P3 component of the visual EP at Fz, Cz, Pz, O1, and O2. The N2 and P3 component was more greatly reduced in the right hemisphere than in the occipital region. In contrast, highs who were asked to experience anosmia to odors showed olfactory EP P300 amplitude increases rather than decreases in hypnosis but not waking, whereas lows showed no changes in P300 amplitudes in the temporal region (T3 and T4) (A. F. Barabasz & Lonsdale, 1983). The instructions in the Barabasz and Lonsdale study may have induced a surprise factor, and thus subjects generated greater, not lesser, P300 amplitude when given suggestions of anosmia (D. Spiegel & Barabasz, 1987, 1988).

Using electrical tooth pulp stimulation, Sharav and Tal (1989) found that suggestions of hypnotic anesthesia blocked cognitive awareness of pain without interrupting the initiation of the early component of the masseter inhibitory period, but suppressing its late component. Cutaneous reactivity against histamine prick tests to the arms in highly hypnotizable volunteers was evaluated in nonhypnotic and hypnotic analgesia conditions by Zachariae and Bjerring (1990). During hypnotic analgesia, pain-related EPs accompanying argon laser stimulations and the flare reaction to the prick tests were significantly reduced. Arendt, Zachariae, and Bjerring (1990) evaluated hypnotically suggested hyperaesthesia and analgesia to painful laser stimulation in highly hypnotically susceptible subjects. The amplitude of the EPs increased during hyperaesthesia and decreased during analgesia, while the latency of the potential remained unchanged.

Mean integrated amplitude power within various hertz bands in fronto-parietal bipolar recordings was examined in a patient undergoing dental surgery with hypnosis as the sole anesthetic (Chen, Dworkin, & Bloomquist, 1981). Total energy output of the left and right hemispheres diminished during hypnosis, with a greater diminution in the left hemisphere in alpha and theta bands. Karlin et al. (1980) reported on a preliminary investigation of hemispheric EEG changes during experimentally produced cold-pressor pain during waking and hypnotic analgesia. Evidence tentatively suggested a shift toward greater overall right-hemisphere involvement at bipolar parieto-occipital derivation that correlated with degree of pain reduction during suggested analgesia.

Crawford (1990a,b, 1991a,b) compared four high hypnotizable individuals, who could eliminate completely the perception of pain (thereby producing anesthesia) induced by a cold-pressor task, with seven low hypnotizable individuals who were unable to reduce pain perception greatly. Unipolar recordings at frontal (F3, F4), temporal (T3, T4), parietal (P3, P4), and occipital (O1, O2) regions with references to balanced ear-lobes was done in nonhypnotic and hypnotic sessions on the same day. Conditions within each were prerest baseline, pain dip with no analgesia, suggested hypnotic analgesia without pain, suggested hypnotic analgesia with pain dip, and postrest baseline. The left hand and lower arm were held in cold water (1°C) for 60 seconds with EEG recording after 10 seconds of immersion. During prerest, from 13 to 19 Hz (low beta) and 37 to 42 Hz (high beta, like the 40-Hz band discussed earlier), there was more mean power in hypnosis than in waking for all subjects. Highs generated more mean theta power than lows during pain and hypnotic analgesia con-ditions in hypnosis across all locations (see Figure 9.5). During pain and suggested analgesia dips, lows showed no significant theta power asymmetries between the left and right hemispheres at the four regions, whereas the highs showed significant asymmetries in some regions. In the temporal and parietal regions, especially the temporal, the highs were significantly more left-hemisphere-dominant in the pain dip while ex-periencing pain, and then demonstrated a shift in hemispheric dominance during hypnotic analgesia. There was a significant decrease in left-hemisphere theta power and a significant increase in right-hemisphere theta power. Such shifts may be indicative of dramatic changes in atten-tional focusing and defocusing upon the painful stimuli, which involved shifts from left- to right-hemisphere functioning. While pain was being felt, attention was focused in a more analytical, left-hemispheric style, but while pain was being eliminated, the highs were now internally attending to self-generated, right-hemisphere-maintained imagery (for a discussion, see Crawford, 1991b). As discussed in an earlier section on theta, the shifts in hemispheric dominance of theta among the highs may be indicative of greater cognitive flexibility and greater disattentional abilities. Crawford and her associates are investigating this further.

Quite similar findings were reported by Larbig and his associates (Larbig, 1989; Larbig, Elbert, Lutzenberger, Rockstroh, Schneer, & Bir-baumer, 1982), but without consideration of the biological significance of theta. They reported substantially higher theta power in the parietal (Pz), but not the central (Cz), derivation in a fakir (an individual from India who could insert pins into his skin and hang from hooks without experiencing pain), in comparison to controls who showed no change when asked to reduce their pain perception to experimentally induced pain (shock to leg).

Deep Cortical and Subcortical EEG Recordings

Deep electrode implants in inner structures of the brain have been carried out as a neurosurgical diagnostic procedure in medically resistant epileptic patients. De Benedittis and his colleagues at the University of Milan

FRONTAL: HIGH THETA

TEMPORAL: HIGH THETA

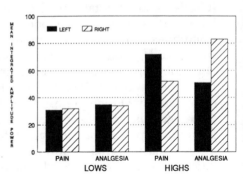

PARIETAL: HIGH THETA

OCCIPITAL: HIGH THETA

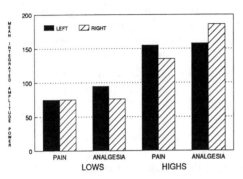

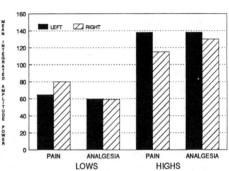

FIGURE 9.5. Mean theta power of the left (solid bars) and right (hatched bars) hemispheres at frontal (F3, F4), temporal (T3, T4), parietal (P3, P4), and occipital (O1, O2) locations for low and high hypnotizable subjects during cold-pressor pain in hypnotic conditions when pain would normally be felt and after suggestions of analgesia. Adapted from *Cold Pressor Pain with and without Suggested Analgesia: EEG Correlates as Moderated by Hypnotic Susceptibility Level* by H. J. Crawford, 1990, July, paper presented at the 5th International Congress of Psychophysiology, Budapest. Adapted by permission of the author.

Medical School, Italy, have taken advantage of these in-depth electrodes to study neurophysiological mechanisms associated with hypnosis (for a review, see De Benedittis & Carli, 1990). An anecdotal report by Crasilneck, McCranie, and Jenkins (1956) first drew attention to this possibility by reporting that in one hypnotized patient hypnosis was terminated each time the hippocampal region was electrically stimulated during brain surgery for the removal of an epileptogenic focus. They hypothesized that the limbic system mediates the neural circuits involved in hypnosis, in view of the role of the hippocampus in maintaining attention.

In one epileptic patient who tested as highly hypnotizable, De Benedittis and Sironi (1986) recorded from seven electrodes each with three limbic leads and three cortical leads. Electrodes were implanted in the limbic structures (the hippocampus and the amygdala bilaterally) and superficial cortices (anterior and posterior temporal cortices; frontal and fronto-orbital cortices). Six were on the left side, the site of the focus. EEG recordings were examined in resting baseline, after imaging instructions in waking, hypnosis, and posthypnosis. During hypnosis background EEG showed an increase in alpha, and to a lesser extent in the beta sensorimotor rhythm, as well as a reduction of focal interictal abnormalities.

In another epileptic patient who tested as moderately hypnotizable, De Benedittis and Sironi (1988) stimulated electrodes deeply implanted in the amygdala and other cerebral structures. During hypnosis, repeated stimulations of the left and right amygdala aroused the subject from hypnosis, whereas stimulation of the temporal neocortices and the right hippocampal Ammon's horn did not alter the hypnotic trance. These authors "postulate that hypnotic behavior is mediated, at least in part, by a dynamic balance of antagonizing effects of discrete limbic structures—the amygdala and the hippocampus. In fact, the trance state is associated with hippocampal activity, concomitant with a partial amygdaloid complex functional inhibition" (De Benedittis & Sironi, 1988, p. 104).

Blood Flow Studies as Indicators of Cerebral Metabolism

Direct evaluation of brain function and cerebral organization can be obtained through the use of recent imaging techniques that employ low-level radioactively labeled emitters to assess regional brain metabolism, cerebral blood flow, and receptor location and concentration. Energy metabolism in the brain is considered to be indicative of cognitive activity, effort and arousal. Three of these approaches—the two-dimensional rCBF, the three-dimensional PET, and SPECT—have been used to compare nonhypnotic and hypnotic conditions.

In the first study to be conducted, Crawford, Ruben Gur, and their associates (Crawford et al., 1985; Crawford, Gur, et al., 1986; see also Crawford, 1989) studied the effects of rest, ischemic pain without suggested analgesia, and ischemic pain with suggested analgesia, all in sessions with and without hypnosis. rCBF was measured by the xenon inhalation method. Subjects were stringently screened on the HGSHS (Shor & Orne, 1962), the more cognitively oriented SHSS:C (Weitzenhoffer & Hilgard, 1962), and the highly cognitively oriented Revised Stanford Profile Scale of Hypnotic Susceptibility, Form I (Weitzenhoffer & Hilgard, 1967); they were also screened for strong right-handedness, low anxiety, no depression, and a lack of medical and psychiatric disorders. Six men very low in hypnotizability and six men very high in hypnotizability participated. An additional requirement of the highs was the demonstrated ability to use suggested hypnotic analgesia to eliminate all pain perception completely in two preliminary training sessions, one with cold-pressor pain and one with ischemic pain.

The hypnotic and nonhypnotic sessions were conducted on separate days, with the order of sessions counterbalanced across subjects. Measurements of rCBF were made in each of three conditions in the two sessions: rest, ischemic pain, and ischemic pain with analgesia suggestions. Subjects lay in a supine position with their eyes closed. The rCBF was measured in 32 regions of both hemispheres by the conventional 133-xenon inhalation technique (Obrist, Thompson, Wang, & Wilkinson, 1975; Risberg, Ali, Wilson, Wills, & Halsey, 1975). Trace amounts of 133-xenon mixed with air were inhaled during 1 minute, followed by 14 minutes of normal air breathing by means of a face mask and a spirometer system. Clearance of the tracer's gamma radiation was recorded by 32 stationary scintillation detectors, placed anteriorly to posteriorly over 16 homologous regions of each hemisphere. The recording of the arrival and disappearance of the diffusible tracer forms the basis for the initial slope index (ISI) of grey matter flow (Obrist et al., 1975; Risberg et al., 1975), which is the initial slope at time 0 of the mathematically equivalent instantaneous bolus injection.

There was a significant interaction (see Figure 9.6) between the two conditions (nonhypnotic and hypnotic) and hypnotic susceptibility level ($p < .05$), of a similar nature in rest alone or across all three conditions of rest, or ischemic pain with or without suggested analgesia. During the nonhypnotic condition, low and high hypnotizable men had quite similar overall ISI mean blood flows. In the hypnotic conditions, the lows remained the same, while the highs showed a dramatic increase in rCBF. This was not due to differences in breathing rates or CO_2 consumption.

In all four regions—anterior, parietal, temporal, and temporo-posterior—the highs demonstrated enhanced rCBF, ranging from 13% to 28% during rest, whereas the lows showed nonsignificant changes. It was the temporal region during hypnotic rest that showed the largest increase in glucose metabolism within the highs. During pain with hypnotically suggested analgesia, all regions discriminated between the lows and highs. The highs showed greater glucose metabolism in the temporal region during hypnosis. It is believed that the enhanced rCBF in hypnosis among the highs is indicative of increased cognitive effort and focused attention.

In a similar study of the effects of hypnosis on rCBF with the 133-xenon inhalation method in 12 men, Meyer, Diehl, Ulrich, and Meinig (1989) reported a global increase of rCBF in both hemispheres, as did Crawford, Gur, and their associates (Crawford et al., 1985, Crawford, Gur, et al., 1986; Crawford, 1989), accompanying hypnotically suggested arm

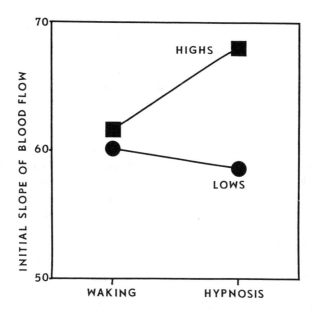

FIGURE 9.6. Overall mean initial slope of blood flow during nonhypnotic and hypnotic sessions, collapsed across rest, ischemic pain, and ischemic pain with suggested analgesia for low and high hypnotizable subjects. From *Regional Cerebral Blood Flow and Hypnosis: Differences between Low and High Hypnotizables* by H. J. Crawford, R. Gur, B. Skolnick, R. Gur, and D. Benson, 1986, July, paper presented at the 3rd International Congress of Psychophysiology, Vienna. Reprinted by permission of the authors.

levitation. In addition, "a global increase of cortical blood flow was found, together with a regional activation of the temporal centers for acoustic attention. Moreover, under hypnotically narrowed consciousness focus, an unexplained deactivation of inferior temporal areas occurred" (Meyer et al., 1989, p. 48).

Halama (1989) used SPECT to study changes in cortical perfusion before and during hypnosis in 17 patients (16 with neurotic depression, 1 with epilepsy), all of whom appeared to be responsive to hypnotic suggestions, although no standardized testing was performed. As in the two studies described above, there was a global cortical perfusion increase in hypnosis. As patients entered hypnosis, there was a significant decrease in brain metabolism in the left hemisphere in the gyrus temporalis and inferior region, as well as in areas 39 and 40. In the right hemisphere there was a cortical "frontalization," particularly in the higher areas (7 cm above the meato-orbital level) more than in the deeper ones (4 cm above the mean meato-orbital level). Thus, during hypnosis there was a shift toward greater right-hemisphere involvement in certain parts of the anterior region, but not elsewhere. In another SPECT study, De Benedittis and Longostreui

(1988; De Benedittis & Carli, 1990) evaluated 5 low and 5 high hypnotizable subjects in hypnosis, and 10 additional subjects in nonhypnotic rest and during hypnotic analgesia. They too reported increases in brain metabolism only among the highs during hypnosis.

The four studies suggest the utility of cerebral blood flow methodology in the analysis of glucose metabolism in both cortical and subcortical brain regions during waking and hypnosis. Only Crawford et al. (1985) and De Benedittis and Longostreui (1988) assessed the hypnotic susceptibility level of their subjects with standardized tests and compared individuals low and high in hypnotizability. The studies of Meyer et al. (1989) and Halama (1989) only used hypnotically responsive individuals. Substantial increases in global blood flow were found during hypnosis in the hypnotically responsive subjects, whether they were normal subjects or psychiatric patients. Halama (1989) demonstrated that with the use of the three-dimensional SPECT, as with the PET, one can obtain precise information about both cortical and subcortical brain structures. Because of practical limitations that restrict rCBF and PET studies to larger medical facilities, as well as the higher levels of administered radioactivity required by them, the much safer and less expensive SPECT may be more accessible to researchers desiring to pursue this field of research.

Electrodermal Activity

Early research with measures of palmar sweating, an autonomic measure under the control of the sympathetic branch of the autonomic nervous system, produced generally inconclusive results concerning the direction of change in activity with the induction of hypnosis (O'Connell & Orne, 1962, 1968; Pessin, Plapp, & Stern, 1968; J. A. Stern, Edmonston, Ulett, & Levitsky, 1968). Possible exceptions were reports of reductions in spontaneous or nonspecific responses during hypnosis (Pessin et al., 1968; Ravitz, 1950; O'Connell & Orne, 1962; Tebecis & Provins, 1976).

In a reinvestigation of this issue using a tone habituation paradigm, whereby orienting responses were measured to incidental moderate-intensity tones, Gruzelier and Brow (1985) found faster habituation to tones with hypnosis than with control conditions consisting of baseline, relaxation, and listening to a story read by the hypnotist (the last of these was introduced as a control for the deployment of attention). As is seen in Figure 9.7, faster habituation was obtained in high susceptible subjects and the reverse was found in low susceptible subjects (i.e., habituation was retarded after instructions of hypnosis). During the hypnotic induction, prior to the tones, highs also had lower levels of activity and fewer nonspecific responses. In order to explore hemispheric influences, activity was recorded bilaterally. When nonhypnotic baseline and hypnosis recordings were compared, only highs showed a shift in lateralization from higher left-hemispheric influences in nonhypnotic baseline to higher right-hemispheric influences with hypnosis, despite a reduction in overall activity (Figure 9.8). The laterality results are in keeping with right-hemispheric involvement in hypnosis, and also lead to the hypothesis that highs have greater left- than right-hemisphere involvement in the nonhypnotic baseline state (Gruzelier et al., 1984).

In a subsequent investigation involving unilateral recording, the effects of hypnosis on habituation were replicated, as was the decline in levels of activity with hypnosis. The facilitation of habituation was not observed in subjects instructed to simulate hypnosis (Gruzelier, Allison, & Conway, 1988). A decrease in sympathetic activity with hypnotic relaxation has also been recently reported by G. De Benedittis (personal communication, August 1991) and colleagues through a spectral analysis of the electrocardiogram.

Dichotic Listening Tests

Numerous studies have demonstrated a mean right-ear (left-hemisphere) advantage for dichotically presented verbal material and a mean left-ear (right-hemisphere) advantage for dichotically presented nonverbal material (for an excellent review, see Hugdahl, 1988), although the usefulness of dichotic listening scores as an index of functional asymmetry between the cerebral hemispheres has been questioned (e.g., Teng, 1981). Accepting the hypothesis that hypnosis more strongly activates the right hemisphere, several studies have investigated hypothesized shifts toward greater left-ear advantage (LEA) during hypnosis. The findings are mixed.

Frumkin, Ripley, and Cox (1978) presented 60 pairs of consonant–vowel–consonant (CVC) syllables dichotically to 20 medium to high hypnotizable (scores of 3, 4, or 5 on the Stanford Hypnotic Clinical Scale) college students in nonhypnotic, relaxed hypnotic, and nonhypnotic conditions. The laterality index used was a ratio, $[(R - L)(R + L)] \times 100$, between the correct scores of the left and right ears. Although subjects maintained a right-ear advantage (REA) in all conditions, there was a significant decrease in REA during hypnosis, in support of a shift in favor of right-hemisphere involvement. Reporting on the same subjects, Frumkin, Ripley, and Cox (1979) found a significantly negative correlation between hypnotic susceptibility and a linguistic right-ear score; this finding suggests that within this restricted range (three scores) of hypnotizability, highs are less right-ear-dominant than mediums. A limitation of this study is that laterality ratios do not permit interpretation of absolute hemispheric involvement; for instance, a decrease in left-hemisphere activity or an increase in right-hemisphere activity could lead to greater REAs. Using the

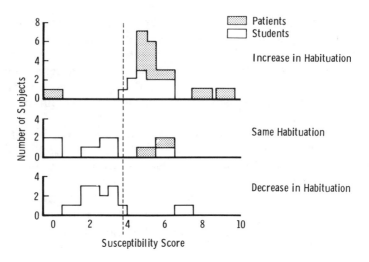

FIGURE 9.7. The majority of subjects who showed an increase in habituation, and therefore fewer orienting responses when hypnosis was compared with baseline, had high susceptibility scores during the induction, whereas the opposite effect was found in low susceptible subjects. Habituation changes were obscured in a minority of subjects by floor and ceiling effects and hence habituation was the same on both occasions. From "Psychophysiological Evidence for a State Theory of Hypnosis and Susceptibility" (p. 293) by J. H. Gruzelier and T. D. Brow, 1985, *Journal of Psychosomatic Research, 29,* 287–302. Copyright 1985 by Pergamon Press. Reprinted by permission.

same methodology, Pagano, Akots, and Wall (1988) replicated these findings in a sample of 15 medium to high hypnotizable subjects.

In a study of 29 college students stringently screened on both the HGSHS and SHSS:C, as well as for right-handedness and normal hearing, Crawford, Crawford, and Koperski (1983) presented 30 pairs of consonant–vowel (CV) syllables during nonhypnotic, alert hypnotic, and nonhypnotic conditions. Unlike the subjects in Frumkin et al.'s research, subjects were encouraged to report both syllables. Although the majority of subjects showed strong REA, some showed an LEA. On a laterality index consistent with that of Frumkin et al. (1978), neither highs nor mediums showed significant REA shifts across conditions. Unexpectedly, low hypnotizable subjects showed a significant decrease in REA during hypnosis. Other laterality indices (percentage of errors, percentage of correct responses, laterality coefficient) yielded very similar patterns. Because methodological changes may have affected the results, Crawford and Mac-Leod-Morgan (1986) compared the effects of alert versus passive hypnosis inductions, as well as of reporting the dominant-ear CVs versus both sets of CVs, in low, medium, and high hypnotizable subjects. Their findings

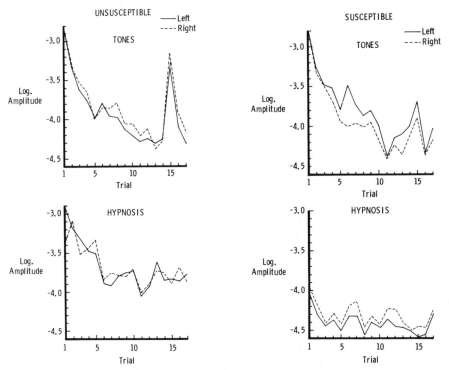

FIGURE 9.8. Lateral asymmetries in the amplitude of orienting responses across trials showing opposite asymmetries in low and high susceptible subjects with baseline tones and hypnosis. No consistent bilateral differences were found in low susceptible subjects. From "Psychophysiological Evidence for a State Theory of Hypnosis and Susceptibility" (p. 298) by J. H. Gruzelier and T. D. Brow, 1985, *Journal of Psychosomatic Research, 29,* 287–302. Copyright 1985 by Pergamon Press. Reprinted by permission.

too failed to support the hypothesized shift to right-hemisphere dominance during hypnosis. Finally, Levine, Kurtz and Lauter (1984, Study 2) reported no significant shifts in REA during hypnosis when lows, mediums, and highs were presented with CVs, with instructions to attend to one or the other ear (a difference from other studies), in counterbalanced nonhypnotic and hypnotic conditions. By contrast, Watterson (1991) reported that highs showed the hypothesized shifts toward right-hemisphere dominance in conditions of attending to one ear only (focused-attention task), but failed to produce the shift in conditions of attending to both ears (ambient-attention task).

Spellacy and Wilkinson (1987) presented a dichotic task that required a verbal recall of a whole word to low and high hypnotizable subjects (assessed by the HGSHS and SHSS:C). There was a significant increase in

REA during hypnosis. Lows showed the usual REA in both nonhypnotic and hypnotic conditions. Of the highs, half showed LEA in the nonhypnotic condition, and all showed REA during hypnosis. Thus, highs may demonstrate a shift in cognitive strategy toward more verbal processing when given a verbal task in hypnosis.

Levine et al. (1984, Study 1) administered six pitch pattern sounds (e.g., "do-re-mi") of contiguous pure tones with instructions to attend to one or the other ear (a difference from other studies). An increase in LEA, as correlated positively with hypnotic susceptibility, during hypnosis provided support for a shift in hemispheric involvement toward greater relative right-hemisphere participation. Thus, although Levine et al. (1984) did not find shifts in REA for verbal stimuli (Study 2), they did for nonverbal stimuli (Study 1). B. L. Sanders (1979) reported that only when extremely hypnotizable subjects were compared against moderately high and low hypnotizable subjects did shifts in laterality toward right-hemispheric functioning on verbal and nonverbal listening tasks emerge. This finding reinforces our view that inadequate screening of hypnotizability, particularly for extremely highly hypnotizable individuals, may account for inconsistent findings.

Laterality ratio scores, which can unknowingly be influenced by the amount of errors present, have been greatly criticized because the relative contribution of left- and right-hemisphere activity cannot be determined (e.g., Beaumont et al., 1984). The percentage of correct responses and percentage of errors have also been criticized as indices, since they do not adequately correct for differences in accuracy when overall performance is, respectively, above or below 50% (Bruder, 1991). Several other measures that adjust for these biases have been proposed, but each has advantages and disadvantages (Bruder, 1991). An awareness of these difficulties and the application of alternative methods of analysis are necessary in future research in this area.

A variety of verbal (digit tests, nonsense syllable tests, fused-work tests, and monitoring tests) and nonverbal (melodies, musical chords, environmental sounds, tone contours, and complex tones) tasks have been shown to be valid measures of hemispheric differentiation (Hugdahl, 1988; Bruder, 1991). Any researcher must employ these tests cautiously, however, because they correlate poorly with one another, reflect different cognitive processes, and involve different functional systems of the brain (Bruder, 1991). In addition, they "differ in memory load, [in] meaningfulness of items, in the use of natural versus synthetic speech, in the extent of fusion or competition of dichotic pairs, and in susceptibility to attentional bias" (Bruder, 1991, p. 220). Despite such limitations, when dichotic listening tests are chosen and evaluated correctly, they can be of value in the assessment of hypothesized shifts in hemispheric dominance during hypnosis. Specifically, the use of verbal and nonverbal dichotic tasks can help determine which cognitive processes and regions of the brain may be differentially affected during hypnosis.

Divided-Visual-Field Research

Utilizing lateralized anatomical connections in the visual system, whereby the temporal hemiretina transmits information to the homolateral visual cortex before transversing the corpus callosum, McCormack and Gruzelier (in press) have investigated hemispheric influences of hypnosis. They examined brightness discriminations in the left and right temporal hemifields, applying psychophysical signal detection procedures to obtain independent estimates of sensory sensitivity (d') dependent on hemispheric activation of judgmental criteria (beta scores), as influenced by subjects' attitudes. Comparisons were made between medium and high hypnotizable subjects in three conditions: nonhypnotic baseline (control), hypnosis, and nonhypnotic baseline (control). Sensory sensitivity was enhanced as a result of an increase in signal-to-noise ratio in the hypnosis condition, whereas discriminability remained the same in the nonhypnotic baseline conditions. However, whereas the effects were bilateral in medium subjects, they were unilateral and of significantly higher magnitude in high subjects (see Figure 9.9). In the highs, the unilateral increase was in the right hemisphere, providing further support for the hypothesis that right-hemispheric processing distinguishes highs from lows in conditions of hypnosis. Attitudinal criteria (beta scores) remained invariant across sessions, which incidentally provides added support for state rather than nonstate underpinnings of hypnosis.

Haptic Tactile Discrimination

To investigate lateralized processing in the tactile modality, Gruzelier and his colleagues have conducted three studies (Gruzelier et al., 1984; Cikurel & Gruzelier, 1990) that involved distinguishing letters and numbers by touch while blindfolded. Left- and right-hand sorting times were compared after correcting for movement times. Processing times have been shown to be independent of movement times and are increased in states of fatigue, as shown in young doctors on night duty (Orton & Gruzelier, 1989).

In the first study (Gruzelier et al., 1984), medical students showed a slowing in right-hand sorting times after the induction of hypnotic relaxation compared with a prehypnosis baseline, whereas left-hand processing times remained unchanged. Susceptibility scores on a scale obtained concomitantly with the hypnotic induction correlated with right- but not

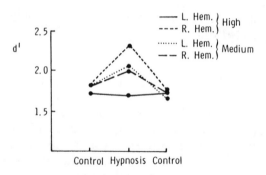

FIGURE 9.9. Divided-visual-field processing showing a unilateral increase in sensitivity with hypnosis in the right hemisphere of high susceptible subjects and bilateral increase in medium susceptible subjects. From "Cerebral Asymmetry and Hypnosis: A Signal Detection Analysis of Divided Visual Field Stimulation" by K. McCormack and J. H. Gruzelier, in press, *Journal of Abnormal Psychology*. Copyright by the American Psychological Association. Reprinted by permission.

left-hand processing times, such that the higher the susceptibility score, the greater the slowing in right-hand times in hypnosis after scores were subtracted from baseline. The second study (Gruzelier et al., 1984) involved middle-aged subjects. Unlike students, they exhibited marked practice effects in hypnosis compared with nonhypnotic baseline. However, this facilitation in processing time with practice was not seen in high susceptible subjects in right-hand processing times, thereby replicating the laterality result of the first study. In view of the contralateral mediation of tactile discriminations involving active as distinct from passive touch, these results suggest a primary role for left-hemispheric inhibition in the induction procedure.

The third study (Cikurel & Gruzelier, 1990) employed an active alert induction procedure (Bányai & Hilgard, 1976) in order to clarify influences of hypnosis as distinct from relaxation. Subjects were hypnotized while pedaling a stationary bicycle ergometer, and were given suggestions of alertness and freshness instead of tranquility and relaxation. The susceptibility scores of active alert and traditional hypnotic inductions were correlated highly. In replication of the previous experiments, a slowing in right-hand sorting times in hypnosis compared with prehypnosis baseline was observed in high susceptible subjects, and occurred similarly in both types of induction procedures. Medium susceptibles showed bilateral slowing, echoing the bilateral changes that occurred in mediums in the divided-visual-field study discussed in the preceding section. The left-hemispheric inhibitory influences in the active/alert induction were, if anything, greater than in the traditional relaxation induction, providing further evidence that hypnosis is as different from relaxation as it is from other quiescent states such as sleep.

Clinical Neuropsychological Tests and the Neuropsychophysiological Model

Continuing our neuropsychophysiological frame of reference, tests validated on neurological patients with focal lesions have been used to substantiate further the neuropsychophysiological model of hypnotic induction. Work by Crawford and her associates has shown that only high hypnotizable individuals demonstrate significant performance enhancements during hypnosis on visual memory tasks (Crawford & Allen, 1983), tasks involving spatial memory for location (Crawford et al., 1985), and eidetic-like imagery memory for Julesz stereograms (Crawford, Wallace, et al., 1986). In addition, high hypnotizable subjects report a substantial increase from detail-oriented to holistic strategies during hypnosis, whereas low hypnotizable subjects do not change (Crawford & Allen, 1983). All of these studies suggest greater right-hemispheric involvement during hypnosis among high hypnotizable subjects. Extending this work, Gruzelier and his associates have examined tasks known to specifically access focal lesions of either the left or right hemisphere.

In one study previously discussed with regard to EEG topographical mapping (Gruzelier et al., 1991), the Warrington Recognition Memory Test (Warrington, 1974) of words and unfamiliar faces was administered to stringently screened low and high hypnotizable individuals. Patients with lateralized temporal and parietal lobe lesions show double dissociations on the two tests, such that left-sided lesioned patients have relatively well-preserved memory for faces and are impaired in memory for words, whereas right-sided lesioned patients have normal verbal memory but are impaired in memory for faces. Our model predicts a reduction in verbal memory in high susceptibles, as a result of the primary left-hemispheric inhibitory influences that are instigated by instructions of hypnosis; this may be accompanied by an increase in right-hemispheric functional activity, mirrored in improved memory for faces.

The results (see Figure 9.4) showed support for the first hypothesis: Word recognition memory was poorer in the hypnosis condition than in a nonhypnotic baseline condition for hypnotically responsive individuals. Memory for faces remained unchanged, supporting the specificity of the left-sided inhibition with hypnosis, but providing no support for an improvement in right-hemispheric processing as assessed with face recognition memory.

The neuropsychophysiological model also posits that low susceptibles will have a bias toward right-hemispheric activity in nonhypnotic baseline conditions—a bias that subserves broadened attention with a lesser ability to disattend to irrelevant stimuli (Crawford, 1991b; Dimond, 1980; Gruzelier, Eves, & Connolly, 1981), that is also moderated by levels of anxiety (Gruzelier, 1987; Gruzelier & Phelan, 1991), both of which militate against the induction of hypnosis. Nevertheless, at least some left-hemispheric activation will occur as lows attempt to focus on the hypnotist's induction, which is typically verbal and will normally engage the temporal lobe of the left hemisphere. At the same time, lows will fail to succumb to the inhibition originating from anterior frontal regions, which is posited to underpin the experience of letting go and giving up reality testing. To return to the results of the memory experiment, lows shifted from a relative superiority in memory for faces over words in the nonhypnotic baseline to the opposite memory advantage in hypnosis; in other words, hypnosis produced in them left-hemispheric activation in temporal regions (Gruzelier et al., 1992).

To turn now to within-hemisphere dynamics, it is posited (as just mentioned) that hypnosis involves an inhibition of frontal functions, as seen in the handing over by the subject to the hypnotist of executive and planning functions of the anterior frontal region, as well as in the suspension of critical analysis and reality testing (e.g., Crawford, 1991b; Gruzelier, 1990). Coincidental with this are heightened awareness or involvement, and greater flexibility in sensory and emotional receptive functions (depending on the nature of the instructions given by the hypnotist). An enhancement of posterior visual discriminations was in fact observed in the previously discussed divided-visual-field study (McCormack & Gruzelier, in press). Furthermore, in high susceptible subjects this anterior-to-posterior shift will be coupled with a left-to-right shift. Complementary to such a hypothesis are EEG hemispheric specificity differences between the anterior and posterior regions of the brains in low and high hypnotizable subjects (Crawford, 1989; Mészáros et al., 1989). In addition, the greater right posterior EEG hemispheric power associated with imaginal tasks in the high hypnotizable subjects provides further support (e.g., Crawford, 1989; Mészáros et al., 1989).

Gruzelier and Warren (1992) investigated lateralized frontal functions with tests of word fluency, design fluency, and motor dexterity. In high susceptible subjects, reductions in performance with hypnosis were found in fluency for letter categories (an anterior frontal function), whereas this was not found in fluency for semantic categories (which involves temporal lobe as well as frontal functions). The left temporal lobe is presumed to remain functionally active as it tracks the hypnotist's induction, as seen in a preliminary auditory EP study (Gruzelier, Thomas, Conway, Liddiard, Jutai, McCormack, Golds, Perry, Rhonder, & Brow, 1987; Jutai, Gruzelier, Golds, & Thomas, in press). Design fluency, a right frontal task, showed improvements in fluency with hypnosis in contrast to the impairment or no change in verbal fluency. Finger-tapping dexterity showed reductions in activity bilaterally. Thus, considered together, the results indicated some bilateral inhibition of anterior functions but a bias toward greater left- than right-sided inhibition.

Final Comments on Our Neuropsychophysiological Working Model

Throughout the 1980s and into the 1990s, we have been building a neuro-psychophysiological model of hypnosis in our two laboratories to help explain neuropsychophysiological findings in the literature that have not in general been meaningfully interpreted by the researchers, as well as to guide us in the development of new experiments to test and refine our model. The exciting results now coming from our own work, as well as from that of a growing number of psychophysiologists, have greatly helped us in the model's evolution. We are now quite confident that the behavioral differences related to hypnotic susceptibility are correlated with and influenced by neurophysiological mechanisms, thus providing some support for a trait view of hypnotizability, accompanied by perhaps even a heritability component (e.g., Morgan, 1973).

Our review of results indicates that neuropsychophysiological evidence may assist in resolving the classical conundrum of distinguishing hypnotically susceptible from unsusceptible individuals in the baseline, nonhypnotic state. Crawford (1989; Crawford & Allen, 1983) earlier concluded that high susceptible individuals show greater cognitive flexibility and are better able to shift their attention and cognitive strategies and to comply with the instructions of the hypnotist. We have outlined comparisons of lateral brain functions of high and low susceptibles; these have shown that, contrary to the view that highs are characterized by right hemisphericity (e.g., Gur & Gur, 1974; Graham, 1977), highs exhibit greater hemispheric specificity (left or right), depending on task demands (e.g., Crawford, 1990a,b, 1991a,b; Karlin et al., 1980; MacLeod-Morgan & Lack, 1982; Mészáros & Bányai, 1978; De Pascalis et al., 1989).

Gruzelier and colleague's recordings of bilateral electrodermal orienting activity and bilateral haptic processing have indicated that high susceptibles have imbalances of activity favoring the left hemisphere. Performance on validated neuropsychological tests contrasting left- and right-hemisphere processing, such as word versus design fluency and word versus face recognition memory, has also disclosed left-hemispheric processing advantages in highs (Gruzelier et al., 1991; Gruzelier & Warren, 1992). In line with our neuropsychophysiological model of hypnosis, which describes the engagement of anterior inhibitory functions that extends bilaterally, the left hemisphere is more involved than the right in the first stage of the hypnotic induction process. We argue that left-hemispheric advantages in high hypnotizable individuals may be seen to facilitate hypnosis.

In some studies that have demonstrated left-hemispheric frontal advantages in highs, lows have been shown to possess the opposite asymmetry, as distinct from no asymmetry at all. In other studies, lows show a hemispheric balance in EEG activation regardless of task, whereas highs shift hemispheric activation dependent upon the task. This may shed light on factors that hamper the induction of hypnosis.

Right-hemispheric functional biases in activity have been found to accompany states of moderate anxiety (Gruzelier, 1987). The influence of anxiety was investigated in medical students by examining them on two occasions, one of which was the day before an examination, and the other a month before or after. The ecological validity of the examination stressor was corroborated through questionnaire measures of anxiety, which disclosed increases in frustration and tension. Autonomic measures of electrodermal activity indicated retarded rates of habituation of the orienting response, as well as a raised incidence of spontaneous fluctuations of skin conductance, during the examination time. In the cognitive domain of lexical processing (assessed with the divided-visual-field procedure), a right-hemispheric advantage, in contrast to the expected left-hemispheric advantage for verbal processing, was found during the examination period. By contrast, left-hemispheric advantages were obtained during the nonexamination control period. Thus, anxiety produced a lateral shift in functional activity in the brain. Evidence in low hypnotizable individuals of an imbalance of function favoring the right hemisphere, both in nonhypnotic baseline conditions and, importantly, during hypnosis induction (Gruzelier & Warren, 1992; Gruzelier et al., 1991), coupled with retarded habituation of electrodermal responses (Gruzelier & Brow, 1985; Gruzelier, 1987), is compatible with possible anxiety and/or generalized, nonfocused attentional processing in lows. This anxiety and this type of processing are inferred to militate against hypnotic induction—an inference not simply based on clinical acumen, but here shown to have a neuropsychological counterpart that distinguishes lows from highs.

Although the enhancement of hypnotizability in low susceptibles has met with failure on many occasions (for a review, see Perry, 1977), several studies that have emphasized the reduction of anxiety and a reorganization of cognitive functioning suggest the possibility of enhancing hypnotic responsiveness under certain conditions. M. J. Diamond (for a review, see M. J. Diamond, 1977) found that hypnotic responsiveness was enhanced after therapy that emphasized enhanced interpersonal relationships (reduction of social anxiety). More germane to our psychophysiological studies, A. F. Barabasz found that extended REST experiences enhanced responsiveness in Antarctica (A. F. Barabasz, 1982) as well as in the laboratory (A. F. Barabasz, 1982; A. F. Barabasz & Barabasz, 1989). It is hypothesized that the cognitive disorganization that occurs in REST, coupled with reduced anxiety, sets the stage for cognitive reorganization so that enhanced hypnotic responsiveness, as well as increased theta production (A. F. Barabasz, 1990d), is evident. The importance of assessing the hypnotic susceptibility level of individuals participating in REST experiments has yet to be considered systematically, but is of value (e.g.,

Crawford, 1992). The long-lasting effects of REST experiences also have yet to be investigated systematically.

One of the most robust electrophysiological findings is the greater theta power found in highs in comparison to lows in both nonhypnotic and hypnotic conditions (e.g., Crawford, 1990a,b, 1991a,b; Sabourin et al., 1990). Combined with studies of differential hemispheric specificity and habituation, the evidence strongly supports the view that hypnotic susceptibility reflects an important attentional ability (e.g., Crawford et al., 1991). Only when one can focus attention and ignore certain stimuli completely can absorption and the giving up of reality testing, or even responsiveness to hypnotic suggestions, follow. This was exemplified in experiments involving habituation of the orienting response, a process that reflects the ability to focus attention on a stimulus and is a prerequisite for the redirection of attention elsewhere: Habituation was found to be facilitated in highs during hypnosis and to be retarded in lows (Gruzelier & Brow, 1985). EP studies (e.g., Corby et al., 1980; Dragutinovich & Sheehan, 1986) support neurophysiological differences, reflective of differences in sustained attentional ability between lows and highs instructed to attend or disattend to sensory stimuli. Highs can often reduce or eliminate the perception of pain after hypnotically suggested analgesia and anesthesia—an extreme example of disattention to pain and the redirection of attention elsewhere. Of importance is that there is a shift in theta power dominance from the left to the right hemisphere when highs shift their attention away from painful stimuli (Crawford, 1990a,b, 1991a,b). Thus, the ability to disattend to irrelevant stimuli (to habituate) provides a major clue as to what contributes to the development of dissociative behavior, a topic considered further elsewhere (Crawford, 1991b; Crawford & Barabasz, in press).

The studies of haptic processing have underscored still further the importance of left-hemispheric dynamics in hypnosis: It was the changes in left-hemispheric tactile discriminations, not right-, that related to the depth of hypnosis (Gruzelier et al., 1984). Although there is good agreement on primary right-hemispheric involvement in the hypnotic trance per se, it is our contention that this right posterior activation may give way to focal left posterior activation, according to the demands required of the hypnotic subject (e.g., Crawford, 1986). With hindsight, what may be more central to hypnosis is the inhibition of anterior frontal lobe functions.

Accordingly, instructions of hypnosis can be seen to trigger a process that alters brain functional organization—a process that at the same time is dependent on individual differences in existing functional dynamics of the central nervous system. Our neuropsychophysiological approach validates not only the nature of the underlying functional organization that characterizes the susceptible individual, but also the development of the hypnotic process. By virtue of the fact that our chosen perspective is a neuropsychophysiological one, this approach informs our understanding of the phenomenology of the hypnotic experience. This will lead not only to further elucidation of the induction process, but also to advances in the efficacy of hypnotic induction procedures, and ultimately to an enrichment of the applications of hypnosis. Finally, it should lead us to further understanding of the neurophysiology of individual differences in attentional and cognitive processing.

Acknowledgments

We gratefully acknowledge Arreed F. Barabasz's critical review of an earlier version of this chapter. Portions of the research from Helen J. Crawford's laboratory were supported by grants from The Spencer Foundation and a National Institute of Health Biomedical Research Support Grant. Research from John H. Gruzelier's laboratory was supported by grants from the Medical Research Council of Great Britain.

CHAPTER TEN

Situational and Personality Correlates of Hypnotic Responsiveness

IRVING KIRSCH
JAMES R. COUNCIL

People differ considerably in their responsiveness to hypnosis. Levels of responsiveness are more or less normally distributed and are as stable as most personality traits (E. R. Hilgard, 1965a; Morgan, Johnson, & Hilgard, 1974; Piccione, Hilgard, & Zimbardo, 1989). One of the most important tasks of research on hypnosis is to establish the determinants of these differences in responding.

The dependent variable in this body of research is often termed "hypnotizability" or "hypnotic susceptibility." To some extent, however, these terms beg the question. "Hypnotizability" and "susceptibility" imply personal traits that are not influenced by situational variables. Yet it is the purpose of research to establish the degree to which responsiveness is influenced by situational factors, as well as the degree to which it is due to an ability or predisposition. As a matter of convenience, we continue to use the conventional terms in this chapter. We do so, however, with some misgivings, and we ask the reader to understand that we are not making the *a priori* assumption of some highly stable trait underlying responsivity to hypnosis. What we mean by "suggestibility" is simply the degree to which suggested responses were observed or reported in the specific situation in which the research was conducted. We use the term "hypnotizability" to mean suggestibility following the administration of a hypnotic induction.

We begin with a review of the literature on personality correlates of hypnotizability. This is followed by a section on situational influences on suggestibility. Finally, we consider the interface of person and situation, as manifested by situation-specific person variables.

Personality Correlates of Hypnotic Responsiveness

The possibility that one or more dimensions of personality underlie hypnotizability has stimulated theory and research since the 19th century (E. R. Hilgard, 1967). Tests of hypnotizability show remarkably high test–retest correlations and high intercorrelations (E. R. Hilgard, 1965a; Morgan, Johnson, & Hilgard, 1974; Piccione et al., 1989). Although these findings indicate that hypnotic responsiveness is "trait-like" in its consistency, attempts to find other personality attributes with which hypnotizability is correlated have been largely unsuccessful.

Weitzenhoffer (1953), Deckert and West (1963b), T. X. Barber (1964), and E. R. Hilgard (1965a, 1967) reviewed over 70 studies using standard measures of personality that were published between 1930 and 1964. The general pattern of these studies was that of an initial report of a significant relationship, followed by failures to replicate in subsequent studies. For example, Rosenzweig and Sarason (1942), using the Picture–Frustration test and a behavioral task involving failure, reported high correlations between hypnotizability on the one hand and impunitiveness and repression on the other, but five subsequent studies by other investigators failed to confirm these findings (T. X. Barber, 1964). Similarly, significant relationships were initially reported between hypnotizability and the Guilford–Zimmerman Temperament Survey, the Maudsley Personality Inventory, the Minnesota Multiphasic Personality Inventory (MMPI), and the Edwards Personal Preference Schedule, but later research did not replicate these findings (T. X. Barber, 1964; Deckert & West, 1963b).

Inconsistent or nonsignificant results were also obtained with the Thurstone Personality Schedule, the Bernreuter Personality Inventory, the Rorschach, the Thematic Apperception Test, the Leary Interpersonal Checklist, the California Psychological Inventory, and other personality measures (T. X. Barber, 1964; Deckert & West, 1963b; E. R. Hilgard, 1965a, 1967; Weitzenhoffer, 1953). Such findings, as well as the poor methodology of some studies, led these reviewers to conclude that there was no evidence of strong or consistent relationships between hypnotic susceptibility and personality factors.

Since the 1960s, research on personality correlates has been focused primarily on absorption, imaginative involvement, and fantasy proneness—concepts so closely related to one another that it is not clear that they represent different constructs. These traits have been of interest to researchers because they represent a point of convergence between otherwise disparate theories of hypnosis (e.g., J. R. Hilgard, 1970; S. C. Wilson & Barber, 1981). Also, in marked contrast to earlier research, research on these variables has produced replicable correlations with hypnotizability. More recently, research examining the association between hypnotizability and various measures of dissociative capacity has appeared, stimulated by E. R. Hilgard's (1977a) highly influential proposal of neodissociation theory. In this section, we review studies examining these variables as predictors of hypnotizability.

Absorption

"Absorption" can be defined as a predisposition or openness to experience alterations of cognition and emotion over a broad range of situations (Roche & McConkey, 1990). The evolution of absorption as a personality construct started in the early 1960s with the development of the Personal Experiences Questionnaire (PEQ; Shor, 1960; Shor, Orne, & O'Connell, 1962), which assessed a wide range of naturally occurring "trance-like" experiences. Subsequent measures continued to focus on imaginative experiences occurring in everyday life and shared many items. Ås retained much of the PEQ's content when constructing his Experience Inventory (EI; Ås, 1963; Ås, O'Hara, & Munger, 1962), and Lee-Teng (1965) included items from the EI in her Hypnotic Characteristics Inventory (HCI). The PEQ, EI, and HCI all bore significant correlations with hypnotizability, although most were low to moderate.

Continuing the development of such scales, Tellegen and Atkinson (1974) used items from the earlier questionnaires in the construction of a 71-item research questionnaire. This questionnaire was used in a factor-analytic study, which reported evidence that absorption was a personality trait related to hypnotizability and orthogonal to other major dimensions of personality. The research questionnaire has since been refined into a 34-item measure known as the Tellegen Absorption Scale (TAS; Tellegen, 1981, 1982). The TAS has become the most widely used measure of absorption and has significantly predicted hypnotic responsiveness in numerous studies (e.g., Council & Huff, 1990; Council, Kirsch, Vickery, & Carlson, 1983; Crawford, 1982a; Farthing, Venturino, & Brown, 1983; Finke & Macdonald, 1978; Frischholz, Spiegel, Trentalange, & Spiegel, 1987; Kumar & Pekala, 1988; Nadon, Laurence, & Perry, 1987; Radtke & Stam, 1991; Roberts, Schuler, Bacon, Zimmerman, & Patterson, 1975; Roche & McConkey, 1990; Spanos, Brett, Menary, & Cross, 1987; Spanos & McPeake, 1975a,b; Spanos, Radtke, Hodgins, Bertrand, Stam, & Moretti, 1983; Spanos, Rivers, & Gottlieb, 1978; Spanos, Steggles, Radtke-Bodorik, & Rivers, 1979; Tellegen & Atkinson, 1974; Yanchar & Johnson, 1981).

Correlations between the TAS and hypnotic susceptibility scales, though generally significant, have been modest, explaining about 10% or less of the variance in hypnotizability scores. Although some investigations have obtained higher correlations, these have tended to have smaller samples, more difficult hypnosis scales, and greater proportions of female subjects (de Groh, 1989). In general, studies using hypnosis scales (e.g., the Barber Suggestibility Scale [BSS], the Harvard Group Scale of Hypnotic Susceptibility [HGSHS]) that consist primarily of ideomotor tasks and comparatively easy cognitive suggestions have yielded less impressive correlations than those using scales that contain a greater number of more difficult cognitive suggestions (e.g., the Stanford Hypnotic Susceptibility Scale, Form C [SHSS:C]) (de Groh, 1989; Roche & McConkey, 1990). The dream, age regression, and hallucination items on the SHSS:C, as well as other cognitive items common to Forms A and C of the SHSS, were reported to correlate most highly with the HCI (Lee-Teng, 1965), suggesting that these items may also be mainly responsible for significant relationships between the TAS and hypnotizability. Similarly, Balthazard and Woody (1992) reported that absorption was unrelated to passing ideomotor and easy cognitive items on the HGSHS, but successfully predicted performance on more difficult items. Taken together, these data support the hypothesis that absorption may be a reasonably good predictor of responses to difficult cognitive suggestions (e.g., suggested hallucinations), but not of ideomotor responding. It is worth noting that in their classic presentation of absorption, Tellegen and Atkinson (1974) modified their measure of hypnotic responsiveness to include a higher proportion of such cognitive–imaginative items.

The TAS and most other measures of absorption are transparent and positively keyed, which makes them vulnerable to biased responding and reactive effects (Council, Kirsch, & Hafner, 1986). In fact, there is evidence that an acquiescence response set could be partially responsible for the significant correlations of these scales with measures of hypnotic susceptibility. Lee-Teng (1965) found that HCI scores correlated significantly with sum-true scores on the MMPI, and reported a factor analysis showing that the sum-true score was most characteristic of the inventory items. With the HCI rescored for sum-yes answers, the correlation with hypnotizability increased (E. R. Hilgard, 1965a). Although no studies have directly investigated the TAS for acquiescence response bias, these findings caution against interpreting TAS scores too literally on the basis of item content.

Context Effects and the Tellegen Absorption Scale

Regardless of the problems noted above, the long search for reliable personality correlates of hypnotizability had seemingly yielded success with the discovery of the relationship between absorption and hypnotizability. The association of hypnotic responsiveness with absorption made sense from virtually all theoretical perspectives, and provided a rare consensus among hypnosis theorists (Spanos & Barber, 1974). However, some recent research suggests that the relationship may have been affected by a measurement artifact.

In the first of a series of studies on "context effects," we (Council et al., 1986) administered standard measures of absorption and hypnotizability in two different contexts. One condition duplicated the usual method: Subjects who volunteered to participate in a hypnosis experiment first filled out the TAS and were then tested on a group adaptation of the SHSS:C. In the second condition, each test was given in separate contexts, so that subjects would not be aware that the two scales were part of the same study. We found the usual modest correlation between hypnotizability and absorption only when subjects completed both measures in the same context. When subjects were unaware that tests of absorption and hypnotizability were part of the same study, the correlation was close to zero.

The hypothesis that the relationship between hypnotizability and absorption is context-dependent has now been tested in at least seven subsequent studies (de Groot, Gwynn, & Spanos, 1988; Drake, Nash, & Cawood, 1990–1991; Green, Kvaal, Lynn, Mare, & Sandberg, 1991; Nadon, Hoyt, Register, & Kihlstrom, 1991; Rhue, Lynn, & Jacquith, 1989; Perlini, Lee, & Spanos, 1992; E. Z. Woody, Bowers, & Oakman, 1990). Two issues are raised in these studies. One relates to the reliability, magnitude, directionality, and cause of context effects. The other concerns whether there is a relation between hypnotizability and absorption that can be found independently of any artifacts that may be produced by contextual cues. Although the first issue is quite complex, the second is our present concern, and it can be answered relatively straightforwardly. All that is required is an examination of the correlations between absorption and hypnotizability with context controlled, so that subjects are unaware that the two constructs are being measured as part of the same study.

Of the eight studies in which context effects were controlled, only two reported significant associations when absorption and hypnotizability were assessed in totally separate contexts. Nadon, Hoyt, et al. (1991) found a small significant correlation ($r = .18$) between the TAS and behavioral scores on the HGSHS, but a negligible nonsignificant correlation between absorption and subjective scores on the HGSHS.[1] With separate testing contexts, Perlini et al. (1992) reported small ($r = .19$) to moderate ($r = .31$) correlations between an abbreviated version of the TAS and both behavioral and subjective scores on the Carleton University Responsiveness to Suggestion Scale (CURSS). This is the only report of a context-independent correlation between absorption and subjective responses to hypnosis, and it is all the more remarkable because the absorption items were embedded among an equal number of filler items, thus making context effects less likely.

In contrast to these two reports, nonsignificant, near-zero correlations between the TAS and all measures of hypnotizability were reported in the remaining six studies in which the two constructs were measured in separate contexts (Council et al., 1986; de Groot et al., 1988; Drake et al., 1990–1991; Green et al., 1991; Rhue et al., 1989; E. Z. Woody et al., 1990). Given the fairly large samples used in some of these studies, one is left with the conclusion that if there is a relation between absorption and hypnotizability, it is very small and unreliable.

The validity of the TAS as a predictor of hypnotizability is also called into question by studies indicating that the association between the two can be affected by other contextual factors. For example, when administered in disguised versions with filler items, the TAS has failed to predict hypnotizability in two studies (Chiofalo & Coe, 1982; Spanos, McPeake, & Churchill, 1976), although two studies have reported positive relationships (Balthazard & Woody, 1992; Perlini et al., 1992). Spanos and McPeake (1975a) reported that positive labeling of hypnosis enhances the correlation between the TAS and hypnotizability, while negative labeling diminishes it. Rhue et al. (1989) also found that labeling the TAS strongly influenced its correlation with hypnotizability. Calling the TAS a "hypnotic experience inventory," for example, resulted in correlations with hypnotizability ranging from .43 to .80.

Findings of context effects have understandably evoked consternation among hypnosis researchers. For example, Kihlstrom, Hoyt, Nadon, and Register (1987) stated that these findings, if confirmed, "would undercut both the empirical and construct validity of absorption, and leave us with no reliable individual difference correlates of hypnotizability." Unfortunately, the problem of context effects has since been shown to generalize beyond the relationship between absorption and hypnotizability. Context-dependent relationships have also been reported between hypnotizability and measures of dissociation, bulimia, mysticism, daydreaming frequency, and beliefs in paranormal phenomena (Green et al., 1991; Lynn, Predieri, Green, Mare, & Williams, 1990; de Groot et al., 1988). These findings suggest that investigators who use transparent questionnaires and do not control for context effects may find significant relationships that are actually the results of a methodological artifact.

Imaginative Involvement

J. R. Hilgard (1970) defined "imaginative involvement" as an "almost total immersion" in an activity, accompanied by disattention to irrelevant stimuli. On the basis of extensive interviews before and after hypnotizability assessment, she concluded that there are multiple pathways into hypnotic responding, but that imaginative involvement is a major underlying factor. Most of the highly hypnotizable persons in her study reported a variety of involvements in everyday imaginative experiences. This construct is closely related to absorption, and findings with the TAS and related scales have been taken to support the construct validity of imaginative involvement and its relationship to hypnotizability (J. R. Hilgard, 1979b; Drake et al., 1990–1991; Tellegen & Atkinson, 1974).

More direct support for the construct of imaginative involvement is found in studies that have used measures directly related to J. R. Hilgard's

(1970) interviews. Baum and Lynn (1981) and Fellows and Armstrong (1977) reported a relationship between involvement in reading and hypnotizability. Similarly, Snodgrass and Lynn (1989) reported that high hypnotizable subjects reported significantly greater involvement in music than low hypnotizable subjects did. LeBaron, Zeltzer, and Fanurik (1988) interviewed samples of children, and reported that involvement in stories, games, and pretend play correlated significantly with hypnotizability. S. Davis, Dawson, and Seay (1978) used a questionnaire based on J. R. Hilgard's (1970) interviews, and found that high scorers on this measure were significantly more hypnotizable than were low scorers.

All of these findings have been supportive, but the identification of imaginative involvement with absorption has led one group of investigators to readminister J. R. Hilgard's interview while controlling for context effects. Although they did not find a significant difference in correlations between conditions, Drake et al. (1990–1991) reported that when the interview was administered in contexts separated from an assessment of hypnotizability, correlations were not significant. This final result, like those on absorption, casts some doubt on imaginative involvement as a predictor of hypnotizability.

Fantasy Proneness

The "fantasy-prone" personality was first described by S. C. Wilson and Barber (1981, 1983a), on the basis of interviews comparing excellent to average hypnotic subjects. Highly hypnotizable subjects appeared to comprise a type characterized by deep involvement in a private world of fantasy, vivid daydreams, and seemingly paranormal experiences. Research on fantasy proneness has been facilitated by a self-report measure based on S. C. Wilson and Barber's (1981, 1983a) interview procedure, the Inventory of Childhood Memories and Imaginings (ICMI; S. C. Wilson & Barber, 1983b). Other researchers have continued to investigate the fantasy-prone personality, and Lynn and Rhue in particular have conducted an impressive program of research on fantasy proneness and its relation to hypnotizability (Lynn & Rhue, 1986, 1988; Rhue & Lynn, 1987). Their findings (summarized in Lynn & Rhue, 1988) have been generally supportive of S. C. Wilson and Barber's (1981, 1983a) description of the fantasy-prone person, but the relationship between hypnotizability and fantasy proneness appears to be more modest than that reported by Wilson and Barber.

Although an earlier study (Lynn & Rhue, 1986) found that high fantasizers were significantly more hypnotizable than other groups, Rhue and Lynn (1989) and Council and Huff (1990) reported that high and medium fantasizers did not differ in hypnotizability. Although these data fail to confirm S. C. Wilson and Barber's hypothesis that fantasy proneness is a marker of exceptionally high hypnotizability, all three studies reported significant, though moderate, correlations between hypnotizability and fantasy proneness.

The possibly contaminating effects of context have been controlled in at least two studies of fantasy proneness and hypnotizability. Green et al. (1991) reported that the ICMI was significantly associated with measures of hypnotizability, although at a low level (r's = .13 to .18). Unfortunately, the ICMI contains two items that refer explicitly to hypnosis, which may provide cues about the experimenter's hypothesis similar to those provided by assessing both variables in the same context. Silva (1990) removed those two items from the ICMI, administered it in one context, and tested hypnotizability in another. Despite these controls, he obtained a significant correlation between fantasy proneness and scores on the CURSS. This suggests that in contrast to the TAS and J. R. Hilgard's measure of imaginative involvement, the ICMI may have a relationship to hypnotizability that is not context-dependent. On the other hand, there is considerable conceptual overlap among these constructs, and all three measures are highly correlated with one another (Drake et al., 1990–1991; Green et al., 1991). In addition, the ICMI's content is quite heterogeneous, and the component(s) responsible for the reported context-independent correlations have not yet been determined.

Imagery Vividness

Though it is not, strictly speaking, a personality trait, imagery vividness may be a relatively stable capacity along which individuals differ; given its conceptual relation to absorption, imaginative involvement, and fantasy proneness, this seems the appropriate place to consider its relation to hypnotizability. This has been assessed in a number of studies (reviewed by de Groh, 1989), and moderately positive correlations are generally reported. However, context effects were not controlled in any of the studies cited in de Groh's review. Perlini et al. (1990) failed to find significant correlations between hypnotizability and imagery vividness when both were measured in separate contexts. However, the correlations they reported ranged from −.01 to .22, and the higher correlations came from a relatively small sample. Therefore, the most one can conclude is that a context-independent relation between imagery vividness and hypnotizability has not yet been definitively established.

Dissociation

If anything, "dissociation" has figured more pervasively in theories of hypnosis than absorption has. This concept was prominent in early theories of Charcot, James, Janet, Freud, and Prince (Breuer & Freud, 1893–

1895/1955; Charcot, 1889; Freud, 1893/1959; E. R. Hilgard, 1977a; James, 1890/1981; Janet, 1901; Kihlstrom & McConkey, 1990; Prince, 1939). Although interest in dissociation was low from the early part of this century to the 1960s, the publication of *Divided Consciousness: Multiple Controls in Human Thought and Action* (E. R. Hilgard, 1977a) has stimulated much contemporary hypnosis theory and research.

Even researchers who are sympathetic to dissociation find the concept difficult to define (Frankel, 1990; Gruenewald, 1986; Margolis & Margolis, 1979). According to neodissociation theory (E. R. Hilgard, 1977a), information processing involves multiple parallel paths or systems. Dissociation consists of one or more of these systems' operating outside of awareness and influencing cognition, affect, or behavior. Hypnosis is just one means by which systems may be split off from conscious awareness. E. R. Hilgard discusses dissociation as a normal aspect of information processing and treats the capacity for dissociation as a trait underlying hypnotic responsiveness (E. R. Hilgard, 1977a).

Most researchers attempting to link hypnotizability with dissociation adhere more or less closely to E. R. Hilgard's (1977a) neodissociation theory. Bartis and Zamansky (1986) define dissociation more operationally as an inconsistency between an individual's perception of an event and other concurrent behavioral and/or cognitive aspects of the same event. D. Spiegel (1986), from a more clinical standpoint, defines dissociation as a condition in which specific subsets of material exclude other subsets of material from conscious awareness. Perhaps because of the widespread acceptance of neodissociation theory, many papers have treated dissociation without defining it. After all, as Gruenewald (1986) has observed, "everyone knows" what is meant by dissociation, even though its specific nature is difficult to describe. This trend is unfortunate, since the concept of "dissociation" has become so diffuse that it is in danger of going the way of "hysteria" (Frankel, 1990).

The theory that dissociative processes may form the basis of hypnotic responding has led some workers to hypothesize that individual differences in hypnotic responsiveness are the results of stable differences in dissociative capacity or ability. Thus, dissociation has been treated both as a process or "state" responsible for hypnotic behavior, and as an individual difference or "trait" underlying hypnotizability. The discussion in this chapter focuses on dissociation in the latter sense, and begins by considering two self-report measures that have been related to hypnotizability.

Dissociative Experiences Scale

Bernstein and Putnam (1986) defined dissociation as a continuum that includes normal and abnormal experiences. However, they specifically identified the Dissociative Experiences Scale (DES) as a measure of pathological dissociation, and intended it for use with clinical populations. DES item content was developed through consultations with clinicians specializing in dissociative disorders and interviews with patients diagnosed as having *Diagnostic and Statistical Manual of Mental Disorders,* third edition (DSM-III) dissociative disorders. The DES is heavily loaded with content related to amnesia and depersonalization, and some items might connote psychopathology to test takers. Carlson and Putnam (1988) reported a factor analysis that found three main factors accounting for about 63% of the variance in DES items. The first two were interpreted as representing amnesia and depersonalization/derealization. The third, on which about a third of the items loaded, was seen as related to absorption and imaginative involvement. Carlson and Putnam (1988) presented evidence that the DES could discriminate between patients diagnosed with and without dissociative disorders, and concluded that it might prove useful as a diagnostic screening device, but did not discuss the DES with regard to hypnosis.

Although the DES is relatively new at the time of this writing, several studies have examined its relationship to hypnotizability. An unpublished study by Perry (described in Carlson & Putnam, 1989) found a high correlation ($r = .61$) between the DES and the SHSS:C; but his sample contained equal numbers of subjects low, medium, and high in hypnotizability, and this may have inflated the correlation. Four studies have employed more representative samples and have reported more modest correlations (r's = .18 to .24; Green et al., 1991; Nadon, Hoyt, et al., 1991; Silva, 1990; E. Z. Woody et al., 1990). All of these investigators controlled for context effects, and all found that the correlation between hypnotizability and the DES was only significant when the two measures were administered in the same context.

Taken together, these data indicate that, at best, the DES has a small relationship with hypnotizability. Furthermore, if such a relationship exists, it is likely to reflect the overlap between the DES and absorption. Correlations between the DES and the TAS ranging from .40 to .75 have been reported (Green et al., 1991; Nadon, Hoyt, et al., 1991; E. Z. Woody et al., 1990), and this level of relationship is maintained even when the scales are administered in separate contexts (Council, Waters, Sanderson, & Svenby, 1991). The DES is also significantly correlated with fantasy proneness as measured by the ICMI (Green et al., 1991; Silva, 1990). It would be interesting to determine whether significant correlations between the DES and hypnotizability are confined to the absorption factor found in Bernstein and Putnam's (1986) factor analysis, or whether they can be found for the amnesia and depersonalization/derealization factors as well.

Perceptual Alteration Scale

The Perceptual Alteration Scale (PAS; S. Sanders, 1986) was developed specifically for research on hypnotic susceptibility. E. R. Hilgard's (1977a) neodissociation theory was used to guide the selection of 22 items from the MMPI item pool, and to generate additional items to form a final scale consisting of 60 items. S. Sanders (1986) reported data indicating satisfactory internal consistency within three subscales assessing modifications of affect, control, and cognition, as well as evidence of discriminant validity. Although Sanders did not present data on the relationship of the PAS to hypnotizability, it was used along with the DES in the Nadon, Hoyt, et al. (1991) and Green et al. (1991) studies described above. Nadon, Hoyt, et al. (1991) reported a small but significant association between the PAS and hypnotizability, but as described earlier (see Note 1), testing contexts were not kept separate in this part of their study. Green et al. (1991) reported a significant correlation, but only when the PAS was administered in a hypnotic context; when testing contexts were kept separate, correlations between the PAS and hypnotizability were nonsignificant, despite a relatively large sample ($n = 240$).

Behavioral Measures of Dissociation

Instead of using a pencil and paper inventory to measure dissociative capacity, Stava and Jaffa (1988) assessed the relations between hypnotizability and various behaviors that could be interpreted as examples of dissociation in nonhypnotic contexts. Subjects were assessed for their ability to attend simultaneously to two different tasks (divided attention), to attend to a single task while ignoring other stimuli (selective attention), and to recall information that they had been told to ignore (incidental learning). None of these abilities was related to hypnotizability.

Summary

Consistent with previous reviews (T. X. Barber, 1964; Deckert & West, 1963b; E. R. Hilgard, 1965a, 1967; Hull, 1933; Weitzenhoffer, 1953), our survey of the literature indicates that the search for dispositional correlates of hypnotizability continues to yield surprisingly meager results for a behavior that appears to be relatively stable. The exceptions are a cluster of intercorrelated scales that measure the tendency to have imaginative and dissociative experiences in nonhypnotic contexts. These correlations, however, appear to be at least partially dependent on the subjects' knowledge that the scales are being investigated in relation to hypnosis, and the magnitude of the association is quite small, leaving most of the variance in hypnotizability unexplained.

The only "personality" correlate of hypnotic responsiveness that has been found to be highly predictive of hypnotic responsiveness is the person's responsiveness to the same suggestions administered in a nonhypnotic context (E. R. Hilgard & Tart, 1966; Hull, 1933). Waking suggestibility typically accounts for about 45% of the variance in hypnotic suggestibility. This does not explain hypnotizability, however. Instead, it is a consequence of the relatively small effect that hypnotic inductions have on response to suggestions. It is an indication that suggestibility, rather than hypnotizability, is what needs to be explained.

Situational Correlates of Suggestibility

In this section, we review studies of situational determinants of suggestibility. In our examination of dispositional correlates, the dependent variable has been "hypnotizability," defined as responsiveness to suggestions made after the administration of a hypnotic induction. Here, in examining the effects of situational variables, we look at "suggestibility" rather than "hypnotizability" as the dependent variable. In the absence of a hypnotic context, it is not proper to refer to responsiveness to suggestion as "hypnotizability." Thus, by looking at "suggestibility" as the dependent variable, we can include hypnotic inductions and their components as situational independent variables that may influence responsiveness to suggestion.

Hypnotic Inductions and Suggestions

Tests of hypnotic responsiveness are generally preceded by hypnotic inductions that define the situation as "hypnosis" and administer relaxation instructions. Additional procedures include suggested visual imagery and various ideomotor suggestions, the most common of which is suggested, nonvolitional eye closure. These inductions produce significant but modest enhancement of responsiveness to suggestion (T. X. Barber & Glass, 1962; Weitzenhoffer & Sjoberg, 1961; E. R. Hilgard & Tart, 1966; Hull, 1933). The effect of induction procedures is surprisingly small, however. People display a wide range of responsiveness to suggestion without any induction at all.

Each of the components of conventional inductions has been shown to produce a small effect on response to suggestion. Suggestibility is enhanced when the situation is labeled "hypnosis," with no other induction components preceding the administration of test suggestions (T. X. Barber & Calverley, 1964d, 1965a). Similarly, the provision of relaxation instructions enhances suggestibility regardless of whether the situation has (T. X. Barber & Calverley, 1965a,b; Starr & Tobin, 1970) or has not (F. J. Evans, 1967) been defined as hypnotic. G. P. Mitchell and Lundy (1986) evaluated the effects of three induction procedures: relaxation instructions without suggested imagery, suggested imagery without relaxation, and an induction that combined relaxation and guided imagery. Although behavioral scores were not significantly different across the three inductions,

inductions containing relaxation instructions elicited higher subjective scores than the imagery-only induction, and the combined procedure elicited reports of greater depth and involuntariness than the relaxation only induction.

Although relaxation instructions facilitate hypnotic responding, they do not appear to be an essential component of hypnotic inductions; alert inductions, in which relaxation is replaced by instructions to remain alert (Gibbons, 1975, 1976; Kirsch, Mobayed, Council, & Kenny, 1990) or in which relaxation is inhibited by vigorous physical activity (Bányai & Hilgard, 1976), result in levels of responsiveness as great as those produced by traditional relaxation inductions. Also, equivalent levels of hypersuggestibility can be produced by credible expectancy manipulations, such as the administration of placebo pills (Glass & Barber, 1961) and noncontingent biofeedback (Council et al., 1983). It seems likely that the role of relaxation instructions is to enhance the credibility of the definition of the situation as hypnotic. Because of culturally transmitted information about hypnosis, subjects expect hypnosis to occur only if some special procedure is used, and relaxation instructions are particularly consistent with hypnotic inductions as portrayed in the mass media.

It is important to note that defining the situation as hypnosis increases suggestibility for most subjects, but it may have the opposite effect with people who score on the low end of hypnotic susceptibility scales. Spanos, Perlini, and Robertson (1989) reported that in response to an analgesia suggestion, low hypnotizable subjects indicated as much pain reduction as did high hypnotizable subjects, but only when the suggestion was neither defined as hypnosis nor preceded by an induction procedure (see also Spanos, Kennedy, & Gwynn, 1984).

"Advanced" Hypnotic Techniques

Standard induction procedures are quite simple and can be learned through brief instruction or simply through reading sample inductions in books. Similarly, most hypnotic suggestions are straightforward requests for the subject to have a particular subjective experience. However, many clinicians believe that suggestibility can be enhanced even more by specialized inductions and other complex techniques. Procedures advocated by followers of Milton Erickson, and taught in workshops on "Ericksonian hypnosis," are quite popular at present. Ericksonian techniques include inductions tailored to the characteristics of the individual subject, confusion inductions, permissively worded suggestions, and indirect inductions and suggestions (Erickson, Rossi, & Rossi, 1976; Lankton & Lankton, 1983).

Only some of these procedures have been evaluated in controlled empirical tests, and these have not fared well enough to justify the emphasis that is placed on them in the books and workshops in which they are taught. T. X. Barber and Calverley (1966) reported greater responsiveness to permissively worded suggestions than to authoritatively worded suggestions. However, their permissive wording involved instructing subjects to try to generate the response, rather than directly suggesting the experience. It is possible that their findings resulted from the encouragement of active effort, rather than from the permissiveness of the suggestion. In any case, the permissive wording they used is hardly representative of the procedures advocated by Ericksonians.

The effects of indirect and permissive wording of inductions and suggestions on hypnotizability have been assessed in at least four studies (Alman & Carney, 1980; Lynn, Neufeld, & Matyi, 1987; Matthews, Bennett, Bean, & Gallagher, 1985; Spinhoven, Baak, Van Dyck, & Vermeulen, 1988). No significant differences in hypnotizability scale scores were found in any of these studies. In the Alman and Carney (1980) study, permissive and indirect wording elicited greater responding to a posthypnotic suggestion, and in the Matthews, Bennett, et al. (1985) study, subjects reported feeling more deeply hypnotized following the indirect induction. Conversely, Lynn, Neufeld, and Matyi (1987) reported that direct suggestions elicited significantly greater reports of subjective involvement and of feelings of involuntariness. In sum, these studies indicate that neither directiveness nor permissiveness has much of an effect on hypnotic responsiveness.

The effects of J. Barber's (1977) "rapid-induction analgesia" (RIA), which is an indirect Ericksonian procedure, have been compared to those of a conventionally worded induction and suggestion in two studies (Fricton & Roth, 1985; Van Gorp, Meyer, & Dunbar, 1985). Fricton and Roth (1985) reported that the RIA technique was more effective than a directly worded counterpart. In strong contrast to these findings, Van Gorp et al. (1985) reported that a conventional induction and analgesic suggestion was significantly more effective than the RIA procedure in reducing self-reported pain. In fact, RIA failed to produce any analgesic effect whatsoever in their study.

Matthews, Kirsch, and Mosher (1985) compared the effects of a "double induction," developed by Bandler and Grinder (1975) on the basis of Erickson's therapeutic techniques, to those of a conventional induction. The double induction is a complex procedure involving two hypnotists, each speaking into a different ear of the subject. No differences were found between the two procedures.

Finally, Van Der Does, Van Dyck, Spinhoven, and Kloosman (1989) asked 12 experienced hypnotherapists—of unspecified theoretical orientations—to "use whatever induction procedures and wording of suggestions seemed appropriate for a particular [subject]" (p. 2) and compared the effects of their efforts to those of experimenters who had memorized the induction contained in the Stanford Hypnotic Clinical Scale. No significant differences were found.

Taken together, these studies suggest that advanced training in specialized inductions and suggestion procedures may not be particularly useful as a means of enhancing subjects' suggestibility. Instead, responsiveness is optimized by a conventional induction including both relaxation and imagery, followed by direct suggestions delivered with a forceful tone of voice (T. X. Barber & Calverley, 1964d). The effects of suggestions can also be enhanced by wording suggestions so that they include instructions to intentionally imagine events consistent with the suggestion (Bartis & Zamansky, 1990). Whether suggestions are presented live or via audiotape seems to make little or no difference (T. X. Barber & Calverley, 1964f; L. S. Johnson & Weise, 1979).

Enhancing Suggestibility without a Trance Induction

Induction procedures are aimed at producing an altered state of consciousness (trance), of which hypersuggestibility is thought to be one characteristic (E. R. Hilgard, 1977a). In challenging the hypothesis that hypnosis is an altered state, T. X. Barber and his colleagues developed procedures for enhancing suggestibility without producing other alterations in conscious state. These include task-motivational instructions (T. X. Barber, 1969) and imagination training (Comins, Fullam, & Barber, 1975).

Task-Motivational Instructions

Subjects given task-motivational instructions are told that their abilities to imagine and visualize are being tested, that how well they do depends on their willingness to imagine as requested, and that "everyone passed these tests when they tried." They are asked to cooperate by imagining vividly, so as to help the experiment by scoring as highly as they can. Combining the data from three studies conducted with his colleague D. S. Calverley, T. X. Barber (1969) reported that these instructions were as effective as a traditional trance induction in enhancing both behavioral and subjective responses to suggestions. Other data, however, suggest that task-motivational instructions may generate particularly strong pressure on subjects to comply with the experimenter's wishes by faking hypnotic responses. These data indicate that increases in responsiveness produced by task-motivational instructions may be reversed by a strongly worded request for honest reporting (K. S. Bowers, 1967; Spanos & Barber, 1968).

Imagination Training

Imagination training, which has also been referred to as a "cognitive skill induction" (N. Katz, 1978), is another method developed by T. X. Barber and his colleagues for enhancing suggestibility (Comins et al., 1975). On the face of it, imagination training seems less vulnerable than taskotivational instructions to the charge of pressuring subjects to dissemble. Not to be confused with simple imagination instructions that have been used to gather base rate estimates of suggestibility (e.g., E. R. Hilgard & Tart, 1966), imagination training involves teaching subjects to generate "goal-directed fantasies" in order to produce hypnotic responses. Goal-directed fantasies are images of situations that would produce the desired response. For example, to experience arm levitation, people might imagine helium-filled balloons attached to their arms.

Imagination training procedures typically begin with the provision of information aimed at dispelling myths about hypnosis (e.g., that a hypnotized person loses control over his or her behavior) that may inhibit people from cooperating with hypnotic procedures. This is followed by a description of hypnosis as a learnable cognitive skill that is under the subjects' control. Subjects are then told that they can generate hypnotic responses by becoming absorbed in goal-directed imagery, and are provided with practice in generating appropriate images. Research on these skill inductions has shown them to be as effective as, or slightly more effective than, traditional trance induction procedures in enhancing suggestibility (Comins et al., 1975; Council et al., 1983; N. Katz, 1978, 1979; Vickery, Kirsch, Council, & Sirkin, 1985). Unlike the effects of task-motivational instructions, these effects are obtained even when strong demands for honesty are included in the instructions given to subjects (Council et al., 1983; Vickery et al., 1985).

Expectancy-Altering Information

Small but reliable gains in responsiveness can be produced by providing verbal information indicating that responding to suggestions is easy (T. X. Barber & Calverley, 1964d). Similarly, telling subjects that people are either more or less responsive on a second test of hypnotizability produces corresponding changes in responsiveness (Vickery & Kirsch, 1985). Also, having subjects view a model who responds successfully to suggestions enhances the subjects' responsiveness (Botto, Fisher, & Soucy, 1977; Coe & Steen, 1981; Klinger, 1970), and this enhancement appears to be mediated by its effects on subjects' response expectancies (Coe & Steen, 1981).

The use of bogus feedback from personality tests as an expectancy manipulation has also been studied. Subjects given feedback indicating that they were likely to be highly susceptible to hypnosis achieved higher hypnotic response scores than controls in three of these studies (Gregory & Diamond, 1973; Johnston, Chajkowaski, DuBreuil, & Spanos, 1989; Wickless & Kirsch, 1989), but such feedback had no significant effect on responsiveness in two others (Goebel & Stewart, 1971; Saavedra & Miller, 1983). Bogus feedback indicating low hypnotizability produced a decrement in response rates in one study (Saavedra & Miller, 1983), but had no significant effect in two others (Goebel & Stewart, 1971; Johnston et al., 1989).

When subjects are given transparent personality measures prior to being evaluated for hypnotizability, their responses to those measures may alter their expectancies about their hypnotizability, which in turn can affect their responsiveness. Evidence of this process is provided by studies showing a "context effect," in which administering transparent questionnaires in the same context in which hypnosis is later assessed results in inflated correlations between the questionnaire and hypnotizability (Council et al., 1986; de Groot et al., 1988; Green et al., 1991; Nadon, Hoyt, et al., 1991).[2] Similarly, giving a questionnaire a label that emphasizes its connection to hypnosis can inflate correlations (Rhue et al., 1989). However, like the effects of false feedback, these effects are weak and inconsistent (Perlini et al., 1992).

Whereas context effects and the effects of false feedback are weak and variable, substantial effects on suggestibility have been obtained through the use of experiential feedback as an expectancy modification procedure (Wickless & Kirsch, 1989; Wickless, Kirsch, & Moffitt, 1991; D. L. Wilson, 1967). In these studies, experimenters suggested various perceptual phenomena and provided surreptitious confirmation of the suggested effects via hidden lights and audiotape recordings. Suggestibility was then assessed on standard hypnotizability scales. Not only were substantial mean differences in hypnotizability found in these studies, but also the effect of these procedures was great enough to alter the shape of the distribution of hypnotizability scores. In contrast to control subjects, among whom a normal distribution of suggestibility scores was obtained, a J-shaped distribution of hypnotizability scores was found among subjects who had been exposed to surreptitious experiential feedback. A majority of these subjects scored in the high range, and almost none scored in the low range.

The Modification of Hypnotizability

A variety of methods have been used in successful efforts to enhance hypnotizability, including reinforced practice, modeling, poetry, music, sensory restriction, brain wave feedback, electromyographic feedback, personal growth training, encounter group training, and imagination training (DeVoge & Sachs, 1973; M. J. Diamond, 1972; M. J. Diamond, Steadman, Harada, & Rosenthal, 1975; Kinney & Sachs, 1974; London, Cooper, & Engstrom, 1974; Sachs & Anderson, 1967; R. S. Sanders & Reyher, 1969; Shapiro & Diamond, 1972; Talone, Diamond, & Steadman, 1975; Shor & Cobb, 1968; Silber, 1980; Tart, 1970a; Vickery et al., 1985; Wickramasekera, 1969, 1970, 1973). These effects are rather small, however, and the sheer variety of successful enhancement procedures suggests something akin to a placebo effect. Similar levels of suggestibility enhancement have been produced by "hypnotic placebos" (Council et al., 1983; Glass & Barber, 1961; Shor & Cobb, 1968), and the effects of imagination training have been duplicated by simply misinforming subjects that people are generally more responsive on a second test of hypnotizability (Vickery & Kirsch, 1985).

The newest and most thoroughly tested hypnotizability modification procedure is the Carleton Skill Training Program (CSTP) developed by Spanos and his colleagues (Bates & Brigham, 1990; Bates, Miller, Cross, & Brigham, 1988; Gearan, 1990; Gfeller, Lynn, & Pribble, 1987; Gorassini & Spanos, 1986; Spanos, Cross, Menary, Brett, & de Groh, 1987; Spanos, de Groh, & de Groot, 1987; Spanos, Robertson, Menary, & Brett, 1986; Spanos, Robertson, Menary, Brett, & Smith, 1987). The CSTP includes the cognitive training procedures described earlier as a "skill induction," which has been shown to be moderately effective in enhancing hypnotizability (M. J. Diamond, 1972; M. J. Diamond et al., 1975; Vickery et al., 1985). In addition, subjects are encouraged to emit the suggested response physically, while at the same time using goal-directed imagery to help themselves experience the response as occurring nonvolitionally. In most of these studies, the increase in suggestibility produced by the CSTP has been substantial, although more modest results have been reported in some studies (Bates et al., 1988; Gearan, 1990).

The most troublesome aspects of the CSTP are the instructions for behavioral compliance that are part of the training package (Bates, 1990; Bates & Brigham, 1990). Subjects are instructed to intentionally enact suggested responses behaviorally and to "make believe" that these are occurring nonvolitionally. For example, subjects are told that following an arm levitation suggestion, "Your arm will not really go up by itself; you must raise it." These instructions may lead at least some subjects to fake high hypnotizability, whereas untrained responsive subjects ("natural highs") generally do not simply fake their responses (Kirsch, Silva, Carone, Johnston, & Simon, 1989).

Spanos and Flynn (1989a) countered the compliance hypothesis with data showing that the hypnotizability scores of trained subjects are lower than those of simulators (subjects who have been instructed to act as if they had been transformed by training into excellent hypnotic subjects). The problem with this argument is that training is not effective for all subjects. As a result, trained subjects have lower hypnotizability scores than *nonsimulating* highly hypnotizable subjects. For example, Spanos and Flynn (1989a) reported a mean SHSS:C behavioral score of only 6.80 for their trained subjects. Rather than showing that trained subjects are not simulating, this merely indicates that they are not all transformed into hypnotic virtuosos. It is possible that those subjects whose hypnotizability scores are substantially enhanced by training are merely faking, whereas those who do not fake remain as unsuggestible as they were prior to training. If this were occurring, it would lead to the same pattern of results as that reported by Spanos and Flynn (1989a).

Even if successfully trained subjects are not merely simulating (and we suspect that they are not), it is possible that the means by which they are taught to generate responses are different from the means by which most natural highs generate responses. The CSTP instructs subjects to interpret hypnotic suggestions as requests for voluntary physical enactment combined with goal-directed imagery. However, very few untrained subjects report interpreting responses in this way (Katsanis, Barnard, & Spanos, 1988-1989; Silva, 1990). Therefore, either trained highs are adopting an interpretational set that is different from that of natural highs, or they are ignoring that aspect of the CSTP instructions and are responding to some other components of the training program.

Summary

Whereas our review of personality correlates of suggestibility has yielded meager results, the search for situational correlates has been more productive. Suggestibility can be enhanced by defining the situation as hypnosis, providing disinhibiting information, enhancing expectations of successful responding, teaching subjects to generate goal-directed imagery, administering a credible induction ritual, delivering direct suggestions in a forceful tone of voice, wording suggestions so that subjects are asked to "try" instead of telling them that they "will" experience suggested effects, and including instructions for goal-directed imagery in the suggestions (e.g., "Imagine that a helium-filled balloon is tied to your wrist").

Although the number of situational correlates of suggestibility is large, in most cases the magnitude of their effects is relatively small. Notable exceptions are the provision of an experiential expectancy manipulation (Wickless & Kirsch, 1989) and instructions to intentionally generate the suggested behavior (Gorassini & Spanos, 1986), both of which produce substantial increments in responsiveness. The degree to which various combinations of these procedures are more effective than their use individually remains to be established.

Situation-Specific Person Variables: The Interface of Person and Situation

Although personality variables considered in isolation and situational variables considered in isolation leave much of the variance in responsiveness unexplained, perhaps the interaction of these variables can provide a more comprehensive account of suggestibility. Situations and personality traits interact to produce situation-specific person variables, such as attitudes, values, cognitive sets, intentions, and expectancies. These differ from personality variables in that they lack cross-situational consistency. Situation-specific person variables may mediate the effects of traits and situations on suggestibility (M. J. Diamond, Gregory, Lenney, Steadman, & Talone, 1974). Some support for this supposition is provided by the fact that the two situational interventions that have been shown to have a substantial impact on suggestibility were aimed at altering person variables: expectancy in one case (Wickless & Kirsch, 1989) and interpretational set in the other (Gorassini & Spanos, 1986).

Attitudes and Expectancies

It is reasonable to assume that people with positive attitudes toward hypnosis would be more cooperative and therefore more likely to respond successfully. Supporting this hypothesis are a number of studies showing moderate correlations between attitudes and hypnotizability (M. J. Diamond et al., 1974; Melei & Hilgard, 1964; Rosenhan & Tomkins, 1964; Saavedra & Miller, 1983; Spanos, Brett, Menary, & Cross, 1987; Spanos & McPeake, 1975b; Yanchar & Johnson, 1981). Significant correlations have also been reported between subjects' predictions of their hypnotizability and their subsequent responsiveness to suggestion (Council et al., 1983, 1986; Derman & London, 1965; Johnston et al., 1989; Katsanis et al., 1988–1989; Kirsch, 1991; Melei & Hilgard, 1964; Saavedra & Miller, 1983; Shor, 1971; Shor, Pistole, Easton, & Kihlstrom, 1984). The magnitude of these correlations varies substantially. Though some are modest, others are high enough to account for much of the variability in hypnotic responsiveness (e.g., Council et al., 1983; Council et al., 1986; Johnston et al., 1989; Kirsch, 1991).

Expectancies appear to at least partially mediate the relationship between personality variables and hypnotizability. Hypnotic response expectancies are significantly correlated with absorption (Council et al., 1983) and fantasy proneness (Silva, 1990). We (Council et al., 1983) reported that with expectancy statistically controlled, partial correlations between absorption and hypnotizability were nonsignificant. In contrast, Silva (1990) found that fantasy proneness predicted subjective (but not behavioral) responses to hypnosis, even with expectancy partialed out. Nevertheless, the same analysis suggested that even the association between subjective responses and fantasy proneness was partially mediated by expectancy.

Expectancies are conventionally defined as subjective probabilities. However, most hypnotic "expectancy" scales ask subjects to estimate their levels of responsiveness, rather than their subjective probabilities of achieving particular levels of responsiveness. For many subjects, these predictions may amount to mere guesses; hence their correlations with hypnotic behavior are likely to be underestimates of the association between expectancy and response.

Saavedra and Miller (1983) took this possibility into account by assessing subjects' levels of confidence in their predictions and then computing a prediction × confidence analysis of variance, with hypnotizability scores as the dependent variable. This resulted in a highly significant interaction (accounting for more than 20% of the variance), explained by the finding that as confidence increased, predictions were more accurate. Similarly, Johnston et al. (1989) assessed confidence as well as predicted responsiveness and reported a correlation of .71 between expectancy and behavioral scores on the BSS among subjects whose reported confidence levels were above the median for the sample. However, a similar effect was not found for self-predictions of scores on the CURSS. Finally, these findings were replicated by Kirsch (1991), who reported that correlations between self-prediction and hypnotizability scores were significantly higher among subjects expressing greater confidence in their predictions. Thus, the relation between predicted and actual suggestibility appears to be moderated by subjects' level of confidence in their predictions. Confidently held expectations are fairly good predictors of hypnotizability, but guesses are not.

This leaves open the question of what determines hypnotizability among subjects who do not have confidently held expectations about their suggestibility. Kirsch (1990) hypothesized that weakly held expectations are likely to be changed by the experience of a trance induction. Depending on the degree to which subjects experience various changes in conscious state (e.g., relaxation), and on their criteria for concluding that they have been hypnotized (e.g., whether they understand hypnosis to be a greatly altered state of awareness), the subjects reach a conclusion about the degree to which they are hypnotized, and this conclusion elicits altered and more confidently held expectations about their responses to subsequent suggestions.

In support of this hypothesis, we (Council et al., 1986) reported that postinduction response expectancies were related only moderately to preinduction expectancies (indicating substantial change as a function of the experienced induction), and that the latter were significantly better predictors of hypnotizability. These results were replicated by Kirsch (1991), who also found that postinduction expectancies were held with greater confidence than were preinduction predictions. It should be noted that postinduction expectancies are strong predictors of hypnotizability even with self-reported depth of trance partialed out (Council et al., 1986). This indicates that the relationship between these expectancies and subsequent responding is not merely epiphenomenal.

Interpretational Sets and Active Responding

People have different interpretations of what is being requested of subjects in a hypnotic situation. Some interpret the situation as one calling for complete passivity, in which they are merely to wait for suggestions to affect them, without doing anything to help or hinder the process. Others interpret hypnosis as a situation in which they are being asked to actively generate suggested experiences and/or their behavioral counterparts. It should be easier to experience a suggested phenomenon when one actively tries to do so; therefore, an active interpretational set of this sort ought to facilitate successful responding (Katsanis et al., 1988–1989).

A variety of data strongly support the hypothesis that actively imagining events that are congruent with suggestions (i.e., engaging in goal-directed fantasies) facilitates hypnotic responding. Spanos and his colleagues asked subjects to report retrospectively on their thoughts and imaginings while they were responding to various hypnotic suggestions (Spanos, 1971; Spanos & Barber, 1972; Spanos & Ham, 1973). In these studies, subjects who had spontaneously generated goal-directed fantasies were far more likely to pass hypnotic test suggestions. Convergent evidence is provided by studies discussed earlier, in which instruction in goal-directed imagery was used successfully to enhance hypnotic responsiveness.

Although the effect of goal-directed imagery on hypnotizability has been reliably established, some of the data suggest that this effect may be at least partially mediated by subjects' expectations. Highly suggestible subjects are able to generate hypnotic responses while engaging in imagery that is inconsistent with suggestions, provided that they are given information indicating that this is characteristic of hypnotic responding (Bartis & Zamansky, 1986; Spanos, Weekes, & de Groh, 1984; Zamansky, 1977; Zamansky & Clark, 1986). Also, among people who have not been selected for exceptionally high levels of hypnotizability, goal-directed imagery inhibits responding when subjects are told that this will be its effect (Kirsch, Council, & Mobayed, 1987).

The most convincing evidence of the mediational role of expectancies was reported by Lynn, Snodgrass, Rhue, and Hardaway (1987). Although high hypnotizable subjects were more likely to generate goal-directed fantasies spontaneously, low hypnotizable subjects were able to generate and become very absorbed in similar fantasies when instructed to do so. Unlike the highs, however, the lows did not believe that their fantasies would produce suggested ideomotor movements, a belief that was highly correlated with behavioral responding. As a result, their level of behavioral response did not equal that of the highly hypnotizable subjects, even though their fantasy production was equivalent in both frequency and degree of subjective involvement.

Noting the insufficiency of imagination alone to produce behavioral responses to suggestion, Spanos (1986b) has proposed that subjects intentionally emit the behavioral components of the suggested responses, while using fantasy to experience the responses as occurring nonvolitionally. In support of this hypothesis, Spanos and his colleagues have demonstrated that a training program aimed at teaching this strategy to subjects substantially increases responsiveness (see "The Modification of Hypnotizability," above). However, when untrained subjects are asked to indicate their interpretational sets, very few indicate physical enactment of the behavioral component of the response (Katsanis et al., 1988–1989; Silva, 1990). In Silva's sample of 190 subjects, for example, only 21 indicated using this interpretational set for even one suggestion, and not one reported using it for more than three of the seven suggestions that were administered. The use of goal-directed fantasy was the most frequently endorsed method of responding, although the adoption of a purely passive interpretational set may have been inhibited by the use of the CURSS, in which instructions for goal-directed imagery are imbedded in all suggestions.

Summary and Conclusions

After decades of negative results, a number of conceptually overlapping and empirically correlated scales have been developed that reliably predict hypnotizability. The conceptual and empirical overlap between these scales suggests that the relationship is due to a single underlying trait, related to a capacity and/or propensity toward imagination. Happily, this relationship is consistent with all current theories of hypnosis, and may therefore provide some respite from the contentiousness that characterizes most hypnosis scholarship.

Despite research—including our own—that casts doubt on the relationship between this imaginative trait and hypnotizability, we believe the association to be real. Although its effects, as indexed by measures of absorption, imaginative involvement, or fantasy proneness, appear largely mediated by expectancy, we do not think that they are entirely so mediated. However, the relationship is surprisingly and disappointingly small. In fact, it seems smaller than the typical "personality coefficient" and apparently accounts for far less than 10% of the variance in hypnotizability.

Most situational variables also fail to explain much of the variance in suggestibility. For that reason, the two notable exceptions—experiential expectancy modification (e.g., Wickless & Kirsch, 1989) and the CSTP (Gorassini & Spanos, 1986)—are especially important. The questions to be asked of these procedures are as follows: (1) What are the mechanisms by which they produce changes in response, and (2) are they the same mechanisms that account for naturally occurring differences in hypnotizability? If the mechanisms can be identified, and if they are the same as those responsible for naturally occurring variance in responsiveness, then they should facilitate the construction of scales that will show a substantial multiple correlation with hypnotizability.

Given the temporal stability of hypnotizability scores, the continuing failure to find correlates that account for a substantial portion of the naturally occurring variance is surprising. The single exception is nonhypnotic suggestibility, but that cannot be used to "explain" hypnotizability. Instead, it is that which needs to be explained, and hypnotic inductions (which are the sole operational distinction between the terms "hypnotizability" and "suggestibility") are best seen as merely one situational variable that can affect suggestibility. In fact, traditional inductions may have become somewhat of a fetish, given that equivalent enhancement of suggestibility can be produced without them. Imagination training, for example, renders the relaxation/eye fixation induction redundant (Vickery et al., 1985), and we suspect that its use in testing the effects of the CSTP is mere window dressing, adding nothing to subjects' responsiveness.

It seems likely that no one global variable, be it dissociation, expectancy, or strategic enactment, fully explains suggestibility. Suggestibility is most likely the product of a number of factors, including abilities, propensities, attitudes, interpretations, beliefs, and expectancies. The problem is to identify the specific abilities, beliefs, and so forth that affect suggestibility; to find adequate ways of measuring them; and to construct a theoretical account of how they interact. No theory, including our own, is currently able to provide a complete and convincing solution to this problem. It is to the credit of hypnosis scholars that their theories have changed in response to new data, and it is likely that those theories will continue to evolve as the body of accepted empirical findings continues to grow.

Notes

1. One of the methods that has been used in attempts to control for context effects is to administer the TAS prior to any mention of hypnosis, and then again just before hypnosis is measured (Nadon, Hoyt, et al., 1991, Experiment 1). It is important to note that this procedure does *not* control for context effects. The readministration of the absorption measure provides subjects with the information that absorption and hypnotizability are being assessed as part of the same study, thus making it possible for subjects' responses to the questionnaire to affect their responses to hypnosis. Thus, in the Nadon, Hoyt, et al. study, a condition in which assessment contexts were kept completely separate can be found only in Experiment 2.

2. Though this was not reported in the text of their article, Nadon, Hoyt, et al. (1991) obtained a significant context effect similar to the one we reported (Council et al., 1986). In their second experiment (which was the only part of their study that included a group in which context had been kept strictly separate), the correlation between hypnotizability and an initial assessment of absorption was .24 among subjects whose hypnotizability was assessed after they were made aware that absorption was being related to hypnotizability, whereas it was only .05 among subjects tested for both hypnotizability and absorption only in separate contexts. These correlations were significantly different from each other ($z = 2.02$, $p < .05$).

CHAPTER ELEVEN

The Hypnotizable Subject as Creative Problem-Solving Agent

STEVEN JAY LYNN
HARRY SIVEC

Our charge in writing this chapter was to review and integrate the rather disparate literatures on hypnosis, imagination, fantasy, and creativity. Our chapter addresses a number of questions pertaining to the relations between and among hypnosis, imaginative/fantasy processes, and creativity: Are subjects' nonhypnotic imaginative involvements and their creativity related to hypnotizability? Are patterns of fantasy and imaginative involvements during hypnosis associated with enhanced hypnotic responsiveness and the experience of suggestion-related involuntariness?

In reviewing the literature on hypnosis, imagination, fantasy, and creativity, we argue that whereas these processes and abilities may be important, they provide neither a complete nor a satisfactory account of subjects' responses to hypnosis. To be sure, creativity, as conventionally defined by creativity tests, does not begin to capture the nature and complexity of subjects' creative problem solving during hypnosis. Hypnosis is a very special situation, with unique cultural and personal connotations for subjects. We argue that in order to explain the complex and subtle alterations in subjective experience and responses that are evident in this context, it is not fruitful to reduce subjects' responses to an expression of mere compliance. Furthermore, in isolation, constructs such as expectancy or imagination do not provide a sufficient account of hypnotizability. Rather, we maintain that it is necessary to consider the interaction of multiple variables and processes that promote what amounts to creative problem solving in the hypnotic context.

In order to integrate the diverse literatures we review, we elaborate the metaphor of the hypnotizable subject as a creative problem-solving agent. Our view extends the theorizing of Sheehan and McConkey (see McConkey, 1991; Sheehan & McConkey, 1982; Sheehan, 1991), Sarbin and

292

Coe (Sarbin & Coe, 1972; Coe & Sarbin, 1991), and Spanos (1986b, 1991), who have drawn attention to hypnotized subjects' active and creative participation in the events of hypnosis and the constructive, problem-solving nature of successful responding. Our viewpoint thus stands in contradistinction to theories based on dissociation, ego receptivity, and regression, which do not emphasize the subjects' goal-directed strivings to experience and respond to hypnotic suggestions. When we say that subjects are goal-directed, we do not mean to imply that the subjects' motivations are necessarily consciously articulated, nor do we mean that conscious effort necessarily accompanies subjects' strivings to decipher and fulfill the requirements of hypnotic suggestions. Furthermore, subjects are not necessarily aware of the problem-solving quality of responding to the hypnotic situation. Indeed, many features of the hypnotic context discourage awareness and analysis of the personal and situational factors that influence hypnotic behavior (Lynn & Rhue, 1991). Nevertheless, subjects' wishes, expectancies, and motivation to experience the events of hypnosis, along with the dynamic and often highly personal nature of subjects' intentions, ultimately play an important role in shaping the experience and response to hypnotic communications.

At the outset, it is important to emphasize that we do not use the term "creativity" in the sense that it is used in popular culture to describe breathtaking leaps of imagination or the quality inherent in acts, products, or works of art that are uniquely original, socially valuable, or singularly innovative. Rather, we view creativity as a problem-solving process in which a person devises a novel response (for that person) to a particular problem at hand (see Weisberg, 1986). This process is fueled by the force of the person's motives, expectancies, attitudes, imagination, personal resources, and abilities. Creativity and problem solving, within and apart from the hypnotic context, are thus construed as multifaceted processes that are related to but cannot be reduced to what conventional creativity tests measure. Creativity so construed has much in common with the "creativity of everyday life" that is intimately tied to the resolution of mundane problems.

We begin with a brief overview of the role of fantasy and imagination in modern accounts of hypnosis and hypnotizability. We then present our perspective of the hypnotizable subject as a creative problem-solving agent before we review the literature on hypnosis and imaginative activity, goal-directed fantasy, expectancies, and creativity.

Imagination, Fantasy, and Hypnosis Theories

In 1779, Franz Anton Mesmer published his landmark doctoral dissertation, which many credit as elaborating the discovery of hypnosis. Five years later, the famous investigative commission led by Benjamin Franklin concluded that imagination and imitation could account for the purported effects of animal magnetism (Sheehan, 1982). The crucial role played by imagination in the production of hypnotic phenomena can be seen in the early writings of Braid (1843), Binet (1896), and Bernheim (1884/1971); in Hull's (1933) demonstration of the equivalence of suggested and imagined swaying on physical movements; in Jeness's (1944) finding that vivid imagers are more readily hypnotized than poor imagers; in Arnold's (1946) theory of ideomotor action, which forged a connection between vivid and sustained imagining and suggestion-related responses; and in contemporary theorists', researchers', and therapists' recognition of the role of imaginative processes in a variety of adaptive behaviors (T. X. Barber, 1985; Heyneman, 1990; Sheehan, 1979a; Spanos & Barber, 1974; Weitzenhoffer, 1980; S. C. Wilson & Barber, 1981). Indeed, more than 200 years after Franklin's commission was convened, imagination still occupies a central place in our thinking about hypnosis (Lynn & Rhue, 1987).

Contemporary theorists have accorded imagination and fantasy a prominent role in understanding hypnotic phenomena, whereas researchers have examined imagery and fantasy both in their own right and as correlates of hypnotic responding. So prominently has imagination figured in hypnosis theories that it constitutes one of the few common factors or mechanisms that unite disparate accounts of hypnosis (see Lynn & Rhue, 1991; Spanos & Barber, 1974). Although Spanos and Barber (1974) were the first to argue that state and nonstate theorists agree that "responsiveness to hypnotic suggestions involves a shift in set or orientation away from the pragmatic one that governs our everyday transactions to one that involves imagining" (p. 503), this assessment was recently echoed by Coe and Sarbin (1991).

In this chapter, we adopt the increasingly accepted perspective that daydreaming, fantasy, and imaginative activities are not readily distinguishable. Singer and Pope (1981) have forcefully argued that everyday consciousness can be characterized as consisting of many elements or aspects that are not "secondary-process" or reality-bound. Indeed, daydreaming, fantasy, and related forms of reverie are commonplace, naturally occurring experiences in normal individuals (Singer, 1966, 1975a,b, 1978). In Starker's (1978) opinion, daydreaming and fantasy are difficult to distinguish from other imaginal processes because they are part of a continuum in thought processes ranging from planful problem solving to uninhibited fantasy (E. Klinger, 1971; Gold & Reilly, 1985–1986). Segal, Huba, and Singer (1980) suggest that fantasy can be described as a subset of daydreaming "that usually involves somewhat greater speculation, somewhat more of a thrust toward future possibilities, or a juxtaposition of elements from long-term memory that may have much less probability of occurrence in the external life of the individual" (p. 37). Furthermore, in everyday life these internal events are constantly changing from one to another, with boundaries and transitions that are difficult to mark.

Hypnosis theoreticians have also shied away from making rigid distinctions among daydreaming, fantasy, and imagination. These concepts are rarely clearly defined; sharp boundaries among the constructs are seldom drawn; and they have been operationalized in a variety of ways. Nevertheless, there is keen interest in studying imaginative involvements, fantasy, and daydreaming as correlates of hypnotizability. Moreover, subjects' reports of increased spontaneous and instructed imagery and fantasy during hypnosis have been identified as key markers of alterations in subjective experience that occur during hypnosis (E. R. Hilgard, 1977a). Psychoanalytic theorists (Fromm, 1979; Gill & Brenman, 1959; M. R. Nash, 1991) have drawn upon concepts such as "regression in the service of the ego" to characterize the temporary shift from secondary- to primary-process thinking that is believed to account for the freeplay of fantasy and imaginative activity that many hypnotized subjects report (see M. R. Nash, 1991). According to research conducted by Fromm and her associates (Fromm, Brown, Hurt, Oberlander, Boxer, & Pfeifer, 1981; Fromm & Kahn, 1990; Lombard, Kahn, & Fromm, 1990), imagery is a prominent aspect not only of heterohypnosis but of self-hypnosis as well. In fact, imagery is a hallmark of self-hypnosis, and correlates positively with hypnotic depth. Self-hypnotic imagery was found to be marked by imagery with both a reality-oriented and a fantastic quality (Kahn, Fromm, Lombard, & Sossi, 1989).

Fromm and her colleagues (e.g., Fromm, 1979; Fromm, Lombard, Skinner, & Kahn, 1987–1988) relate the striking changes in subjects' experience and behavior during hypnosis to a construct termed "ego receptivity." Contrasted with a passive or a vigilant and task-oriented mode of ego functioning, ego receptivity permits the subject to temporarily suspend critical judgment, strict adherence to reality orientation, and the deliberate control of behavior and emotional experiences during hypnosis. At the same time, this receptive orientation facilitates the flow of unconscious and preconscious material (e.g., fantasy, imaginings), which emerge with a spontaneous, effortless quality.

Adopting a very different perspective, social-cognitive theorists (Coe & Sarbin, 1991; Lynn & Rhue, 1991; Sarbin, 1950; Sarbin & Coe, 1972) maintain that hypnotic conduct can be thought of as goal-directed action. Consistent with this viewpoint, imagining or fantasizing in response to suggestions involves something other than assuming a passive attitude or stance called for by suggestions. Rather, it is an "active form of conduct, a doing" (Sarbin, 1972, p. 344). Sarbin and Coe (Coe & Sarbin, 1991; Sarbin, 1950; Sarbin & Coe, 1972) hold that successful hypnotized subjects become actively involved in the roles called for by suggestions and behave "as if" the role and imagined scenario were real. Imaginative skills facilitate subjects' engaging in "as if" behavior that lends force and credibility to their attempts to enact the roles implied by the hypnotist's suggestions.

Sheehan (1979a) has endorsed an "as if" formulation of the role of imagery in hypnosis, as evident by his statement that the good hypnotic subject or imager "acts as if the 'hallucinated' object perceived were present." (p. 407), whether or not the image or percept is akin to that of nonhypnotic perception. However, as Sheehan notes, conceptualizing imagery in hypnosis in terms of "as if" behavior is consistent with a variety of theoretical viewpoints, and does not necessarily imply acceptance of a role theory account of hypnosis.

Indeed, this "as if" perspective, along with Arnold's (1946) hypothesis that intense imagining is crucial to convincing hypnotic responses, was adopted by T. X. Barber, Spanos, and Chaves (1974). Arnold contended that intense, sustained uncontradicted imagining of a suggested behavior leads automatically to the occurrence of that behavior. Subjects' reports of nonvolition are viewed as accurate reflections of the supposed automatic nature of ideomotor action. Hence, only if subjects interrupt their imaginings are they able to easily resist suggested behavior. In short, behavioral and subjective responses to suggestions are direct byproducts of absorbed involvement in suggestion-related events.

In a similar vein, T. X. Barber et al. (1974) maintained that "subjects are responsive to test suggestions when they think and imagine with the themes that are suggested" (p. 64). Spanos and his colleagues (Spanos, 1971; Spanos & Barber, 1972; Spanos, Horton, & Chaves, 1975) argued that a pattern of imaginative activity during hypnosis—goal-directed fantasy (GDF)—was intimately connected with both hypnotic responding and reports of suggestion-related involuntariness. Spanos's later writings have edged away from viewing hypnotizability as a direct function of thinking and imagining along with suggestions. Nevertheless, Spanos (1991) continues to maintain that imaginal abilities enhance hypnotic responsivity, even though an active interpretational set is necessary to facilitate the translation of imaginal abilities into subjectively compelling hypnotic enactments.

The Hypnotizable Subject as Creative Problem-Solving Agent

The perspective taken in this chapter is that hypnotizable subjects can be thought of as creative problem-solving agents who use their resources and abilities to respond successfully to suggestions. To do so, subjects must integrate information from an array of situational, intrapersonal, and interpersonal sources, even though they are not necessarily aware of the cognitive and situational determinants of their conduct. As creative agents, they shape their experience and direct their actions in terms of their anticipations, agendas, and perceptions of contextual and interpersonal demands (see Lynn & Rhue, 1991). We view the ability to imagine suggested events and to discern the sometimes subtle implications of suggestions as a creative process, and the ability to experience suggestion-related sensations and to respond to hypnotic suggestions as a form of creative expression. In short, creative problem solving in the hypnotic context is best viewed as a multidimensional process, with different elements and determinants interacting to contribute to the successful resolution of problems posed by individual suggestions and the broader hypnotic context.

Imagery has an important role in hypnosis. It can facilitate the subjective experience of suggested events, and it can legitimize and fortify subjects' suggestion-related responses. It thus constitutes one mechanism or aspect of subjects' creative response to suggestion.

Certain aspects of hypnosis promote the ready availability of imagery and fantasy. Without question, imaginative involvement in suggestion-related fantasy is one of the central demands, if not one of the hallmarks, of the hypnotic situation. The hypnotic proceedings invite subjects to close their eyes and to tune out stimuli that compete for their attention. Subjects are encouraged to focus directly on the hypnotist's communications; to suspend their current concerns and their critical/analytical faculties or to let them recede into the background of awareness; and, most importantly, to engage in fantasy and give free rein to the imagination in line with suggested experiences. Some hypnotic suggestions (e.g., hand levitation) include an unambiguous request for subjects to imagine specific events, whereas other suggestions (e.g., age regression) imply that the subjects are to engage in recalling, imagining, or fantasizing about earlier life events. E. R. Hilgard (1977a) has observed that imagination and memories are closely related, insofar as the features of something imagined are largely derived from previous experience and retained in memory (see also Paivio, 1971).

Yet imagery is only one aspect of creative problem solving in the hypnotic context. For example, if subjects fail to discern that a behavioral response is part and parcel of successfully passing a particular suggestion, there is no guarantee that they will enact an overt response to the suggestion (see Heyneman, 1990; Lynn, Snodgrass, Rhue, & Hardaway, 1987; Spanos, 1986b). This sort of "catching on" to the implications of suggestions, however subtle or tacit they may be, is an important aspect of finding creative solutions to the problem posed by suggestions—the "problem" being to discern what is required of the subjects on an ongoing basis, and to generate subjective experiences and behaviors consistent with successfully passing the suggestions or metaphors offered in a therapeutic context.

The act of imagining can itself be a creative act, whether or not it perfectly captures or represents the object or event imagined. As Sheehan (1979a) has noted, even in hypnosis the processes of imagery and perception are distinguishable, despite certain functional similarities. Furthermore, hypnotized subjects' imaginings do not necessarily correspond to the literal events suggested; subjects often spontaneously elaborate imaginings in response to suggestions, generate novel associations within the hypnotic context, and devise ingenious and idiosyncratic ways of integrating complex task demands (see Sheehan & McConkey, 1982). As E. R. Hilgard (1977a) describes it, hypnotizable subjects can "readily add content to the suggestions of the hypnotist as in elaborating a fantasy or describing the scenes in a hallucinated motion picture" (p. 160). At times, hypnotized subjects experience nonsuggested phenomena, which may reflect their unique fantasies and associations in the hypnotic context (see Brentar & Lynn, 1989, for a review). This creation, elaboration, synthesis, and transformation of images and associations occurs within subjects' creative problem-solving attempts to respond appropriately to suggestions, as they are understood within the framework provided by the hypnotic communications and by the unfolding hypnotic relationship (Coe & Sarbin, 1991; Lynn & Rhue, 1991; McConkey, 1991; Sheehan, 1991; Sheehan & McConkey, 1982; Spanos, 1991).

At this point it is useful to discuss creativity and its interface with imagination and with hypnosis as a problem-solving situation. There are many definitions of "creativity" (Kosslyn & Jolicoeur, 1981). Indeed, creativity has been viewed as a product, a process, a capacity, or an aspect of self-actualization (see Tryk, 1968). However, conceptualizing creative behavior in the matrix of a problem-solving context in which imagination and fantasy play a role is harmonious with contemporary developments in the field of creativity.

Shaw and De Meers (1986–1987) have summarized literature on the relation between imagery and creativity. The authors draw attention not only to subjective accounts of the relation between imagery and creativity among "creative geniuses" such as Einstein, Poincaré, and Nietzsche, but also to theoretical accounts (e.g., Bartlett, 1932; Koestler, 1964; Paivio, 1971; Richardson, 1969) that highlight the use of imagery in the service of creativity. Some investigators believe that a strong relationship exists between vividness of mental imagery and creativity (e.g., Khatena, 1976; Leonard & Lindauer, 1973; Torrance, 1966). The evidence in support of this relationship is mixed, however; some studies have yielded positive findings (e.g., Forisha & Nagy, 1979; Hargreaves & Bolton, 1972; Shaw & De Meers, 1986–1987; Shaw & Belmore, 1982–1983), and other studies have yielded negative findings (Durndell & Wethernick, 1976; Forisha, 1980; Suler & Rizziello, 1987). Research evidence reviewed by Kirsch and Council (Chapter 10, this volume) suggests that there is a low to moderate relationship between imagery ability and hypnotizability.

The idea that problem solving is associated with creativity and imagery is one of the hubs of a number of models of creativity. For example, Torrance (1988), who has underscored the role of productive imagination in creativity, has also contended that creativity involves a sensitivity to problems along with the search for solutions. Gestalt psychologists generally substitute the terms "productive thinking" and "problem solving" for the term "creativity" (see Busse & Mansfield, 1980). Sternberg (1988) has called attention to the important role of the ability to integrate and restructure existing knowledge in arriving at creative solutions to problems. Furthermore, fantasies, daydreams, and imaginings may help persons to identify and cognitively work through life dilemmas and current concerns (E. Klinger, 1971) by way of a process that Sarbin (1972) has described as "muted role taking," which includes imaginal rehearsal. S. Sanders (1978) has described a short-term creative problem-solving approach to psychotherapy which is used in conjunction with hypnosis; this approach involves visualizing the problem, imagining alternative reactions, dreaming about new solutions, and testing their adequacy in real-life situations.

Relatedly, Weisberg (1986) has noted that creative thinking involves the use of imagination in situations in which individuals—whether they be artists, poets, scientists, or sculptors—apply their resources and abilities to solve problems. Creative thinking is not restricted to "geniuses" or individuals who are distinguished by their professional accomplishments or by particularly original thinking. Instead, creativity is inherent in the mundane flow of thought and imagination in relation to problems and challenges. As Gur and Reyher (1976) observe, "As we see it, creativity is one aspect of thinking and problem solving in general" (p. 248). For Weisberg, creative problem solving involves a "person's producing a novel response that solves the problem at hand" (1986, p. 4). For the purposes of the discussion that follows, it is very important to note that this definition implies only that the solution must be novel for the person; it is not necessary that the solution be entirely original in order to qualify as "creative."

The thesis of this chapter is that hypnotizable subjects' goal-directed attempts to respond to and experience suggestions can be framed in terms of creative problem solving. As in other problem-solving situations, the subjects are faced with a variety of choices about what to do or not to do during hypnosis. There is little doubt that hypnotic action and experience are the end results of what subjects think and believe about hypnosis, what they imagine or fail to imagine, what they attend to or do not attend to, what they wish to do or not to do, and how they perceive hypnotic communications and come to evaluate their experience (see Lynn & Rhue, 1991).

For many hypnotizable subjects, the essential agenda or problem to be resolved is how to experience and respond to suggestions. The problem gestalt can be thought of as the constellation of attitudes about hypnosis, demand characteristics, and implicit and explicit expectations and performance standards. Nevertheless, the problem gestalt is typically not experienced by subjects as an externally imposed structure for at least two reasons. First, as Lynn and Rhue (1991) have maintained, many hypnotizable subjects are intrinsically motivated. They may wish to experience hypnotic events just to "see what will happen," or to achieve a hypnotic "state" that is a desirable end in itself, or to feel a sense of mastery at succeeding at the task at hand. Some subjects exhibit a particular wish to please the hypnotist that echoes back to earlier meaningful relationships (see Sheehan, 1980; Sheehan & McConkey, 1982). The wish to be hypnotized often reflects multiple motives that are tacit and complex; like other motives or intentions, once they are formed or engaged, they no longer require much conscious control to proceed (Beckmann, 1987; Heckhausen & Beckmann, 1990).

Second, demands, performance standards, cognitive strategies, and problem-solving sets (see also Tellegen, 1981) are often tacit, are perceived or executed with little effort, and are not ordinarily subjected to conscious introspection in the flow of hypnotic experience. Features of the hypnotic context (e.g., passive wording of communications) also diminish awareness of response antecedents or determinants, and fortify perceptions of suggestion-related involuntariness.

To begin to flesh out the picture of hypnotizable subjects as creative problem-solving agents, we review the literature pertinent to subjects' use of imagination within and apart from the hypnotic context. As we have noted, there is considerable consensus that imaginal activities are of crucial importance during hypnosis, so it stands to reason that individual differences in subjects' tendency to engage in imaginative activities outside the hypnotic situation play at least some role in accounting for individual differences in hypnotic responding.

Hypnosis and Subjects' Capability for Imaginative Activity

Imaginative Involvement

Ever since Shor (1960) first studied the prevalence of "hypnotic-like" experiences in everyday life, workers in the field of hypnosis have been intrigued by the correspondence between hypnotic responsiveness and naturally occurring hypnotic-like experiences. Using special inventories, researchers (Ås, O'Hara, & Munger, 1962; Lee-Teng, 1965; Shor, Orne, & O'Connell, 1966) have documented a relationship between hypnotizability and nonhypnotic experiences characterized by deep absorption and concentration, pleasure, and loss of awareness of external reality.

Josephine R. Hilgard's (1965, 1970, 1979a) pioneering intensive interviews and rating study at Stanford University, in which she attempted to predict hypnotizability in advance of hypnosis, was successful in identifying prominent areas of "imaginative involvements" in hypnotizable subjects' everyday lives (e.g., sensory experiences, reading, music, the dramatic arts, religion, and adventure). She noted that imaginative involvements "permit a temporary absorption in satisfying experiences in which fantasy plays a large role" (1970, p. 483). Those subjects who reported a long history of such involvements tended to be more hypnotizable than those subjects who reported few such imaginative involvements in their background. Nevertheless, J. R. Hilgard (1979a) was careful to acknowledge that the prediction of hypnotizability from subjects' history of imaginative involvements is "far from perfect" (p. 494).

de Groh (1989), in her review of the correlates of hypnotizability, cited a number of potential criticisms of the reliability of J. R. Hilgard's results (e.g., problems in categorizing variables, interview bias). For example, she noted that Drake, Nash, and Cawood (1990–1991) found that the positive relation between imaginative involvement and hypnotizability was dependent on whether the interview was administered in the context of hypnosis or not. de Groh (1989) suggested that this might indicate that the relation between hypnotizability and imaginative involvement is a context-mediated artifact. These potential problems notwithstanding, several studies have buttressed the construct validity of Hilgard's concept of imaginative involvement. S. Davis, Dawson, and Seay (1978) found that subjects who were identified as high in imaginative involvement, on the basis of their responses to a scale that represented different areas of imaginative involvement derived from Hilgard's work, scored higher on Form A of the Stanford Hypnotic Susceptibility Scale (SHSS:A) than did subjects who scored low in imaginative involvement.

Like Shor (1960) and J. R. Hilgard (1970, 1979), T. X. Barber (1979) and Singer and Bonanno (1990) have called attention to the relation between involvement in hypnosis and involvement in specific life situations such as imaginative reading (Shor, 1970). Two studies have examined hypnotizability in the context of reading involvement by exposing subjects to actual stimuli presumed to be conducive to imaginative involvement. In one study, Fellows and Armstrong (1977) found that high hypnotizable subjects became more involved in imaginative reading than low hypnotizable subjects. Baum and Lynn (1981) included nonimaginative reading passages and demonstrated that differences in self-reported involvement between subjects high and low in susceptibility (on the Harvard Group Scale of Hypnotic Susceptibility, Form A [HGSHS:A] and the Creative Imagination Scale [CIS] of S. C. Wilson & Barber, 1978) emerged in response to imaginative reading materials, but not in response to more technical, less imaginative prose. This research suggests that the relationship between imaginative involvement and hypnosis may depend in part upon the nature of the stimulus materials used that engage or fail to engage subjects' imaginative proclivities. In addition, high hypnotizable subjects tended to express greater involvement in high than in low imaginative material, confirming J. R. Hilgard's (1965, 1970) observations derived from interviews.

Snodgrass and Lynn (1989) studied high, medium, and low hypnotizable subjects' (HGSHS:A) involvement in music passages rated as high and low in imaginativeness. This research was inspired by J. R. Hilgard's (1974a) finding that the area of involvement in "savoring of sensory experiences" (i.e., music and nature involvement) was more strongly associated with hypnotizablility than the other areas explored in her research. Snodgrass and Lynn (1989) found that high hypnotizable subjects reported greater absorption in classical music than low hypnotizable subjects. Whereas the medium hypnotizables fell between the high and low subjects on the absorption measure, supporting the relation between hypnotizability and absorption, they were not found to differ from either the high or low susceptible. Furthermore, there was a tendency for hypnotizability to have an effect on subjects' imagery elaboration in response to the high but not the low imaginative passages—an effect paralleling Baum and Lynn's (1981) finding that high and low subjects differed in response to imaginative reading passages but not in response to less imaginative passages on a measure of imaginative involvement.

An important feature of the Baum and Lynn (1981) and Snodgrass and Lynn (1989) studies was that they separated the hypnosis-testing context from the later tasks of reading and music involvement, respectively. It is therefore unlikely that the results were seriously compromised by situation-based expectancies. The studies in the area of imaginative involvement have only begun to cover the full spectrum of antecedents purportedly conducive to imaginative involvement (e.g., enjoyment of nature). There is a need for future research to examine multiple antecedents of hypnotizability in the context of the same investigation, in order to clarify the degree to which diverse involvements are related to hypnotizability.

Absorption

The construct of "imaginative involvement" paved the way for the elaboration of the related construct of "absorption" (Tellegen & Atkinson, 1974). Tellegen (1987) recently defined "absorption" as "a disposition, penchant or readiness to enter states characterized by marked cognitive restructuring," and a "readiness to depart from more everyday life cognitive maps and to restructure . . . one's representation of one's self and its boundaries." Roche and McConkey (1990) believe that imaginative involvement and absorption converge, insofar as they are both associated with "an openness to experience emotional and cognitive alterations across a variety of situations" (p. 93). The link between these constructs and openness to experience is supported by a recent study by Glisky, Tataryn, Tobias, Kihlstrom, and McConkey (1991), which confirmed an appreciable association between absorption and measures of openness to experience.

A good deal of research (see Roche & McConkey, 1990) followed on the heels of the development of Tellegen and Atkinson's (1974) Absorption Scale. Fortunately, within the past few years, two excellent reviews (de Groh, 1989; Roche & McConkey, 1990) of the correlates of hypnotizability have been published. These reviews agree that although many studies report a low to moderate degree of association between absorption and hypnotizability, absorption correlates variably with hypnotizability ($r =$ .13–.89; Roche & McConkey, 1990). Roche and McConkey (1990) attribute this variability to variations in the number and types of subjects in the studies, the disparate emphases of the studies, and the methodological rigor of the studies. Furthermore, attitudes and context-based expectancies may moderate the results obtained across studies. Context effects are thoroughly examined by Kirsch and Council in Chapter 10 of this volume, so they are not discussed further here. However, research indicates that unfavorable information about hypnosis can diminish the relationship between absorption and hypnotizability (Spanos & McPeake, 1975b), and that the association between absorption and hypnotizability is greater for subjects with positive attitudes than for subjects with more negative attitudes about hypnosis (Spanos, Brett, Menary, & Cross, 1987). Nevertheless, as de Groh (1989) notes, the relationship between absorption and hypnotizability is modest even when attitudes are taken into consideration. Research by Nadon, Laurence, and Perry (1987) demonstrates the value of multivariate procedures in helping to understand absorption. The authors discovered that although absorption was important in identifying low hypnotizable subjects, variables such as a preference for imagic thinking and a belief in the supernatural were important in discriminating medium and high hypnotizable subjects.

Fantasy Proneness

A third construct, "fantasy proneness," is intimately related to imaginative involvement and absorption. S. C. Wilson and Barber (1981, 1983a) discovered fantasy-prone persons in the context of their intensive interview study of hypnotizable persons. The researchers found that, with one exception, their 27 excellent hypnotic subjects reported a long-standing history of fantasy involvements, whereas the 25 nonexcellent (poor, medium, and medium–high in hypnotizability) hypnotic subjects with whom they were compared rarely reported a history of profound fantasy involvements.

S. C. Wilson and Barber (1981) drew attention to the parallels between imaginative involvement and fantasy proneness. In fact, the concept of "fantasy proneness" is derivative of and encompasses J. R. Hilgard's construct of "imaginative involvement," and is empirically related to absorption ($r = .75$; Lynn & Rhue, 1986) and positive/constructive daydreaming ($r = .48$; Neufeld, Lynn, Jacquith, Weekes, & Brentar, 1987). Thus, there is considerable overlap among all of these constructs.

S. C. Wilson and Barber contended that fantasizers' intense imaginal involvements represent manifestations of adaptive fantasy abilities at the extreme end of the continuum of the trait of fantasy proneness. The researchers estimated that fantasy proneness is evident in as much as 4% of the general population. Wilson and Barber (1981) reported that fantasizers' most outstanding feature is their profound involvement in fantasy. Many of their subjects reported spending at least half of their waking life fantasizing. The fantasizer subjects also reported the ability to hallucinate objects and to experience what they fantasized "as real as real." This included rich and vivid imagery before sleep, vivid recall of personal experiences, the achievement of orgasm in the absence of physical stimulation, and physical reactions (e.g. anxiety, and nausea) to observed violence on television. Fantasizers also reported psychic and out-of-body experiences, as well as occasional difficulty in differentiating fantasized events and persons from nonfantasized ones. Finally, the fantasizers exhibited a sensitivity to social norms, which resulted in a secret fantasy life that few were privy to. In short, fantasy appeared to be an integral part of these fantasizers' identities and their everyday lives.

S. C. Wilson and Barber argued that fantasizers' lifetime history of intense fantasy is conducive to their quickly and easily experiencing hypnotic phenomena, such as age regression, visual hallucinations, hand anesthesia, and auditory hallucinations. By this logic, the majority of fantasizers should score as high hypnotizable subjects on conventional hypnosis scales.

As an initial test of this hypothesis, Lynn and Rhue (1986) selected fantasy-prone subjects and tested their hypnotizability. As in each of Lynn and Rhue's studies that selected subjects on the basis of fantasy proneness, the researchers used the Inventory of Childhood Memories and Imaginings (ICMI; S. C. Wilson & Barber, 1983b) as a screening instrument. This questionnaire was adapted by Wilson and Barber from the interview schedule they had used in their research. To conform with Wilson and Barber's estimates of the prevalence of fantasy-prone persons, Lynn and Rhue selected fantasizers who scored in the upper 2% to 4% of the population. The researchers contrasted these subjects with nonfantasizers, who scored in the lower 2% to 4%, and with medium fantasy-prone subjects, who scored in the range between the scores of the fantasy-prone subjects and the nonfantasizers.

In their first study (Lynn & Rhue, 1986), fantasizers outperformed less fantasy-prone subjects on measures of hypnotizability, waking suggestions (CIS; S. C. Wilson & Barber, 1978), and vividness of imagery. However, fantasy proneness was not a perfect predictor of hypnotizability. In fact, more than a third of the nonfantasizers (35.29%) scored as high hypnotizable, and nonfantasizers were just as hypnotizable as medium fantasy-prone subjects. Nevertheless, nearly 80% of fantasizers scored in the high hypnotizable range.

A finding of particular relevance to our discussion was that fantasizers were more creative than medium fantasy-prone subjects and nonfantasizers, as measured by a test of subjects' preference for visual complexity of simple or complex line drawings (Barron–Welsh Revised Art Scale; Welsh & Barron, 1963). In a recent study, Rhue, Lynn, Bukh, and Henry (1991) replicated this finding, and also found that fantasizers outperformed the nonfantasizers with whom they were compared on another test of creativity—the Alternate Uses Test (Guilford, 1959), which taps divergent thinking ability by requiring subjects to generate multiple uses for well-known objects. Thus, fantasizers not only exhibited a facility for responding to suggestions, but they also were found to be creative, as gauged by multiple indices.

In a subsequent study (Rhue & Lynn, 1989), subjects were required to participate only in a single-session experiment rather than an intensive, multisession interview study. Furthermore, subjects were classified as fantasy-prone on the basis of their ICMI scores. Even when the conditions of testing were radically altered from the first study, the majority of fantasizers tested as high hypnotizable, and fantasizers were more hypnotizable than nonfantasizers. However, it was also found that fantasizers were no more hypnotizable than medium fantasy-prone subjects, and that nonfantasizers emerged as the group distinctly lowest in hypnotizability. This pattern of results has been replicated by Huff and Council (1987) and by Siuta (1989) in Poland.

S. C. Wilson and Barber (1981) found that 96% of their highly hypnotizable subjects could be described as fantasy-prone. One reason why the researchers might have secured evidence for an impressive link between hypnotizability and fantasy proneness is that they used a highly select group of fantasy-prone subjects. That is, all of Wilson and Barber's fantasizers were women; many were professionals with postgraduate degrees. Furthermore, many of the women were recruited from the ranks of participants in workshops the researchers conducted, and were acquainted with the researchers by way of personal or professional relationships (e.g., therapy clients). However, another reason why Wilson and Barber might have secured evidence for such a high degree of correspondence between fantasy proneness and hypnotizability was that they selected subjects on the basis of their hypnotic talent rather than on the basis of their fantasy proneness.

To address the question of whether evidence for a link between fantasy proneness and hypnotizability would be documented when subjects were selected on the basis of hypnotizability rather than fantasy proneness, Lynn, Green, Rhue, Mare, and Williams (1990) selected subjects who scored in the upper 5% of hypnotizability. This select group of subjects was required to score 11 and 12 on both the HGSHS:A and the individually administered Stanford Hypnotic Susceptibility Scale, Form C (SHSS:C; Weitzenhoffer & Hilgard, 1962). The investigators compared these subjects' scores on the ICMI with subjects who scored 11 or 12 on the HGSHS:A but were not screened on the SHSS:C. These latter subjects scored within the upper 10% of their population.

Only 2 of the 12 subjects (16.66%) who were screened with both hypnotizability scales scored as fantasizers on the ICMI (upper 4% of the ICMI distribution). A similar frequency of subjects who scored 11 or 12 on the HGSHS:A alone—that is, 12.82% (5 of 39)—scored as fantasizers. Therefore, the authors were unsuccessful in approximating S. C. Wilson and Barber's findings. This indicates that less correspondence between fantasy proneness and hypnotizability exists than Wilson and Barber's preliminary research suggested.

Daydreaming Styles

Investigators have studied everyday imaginative and fantasy involvements in the context of daydreaming research. At least three distinct fantasy styles have been identified (Huba, Singer, Aneshensel, & Antrobus, 1982; Singer & Antrobus, 1972; Starker, 1978): (1) positive/constructive (PC), marked by pleasant feelings and positive attitudes toward daydreaming; (2) guilt/fear of failure (GFF), associated with themes of guilt, fear, sadness, fear of failure, and achievement fantasies; and (3) poor attentional control (PAC), involving anxiety, a tendency toward easy distractibility, and an inability to remain involved in a single task (Huba et al., 1982; Singer & Antrobus, 1972). Three studies (Crawford, 1982a; Hoyt, Nadon, Register, Chorny, Fleeson, Grigorian, Otto, & Kihlstrom, 1989; Neufeld et al., 1987) have found that hypnotizability is related to the PC daydreaming style but not to the PAC or GFF style. Neufeld et al. (1987) also showed that the PC daydreaming style was correlated with subjects' fantasies in response to a hypnotic dream suggestion. Thus, subjects' experience of a hypnotic suggestion was related to their characteristic daydreaming style. Nevertheless, the magnitude of correlations between daydreaming style and hypnotizability was not particularly impressive, ranging from .16 (Hoyt et al., 1989) to .41 (Crawford, 1982a).

Summary of the Research

The available research indicates that whether research is couched in terms of the construct of imaginative involvement, absorption, fantasy proneness, or daydreaming style, many hypnotizable subjects are able to fantasize and imagine in response to nonhypnotic activities that require a temporary diminution of rational, reality-bound, analytical thinking. Furthermore, Lynn and Rhue's research suggests that creativity is related to fantasy proneness. However, these positive findings must be qualified by the fact that nonhypnotic imaginative and fantasy involvements, in and of themselves, are not very successful at predicting hypnotizability.

    This general conclusion is consistent with our view of the hypnotizable subject as creative agent. More than imagery and fantasy ability is required to respond successfully to hypnosis. Individual differences probably exist in the ability to translate suggested images into sensations (e.g., feeling "wet" while imagining oneself swimming); this ability may be independent to some extent of imagery vividness or imaginative involvement. Also important is the ability to decipher task demands, along with the ability to participate fully in a cooperative relationship in which the role of the "good subject" is enacted. It is also clear that negative response sets (e.g., attitudes) and lack of motivation to respond to suggestions dampen responding in even highly imaginative subjects (see Lynn & Rhue, 1991). Finally, subjects' imaginings and fantasies are often woven around their prehypnotic expectancies about hypnosis, the implicit and explicit cues that emanate from the hypnotic relationship, and the wording of the suggestions they receive.

    We next consider how suggestion wording is related to fantasies experienced during hypnosis, and how these fantasies in turn are related to subjects' experience and performance. We also examine how subjects' standards for evaluating their performance may play an important role in creative problem solving. The review of goal-directed fantasy that follows is the first contemporary review of the literature on this topic.

Goal-Directed Fantasy: Patterns of Imaginative Activity during Hypnosis

Review of the Research

Spanos (1971) hypothesized that subjects were most likely to perceive their behavioral responses to suggestion as involuntary when they become absorbed in a pattern of imaginings called "goal-directed fantasy" (GDF). GDFs are defined as "imagined situations which, if they were to occur in reality, would be expected to lead to the involuntary occurrence of the motor response called for by the suggestion" (Spanos, Rivers, & Ross, 1977, p. 211). For instance, subjects administered a hand levitation suggestion are exhibiting a GDF if they report imagining a helium balloon lifting the hand, or a basketball being inflated under the hand. Suggestions worded to stimulate GDFs thus provide subjects with a cognitive strategy for generating and intensifying feelings of involuntariness (see Spanos, 1971; Spanos & Barber, 1972).

    In Spanos's (1971) first study of GDFs, subjects received ideomotor and challenge suggestions taken from the Barber Suggestibility Scale (BSS; T. X. Barber, 1969) and the SHSS:C, in addition to an amnesia suggestion. With few exceptions, subjects who passed suggestions also reported

GDFs. According to Spanos, subjects who failed test suggestions typically indicated that they were unwilling or unable to imagine the suggested events, or they imagined situations that were unrelated to passing the test suggestions (e.g., when given an arm levitation suggestion, a subject who did not pass the suggestion reported "seeing" a green kangaroo hopping around the room).

In a follow-up study, Spanos and Barber (1972) found that hypnotized subjects who reported GDFs rated their responses to an arm levitation suggestion as more involuntary than those who did not report GDFs. Unlike findings in Spanos's (1971) first study, the reports of GDFs were not associated with enhanced overt responding to test suggestions. Subjects who received GDF suggestions reported the most GDFs (100%), followed by subjects who were instructed to imagine the arm rising (40%), by subjects who received a direct suggestion for the arm to lift (20%), and finally by subjects who received a direct command for the arm to lift (10%). Regardless of their test condition, subjects reported that they were equally hypnotized. Because reports of nonvolition varied as a function of group membership, but subjects were equally hypnotizable across the groups, Spanos and Barber concluded that experienced nonvolition cannot be accounted for in terms of differences in level of suggestibility between treatments. Furthermore, the fact that 40% of subjects who did not display GDFs defined their overt behavior as involuntary indicates that these subjects were employing other strategies for defining their behavior as nonvolitional.

Spanos and Ham (1973) showed that GDFs were not limited to hypnotic conditions. That is, hypnotized and awake task-motivated subjects did not differ in the number of GDFs they exhibited. Subjects reported more GDFs when they met a criterion of selective amnesia than when they failed to meet this criterion.

A study by Coe, Allen, Krug, and Wirzmann (1974) repeated Spanos's (1971) procedure, with the exception that they used seven cognitive items historically associated with deep hypnosis taken from the SHSS:C. The authors found evidence for a moderate correlation ($r = .52$) between total objective scores and the number of GDFs reported. However, unlike the clear-cut findings reported by Spanos (1971), only two of the seven individual items (age regression and negative visual hallucination) showed a significant relation between GDFs and objective response to the suggestion. The investigators hypothesized that suggestions worded to encourage GDF use may be particularly important for subjects who are lower in fantasy ability.

Buckner and Coe (1977) examined this hypothesis in an experiment in which they tested three groups of 20 subjects who were categorized in terms of imaginative capacity (upper, middle, and lower third of scores) on the basis of a test that required subjects to vividly imagine eight items (e.g., "being unable to stand up—stuck to your chair"), and then to report what sorts of things they thought, felt, imagined, and said to themselves in achieving each sensation. For the experiment proper, subjects were administered either a hypnotic susceptibility scale (seven-item SHSS:A) containing item wordings that suggested GDFs, or they were administered a scale modified so that it was not worded to suggest GDFs.

This research did not support the hypothesis that subjects' prehypnotic tendency to use GDFs is related to hypnotic susceptibility or the production of GDFs during hypnosis. Although subjects who received the hypnotic scale designed to increase GDFs reported more GDFs than subjects who received the non-GDF scale, this increase in GDF reports did not result in a corresponding increase in hypnotic responsiveness. Nevertheless, for the total sample, there was a significant relationship ($r = .36$) between GDF reports during hypnosis and hypnotic susceptibility. Unfortunately, no attempt was made to measure subjects' experience of suggestion-related involuntariness.

Spanos, Spillane, and McPeake (1976) extended Spanos and Barber's (1972) earlier research by using more suggestions (i.e., arm levitation, arm catalepsy, and amnesia) and by comparing subjects' responses to task motivation instructions versus an hypnotic induction. The three suggestions were worded so as either to encourage GDFs, or not to provide an explicit GDF strategy. In response to two (arm levitation and arm catalepsy) out of the three suggestions that were administered, subjects provided with a GDF strategy were more responsive behaviorally and subjectively (i.e., experienced greater involuntariness) than subjects who did not receive GDF suggestions. The results were equivalent in the hypnotic and task-motivated conditions, suggesting that GDF is a useful strategy in both hypnotic and nonhypnotic conditions. The authors note, however, that one limitation of the research was that GDF suggestions were somewhat longer than the nonstrategy suggestions.

Spanos, Rivers, and Ross (1977) administered a 40-second arm catalepsy suggestion (taken from Spanos & McPeake, 1977) to subjects. The researchers found that subjects' rated absorption in the suggestion correlated both with their expectancy of arm bending and with the number of sensations they reported in the arm. The GDFs reported by subjects were related to their reports of suggestion-related involuntariness.

Spanos and McPeake (1977) tested the idea that strategies other than GDF can augment responsiveness to test suggestions. For instance, some suggestions (such as that for arm catalepsy, in which it is suggested that the arm feel stiff and rigid) encourage subjects to experience sensations that are consistent with suggested effects. To test the relative effectiveness of cognitive strategies, subjects were hypnotized (T. X. Barber, 1969) and then received arm immobility and arm catalepsy suggestions with one of three strategies: (1) GDF; (2) focus on bodily sensations; or (3) information about effects (subjects were told that they would not be able to bend the arm; i.e., they were informed of overt behavior and subjective effects expected).

The major finding was that GDF suggestions were no more effective than suggestions with alternative strategies in increasing either GDF reports or responsiveness to suggestions. However, the reports of GDF (assessed independently of suggestion strategy) were associated with greater suggestion-related involuntariness scores than were non-GDF reports (consistent with Spanos, 1971; Spanos & Barber, 1972; Spanos, Rivers, & Ross, 1977), as well as with overt responding to the suggestions. These findings, taken together with Spanos and Barber's (1974) finding that 40% of their subjects who passed items and also experienced involuntariness in their responses did not report GDFs, suggests that some other important factors are involved in responding to suggestions.

The effects of GDFs on subjects' ability to control experimental pain have also been examined. Chaves and Barber (1974) used a heavy weight applied to the finger for 2 minutes as a pain stimulus. The researchers obtained pain reports from subjects during a baseline pretest and during a posttest in which one of several experimental treatments was administered. During the posttest, subjects who had been asked to utilize GDFs for reducing pain (i.e., to imagine pleasant events, or to imagine the finger as insensitive) showed a reduction in pain as compared to uninstructed control subjects. Subjects who were merely led to expect pain reduction, but not provided with cognitive strategies, also reported reduced pain during the posttest as compared to control subjects. This reduction, however, was smaller than for subjects using cognitive strategies. Finally, the degree of pain reduction was found to be related to the proportion of time that subjects used the cognitive strategies ($r = -.67$).

The hypothesis that it is not the specific content of a fantasy, but rather the fact that it is of a goal-directed nature, that matters was tested by Spanos, Horton, and Chaves (1975). The investigators secured support for this hypothesis in an analgesia study in which subjects immersed one of their arms in ice water and (1) were asked to imagine a situation that, if real, would be inconsistent with pain (relevant strategy); (2) were asked to imagine a situation unrelated to pain (irrelevant strategy); or (3) were not given special instructions (control group). Whether subjects used a relevant or irrelevant strategy did not alter the pain thresholds for subjects with low pretest thresholds. However, among those subjects with high pretest thresholds, a relevant GDF strategy was more effective than an irrelevant strategy, which in turn was more effective than the control condition. Under both strategy conditions, subjects who were highly involved in their imaginings were better able to tolerate pain than subjects who were not.

Spanos and Gorassini (1984) conducted an investigation to determine whether involuntariness ratings were moderated by the structure of the communications administered. In contrast with directives, which instruct subjects to make specific responses (e.g., "Please lower your arm"), passively worded suggestions imply that overt behaviors occurring in response to imagined events occur involuntarily (e.g., "Imagine a force moving your arms apart"). The authors found that subjects responded more to directives than to suggestions, but they rated their responses to suggestions as more involuntary than their responses to directives. Not only were more GDFs reported in response to suggestions than directives, but GDFs were correlated with rated involuntariness and hypnotizability. The finding that hypnotic and task motivation procedures produced equivalent degrees of overt responding and involuntariness in response to both suggestions and directives was interpreted as evidence against the idea that hypnotic procedures facilitate a "dissociation" in cognitive processing that leads to the loss of control over everyday behaviors.

Spanos and de Groh (1983) essentially replicated these results. Although they did not measure GDFs, they showed that even though hypnotic and task-motivated subjects moved less in response to a suggestion than in response to a directive or instruction, they rated their responses to a suggestion (e.g., "Imagine a force moving your arm to the right") as more involuntary than their responses to a directive (e.g., "Move your arm") or instructed action (e.g., "Reach for a pencil").

Summary and Questions

Whereas some studies have shown that GDFs enhance overt responding (e.g., Coe et al., 1974; Spanos, Spillane, & McPeake, 1976), and suggested pain reductions (Chaves & Barber, 1974; Spanos, Horton, & Chaves, 1975), subjects who report GDFs do not invariably respond to suggestions (Buckner & Coe, 1977; Coe et al., 1974; Lynn, Snodgrass, Rhue, & Hardaway, 1987; Spanos, 1971; Spanos & Barber, 1972; Spanos & McPeake, 1977; Spanos, Spillane, & McPeake, 1976). Indeed, even within the same study, the results are at times contradictory: Some suggested responses are found to be associated with GDFs, whereas others are not found to be associated with GDFs (e.g., Coe et al., 1974; Spanos, Spillane, & McPeake, 1976).

Inconsistencies across studies cannot be attributed to the type of suggestion studied; no definitive pattern emerges with respect to suggestion type. That is, in Spanos, Spillane, and McPeake's (1976) research, GDFs were associated with an arm levitation and an arm catalepsy suggestion, but not with a so-called cognitive suggestion (amnesia). However, Coe et al. (1974) found that GDFs in relation to several cognitive items (i.e., negative hallucination and age regression) were associated with behavioral response to the suggestion.

The findings with respect to hypnotic involuntariness are more clearcut. The link between GDFs and reports of involuntariness has been substantiated by numerous studies indicating that GDFs are related to subjects' tendency to define their overt responses to suggestions as involuntary occurrences (e.g., Lynn, Snodgrass, 1987; Spanos, et al., 1971; Spanos, Spillane, & McPeake, 1976; Spanos & Barber, 1972; Spanos & Gorassini, 1984; Spanos & McPeake, 1977; Spanos, Rivers, & Ross, 1977). The research reviewed is thus strongly supportive of the hypothesis that cognitive strategies—GDFs—foster the perception of actions as involuntary happenings.

It is also noteworthy that the GDF–involuntariness association is not limited to hypnotic conditions. A number of studies (Spanos, Spillane, & McPeake, 1976; Spanos & Gorassini, 1984) demonstrate quite clearly that hypnotized and task-motivated subjects' report GDFs at equivalent rates, and that the link between GDFs and reports of involuntariness holds for task-motivated as well as hypnotized subjects. This suggests that the structure of communications, rather than the testing context (hypnotic vs. nonhypnotic), is a crucial determinant of involuntariness reports.

This brief literature review raises a number of important questions. First, what can account for the inconsistent findings regarding the relation between GDF and overt response to suggestion? One possibility is that it is not the mere presence or absence of GDFs that is associated with hypnotic responding; rather (or in addition), subjects' degree of absorption in fantasized events moderates overt responding. That is, subjects whose concentration on the suggested imagery is poor, who experience cognitive intrusions, or whose stream of consciousness diminishes the credibility of suggested events may be less likely to respond to suggestions than subjects who truly experience the imagined events as "real."

Unfortunately, the majority of studies we have reviewed used crude measures of the presence or absence of GDFs. Two studies (Spanos & Ham, 1975; Spanos & McPeake, 1975b) that did not examine GDFs per se, but did use more sensitive, continuous measures related to imaginative involvement, suggest that degree of involvement is an important variable. In the Spanos and McPeake (1975b) study, ratings of imaginative involvement were associated with experienced involuntariness, degree of credibility assigned to imaginings, and hypnotizability. In the Spanos and Ham (1975) study, which used a hypnotic dream as the target suggestion, subjects' involvement in their imaginings was correlated with ratings of involuntariness of imagining ($r = .73$) and with hypnotizability scores. Subjects' involvement in their dreams was also related to the degree of implausibility and fearfulness expressed in their dreams. These findings are consistent with the hypothesis that individual differences in response to hypnotic suggestion reflect individual differences in subjects' willingness and ability to become involved in their imagining.

Studies designed to examine the link between imagination during hypnosis and hypnotizability have generally failed to assess diverse yet potentially interrelated aspects of imaginative involvement (e.g., degree of involvement, intrusive cognitions, credibility and vividness of imagining). Their relative independence of one another remains to be ascertained, as does the particular influence of certain aspects of imaginative involvement.

Another reason why no intimate connection between hypnotic responding and GDFs could conclusively be demonstrated is that "many subjects who pass suggestions totally disregard the suggested fantasies and instead construct other imaginary situations which do not necessarily imply the performance of the correct response" (Spanos, 1971, p. 91). Spanos and McPeake (1977), for example, noted that a quarter of the subjects who received an arm catalepsy suggestion reported a GDF that differed from the suggested GDF. Spanos and Ham (1975) commented that the content of some subjects' hypnotic dreams "depicted such highly charged emotional events as strangulations, bloody accidents, sexual innuendos, and cardiac arrests" (p. 48). Others involved the unintegrated juxtaposition of unrelated events, and some contained highly implausible or patently impossible happenings (e.g., flying people). In the Chaves and Barber (1974) research, some subjects reported that they used the suggested cognitive strategy; however, they also commented that they would have preferred to use their own strategies. Even when GDFs are not explicitly suggested, subjects who respond overtly to suggestions often spontaneously devise and carry out self-directed GDFs (Spanos, 1971; Spanos & Barber, 1972; Spanos & Ham, 1973; Spanos & McPeake, 1975b; Spanos, Spillane, & McPeake, 1976).

The research on GDFs indicates quite clearly that some subjects creatively elaborate suggestions. These subjects view suggestions as "convenient guides" around which to weave fantasy situations (Spanos & Ham, 1973). Just how goal-directed yet nonsuggested imagery relates to hypnotizability is a viable focus for future research. Also, it is apparent that some subjects appear to use cognitive strategies such as GDFs to facilitate their responses to suggestions, whereas other subjects' use of cognitive strategies is less obvious or not apparent in their reports (see McConkey, 1991). Examining the attitudinal and cognitive characteristics of strategy-using versus non-strategy-using responders would also be a worthwhile focus of research efforts.

Are GDFs valid correlates of hypnotizability? Spanos and McPeake (1977) observe that GDFs may simply be artifacts of hypnotic suggestions because they are embedded in the suggestion's content. So highly hypnotizable subjects may simply respond to GDF suggestions just as they respond to other suggestions, thereby creating the false impression that GDF (another suggested response) is responsible for high hypnotizability.

In Chapter 1 of this volume, Woody, Bowers, and Oakman make a similar argument. They contend that even though many hypnotized subjects who receive an analgesia suggestion report cognitive strategies along with reduced pain, it does not necessarily follow that the cognitive strategies mediate the pain reduction. Instead, the strategies and analgesia experienced could be independent responses that co-occur because they are both suggested as part of the initial analgesia suggestion. Of course, this is only one possibility, but it suggests that much needs to be learned about the extent to which cognitive strategies directly mediate suggested responses.

One reason why cognitive strategies might fall short of facilitating behavioral responses has to do with the performance standards that subjects set for themselves. As in any problem-solving situation, subjects approach the hypnotic situation with different personal standards for evaluating the adequacy of their experiences and responses. Hypnotizable subjects ordinarily do not engage in a great deal of conscious self-analysis or self-monitoring of their actions or experience in relation to performance standards. Unless derailed, the free-flowing quality of hypnotic experience is maintained, and subjects are not likely to question that they are hypnotized or responding adequately. Subjects' tacit understanding that they are "good subjects" makes response expectancies firmer and perpetuates the perception of hypnotic action as effortless (see Lynn & Rhue, 1991).

Yet this process can be undermined. For instance, subjects may lack requisite imaginal abilities. No matter how hard they attempt to access memories and events of childhood, for example, they may nevertheless be unable to have a personally compelling experience of age regression. Another possibility is that subjects adopt performance standards that are so difficult to meet that they are dissatisfied and frustrated with their response.

This latter hypothesis was supported by research conducted by Lynn, Jacquith, Green, Mare, and Gasior (1991). In their study, one group of subjects was provided with information designed to lead them to adopt a performance standard that was difficult to achieve. That is, they were informed that hypnotized subjects who respond to more than a few suggestions imagine suggested events "as real as real" and respond immediately to suggestions. When compared to a group of subjects who received prehypnotic information contained in the standard HGSHS:A, the subjects who adopted a stringent performance standard responded to fewer hypnotic suggestions and rated their responses as less involuntary. Subjects apparently engaged in a matching-to-standard process that generated performance-based concerns and attenuated hypnotic involvement. Thus, the standards that subjects adopt to evaluate their experience and performance may be as important as their imaginative ability (see Sheehan & McConkey, 1982). Subjects' interpretation of hypnotic behavior is dependent not only on their abilities to experience hypnotic events, but also on the criteria they use to evaluate their responses and experiences. In the next section, we examine the role of expectancies and subjects' interpretations of their behaviors in greater depth. We argue that expectancies work in tandem with imaginative processes and subjects' motivation to respond to shape hypnotic behavior and experience. That is, expectancies provide implicit and explicit goals toward which subjects direct their creative efforts to generate psychological experiences in the hypnotic context.

Hypnotic Responding, Imaginative Activity, and Expectancies

As we have discussed earlier, Arnold (1946) has emphasized the importance of imaginative processes in determining the subject's response to suggestion. The role of expectancies, and Arnold's hypothesis that there is an intimate connection between responding with an involuntary quality and imaginative activity, were examined in a series of countersuggestion studies conducted in Lynn's laboratory. In the first study (Lynn, Nash, Rhue, Frauman, & Stanley, 1983), hypnotic, simulating, and imagination control subjects were instructed to attend to, imagine, and think about described actions, but to resist engaging in movements. In this context, support for Arnold's position would be secured if hypnotic and imagination subjects, both instructed to sustain suggestion-related imaginings, responded to suggestions and reported involuntariness. In contrast, imaginative processes would be of secondary importance if imagining subjects, in contrast to hypnotic subjects, resisted suggestions while they continued to imagine and be absorbed in suggestions.

That imagining subjects reported feeling as absorbed and involved in imaginings as hypnotic subjects but resisted responding does not support Arnold's (1946) position that imaginative processes are a crucial link between suggestion and involuntariness. The results are more consistent with the position advanced by Spanos (1991) that subjects' imaginings do not directly cause their actions. Nevertheless, the hypnotic induction may be instrumental in translating imaginative involvements into behavior. This role could perhaps be one of legitimizing change. However, the relationship is not simple, because simulators also behaved like subjects with imagination instructions.

The importance of how subjects interpret their experience is illustrated by a number of studies that either tacitly or explicitly manipulated subjects' expectancies regarding the relation between imagination and involuntariness. Lynn, Nash, Rhue, Frauman, and Sweeney (1984) found that imaginative involvement was secondary to expectancies in engendering perceptions of involuntariness. Prior to hypnosis, and prior to subjects' being instructed to resist suggestions, an experimental assistant informed the subjects either that other "good" hypnotic subjects could successfully resist suggestions and retain control over their movements, or that other "good" subjects fail to resist suggestions and experience loss of voluntary control over their actions during hypnosis. This information affected hypnotizable subjects' ability to resist the hypnotist and tended to affect subjects' report of suggestion-related involuntariness in line with induced expectancies about appropriate responding. Furthermore, subjects who successfully resisted suggestions and subjects who failed to do so reported comparable levels of hypnotic depth and imaginative involvement in suggestions.

Spanos, Cobb, and Gorassini (1985) conducted a similar experiment, in which they found that hypnotizable subjects who were instructed that they could become deeply involved in suggestions and yet resist them successfully resisted 95% of the suggestions and rated themselves as maintaining voluntary control over their behavior. Thus, subjects are able to resist nearly all of the suggestions when resistance is facilitated by situational demands. It is worth noting that subjects in this research who resisted hypnotic suggestions rated themselves as just as deeply involved in the suggestions as subjects who failed to resist suggestions after being informed that deeply hypnotized subjects were incapable of resisting suggestions.

Lynn, Snodgrass, et al. (1987) hypothesized that in the first countersuggestion study (Lynn et al., 1983), in which hypnotizable subjects resisted fewer suggestions than imagining subjects, the imagining subjects did not make a connection between imagining a suggested action and responding involuntarily, as did subjects in the hypnotic condition. What if imagining subjects came to associate or connect imagined responses to suggestion with "involuntary" responding? Would they then move in response to suggestions, despite instructions to resist, as did hypnotizable subjects in the first countersuggestion study?

The answer to this question was "Yes." In an initial hypnosis screening session, subjects were informed that hypnosis was actually a "test of imagination." To fortify the link between imagination and involuntariness, the hypnotic induction was administered along with other imagination measures. In a second session, high and low hypnotizable subjects were instructed to imagine along with suggestions, but to resist responding to motoric suggestions. Under these test circumstances, the responses of hypnotizable imagining subjects were comparable to that of hypnotized subjects in Lynn et al.'s (1983) earlier countersuggestion research. That is, imagining subjects tended to move in response to suggestion, despite being instructed to resist.

In this study, half of the subjects received explicit instructions that defined GDFs and invited subjects to use GDFs to enhance their experience of the suggestions; the remaining half of the subjects received no explicit priming instructions. As in many of the GDF studies we have reviewed, correlational analyses revealed that GDFs were associated with the experience of involuntariness; however, GDFs were not associated with responding to suggestions. With instructions designed to increase the use of GDFs, low and high hypnotizable subjects reported equivalent GDF absorption and frequency of GDFs. However, highs responded more and reported greater involuntariness than lows, even when their GDFs were equivalent.

Lynn and his colleagues therefore found no support for the hypothesis that sustained, elaborated suggestion-related imagery mediates response to suggestion (Arnold, 1946). The researchers also failed to find support for Zamansky and Clark's (1986) hypothesis that low hypnotizable subjects, lacking the capacity to dissociate incompatible cognitions from relevant ones, are able to pass suggestions only when it is possible to become absorbed in them. Even when lows and highs were absorbed in GDFs to a comparable extent, lows were not as responsive to suggestions as highs. One of Lynn et al.'s most interesting findings was that highs and lows held very different expectancies about imagining and hypnotic responding: Highs believed that imaginative subjects responded to more suggestions, and believed that a greater correspondence existed between imagining and responding. These measures of expectancy predicted both responding and involuntary experience.

The fact that high and low hypnotizable subjects construe the relation between imagining and the occurrence of suggested responses in very different ways suggests the following interpretation of the relation between overt response to suggestion and imagination: When instructed to do so, lows respond to suggestion by engrossing themselves in suggestion-related imagery. However, they fail, for the most part, to perceive or construct a connection between their suggestion-related imaginings and moving in response to suggestion. This suggests that despite being absorbed in imagery, lows wait passively for suggested events to occur. Not surprisingly, nothing happens. In contrast, highs take a much more active and constructive approach to the situation. They are successful in creating role-related experiences and behaving as suggested, while simultaneously generating imagery of a kind that qualifies their responding as an involuntary happening.

A number of other studies have examined the effects of expectancies on imaginings and hypnotic behavior. Spanos, Weekes, and de Groh (1984) informed subjects that deeply hypnotized individuals could imagine an arm movement in one direction while their unconscious caused the arm to move in the opposite direction. Even though subjects so informed moved in the opposite direction, they imagined suggested effects and described their countersuggestion behavior as involuntary.

Kirsch, Council, and Mobayed (1987) documented stronger effects for expectancy than for involved imagining. The researchers showed that subjects who imagined along with suggestions responded to suggestions when they were led to believe that imagery would enhance suggestions. However, subjects also responded to suggestions when they were led to believe that imagining events incompatible with suggestions enhanced responding. Unfortunately, Kirsch et al. did not assess involuntariness, and did not evaluate the extent to which subjects engaged in GDFs. However, their findings were consistent with the hypothesis that GDFs enhance response to suggestions by virtue of their influence on response expectancies (Kirsch, 1985). Their research was also consistent with studies showing a stronger effect for expectancy than for involved imagining (Lynn et al., 1984; Spanos, Cobb, & Gorassini, 1985; Zamansky, 1977).

B. Wallace's (1990a,b) research suggests that low hypnotizable subjects may have the capacity to use imagery during hypnosis, yet fail to do so because they do not choose to use imagery. According to B. Wallace (1990a), when compared to lows, highs are better at gestalt closure tasks (Crawford, 1982a), and at discovering embedded objects in pictures (Priebe & Wallace, 1986) and in letter arrays (B. Wallace & Patterson, 1984). Wallace and Patterson (1984) attributed this to the more efficient cognitive strategies used by highs. Crawford and Allen (1983) have maintained that highs make greater use of imagery than lows do when performing a visual search. When B. Wallace (1990b) taught low hypnotizable subjects efficient search strategies for finding objects embedded within an array of pictorial scenes, their task performance improved and equaled that of high hypnotizable subjects. The majority of low subjects acknowledged that their posttraining search behavior was the result of using imagery, which they typically did not use. Thus, differences between highs and lows may not reside so much in their imaginative *capacity* as in whether they use imagination during hypnosis. To be sure, if subjects fail to associate creating a vivid imaginal experience with successfully responding to suggestions, or if they do not wish to create such an imaginative scenario, it is not surprising that they do not imagine to the best of their ability (see Spanos, 1986b).

The studies we have reviewed highlight the importance of subjects' expectancies (Kirsch, 1991; Spanos, 1991) and their active cognitive efforts to interpret, understand, and devise creative ways of responding to suggestions (McConkey, 1991; Lynn & Rhue, 1991; Sheehan, 1991). Nevertheless, subjects may miss the import of hypnotic suggestions, fail to imagine suggested events, and test as low in hypnotizability. Alternatively, subjects may imagine suggested events, yet may fail to recognize that an overt behavioral response is required (see Spanos, Cross, Menary, Brett, & de Groh, 1987). Still another possibility is that subjects lack the imaginal skills (Spanos, Cross, et al., 1987) to experience hypnotic events credibly, and thus fail hypnotic suggestions. Hypnotizable subjects are successfully able to integrate and resolve multiple and sometimes conflicting demands, and are able to generate subjective experiences that are consistent with role-appropriate behaviors. In short, hypnotizable subjects are creative problem solvers.

Hypnosis and Creativity

Review of the Research

Even though conventional measures of creativity do not begin to tap the sorts of "problems" faced by the subject in the hypnotic situation, a legitimate question is whether high hypnotizable subjects test higher on conventional measures of creativity than their low hypnotizable counterparts. Another question of interest is whether hypnosis facilitates creative expression above and beyond nonhypnotic conditions.

P. G. Bowers and K. S. Bowers conducted the seminal work examining the link between hypnotizability, hypnosis, and creativity. This early research was informed by the ego-analytic theory of psychological regression, which, as we have noted earlier, has been used to explain both creativity (Kris, 1934/1952) and hypnotic phenomena (Gill & Brenman, 1959). In the first experimental investigation of the relationship between creativity and hypnosis, P. G. Bowers (1967) examined the relationship between defensiveness and creativity. She reasoned that hypnosis might be one way of reducing subjects' defensiveness and thus enhancing creativity. Bowers selected subjects who were at least moderately hypnotizable (i.e., passed 7 or more of 10 HGSHS:A suggestions) and randomly assigned them to one of four groups. Subjects either received waking relaxation instructions, listened to music, and performed a time estimation task to maintain alertness, or received the HGSHS:A induction. Half of the subjects in each of these two groups received cognitive set instructions (e.g., the subjects were exhorted to be "clever, original, flexible, and fluent"), and the other half received defense-reducing instructions (e.g., the subjects were informed that they had the ability to be creative, exhorted to perceive in unconventional ways, and encouraged to notice aspects of the task overlooked previously). Bowers's (1967) "creativity battery" consisted of six measures of divergent thinking adopted from Guilford's (1959) tests.

After subjects received the first half of each of these tests (pretest), they were then hypnotized or given waking relaxation instructions and given the cognitive set or defense-reducing instructions, as appropriate to their condition. Subjects were then posttested on the second half of the creativity measures. The waking and hypnosis groups did not differ on the pretest measures. Although the type of instructions that subjects received was immaterial, hypnosis, relative to waking instructions, was found to increase divergent thinking. The measure of originality, the Consequences Test (Guilford, 1959), was most effective in differentiating subjects in the hypnosis and waking conditions.

The results cannot be regarded as strong support for the facilitative effects of hypnosis; hypnotized subjects were superior to waking/motivated subjects on only one of six creativity measures. Furthermore, P. G. Bowers (1967) cautions that inferences based on her research should be limited, because it was possible that the fact that the situation was defined as hypnotic, along with the experimenter's knowledge of subjects' group assignment, could have contributed to group differences in creativity. The former hypothesis is supported by the fact that in a follow-up study, K. S. Bowers (1968) found that unhypnotizable simulating subjects' performance equaled that of hypnotized subjects on the originality measure.

In order to further contrast the responses of hypnotic and nonhypnotic subjects on creativity tests, and to test the theory of psychological regression, K. S. Bowers and van der Meulen (1970) compared hypnotizable subjects (i.e., passed 8 or more HGSHS:A suggestions) and unhypnotizable (i.e., passed 3 or fewer HGSHS:A suggestions) subjects who were assigned to waking/motivated (i.e., told to relax, listened to soothing music, performed time estimation task), hypnotized (i.e., standard SHSS induction), or hypnosis-simulating treatment groups. As in P. G. Bowers's study (1967), subjects received defense-reducing instructions. To facilitate comparison with P. G. Bowers's earlier work on creativity, Guilford's (1959) Consequences Test was included in the test battery, along with 10 cards of the Holtzman Inkblot Technique (HIT; Holtzman, Thorpe, Swartz, & Herron, 1961) that have a low pull for Human Movement responses, and the Free Association Test (Gardner, Holzmann, Klein, Linton, & Spence, 1959).

The data revealed that high hypnotizable subjects, regardless of their experimental condition, were invariably more creative than less hypnotizable subjects: Out of a total of nine comparisons, eight were significant "beyond or near the .05 level" (1970, p. 251). However, creativity performance did not vary as a function of whether subjects were assigned to hypnotic or nonhypnotic conditions. Thus, hypnosis does not facilitate creativity above and beyond conditions that provide subjects with motivational instructions to perform successfully on creativity tasks.

Providing further support for a relationship between hypnotizability and creativity, K. S. Bowers and van der Meulen (1970) obtained a correlation of .45 between HGSHS scores and a measure of overall creativity. However, when only high hypnotizable subjects were considered in the analysis, the correlation dropped to nearly zero. In explaining these findings, the authors suggested that the attenuated correlation might eventuate from the fact that the HGSHS does not discriminate among highs very well: Several of the tasks are simple motoric suggestions and offer little challenge in terms of the cognitive demands they impose. When subjects were retested on the SHSS:C, which contains more cognitively demanding suggestions, the correlation with the creativity composite increased to .31. Furthermore, the correlation between the creativity composite and a modified hypnotizability scale that included only cognitive items of the SHSS:C was .37.

The authors maintained that their results support the adaptive regression theory for a number of reasons. First, on posthypnotic rating scales, high hypnotizable subjects reported more nonsuggested unusual and unrealistic experiences (e.g., "floating, blacking out, dizziness, changes in body size") than low hypnotizable subjects. Second, the authors maintained that cognitively challenging hypnotizability items (e.g., age regression) produced higher correlations with the creativity composite. Unfortunately, the investigators did not conduct a statistical analysis to document that the correlation of .37 was in fact greater than the correlation of .31.

K. S. Bowers and van der Meulen (1970) secured an interesting post hoc finding that was explored in later research: On four of the creativity measures, women were more creative than men. To explore the intriguing possibility that sex may serve as a moderator variable, K. S. Bowers (1971) compared the responses of men and women, rectangularly distributed across the entire range of the HGSHS:A (three males and three females for each level of hypnotizability, 1–12), on five creativity tests: the HIT (Holtzman et al., 1961); the Free Association Test (Gardner et al., 1959); the Consequences Test (Guilford, 1959); the Remote Associates Test (Mednick & Mednick, 1967); and the Revised Art Scale (Welsh & Barron, 1963). The Wechsler Adult Intelligence Scale (WAIS) Vocabulary subtest, and a measure of spontaneous trance-like experiences the Personal Experiences Questionnaire [PEQ]; Shor, 1960), were also administered.

The Revised Art Scale, the PEQ, and the WAIS Vocabulary subtest were given first, followed by the remaining four tests in the battery either in the same session or at another time. However, before subjects took the remaining four tests, they received the defense-reducing instructions (P. G. Bowers, 1967) previously described. A preliminary analysis revealed that subjects high (9–12 suggestions passed), medium (5–8 suggestions passed), and low (0–3 suggestions passed) in hypnotizability failed to differ from one another on any of the eight creativity measures. Nor were sex differences secured. It was only when highs and lows were compared, to directly parallel the analysis of K. S. Bowers and van der Meulen (1970), that high women outscored both low men and women, and high men on a composite creativity measure.

The second part of the analysis involved correlating the creativity composite with the rectangularly distributed levels of hypnotizability. Women's HGSHS:A scores correlated .41 with overall creativity, and men did not achieve a significant correlation. A subset of men and women returned for administration of the SHSS:C. When the SHSS:C was used as the criterion measure, the correlations were no longer significant and dropped to .25 for women and .02 for men. This stands in contrast with the findings of K. S. Bowers and van der Meulen (1970), who found evidence for a significant relationship between scores on the SHSS: C and a composite creativity measure. However, when only high susceptible subjects were used in the analysis (>7 on the SHSS:C), then the correlation for women increased to .55 (vs. a correlation of –.11 for men). Similarly, when only the highs were considered, the correlation between hypnotizability and PEQ intensity was .45 for women versus .16 for men. K. S. Bowers (1971) concluded that both sex and hypnotizability served as moderating variables.

Following the lines of earlier suggestions (Ås, 1962) that men's fantasy tends to be organized around impulses and drives, in contrast to women's fantasy, which is more attuned to environmental stimulation, K. S. Bowers (1971) hypothesized that the sex differences observed in his research reflected women's tendency to respond to external stimulation (i.e., hypnotic suggestions) and engage in perceptual distortions to a greater extent than males. Thus, sex differences may reflect "basic differences in the organization of imagination" (p. 93).

Perry, Wilder, and Appignanesi (1973) attempted to extend the work of P. G. and K. S. Bowers by adopting a multidimensional factor-analytic approach to study the creativity–hypnosis relationship. The rationale for this design rested on the assumption that a battery of tests measuring diverse conceptualizations of creativity (i.e., product criterion tests, process tests of degree of control of primary process, capacity tests of divergent thinking) would provide a more sensitive means of discerning relationships between hypnotizability and creativity. The authors employed a battery of 14 creativity tests that included 19 measures. Subjects were administered the SHSS:C (with the anosmia-to-ammonia item omitted) following two sessions of creativity testing. All of the measures were entered into a factor analysis using a varimax procedure.

Compared to low hypnotizable subjects, high hypnotizable subjects scored consistently above the mean across all the creativity measures. High (9–11 SHSS:C suggestions passed) and medium (3–8 SHSS:C suggestions passed) subjects, however, were indistinguishable by this consistency criterion (sum of scores above the mean on the creativity tests), although it discriminated both groups from low (0–2 SHSS:C suggestions passed) subjects. This would suggest that it was the lows rather than the highs who were uniquely different.

Only six of the measures of creativity correlated significantly with the SHSS:C: two of the Barron–Welsh scales, and Torrance (1966) Verbal Fluency (the highest, with $r = .40$) Verbal Flexibility, Object Synthesis, and Figural Creativity. Torrance's measures of fluency and flexibility provided the sole consistent relationship between hypnotizability and creativity, such that they correlated significantly with hypnotizability and differentiated the three hypnotizability groups. As Perry et al. (1973) stated, "in terms of individual creativity tests, the relationship between hypnotic susceptibility and creativity is not a robust one" (pp. 178–179). As in the previous research reviewed, the burden of the significant relationships was carried by the women.

Although the magnitude of the individual correlations was not great, on six factors extracted by the factor analysis, four loaded jointly on hypnotic and a number of creativity variables. The authors urged caution when interpreting these data, because the initial intercorrelations for the factor analysis were modest and, as such, the strong factor loadings may simply have reflected spurious relationships. In any event, highs performed consistently better across various measures of creativity.

The question of whether hypnosis enhances figural or verbal creativity was investigated by Gur and Reyher (1976). High hypnotizable male subjects (9–12 HGSHS:A suggestions passed) were divided into three different groups: hypnosis, simulation, and waking. The investigators took precautions to ensure that control subjects were not spontaneously hypnotized, although no manipulation check was used. Subjects were tested with the Torrance Tests of Creative Thinking (Torrance, 1966), modified in the following way: (1) Visual imagery was used to represent meaning rather than language because imagery is theoretically more conducive to tapping primary-process ideation; (2) unlike the previous studies, the tasks were not identified as measures of creativity; (3) the instructions emphasized "waiting for ideas to come rather than pursuing them"; and (4) a free-imagery phase was included to enhance "primary-process thinking." Gur and Reyher also included an additional group of 12 randomly selected male volunteers who were not hypnotized and received the standard Torrance instructions.

Unlike K. S. Bowers (1968) and K. S. Bowers and van der Meulen (1970), Gur and Reyher (1976) found that the hypnotized group scored higher than nonhypnotic controls on a measure of creativity (i.e., Torrance's [1966] measure of Figural Creativity). The reasons for the disparity across studies are unclear; however, in addition to the fact that Gur and Reyher administered the Torrance tests under nonstandard conditions, a number of methodological differences ought to be considered. First, the simulators in Gur and Reyher's (1976) research may not have been as motivated to deceive the hypnotist and enact a convincing role play as were the simulators in previous studies, in which the importance of simulators behaving in a "convincingly hypnotic way" was underscored in a manner more consistent with standard (Orne, 1959, 1979a) simulating instructions (see K. S. Bowers & van der Meulen, 1970). Second, the defense-reducing instructions in previous studies might have minimized differences between hypnotic and nonhypnotic treatments.

Gur and Reyher (1976) suggest that enhanced figural creativity compared to verbal creativity is commensurate with the adaptive-regression formulation of hypnosis and its relationship to creativity. This conclusion was derived by comparing their data with an operational definition of adaptive regression given by Wiseman and Reyher (1973): "Adaptive regression is defined by independent measures showing an increase in blatancy of drive representation and primary process thinking, while secondary process monitoring and reality contact remain unimpaired" (cited in Gur & Reyher, 1976, p. 247). The data obtained from this study conformed to this criterion. That is, the hypnotized group scored higher on drive presence and blatancy (primary-process component) than the other groups, and they achieved higher scores on the Torrance Tests of creativity, suggesting that secondary process functioning was intact. The authors also implicated activation of the right cerebral hemisphere in enhancing creativity via hypnosis, given the enhancement of figural creativity.

The Russian psychologist Vladimir Raikov published an intriguing series of reports (1976, 1977) describing "developing latent creative potentials" (Raikov, 1976, p. 259) in what he termed the "active stage" of hypnosis. Subjects in these studies were instructed to complete tasks during hypnosis while they received instructions that they were famous persons such as musicians or artists, endowed with the requisite skills to perform creatively on musical or artistic tasks. Raikov reported favorable and enduring improvements in subjects' creative abilities, and postulated that an "attitude set" was activated during hypnosis that promoted the improvement in performance.

Although Raikov stated that hypnosis is particularly suited to help achieve creative breakthroughs, his reports contain insufficient information to permit others to evaluate the specific role of hypnosis in accounting for behavioral changes during and following hypnosis. Even though he alluded to a number of studies describing improvements in hypnotic conditions above and beyond those in simulating and waking control conditions, he did not describe the instructions to subjects and experimental conditions in sufficient detail for any evaluation of methodological integrity. Nor did he present statistical analyses and procedures to document treatment effects. In short, although Raikov's reports are interesting and provocative, they provide no basis for concluding that the improvements in creativity he described were associated with a special state of consciousness or even with the induction of hypnosis.

P. G. Bowers (1978, 1982–1983) and K. S. Bowers (P. G. Bowers & Bowers, 1979) added a new dimension to the study of the relationship between hypnosis and creativity by examining the role of effortless experiencing as an element common to both phenomena. Theorists agree (see Stein, 1974) that creative experiences are most likely to occur when an individual is relaxed and passively receptive to associations, and hence experiences creative inspiration as effortless and nonvolitional. P. G. Bowers (1978) suggested that receptiveness to subconscious work accounts for effortless experiences in both creative problem-solving and hypnotic contexts. It bears mention that social-cognitive hypnosis theorists (Lynn & Rhue, 1991) and psychoanalytic theorists (Eisen, in press; Fromm, 1979; M. R. Nash, 1991) converge in acknowledging the importance of a receptive set toward experiencing hypnotic suggestions, insofar as a vigilant, critical, and analytical posture is anathema to the play of creative imagery, the subject's ability to focus on images and related sensations in a sustained manner, and the experience of suggestion-related nonvolition.

To test the hypothesis that aptitude for effortless experiencing accounts for the relationship between hypnotizability and creativity, P. G. Bowers (1978) analyzed the interrelationships between and among hypnotizability, creativity, absorption, vividness of imagery, and effortless experiencing. Rothenberg's (1976) Imagery and Fantasy tasks and Guilford's (1959) Consequences Test were assessed for degree of associated effortlessness, vividness, and absorption. Marks's (1973) Scale of Vividness of Visual Imagery was used to measure the level of vividness, and an absorption questionnaire was employed to determine the level of absorption versus distraction in the tasks. In order to evaluate creativity, subjects rated their own level of creativity compared to that of their peers; they listed recent creative activities, which were rated by judges for level of creativity; and they completed Guilford's (1959) Consequences Test as noted above, with half of the items administered with standard instructions and half of the items administered with additional instructions to allow consequences to occur effortlessly.

Subjects were selected on the basis of their performance on the HGSHS:A and separated into two groups: high (predominantly in the 10–12 suggestions passed range) and low (predominantly in the 1–3 suggestions passed range) hypnotizability, with equal numbers of males and females in each group. Composite scores were computed for vividness, effortlessness, and creativity by adding the mean z scores for each particular measure. For absorption, only the questionnaire was used.

As P. G. Bowers predicted, effortless experiencing, creativity, and high hypnotizability were interrelated. For example, the effortless-experiencing composite was related to high hypnotic ability ($r = .61$) and to the creativity composite ($r = .62$). Hypnotizability and creativity were related as well ($r = .55$). These results were replicated in a follow-up study (P. G. Bowers, 1979, Study 2) using small-group testing procedures. The magnitude of correlation among composite indices of effortless experiencing, creativity, and hypnotizability remained stable at about .50.

In a third study (P. G. Bowers, 1979, Study 3), effortless experiencing was again related to creativity ($r = .29$, $p < .05$). However, vividness of imagery during various tasks was related to hypnotizability ($r = .45$) only for subjects above the mean on the effortless-experiencing composite. Furthermore, gestalt closure performance, hypothesized to be related to right-hemisphere preference or functioning, was associated with both hypnotizability and absorption. In the final study in this series, P. G. Bowers (1982–1983) computed correlations between the effortless experiencing composite, hypnotizability (SHSS:C), and creativity (Consequences Test). The composite correlated with the SHSS:C ($r = .48$) and with the fluency ($r = .56$) section of the Consequences Test.

Combined, these findings lend support to the hypothesis that effortless experiencing of imagery, fantasy, and original ideas are related to both creativity and high hypnotizability. The data lend force to P. G. Bowers's (1979) contention that the "missing link" between hypnosis and creativity is that both phenomena rely on nonvolitional fantasy processes cued by a task. In addition to effortless experiencing, P. G. Bowers and Bowers (1979) have maintained that another element bonding creativity and hypnosis is a preference for cognitive complexity.

Ashton and McDonald (1985) conducted a well-controlled study that extended earlier research in a number of important ways. They examined the differential effects of hypnotic versus nonhypnotic conditions by carefully selecting female subjects high (9–12 range, HGSHS:A and SHSS:C) and low (0–4 range, HGSHS:A; predominantly 0–4 range, SHSS:C) in hypnotizability, and assigning them to hypnotic, simulation, and waking control (listening to relaxing music) conditions. To test Gur and Reyher's (1976) hypothesis that hypnosis enhances figural rather than verbal creativity, subjects received the Torrance Tests of Creative Thinking, Form B (Torrance, 1974), which tap creative functioning in both the visual-perceptive and the verbal-associative domains, along with the Sounds and Images Test (SIT; Cunnington & Torrance, 1965), which assesses the originality of imaginative, associative responses to auditory stimuli. The authors also employed a rating scale for effortlessness and an absorption questionnaire in order to attempt to replicate P. G Bowers's (1978) earlier findings. Composite scores were computed for each measure by computing the average z scores across verbal, figural, and overall (verbal, figural, and SIT) creativity. Hypnotizable subjects outperformed unhypnotizable subjects on the Torrance measures of Verbal Flexibility and Figural Elaboration, the SIT, effortlessness, and absorption. Moreover, the overall creativity composite yielded a significant effect for hypnotizability.

However, only one measure—Figural Creativity—discriminated hypnotic and nonhypnotic control groups. Although hypnotized subjects scored higher than simulating subjects, hypnotized and waking control subjects responded comparably. Thus, as in previous studies (K. S. Bowers, 1968; K. S. Bowers & van der Meulen, 1970), reliable differences between hypnotic and nonhypnotic groups were not secured. These results are not compatible with those of Gur and Reyher (1976), who found enhanced hypnotic performance on the Figural Creativity measure in hypnotizable males, relative to both simulating and waking control subjects. Ashton and McDonald (1985) commented that these differences between studies might be attributable to the fact that Gur and Reyher made significant modifications in the standard instructions administered to subjects, and examined the performance of males with respect to the entire test battery.

L. M. Jackson and Gorassini (1989) wondered whether the conditions of testing in P. G. Bowers's (1978, 1979, 1982–1983) research might have inflated the relation between creativity and hypnotizability secured in her studies. Ashton and McDonald (1985) failed to replicate P. G. Bowers's (1978) robust findings concerning the substantial relationship between effortless experiencing and creativity. The correlation between creativity and effortless experiencing was only .13 (n.s.) when performance-based measures of creativity were used. Bowers, in contrast, relied on self-estimates of creativity that were entered into her composite creativity measure.

L. M. Jackson and Gorassini (1989) suggested that global self-assessments of creativity may be influenced as follows: Subjects who are initially selected for high or low hypnotizability may come to believe that hypnotizability and creativity are positively related, and may base their self-assessments of creativity on their pretested hypnotizability level. Subjects who test as high hypnotizable presumably recognize the connection between their performance and the creativity tests during hypnosis, thus inflating the relation between hypnotizability and subjective indices of creativity, relative to performance-based measures. Waking subjects should have no reason to connect the earlier hypnotizability testing with creativity performance, because efforts will have been made to disguise the purpose of the creativity testing and to sever its link with the initial hypnotizability testing session. Jackson and Gorassini's hypothesis assumes that subjects are, for the most part, uncertain about how creative they actually are, and rely on situational cues and information to infer their level of creativity via a social comparison process (Festinger, 1954; Suls & Miller, 1977).

Consistent with L. M. Jackson and Gorassini's (1989) prediction, when their high and low hypnotizable subjects received explicit feedback (i.e., score, descriptive label, and percentile equivalents) about their hypnotizability level prior to completing creativity tests during hypnosis, a relationship between hypnotizability and self-estimated creativity emerged. No such relationship emerged when subjects were tested in a nonhypnotic waking condition. In fact, in the waking condition, the lows rated their creativity as higher than the highs did. Furthermore, differences did not emerge as a function of hypnotizability when a performance-based measure of creativity—the Torrance Tests of Creative Thinking, Form B (Torrance, 1974)—was used as the criterion index. On the basis of these findings, Jackson and Gorassini conclude that "a global self-report measure of creativity can lead to an apparent but invalid suggestibility–creativity relationship" (1989, p. 342)

Consistent with Gur and Reyher's (1976) research, Figural Creativity, but not Verbal Creativity, was enhanced in the hypnotic versus the nonhypnotic group. However, L. M. Jackson and Gorassini (1989) maintain that if a state of hypnosis (i.e., characterized by regressive or primary-process thinking) is responsible for creativity enhancement, as Gur and Reyher intimated, the effect should be limited to high hypnotizable subjects who are capable of attaining this state. Because Jackson and Gorassini's high and low hypnotizable subjects showed improved figural performance during hypnosis, they contend that the improvement was a result of some correlate of the induction process, such as relaxation, and not of hypnosis per se.

Summary and Integration

The results of the studies we have reviewed are difficult to compare because of the inconsistent measurement and often ambiguous definition of creativity adopted by various researchers (see Ashton & McDonald, 1985). Nevertheless, it is possible to conclude that hypnotized and nonhypnotized subjects cannot be reliably differentiated from one another on measures of creativity. Whereas several studies (Gur & Reyher, 1976; L. M. Jackson & Gorassini, 1989) have shown that hypnotized subjects score higher on creativity measures than subjects in nonhypnotic conditions, the majority of studies (Ashton & McDonald, 1985; P. G. Bowers, 1967; K. S. Bowers, 1968; K. S. Bowers & van der Meulen, 1970) have failed to show that hypnotized subjects' creativity performance is generally superior to nonhypnotic subjects' performance.

L. M. Jackson and Gorassini's study did not unambiguously support the superiority of hypnosis, inasmuch as hypnotized low hypnotizable subjects, who would not be expected to be responsive to hypnosis per se, were also more creative than nonhypnotized low hypnotizable subjects. And, as noted above, differences between hypnotic and simulating conditions in Gur and Reyher's study might be attributable to the fact that simulators did not receive simulating instructions along the lines recommended by Orne (1959, 1979a).

The available evidence does, however, suggest that high hypnotizable subjects tend to score higher than low hypnotizable subjects on a number of measures of creativity (e.g., Ashton & McDonald, 1985; P. G. Bowers, 1967, 1979; P. G. Bowers & Bowers, 1979; K. S. Bowers & van der Meulen, 1970; Perry et al., 1973). The corpus of data thus supports the view that elements of the domain of hypnotizability and creativity intersect—a conclusion that is consistent with our view of the hypnotizable subject as a creative problem-solving agent.

This positive evidence is tempered by the fact that high hypnotizable subjects do not necessarily outperform medium hypnotizable subjects (K. S. Bowers, 1971; Perry et al., 1973), and one study showed that lows were more creative than highs tested in a waking condition (L. M. Jackson & Gorassini, 1989). It is important to clarify the role that medium subjects play in accounting for the hypnosis–creativity relationship (Perry et al., 1973). Indeed, it may be the case that low subjects are distinctly less creative than their medium and high counterparts, rather than that highs are particularly creative.

The superior performance of high versus low subjects is theoretically attributable to their nonhypnotic imaginative and fantasy involvements, their ability to suspend critical judgment, and their effortless experiencing ability (see Ashton & McDonald, 1985). However, even when research has documented an association between hypnotizability and creativity, it has not been of impressive magnitude. Gur and Reyher (1976) have noted that the data suggesting a link between hypnotizability and creativity constitute support for the joint application of the concept of adaptive regression to hypnosis and creativity only "in the very weak sense," insofar as the correlations between measures of creativity and hypnotizability are "rather small" (p. 238). P. G. Bowers (1979) also has observed that the relationship between hypnotizability and creativity is "moderate, rather than strong" (p. 564).

In addition, this relationship is not stable across male and female subjects. Several studies have shown that hypnosis and creativity are related in female but not male samples (K. S. Bowers, 1971; K. S. Bowers & van der Meulen, 1970; Perry et al., 1973). However, at least one study (P. G. Bowers, 1978) has failed to find evidence for sex as a moderator variable. As noted earlier, K. S. Bowers (1971) made the interesting proposal that these sex differences have their roots in a sex-specific organization of imagination. In the absence of confirming data, with independent measures supporting the idea that women's imaginations are more "excitable" by way of external stimulation than men's, this hypothesis ought to be regarded as highly tentative. An equally plausible explanation of sex differences is that males respond in line with sex-role stereotypes, such that the correlation between hypnotizability and creativity in males is attenuated by a reluctance to report unconventional responses (see Lynn & Rhue, 1988).

Comparison between and among hypnosis studies is complicated by the fact that creativity measures have been so diverse (e.g., word associations, self-ratings, inkblot responses, standardized tests) that caution must be exercised in making inferences about the effects of hypnosis on creative functioning (Ashton & McDonald, 1985). Even performance on the Torrance tests, which have been used in a number of studies, is inconsistent: Some research has shown enhanced performance among hypnotized subjects (relative to waking subjects) on the Figural Creativity test (e.g., Gur and Reyher, 1976); other research has shown no such hypnotic enhancement (Ashton & McDonald, 1985); and one study (L. M. Jackson & Gorassini, 1989) has shown increments on the part of both high and low hypnotizable subjects in a hypnotic versus a waking condition. Also clouding the picture is the fact that the test instructions that have been used in hypnosis–creativity research have sometimes departed in radical ways from standard instructions (e.g., Gur & Reyher, 1976).

L. M. Jackson and Gorassini's study (1989) raises the possibility that disparate findings across studies may eventuate not so much from differences in stable attributes of the subjects as from differences in the circumstances of testing across investigations. According to P. G. Bowers (1979), the highest relations between measures of creativity and hypnotizability have come from studies in which composite scores of creativity, combining scores from diverse measures of that concept, have been utilized (K. S. Bowers, 1971; P. G. Bowers, 1978; K. S. Bowers & van der

Meulen, 1970). However, Jackson and Gorassini's (1989) research provides grounds for questioning the validity of studies that combine self-estimates of creativity with performance-based measures in a single index, in research designs that permit subjects to gauge their level of creativity on self-observations of their hypnotizability level. To minimize the effects of context-based expectancies and social comparison influences, it is necessary to separate self- and performance-based creativity measures, and to separate the hypnotizability-testing and creativity-testing phases of the experiment as well.

Comparisons across studies are also rendered problematic because different measures of hypnotizability are used, with different criteria for hypnotizability levels adopted. For instance, P. G. Bowers (1967, 1978), and K. S. Bowers and van der Meulen (1970) required that their subjects considered "moderate" or "high" hypnotizable pass 7–8 and 10–12 HGSHS:A suggestions, respectively. Perry et al. (1973) required that their "high" hypnotizable subjects pass 9–11 SHSS:C suggestions, and Ashton and McDonald (1985) used the most stringent criteria for high hypnotizability, requiring that subjects pass at least 9 HGSHS:A and 9 SHSS:C items. L. M. Jackson and Gorassini (1989) did not specify how many suggestions their "high" and "low" subjects passed, and they used an index of hypnotizability (the Carleton University Responsiveness to Suggestion Scale; Spanos, Radtke, Hodgins, Stam, & Bertrand, 1983) that differed from the hypnotizability scales used in previous creativity research.

If P. G. Bowers is correct that cognitively challenging hypnotizability items produce higher correlations between hypnotizability and creativity, then high hypnotizability may more reliably predict creativity when more stringent hypnotizability-screening procedures are used, along with scales (e.g., SHSS:C) that contain more "cognitive items." To date, this hypothesis has not been adequately tested and awaits more definitive evaluation.

P. G. Bowers and K. S. Bowers hypothesis that high hypnotizable subjects and subjects rated high in creativity are united in their tendency to process certain tasks in a relatively effortless manner suggests that some underlying dynamic or personality characteristic is responsible for these similarities. Hints as to what may be responsible for such effortless responding come from M. Dixon, Brunet, and Laurence's (1990) study of the intriguing hypothesis that high and low hypnotizable subjects process language differently. That is, highs may process information in an effortless, fast, and involuntary manner—in other words, with "automaticity" (Posner & Snyder, 1975; Shiffrin & Schneider, 1977). In contrast, lows' processing of information may require voluntary initiation, may be slower, and may draw on limited cognitive resources (i.e., "strategic processing").

To test this hypothesis, M. Dixon et al. (1990) examined the information processing of high, medium, and low hypnotizable subjects by means of Cheesman and Merikle's (1986) paradigm, which varied cue visibility and probability and assessed automatic and strategic effects on Stroop performance. Compared with the low and medium subjects, high subjects showed significantly greater Stroop effects for both visible and degraded word trials. Strategic differences did not emerge for the three hypnotizability groups. These findings support the contention that highs have particularly strong verbal connection strengths. The authors note that this may account for the propensity of highly hypnotizable subjects to label their responses as "involuntary." More germane to our discussion of imagination, if language processing is more immediate, high hypnotizable subjects may be able to devote more cognitive resources to making creative problem-solving attempts or to visualizing and becoming involved in suggestions.

High hypnotizable subjects' superior ability to process information has also been documented by Saccuzzo, Safran, Anderson, and McNeill (1982). The researchers compared high and low hypnotizable subjects with respect to their ability to identify a briefly exposed informational target stimulus, consisting of a letter when it was preceded (forward masking) or followed (backward masking) by a noninformational mask stimulus. The superiority of the high subjects was apparent but small and subtle in magnitude. The authors tender a number of explanatory possibilities: (1) High subjects may be faster or more efficient in processing input information; (2) they may not evaluate input as carefully at early stages of processing, so that incoming information reaches the cortex more quickly; and (3) they may make better use of the two hemispheres and may be able to transfer information between the two hemispheres more readily than low subjects.

Because the differences in these studies are small, it will be important to learn whether they are of clinical or practical significance. Furthermore, even if high hypnotizable people and more creative people experience experimental tasks as more effortless, P. G. Bowers (1979) cautions that there is no basis for assuming that effortless experiencing affects creative behavior. An alternative possibility is that people who perform tasks successfully experience themselves as completing them effortlessly because they do them well. The direction of cause and effect in this research area will need to be sorted out by future researchers.

P. G. Bowers (1979) makes the further suggestion that the characteristics of a particular problem probably affect the associational processes that lead to a creative solution. The experience of effortlessness may be a function of the degree to which an individual will allow the demands of the task to direct associational processes. Whereas some individuals may interpret the demands of the task as requiring passive associations, which call for less effort, other individuals may perceive the requirements of the task as requiring decision making, which entails substantial effort. In a pilot study (P. G. Bowers, 1979, Pilot Study 2) that involved "promising authors" (part of a prestigious seminar of creative writers), each author was asked to write a story while hypnotized. Whereas some authors were perturbed by the relaxed state of mind because it interfered with their critical thinking and language control, other authors enjoyed the free flow of ideas and welcomed the experience.

Conclusion

The literature on hypnosis and creativity lends support to our view of the hypnotizable subject as a creative problem-solving agent. Hypnosis does not appear to bolster creativity, relative to nonhypnotic conditions. However, the majority of studies that have addressed the issue have documented a relation between hypnotizability and creativity, albeit a more consistent relation for females than for males. Even though the correlations between measures of creativity and hypnotizability are generally small to moderate, they are consistent with the magnitude of correlations secured in research examining the links between and among measures of hypnosis, imagination, fantasy, and daydreaming. The creativity literature we have examined raises fascinating questions about the way information is processed during hypnosis; about how the *quality* of hypnotic experience is related to diverse abilities and personality attributes, including creativity; and about the relationship between contextual factors and performance on hypnosis and creativity tasks.

The disparate literatures we have reviewed indicate that no single factor or variable is a necessary or sufficient determinant of hypnotic conduct and experience. For example, although hypnotizability is related to creativity, hypnotizability is far more than what conventional creativity tests measure. The failure of creativity scores to account for a great deal of variance in hypnotic responding in no way diminishes the appeal of an explanation that emphasizes the problem-solving nature of successful hypnotic performance. This is so because the successful "construction and resolution" of hypnotic experience (see McConkey, 1991) depend on a problem-solving process that is in certain respects unique to the hypnotic context.

As we have seen, neither trait measures of imagination, absorption, or fantasy proneness account for enough variance in hypnotic responding to provide a singular or sufficient explanation of subjects' diverse responses to hypnotic suggestions. Instead, we believe it is important to consider multiple, interactive determinants of hypnotic responding that vary in complex ways from subject to subject to produce a truly individualistic experience of hypnosis. Multivariate research that includes measures of the determinants we have considered in this chapter (e.g., creativity, expectancies, attitudes, imaginative and fantasy abilities), in the context of single studies and across diverse studies, will be necessary to parcel out the variance attributable to single determinants in isolation and in interaction with one another (see Nadon, Laurence, & Perry, 1991).

What emerges from our attempt to integrate diverse bodies of literature is the sense that variability is inherent in subjects' cognitive and behavioral responses to the hypnotic situation. This conceptualization is analogous to P. G. Bowers's view that there are multiple approaches to a problem gestalt. As we have argued, subjects differ in their prehypnotic attitudes and sets toward hypnosis, their imaginings and fantasy activity during hypnosis, their standards for evaluating their experiences and behaviors, and their tacit interpretations of interpersonal and task demands. Hypnotizable subjects are able to generate subjectively compelling (or at least "good enough") experiences of suggestions, while they successfully discern appropriate task demands and behave accordingly. In fact, each suggestion poses a slightly different problem for the subjects to resolve in a satisfactory manner. How the problem of responding to suggestions is resolved will depend on the unique blend of abilities, expectations, self-perceptions, interpretations, and performance standards that are expressed and applied by each subject in the hypnotic situation.

One interesting feature of the creative problem-solving process is that many aspects of the subjects' responses to hypnosis generally (but certainly not always) occur outside the sphere of conscious awareness. So the problem-solving quality of approaching and responding to the hypnotic situation need not be apparent to the subjects. Fantasy, for example, is not necessarily controlled by conscious, analytic processes, but instead is responsive to the problem gestalt (P. G. Bowers, 1982–1983).

This quality of not knowing exactly how problems are solved or creative solutions are reached bridges hypnotic and nonhypnotic situations (e.g., P. G. Bowers, 1982–1983). Although creative solutions are often reached after extensive and deliberate problem-solving attempts, they may also occur with little conscious awareness of the process of creation or via a flash of insight, seemingly *ex nihilo*. Even when a solution to a problem is reached, the steps or cognitive operations involved are often not accessible to conscious awareness or introspection. Lynn, Rhue, and Weekes (1990) have observed, "Just as some people who solve a mathematical puzzle may be unaware of all the cognitive operations involved in solving the puzzle, some hypnotized subjects may be unaware of the strategies involved in responding to suggestions" (p. 172). There is a growing recognition in the field of hypnosis (see Lynn & Rhue, 1991), and among social and cognitive psychologists more generally (see Lewicki, 1986; Pervin, 1990), that cognitive processes, contextual demands, and even intentions that guide or propel behavior do not necessarily reach the threshold of awareness.

The determinants of this lack of awareness are certainly worthy of as much attention as any other feature of hypnosis we have discussed. Yet what is required to capture the complexity of creative problem solving is an approach (see Lynn & Rhue, 1991; Nadon, Laurence, & Perry, 1991) that identifies the multifarious ways in which intrapersonal, interpersonal, and situational determinants of hypnotic behavior interact to produce the unique mix of personal experiences that we call "hypnosis."

CHAPTER TWELVE

Hypnosis and Creativity

VICTOR A. SHAMES
PATRICIA G. BOWERS

When I got to the top of the staircase, there was this tall man with dark hair and dark eyes waiting for me. He gave me a hug and asked me if I wanted to fly.

I said, "Yes, I've always wanted to fly."

He said, "Follow me." We walked to this grassy little hill. It was cold; the wind was blowing. It was a good cold. He jumped into the air and said, "Follow me." So I jumped, too. I just was flying. I was behind him and he was leading the way.

We're flying 500 feet above the ground. We went over a tall, green oak tree and then over this old village with high church steeples and various pointed roofs. We flew through the village and swooped down between houses. We were about 20 feet above ground, flying over a cobblestone street. And then we went higher, over the roofs. . . .

The young woman who described this bird-like flight over trees and rooftops had simply been told by the experimenter to imagine herself climbing a staircase and encountering someone at the top. In general, a hypnotic subject may respond to just a few words of suggestion by becoming immersed in a fantasy world of his or her own creation—as a visitor to extraordinary places or a time traveler, assuming a different identity, engaged in daring adventures. The subject is an active participant in the hypnotic experience who takes advantage of the opportunity to elaborate creatively on the suggestions that are offered.

In the present chapter, we examine the nature of the relationship between hypnosis and creativity. The chapter is organized according to a classification scheme that is widely used in the creativity literature. Our motivation for adopting such a scheme is that the study of creativity in relation to hypnosis has often tended to overlook the fundamental principles that serve to direct creativity research in other domains. By failing to consider these principles, hypnosis researchers have been less than systematic in selecting definitions of creativity, operationalizing constructs, and finding appropriate measures. The structural framework described in the following section provides a format for identifying deficiencies in the literature and for developing a more systematic research program in this area.

The Structure of Creativity Research

The term "creativity" has a growing list of definitions (C. W. Taylor, 1988). Defining creativity has proven to be a challenge because the term is so broad in its usage. It encompasses a wide range of referents, including thoughts, experiences, individuals, behaviors, situations, and products. Rhodes (1961) introduced a classification scheme that has served as an important frame of reference in the study of creative phenomena. The four categories that he described are: "product," "process," "person," and "press."

A product is identified as creative on the basis of two fundamental attributes: "originality" and "appropriateness" (Amabile, 1987). Originality can be interpreted in a number of ways. Thurstone (1952) argued that the product must be novel from the standpoint of the individual who created it, even though society may not regard it as such. According to Perkins (1981), a product must be statistically unusual in order to be considered original. This is consistent with Torrance's (1990) approach, in which the originality of a response is determined by its frequency of occurrence in a normative sample.

Although originality may be considered a necessary criterion for creativity, it is not sufficient. Stein (1953) has claimed that the creativity of a product must be defined relative to the time and place in which it appears. He suggests that for a product to be considered creative, it must be "judged to posses merit by some knowledgeable group of people at some point in time" (Stein, 1974). A number of current definitions of creativity have incorporated Stein's notion that a product must be adaptive to the specific situation in which it was created. Creativity researchers have used terms such as "usefulness," "value," "merit," "quality," and "appropriateness" to describe this criterion for creativity.

A process, unlike a product, can be considered creative without producing anything of social value. One can have the experience of being creative without generating a product that would satisfy any established criteria for creativity. The subjective experience of creativity must therefore be considered separately from the objective creativity of the product. Thurstone (1952) stressed this distinction in his claim that an act is creative if the individual arrives at a solution in a way that would yield a sense of having produced something novel.

Creative individuals are distinguished from the normal population by three criteria: achievement, ability, and disposition or attitude (Barron & Harrington, 1981). Psychological theorists have attributed various patterns of personality traits to creative individuals (Isaksen, 1987), and empirical work has produced a number of creative personality scales (Barron & Harrington, 1981).

A particular situation can be either conducive to or inhibitory of creativity. The term, "press" refers to the interaction between a situation and an individual. Amabile (1984) has described the characteristics of a situation that contribute to the individual's creative experience. For the individual, situational variables can make the difference between an extrinsic motivational orientation, which is detrimental to creativity, and an intrinsic orientation, in which the satisfaction associated with task performance is the critical motivation (Amabile, 1987).

The phenomena of creativity can be approached from each of the four levels described above—namely, product, process, person, and press. This is just as true for the study of creativity in the context of hypnosis as it is for any other context. If hypnosis and creativity are related constructs, as we have already postulated, then the relationship must be detectable on at least one and perhaps all four of the levels specified above. Such a relationship would manifest itself in one of the following ways:

1. Subjects who are highly responsive to hypnosis would share certain personality traits with highly creative people, and there would be a significant correlation between hypnotizability and personality measures of creativity.
2. There would be observable similarities in the subjective experience described by hypnotized subjects and by individuals engaged in the creative process.
3. Hypnotized subjects would generate a more creative product in response to a specific task than would nonhypnotized subjects.
4. Specific situational variables that characterize hypnotic settings would be shown to facilitate creativity.

At each of these four levels, detection of a relationship between creativity and hypnosis requires that appropriate measures of creativity be used (we already possess appropriate measures of hypnosis, in the form of the standardized hypnotic susceptibility scales). Therefore, in this chapter we focus on specific measurement issues related to each particular level of analysis: How does one evaluate the creativity of a product or a person? How does one operationalize the components of the creative process? How does one measure the degree to which an environment demands, or affords, creative expression? Most of the creativity measures that are currently available operate on one of the following two levels: personality and product. From a methodological standpoint, there are inherent difficulties in both the use of creative personality measures to assess creative production, and the use of tests that rely on production to assess personality traits. Later in this chapter, we examine the problems that arise when investigators confound these two types of measures.

Linking Hypnosis and Creativity

The notion that creativity is related to hypnosis has both an observed and a theoretical foundation. In the clinical and experimental setting, hypnotic phenomena that have creative qualities can be observed. A more theoretical link is provided by psychoanalytic theory. The contribution of each of these two influences is considered in this section.

Creative Phenomena in the Experimental and Clinical Setting

Those of us who work with hypnosis on a daily basis have the opportunity to observe a wide range of phenomena that can be considered creative. In administering the Stanford Hypnotic Susceptibility Scale, Form C (SHSS:C; Weitzenhoffer & Hilgard, 1962), researchers frequently receive responses to the age regression, dream, and auditory hallucination items that indicate that the subjects have elaborated on the suggestions in a creative manner.

For instance, one subject in Kihlstrom's laboratory at the University of Arizona gave the following description of the experience she had when she was asked to dream about hypnosis: "I saw a hill which turned into a spiral. The spiral was going into someone's head who was lying down. Then the person started spinning around and the room spun faster and faster until it all disappeared." The subject's response satisfies both types of criteria for a creative product: Not merely is the imagery original, but it is also appropriate to the task that the subject was given.

The clinical hypnosis literature is filled with pertinent examples of creative responses by hypnotized patients. For instance, Levitan (1985) provides a case study of a terminal cancer patient who, in order to address her fear of death and her concern about abandoning her family, was given the chance to rehearse her death during a hypnosis session. She successfully enacted her own death experience and was able to observe the progress of her family after her death. Both of the criteria for a creativity product are satisfied by this patient's response to the researcher's suggestion. Her account of events that had not yet occurred was clearly original; it was also appropriate, in that it facilitated the patient's acceptance of a difficult situation.

Reported cases involving the creation of pseudomemories in the context of a hypnosis session are also pertinent to this discussion. In the case of the "February man" (Erickson & Rossi, 1980), Milton Erickson introduced a fictitious entity into a patient's childhood memories. S. R. Baker and Boas (1983) successfully treated a dental phobia by suggesting to the patient during a hypnotic age regression that a prior unpleasant dental experience had actually been pleasant. This partial reconstruction of the original memory was effective, in that the patient was able to undergo major oral surgery some months later without fear. In both of these cases, the subject's compliance with a creative hypnotic suggestion cannot be considered creative in itself. However, any elaboration that the subject may provide in reconstructing the memory must be viewed as creative, because the subject who is able to embellish the memory with his or her own details has gone beyond the parameters of the suggestion in an original and appropriate manner.

Two other types of phenomena are pertinent to this discussion: hypermnesia and past-life regression. Both classes of phenomena are known to involve some degree of confabulation (Perry, Laurence, D'Eon, & Tallant, 1988). Studies of hypermnesia have consistently found that increases in valid memory obtained through hypnosis are often accompanied by corresponding increases in inaccurate recollection or pseudomemory (Kihlstrom, 1985a). Similarly, reincarnation reports of hypnotized subjects frequently contain anachronisms and other signs of confabulation.

From the standpoint of creativity research, these phenomena raise some interesting questions about what should be considered creative. A memory that is confabulated satisfies one criterion of creativity: it is original material. Even if a subject is merely recalling information from a different context, the transfer of information to a novel context is an original response. But is there any reason to believe that hypnotized subjects, in response to certain tasks, really do generate more of this original material than do waking subjects? Dywan and Bowers (1983) found that hypnotized subjects showed a substantial increase in both accurate and false recall for pictorial material, with the ratio of false to accurate memory being roughly 2:1. Thus, it would seem that hypnotized subjects are able to produce a greater volume of original output than are waking subjects.

Although such output may be original, it is not necessarily creative as long as the criterion of appropriateness fails to be satisfied. The following question must then be answered: Is confabulation an appropriate response to a given task? One view is that confabulated recall in an experiment such as the one conducted by Dywan and Bowers (1983) cannot be considered appropriate, because the experiment called for subjects to provide accurate memory, and subjects who gave confabulated responses failed to do what was asked of them. From this perspective, confabulation can be viewed as an erroneous rather than a creative response.

An alternative viewpoint, however, is that a confabulated response may be viewed as appropriate if it is adaptive to the needs of the subject, independent of the objectives of the experiment. For example, reports of past-life regression in clinical settings indicate that the experiences accessed by patients are usually relevant to the problems that they originally presented. Since there is no evidence that the responses produced by a patient in this context are historically valid, a viable alternative interpretation of past-life regression data is that such a patient is generating original material that provides insight into the nature of his or her problem. This material somehow satisfies the needs of the patient and should therefore be considered appropriate from the patient's perspective.

Psychoanalytic Theory

In his topographic model of the mind, Freud (1900/1953) specified three mental systems, which he called Cs, Pcs, and Ucs. The Cs system, or conscious mind, contains thoughts, feelings, and impulses of which one is presently aware. Although the contents of the Pcs are currently outside of awareness, one can bring them into awareness by turning attention to them. On the other hand, one cannot bring the contents of the Ucs into awareness by fiat or by merely turning attention to them (E. Fromm, personal communication, October 1991).

Within this model, Freud introduced the term "regression" to describe an organism's shift from secondary-process thinking, which is logical and reality-bound, to primary-process thinking, a prelogical, drive-dominated process that can best be seen in dreams and slips of the tongue. Freud maintained that uncontrolled intrusions of primary process into ordinary waking life lead to poor adjustment and to pathology. In contrast to this uncontrolled type of regression, Kris (1934/1952) proposed the notion of "regression in the service of the ego," a type of regression that the ego initiates and terminates for its own benefit rather than for defensive purposes. Creativity, for instance, is termed an "adaptive regression" because it represents a healthy, constructive letting go, accompanied by an increase in primary-process thinking.

Hypnosis first became linked to adaptive regression in a theory proposed by Gill and Brenman (1959). In this theory, the subject's overall ego relinquishes control of its apparatuses to the hypnotist during a hypnotic induction, and a regressive restructuring takes place. The details of this process are described by Gruenewald, Fromm, and Oberlander (1979) as follows:

> Instead of regression occurring in the overall ego, as in regression proper, a subsystem of the ego is triggered into action. . . . In the established hypnotic state, the subsystem becomes reorganized into a temporarily stable structure

that not only regains partial control of the (re-automatized) apparatuses but also is put into the service of the overall ego. . . . The overall ego never loses contact with reality. (p. 625)

Adaptive regression provides a theoretical link between creativity and hypnosis, but it also draws an important distinction between the two processes. Although the regressive aspect is similar in both, only creativity implies any constructive use of the regressive experience. In the hypnotic state, there is increased primary process, but control of it as shown in adaptive-regression scores may not increase (Gruenewald et al., 1979).

Summary

We have so far established that the study of creativity in relation to hypnosis has a basis in both theory and observation. We have also provided an organizational scheme to facilitate our investigation of this relationship. Having laid this groundwork, we can now focus our discussion on the details of how creativity and hypnosis might be related at each of the four levels we have previously described. This discussion encompasses existing theoretical perspectives, empirical findings, and issues that remain to be addressed.

Relationship at the Level of Personality

Creativity is considered a stable personality trait; the same can be said about hypnotizability. A relationship between these traits should manifest itself in two ways: (1) Creative individuals should share specific characteristics with hypnotizable subjects; and (2) personality measures of creativity and hypnotizability should be significantly correlated.

Personality Characteristics

Investigators have studied the characteristics associated with creativity in a wide range of fields, including art, literature, music, and science (Barron & Harrington, 1981). An important consequence of this work is the emergence of a stable set of personality traits that demonstrate consistently high correlations with indicators of creative activity and achievement in various domains. A number of these traits appear on the various creative personality scales that are used in conjunction with Gough and Heilbrun's (1965) Adjective Check List (see Domino, 1970; Gough, 1979; J. M. Smith & Schaefer, 1969; Yarnell, 1971). The following is a selection of adjectives included in the Domino (1970) scale: "absent-minded," "adaptable," "capable," "curious," "disorderly," "egotistical," "enthusiastic," "impulsive," "independent," "outspoken," "rebellious," "sarcastic," "sensitive," "tactless," and "unconventional." The traits identified in the creativity scales for the Adjective Check List are assumed to be core characteristics shared by creative individuals across domains. However, some traits demonstrate field, age, or sex specificity in terms of their degree of correlation with indicators of creative achievement and activity (Barron & Harrington, 1981).

With respect to hypnotizability, findings of stable individual differences have led to the unsuccessful pursuit of personality traits that might be related to this capacity (for a review, see Kihlstrom, 1985a). Hypnotizability has not been found to correlate with the sorts of traits measured by common multidimensional personality inventories such as the Minnesota Multiphasic Personality Inventory and California Personality Inventory. However, investigators have found three interrelated constructs that do correlate significantly with hypnotizability: "absorption," "imaginative involvement," and "fantasy proneness."

Absorption

Shor (1959, 1970) indicated that the experience of hypnosis is characterized by an absence of the subject's usual awareness of the environment and his or her place in it. He referred to this phenomenon as the loss of a "generalized reality orientation" (GRO), which he described as follows:

> In all our waking life we carry around in the background of our awareness a kind of frame of reference or orientation to generalized reality which serves as a context or arena within which we interpret all of our ongoing conscious experiences. Under certain conditions—of which hypnosis is just one—this wide frame of reference or orientation to generalized reality can fade into the very distant background of our minds so that ongoing experiences are isolated from their usual context. When that happens the distinction between imagination and reality no longer exists for us. (Shor, 1970, p. 91)

As this passage suggests, loss of the GRO is by no means confined to hypnosis. Most people report occasional loss of awareness of their environmental frame of reference. For example, Shor described what he called the "book-reading fantasy" to illustrate how a loss of the GRO can be a rather ordinary event for some people:

> When these people read a story, particularly an adventureful novel, they are able to enter the story in imagination so completely that it seems equivalent to living the experience itself. During the time of this fantasy the reader is completely oblivious to the true reality about him. The fantasy world is an encapsulated unit, and it seems totally real. There is nothing else beyond it. (Shor, 1970, p. 92)

Loss of the GRO can occur as a result of simply staring at an object. In a study conducted by Deikman (1963), subjects who were asked to stare at a blue vase for a brief period (usually 15 minutes) reported various types of perceptual distortion. For some of the subjects, the vase become "more vivid" and luminous. The shape of the vase appeared unstable; there were reports of a loss of the third dimension and of a diffusion or loss of the vase's boundaries. One subject said that the outlines of the vase "seem[ed] almost literally to dissolve entirely . . . it [seemed] to be a kind of fluid blue" (Deikman, 1963, p. 208). Another subject made the following observation:

> At one point it felt . . . as though the vase were in my head rather than out there; I knew it was out there but it seemed as though it were almost a part of me. I think that I almost felt at that moment as though, you know, the image is really in me, it's not out there. (Deikman, 1963, p. 206)

This description of a subject–object merging is consistent with the construct of "absorption," which Tellegen and Atkinson (1974) defined as the subject's "full commitment of available perceptual, motoric, imaginative, and ideational resources to a unified representation of the attentional object" (p. 274). In a sophisticated psychometric study, these investigators found that responses to a scale they developed—the Tellegen Absorption Scale (TAS)—loaded on an absorption factor that was related to hypnotizability, but did not load on the two major factors common to personality inventories, which have been labeled "extraversion" and "introversion" (Eysenck, 1947), or "ego control" and "ego resiliency" (Block, 1965). Fromm and Kahn (1990) have shown that absorption is one of the structural factors comprising the essence of self-hypnosis as well (see also Kahn & Fromm, Chapter 14, this volume). Examples of TAS items are "I can sometimes recollect certain past experiences in my life with such clarity and vividness that it is like living them again, or almost so," "I am sometimes able to forget about my present self and get absorbed in a fantasy that I am someone else."

The validity of the absorption construct has been demonstrated in repeated findings of its relation to standardized scales of hypnotic responsiveness (for reviews, see Kihlstrom, Register, Hoyt, Albright, Grigorian, Heindel, & Morrison, 1989; Nadon, Laurence, & Perry, 1987; Roche & McConkey, 1990). Correlations of the TAS with the Harvard Group Scale of Hypnotic Susceptibility, Form A (HGSHS:A; Shor & Orne, 1962) are in the .22 range, whereas slightly higher correlations have been obtained with the SHSS:C (Weitzenhoffer & Hilgard, 1962). Although a study by Council, Kirsch, and Hafner (1986) challenged the generalizability of these correlations, indicating that "the relation of the Absorption Scale . . . and similar measures to hypnotic responsivity is highly reactive to contextual factors" (p. 188), a more recent study by Nadon, Hoyt, Register, and Kihlstrom (1991) failed to replicate the context effect described by Council et al. (1986). From their findings, Nadon, Hoyt, et al. concluded that "the relation between absorption and hypnotic behavior is much more than an artifact of the testing context" (p. 151). Interestingly, a recent study (Balthazard & Woody, 1992) reports that passing difficult hypnotic suggestions is more highly related to absorption than passing easy items.

This relationship suggests that absorption may be a critical ability in terms of facilitating hypnotic experience. Kihlstrom et al. (1989) state that the TAS "seems to measure the individual's capacity for dissociative and holistic experiences involving, respectively, the narrowing and broadening of attentional focus" (p. 259). Tellegen describes absorption as "a disposition, penchant or readiness to enter states characterized by cognitive restructuring" (cited in Roche & McConkey, 1990, p. 92). From these statements, it is evident that absorption is a personality trait that gives hypnotizable subjects the ability to experience characteristic hypnotic behavior. Might absorption also be an important trait of creative individuals?

Although the role of absorption in creativity has not been documented to the same extent as in hypnosis, there is support for the idea that a construct similar to absorption contributes significantly to the creative experience. K. S. Bowers (1984a) suggests that "total immersion of the scientist in his field seems to be an important condition of genuine creativity" (p. 259). The ability to focus attention completely on a specific task has often been cited as a personality trait of creative individuals. Barron (1965) makes the following assertion: "In [creative individuals] I would posit a stronger initial impulse to render experience intelligible, combined with an unusual ability to pay attention and to organize percepts effectively for prediction." The Greek scientist Archimedes embodied such a capacity for focused thought; he was legendary in his preoccupation with his work. In fact, upon discovering a way of measuring the density of gold, he is said to have run naked into the streets shouting, *"Eureka!"* ("I have found it!").

Empirical findings regarding the relationship of absorption and creativity are particularly limited. P. G. Bowers (1978) obtained a correlation of .39 between scores on an absorption questionnaire developed in her laboratory and a composite creativity measure. The latter was obtained by aggregating scores on two self-estimates of creativity and one performance measure—namely, the Guilford Consequences Test (Christensen, Merrifield, & Guilford, 1958). No personality measures of creativity were used.

Imaginative Involvement and Fantasy Proneness

Imagination is a common element of both hypnosis and creativity. Both experiences are often characterized by the ability to form a mental image, to maintain the image in awareness, and to become involved in the image in ways that we describe below. Historically, researchers have interpreted hypnotic behavior in terms of these abilities (Weitzenhoffer, 1980). Durio

(1975) has stressed that creativity and imagery are similar constructs, sharing a constellation of factors that include originality and fluency of responses, spatial abilities, and spontaneous and free associations.

Creative individuals often show exceptional imagery skills. For instance, Nikola Tesla, the inventor of the alternating-current motor, was able to build his inventions without the aid of blueprints, working exclusively from mental images of these devices. The design of the motor came to him while walking through a park with a friend. He described the experience as follows:

> The images I saw were wonderfully sharp and clear and had the solidity of metal and stone, so much so that I told him [his friend], "See my motor here; watch me reverse it." (Madigan & Elwood, 1983, p. 12)

Tesla's ability to construct and modify his invention through mental imagery is an example of what E. R. Hilgard (1981) would call "creative imagination." Of the six categories of imagery included in Hilgard's classification scheme, creative imagination has received the least attention from researchers (Khatena, 1987).

The relation of imagery and hypnosis, on the other hand, has been the subject of great interest. J. R. Hilgard (1970) identified the construct of "imaginative involvement" in a series of interviews that she conducted in her search for personality traits that would be predictive of hypnotizability. She found that high hypnotizable subjects were more likely than low hypnotizable subjects to report a history of satisfying experiences in which they would become engaged in fantasy while reading a book, listening to music, or participating in any of a number of activities in their everyday lives that might allow them to temporarily set aside their ordinary reality.

S. C. Wilson and Barber (1981) formulated a slightly modified version of this construct, which they termed "fantasy proneness." They described fantasy-prone individuals as "living much of the time in a world of their own making—in a world of imagery, imagination, and fantasy" (cited in Lynn & Rhue, 1988, p. 36). Using a measure of this construct developed by Wilson and Barber, Lynn and Rhue (1987) found that fantasy-prone persons score higher than other groups on measures of hypnotizability, vividness of mental imagery, absorption, and creativity. The results of a more recent study by these investigators (Lynn & Rhue, 1988) show that the correlation between hypnotizability and fantasy proneness may be more modest than the values obtained from the earlier study. Although the majority of fantasizers in both studies scored high on measures of hypnotizability, fantasy proneness proved not to be a completely reliable predictor of hypnotizability.

K. S. Bowers (1991b) has suggested that observable correlations of hypnotizability with measures of imaginative involvement and fantasy proneness do not indicate that imagination and goal-directed fantasy mediate hypnotic responsiveness, but rather that they are concomitants of the mechanism by which hypnotic responses occur. A number of findings cited by Bowers demonstrate that hypnotized subjects can respond to suggestions that involve either no imagery or incompatible imagery. Such findings offer persuasive support for the notion that hypnotic response is *not* mediated by imagery-related abilities. On the other hand, the findings that (1) imaginative involvement in activities outside of hypnosis can be predictive of hypnotizability (J. R. Hilgard, 1979a), and (2) some high hypnotizable subjects may require fantasy and imagination in order to achieve hypnotic response (Spanos, 1971), indicate strongly that the capacity to engage in imagery-based thinking contributes to hypnotic responsiveness. If the interpretation of this research is correct, then the ability to engage in imagination and fantasy must somehow serve as an important feature of hypnotic responsiveness without mediating the process by which response occurs.

With respect to creativity, Lynn and his associates have found that fantasy proneness correlates significantly with scores of creativity on the Barron–Welsh Revised Art Scale (Welsh & Barron, 1963) and the Guilford Consequences Test (see Lynn & Rhue, 1986; Rhue, Lynn, Bukh, & Henry, 1991). No known correlational findings for imaginative involvement with creativity are currently available.

Although the constructs of fantasy proneness and imaginative involvement have been treated in this discussion as phenomena related to mental imagery and imagination, they are not truly distinct from the concept of absorption. In fact, Lynn and Rhue (1988) found that measures of fantasy proneness and absorption correlate highly ($r > .70$). These authors conclude that "the constructs of fantasy proneness, imaginative involvement, and absorption are not truly discriminable; they converge in their emphasis on cognitive abilities related to imagination and fantasy that bridge hypnotic and nonhypnotic context" (p. 36).

Correlation of Hypnotizability and Creativity Measures

At the level of personality, the most direct link that can be established between hypnosis and creativity involves the correlation between hypnotic responsiveness and measures of creativity. Several studies have found significant bivariate correlations involving various measures of the two constructs. K. S. Bowers and van der Meulen (1970) administered three tasks related to creativity—the Guilford Consequences Test (Christensen et al., 1958), the Holtzman Inkblot Technique (Holtzman, Thorpe, Swartz, & Herron, 1961), and a free-association test (adapted from Gardner, Holzmann, Klein, Linton, & Spence, 1959)—to high and low hypnotizable subjects, assessing their performance on nine separate measures of creative functioning derived from these tasks. They found that the high hypnotizable subjects attained significantly higher scores on eight of the nine measures. They also observed a gender difference with respect to creative performance, with women scoring significantly higher than men on all measures for all treatment conditions, regardless of their level of hypnotic susceptibility.

This gender difference had a more dramatic impact in a later study by K. S. Bowers (1971), in which male and female subjects were given a battery of creativity tests similar to the one described in the previous study, except for the addition of the Revised Art Scale (Welsh & Barron, 1963) and the Remote Associates Test (Mednick & Mednick, 1967). From this battery, eight measures were derived that generated a composite creativity score for each subject. The findings of this study showed a significant relationship between hypnotic susceptibility and the composite creativity score for female subjects but not for males. Perry, Wilder, and Appignanesi (1973) replicated these findings in an extensive study using a very large battery of psychological tests. However, in a more recent study, P. G. Bowers (1978) obtained an equal correlation ($r = .55$) for both genders.

Using only female subjects, Ashton and McDonald (1985) found that high hypnotizable subjects achieved consistently higher scores than low hypnotizable subjects on the various scoring categories of the Torrance Tests of Creative Thinking (TTCT; Torrance, 1990), as well as on the composite index of overall creativity. L. M. Jackson and Gorassini (1989) were unable to replicate these results when they administered the TTCT to a sample that included both male and female subjects. However, these investigators failed to consider gender effects, and unlike the previous studies, which measured hypnotic susceptibility using both the HGSHS:A and the SHSS:C, theirs relied solely on a single measure of susceptibility— namely, the seven-item Carleton University Responsiveness to Suggestion Scale (CURSS; Spanos, Radtke, Hodgins, Stam, & Bertrand, 1983). As a result of this departure from the methodology used by their predecessors, the findings of Jackson and Gorassini are not directly comparable to those of any of the other investigators.

Directions for Future Research

With respect to personality issues in the study of hypnosis and creativity, a number of deficiencies appear in the literature. The following two research questions, in particular, require further attention:

1. Limited research exists on the correlation of creativity measures with scales of absorption, fantasy proneness, and imaginative involvement. There are no such studies involving the last measure.

2. There has been insufficient use of creative personality measures in the investigations that have been done so far. For instance, the Adjective Check List, which is the primary instrument upon which most creative

personality scales are based, has not been administered in any of the studies reviewed here. If the objective of this research is to compare the personality traits associated with hypnotizable individuals and those who are creative, then personality measures of creativity such as the ones that rely on the Adjective Check List must be incorporated in this work.

As we discuss in the section on creative production, hypnosis researchers have tended to select creativity instruments for use in their studies in an unsystematic way, failing to consider the distinction between measures of personality and production. We suggest that for correlational studies of hypnotizability and creativity, the latter construct be measured using a battery of creative personality measures that might include a scale based on the Adjective Check List, as well as the Barron–Welsh Revised Art Scale and one of the newer instruments such as the Lifetime Creativity Scales (Richards, Kinney, Benet, & Merzel, 1988).

Relationship at the Level of Process

In determining whether or not hypnosis and creativity are related processes, investigators must base their work almost exclusively on individuals' subjective reports of their experience during these processes. As Kihlstrom (1984) has indicated, introspection is a valid form of psychological measurement, but researchers must carefully consider its limitations. Subjective report is susceptible to various forms of distortion, as seen in both the hypnosis literature (e.g., Orne, 1977) and descriptions of creative experiences (Weisberg, 1986).

With these limitations in mind, we shall examine the similarities that have been identified in the subjective experiences reported by creative individuals and hypnotized subjects. The two types of processes appear to be linked by a cognitive restructuring that produces modifications in awareness. A number of related viewpoints concerning the nature of these modifications are included in our discussion.

Absorption Revisited

Tellegen views absorption as a "readiness to depart from more everyday life cognitive maps and to restructure . . . one's representation of one's self and its boundaries" (cited in Lynn & Sivec, Chapter 11, this volume). This restructuring is initiated by the condition that Tellegen and Atkinson (1974) called "total attention" (p. 269). A number of hypnotic suggestions involve a certain degree of "incongruence" (Tellegen, 1978–1979), so that a successful response requires the subject to be able to focus on the information contained in the hypnotic suggestion while ignoring contradictory information. It is not surprising, then, that high hypnotizable subjects also rate highly in absorption. This relation is illustrated in the findings of Bartis and Zamansky (1990), who showed that high hypnotizable subjects can successfully perform suggested tasks when given contradictory information, whereas low hypnotizable subjects cannot.

Absorption may be the doorway through which a hypnotized subject must pass in order to experience the "classic suggestion effect," in which responses appear to the subject to be occurring involuntarily (Weitzenhoffer, 1974). The experience of creative thought may also be facilitated by absorption. In both instances, the role of absorption in initiating a cognitive shift of some type is less than well understood. However, the end result of this process for both hypnosis and creativity is that certain mental representations, as well as the processes that act upon them, undergo changes that affect awareness.

Modifying Awareness

We use the term "awareness" to refer to phenomenal awareness, which is the sum of the mental contents on which an individual is able to introspect and report. Information can remain outside of awareness because it is either permanently unavailable to introspection or temporarily inaccessible (see Kihlstrom, 1987a). Awareness is modified when (1) information that was previously inaccessible is retrieved; or (2) previously accessible information becomes unretrievable. The idea that some type of modification in awareness takes place in the creative process is implicit in Wallas's (1926) four stages: "preparation," "incubation," "illumination," and "verification." In the illumination stage, the individual's awareness seems to be modified to include previously inaccessible information.

Progression through the four stages described by Wallas is marked by a transition from one type of thinking to another. A number of researchers have identified two distinct types of thinking that are part of the creative process. Kris (1934/1952) indicated that this process is marked by a shift from a more secondary-process type of thinking to a more primary-process type of thinking. Osborn (1953) distinguished between "imaginative" and "evaluative" thinking. Deikman (1971) described the following two categories: "passive–receptive" and "active" thought. DeBono (1968) has drawn a distinction between "vertical" and "lateral" thinking. Other researchers have talked of "analytic" versus "holistic" processes, or left- versus right-hemisphere activity. These various theoretical viewpoints are linked by the notions that (1) the creative process involves a cognitive shift, from a more common and familiar mode of thinking to an altogether different form of thought; and (2) this shift contributes to the modification in awareness that is characteristic of creative insight (i.e., the retrieval of previously inaccessible material).

The classic suggestion effect represents a different type of modification, in which previously accessible material becomes temporarily lost to the processes of introspection that are associated with awareness. As we have already discussed, hypnotic response involves the subjective experience of nonvolition in responding to hypnotic suggestions. Although some researchers contend that hypnotized subjects maintain control over their behavior (e.g., Lynn, Rhue, & Weekes, 1990), there is general agreement that subjects nonetheless experience a sense of diminished volitional control during hypnosis. Studies that have employed rating scales to measure involuntariness have consistently found that high hypnotizable subjects are more likely than low scorers to report that their responses to hypnotizability scale items felt involuntary, as if the responses had happened by themselves (see K. S. Bowers, 1981; P. G. Bowers, 1982; Spanos, Radtke, Hodgins, Bertrand, Stam, & Moretti, 1983; P. G. Bowers, Laurence, & Hart, 1988). In this case, the hypnotized subjects appear to lose their normal awareness of volitional control: The responses to suggestions are self-generated, but the persons have no awareness of the generating processes, which would normally be accessible to introspection.

In his neodissociation theory, E. R. Hilgard (1977a) offered a theoretical framework for studying the modifications in awareness that are characteristic of hypnotized subjects. Hilgard proposed that conditions such as those found in the context of hypnosis can disrupt links between the cognitive structures that serve to monitor, organize, and control thought and action. Such a disruption can lead to a condition of divided consciousness, in which percepts, thoughts, feelings, and actions are processed without being represented in phenomenal awareness.

Neodissociation theory provides insight into phenomena in which subjects (1) are unaware of information that is consciously accessible under normal circumstances; or (2) have the subjective experience that a process that is normally intentional is not under conscious control. Most hypnotic phenomena fall into one of these two categories and can therefore be explained by E. R. Hilgard's theory. But is this theory useful in understanding the creative process, particularly as it relates to hypnosis? Neodissociation theory can account for any aspects of the creative process that might involve an element of nonvolition. As we are about to see, such an element can be observed in the creative process. However, Hilgard's theory cannot offer an explanation for aspects of the creative process—or of hypnosis, for that matter—that might result in an enhancement of some ability or an increase in cognitive processing.

Effortless Experiencing

Closely related to the feeling of involuntariness described by hypnotized subjects is the construct that P. G. Bowers (1978) calls "effortless experiencing." Bowers suggests that hypnotized subjects who perceive that their responses are happening without any effort on their part are having a type of experience similar to what takes place in the illumination stage of the creative process. The psychological processes underlying the experience of effortlessness are examined in greater detail later in this section. For now, let us begin the discussion by addressing the phenomenological aspects of this experience.

Creative individuals often describe the experience of having ideas come to them without any conscious control on their part. Although some stages of the creative process involve a great deal of active, disciplined thought, other stages require a more passive approach. Getzels (1975) describes this paradox in the following way: "Despite the self-evident need for strenuous effort, reflection, and rationality in problem solving, creative thinking entails, at least in some degree, surrender to freely rising playfulness, impulse, and a-rationality" (p. 332).

Effortlessness is a predominant theme when well-known writers describe their creative experiences. In fact, the following quotations collected by Madigan and Elwood (1983) are striking in their similarity. For instance, William Thackeray is quoted as saying:

> I have been surprised at the observations made by some of my characters. It seems as if an occult power was moving the pen. The personage does or says something, and I ask, how the dickens did he come to think of that? (p. 283)

George Lichtenberg:

> There is something in our minds like sunshine and the weather, which is not under our control. When I write, the best things come to me from I know not where. (p. 281)

Amy Lowell:

> A common phrase among poets is, "It came to me." So hackneyed has this become that one learns to suppress the expression with care, but really it is the best description I know of the conscious arrival of a poem. (p. 285)

Alfred Russel Wallace:

> No one deserves either praise or blame for the ideas that come to him, but only for the actions resulting therefrom. Ideas and beliefs are certainly not voluntary acts. They come to us—we hardly know how or whence. (p. 284)

The consistent presence of an effortless component in the accounts given by creative individuals of their work, as well as the similarity of these descriptions to the experiences of hypnotized subjects, suggests that a measure of effortless experiencing should correlate highly with measures of both creativity and hypnotizability. In a series of studies conducted by P. G. Bowers (1978, 1979, 1982–1983), subjects were asked to rate the effortlessness with which they performed a variety of imagery, fantasy, and consequences tasks. A 5-point scale was used, ranging from "1. High ease. Image just popped into mind; no effort needed to develop it," to "5. High difficulty. Constantly made effort to get and keep image." For every subject, a composite score for effortless experiencing was constructed, based on the z scores derived from the effortless rating for each task. This composite score produced bivariate correlations of .61 and .62 with hypnotizability and creativity (also a composite score), respectively. Both of these correlations were higher than the .55 value obtained for the relation of hypnotizability and creativity. In one study, the latter correlation dropped to a nonsignificant level—from .55 to .27—when effortless experiencing was held constant, indicating that the relationship of hypnosis and creativity may be mediated by the common variance of effortless experiencing (P. G. Bowers, 1978).

For one of her studies, P. G. Bowers (1979) assembled nine writers, all of whom had been published and were recognized as "promising," for a seminar that involved a series of interviews, administration of the SHSS:C, and session in which the writers were asked to work on a story of their own while hypnotized. The following patterns emerged from this work: (1) The writers ranged in hypnotizability from low to high; (2) mostly, the low hypnotizable writers placed great stress on the "precise and careful control of language" (p. 569), whereas none of the high hypnotizable writers did; (3) for all of the writers, the experience of writing while hypnotized interfered with their careful use of language; (4) this interference proved unpleasant for writers who required control of language; (5) for the remaining writers, the experience felt "similar to writing when a session was going particularly well" (p. 569); and (6) although most of the writers reported that the experience of writing under hypnosis resembled some of their more successful writing sessions, they rated their product as being either average or below average in comparison to material written under ordinary conditions. Bowers concluded that the experience of effortlessness within the creative process does not necessarily guarantee that the product of this process will be creative. She also suggested that the creative *style* of an individual, rather than the degree of creativity that the individual displays, may be related to hypnotizability.

In her writings on the subject of effortless experiencing, P. G. Bowers has provided a theoretical perspective on the relationship of hypnosis and creativity that is unique, in that it blends elements of psychoanalytic theory with concepts from the field of cognitive psychology. The notion of "associative networks" is central to this viewpoint.

According to Bowers, effortlessness is the critical link in understanding similarities between the processes underlying hypnosis and creativity. The mechanism by which either of these experiences becomes effortless involves a transition from one mode of thinking to another. Bowers distinguishes between the active mode of thinking, which is regulated by realistic, logical, sequential rules of association, and the more passive mode, which she terms "fantasy." Of course, activity and passivity may not be discrete categories, and the active–passive distinction may be complicated by other factors such as focused or expanded attention (Fromm, 1979). In the present context, we are concerned only with characterizing one aspect of the creative experience.

The active mode, as described by P. G. Bowers, is accessed during a normal state of arousal. In this condition, awareness is dominated by goals, expectations, and strategies, and information tends to be stored and retrieved in the form of language. These features of the active mode restrict the range of priming that can take place within the associative network. Language, in particular, reduces experience to fit semantic categories and thus limits the number and types of associations that can be drawn from an experience, so that thinking becomes conventional.

In the passive mode, the restricting effects of awareness are bypassed. This has two consequences, which are closely related: (1) Images, rather than words, become the primary form of information storage and retrieval; and (2) a wider associative network is primed. Support for this latter point is found in the work of Spence and Holland (1962), who reported that conscious awareness of a stimulus has restricting effects on associations to the stimulus, in contrast to associations that are made when the stimulus is presented below the awareness threshold. Also of interest is a series of studies by Martindale, who found that low levels of arousal result in increases in creative test performance (e.g., Martindale & Greenough, 1973). MacKinnon (1971) has stated:

> The truly creative person might be distinguished from the non-creative individual by his great ease in moving from more conscious and active to more unconscious and passive states. One might inquire, then, about the ease and speed with which the creative person, as compared with others, falls asleep, enters into a hypnotic trance upon suggestion from another person, or passes into self-induced states of trance or semi-trance. (p. 227)

The creative individual resembles the highly hypnotizable subject in that both have a greater than normal capacity for transition from an active to a passive mode of thinking. According to P. G. Bowers (1979), the creative process "requires a person who can allow an idea or object to influence associations and responses while bypassing temporarily the ordinary ego-controlling, intentional processes" (p. 566). This ability to let the structure of the creative problem determine the types of associations that are made may account for certain characteristics of creative individuals, such as their high level of tolerance for ambiguity and their preference for complexity (see Dellas & Gaier, 1970).

As we have already seen, the highly hypnotizable individual is typically someone who becomes absorbed in nonhypnotic imaginative activities and experiences. Such a person is able to allow the experience simply to take place instead of exerting control over it. For this person, a given stimulus should determine the manner in which the associative network is primed, just as the stimulus should for a creative person. J. R. Hilgard (1970) reported that involvement in stimulus-incited imagination is more predictive of hypnotizability than involvement in impulse-incited imagination.

Individuals who are considered either creative or hypnotizable are able to shift into the passive mode of thinking in response to the appropriate set of conditions, such as those associated with a creative task or a hypnotic induction. Such individuals can allow the circumstances to direct their fantasy processes without competition from conscious decision making, which might otherwise override this response. Effortlessness, then, is experienced to the degree that an individual's task response has been influenced by nonvolitional fantasy associations as opposed to volitional, controlled decision making.

Suggestions for Future Research

The following concerns need to be addressed in future studies of process-related issues:

1. Correlations between effortless experiencing and creativity are influenced by the types of creativity measures that are used. Ashton and McDonald (1985) were unable to replicate P. G. Bowers's (1978) correlation values, obtaining nonsignificant values of .13. It has been suggested that this discrepancy may be due to the fact that two of the three measures used by Bowers were self-ratings, whereas Ashton and McDonald relied on performance-based measures of creativity (L. M. Jackson & Gorassini, 1989). In future studies, it might be appropriate to use either personality or performance measures, depending on the hypothesis that is being tested. The selection of appropriate measures should depend on whether the investigator is interested in the effortlessness with which specific creative responses are produced, or the extent to which a creative individual experiences ideas in an effortless way. The latter is more of a personality issue than the former, and should be measured accordingly.

2. P. G. Bowers's work with creative writers suggests that effortlessness may be a function of an individual's creative style. In order to test this hypothesis, the various styles of creativity must first be identified, and then instruments need to be developed in order to differentiate creative styles. A. N. Katz (1984) has attempted to address the first of these needs by factor-analyzing scores on a battery of creativity instruments. However, until styles can be assessed in a reliable manner, there is no effective way of determining whether effortless experiencing is a function of creative style.

3. To determine whether or not dissociation plays a role in the creative process, it would be useful to obtain correlation values for measures of dissociation and creativity.

Relationship at the Level of Production

Most of the empirical research concerning the relationship of hypnosis and creativity has been aimed at the levels of personality and process, as can be seen in the two basic hypotheses that have received a great deal of the attention in this field. One is that high hypnotizable subjects are also more creative than their low hypnotizable counterparts; the other is that subjects are more creative when they are hypnotized than when they are not. The first hypothesis is directed at the level of personality traits associated with people identified as relatively more creative and more hypnotizable, whereas the second attempts to focus on the processes involved in both creative performance and hypnotic behavior. As P. G. Bowers (1979) has indicated, the two hypotheses converge in that "the characteristic personal qualities of creative or hypnotizable people tend to be aptitudes and/or motivations to engage in the postulated processes" (p. 564). Another very important source of convergence is at the level of production.

Hennessey and Amabile (1988) have stated that "although many contemporary theorists think of creativity as a process and look for evidence of it in persons, their definitions most frequently use characteristics of the *product* as the distinguishing signs of creativity" (p. 13). Creativity can be operationalized most effectively at the level of production, since a creative product is more directly measurable than either a cognitive process or a personality trait.

In this section we discuss measurement issues related to creative production. Such issues have proven particularly relevant in the investigation of the hypothesis that hypnosis enhances creative performance. The selection of appropriate measures, as we shall see, is critical to the effectiveness of research in this area.

Assessment of Creative Products

Most creativity tests require that a product be generated in response to a set of instructions, and then that the product be evaluated according to a specific set of guidelines. The products in these tests tend to be simple and fairly restricted, since the tests themselves are similar to tests of intelligence in their construction and scoring. For instance, in the Remote Associates Test (Mednick & Mednick, 1967), the subject is asked to provide a specific word; the Guilford Consequences Test (Christensen et al., 1958) requires the subject to list possible consequences of improbable events; and the TTCT (Torrance, 1990) figural subtests ask subjects to complete a set of drawings.

A number of attempts have been made to assess the creative attributes of various products (Besemer & O'Quin, 1987). Rating systems for creative products rely on a wide range of criteria, including originality, elaboration, usefulness, and attractiveness. Torrance (1990) developed the following four categories for rating responses to the TTCT: (1) fluency, which is the total number of relevant responses; (2) flexibility, defined as the number of different categories of information represented in a response; (3) originality, a measure of the statistical frequency of a response within a normative sample; and (4) elaboration, or the number of ideas represented in a response. In this rating system, creativity is operationalized in such a way that the amount of information included in a response plays as significant a role in defining the construct as does the quality of the response.

Hypnotic Enhancement of Creativity

Does creative performance increase during hypnosis? Research that has addressed this question has generated a wide variety of responses. K. S. Bowers and van der Meulen (1970), whose study has already been described here, found no treatment effects and a significant treatment × susceptibility interaction on only one (i.e., human movement on the Holtzman Inkblot Technique) of the nine measures of creative performance that they included in their analysis.

In an unorthodox study involving nonstandard administration of the Torrance tests, Gur and Reyher (1976) showed a significant hypnotic treatment effect for figural measures of creativity on the TTCT, but not for verbal measures. Only high hypnotizable male subjects were used in this study. Subjects were assigned to four groups. One group was given the TTCT in a standardized manner and in a waking condition; the other three groups received the TTCT with the following deviations: (1) The test was given orally; (2) the subjects were not told that their creativity was being assessed; (3) the instructions encouraged subjects to wait passively for ideas; and (4) a "free-imagery" phase was included in order to facilitate primary-process thinking. The latter three groups included hypnosis, waking, and simulating conditions.

Although the hypnotized subjects scored higher on the figural subtests than any of the three control groups, there was no significant difference in performance on the verbal subtests between the hypnotized subjects and the group receiving the standardized TTCT instructions. In the absence of hypnosis, the modified instructions resulted in a suppression of verbal creativity and an insignificant increase in figural creativity. The effect of hypnosis in this study was to prevent the suppression of verbal creativity caused by the modified administration procedures, as well as to enhance figural creativity. These findings are weakened by the absence of a comparison group of hypnotized subjects receiving standardized instructions on the TTCT, and by the investigators' failure to account for the suppression of verbal creativity in the control subjects who were given the modified instructions.

Ashton and McDonald (1985) failed to detect any hypnotic treatment effects on the TTCT, except on the elaboration measure of figural creativity. Their study used only female subjects, standardized instructions, and a shortened version of the TTCT consisting of three of the seven verbal subtests and two of the three figural subtests.

L. M. Jackson and Gorassini (1989) also used a shortened version of the TTCT, administered to subjects of both genders in a standardized manner. On three of the four measures of figural creativity (i.e., fluency, flexibility, and elaboration), hypnotized subjects scored significantly higher than waking subjects. Notably, there was no treatment × susceptibility interaction. In other words, the enhancement in figural creativity after hypnotic procedures was equally present for all subjects, and not just the highly hypnotizable ones.

Methodological Limitations

What is most striking about this field of research is the absence of robust findings. A number of methodological differences seem to underlie this discrepancy among researchers. Foremost among these is the selection of assessment procedures to measure creativity. As indicated by Treffinger (1987), measurement issues have become the major stumbling block in the area of creativity research. No fewer than 186 instruments have been listed in the *Journal of Creative Behavior* as being "useful in studying creative behavior and creative talent" (G. A. Davis, 1971; Kaltsounis, 1971, 1972; Kaltsounis & Honeywell, 1980). There are almost as many definitions and theoretical perspectives on creativity as there are instruments to measure it. Furthermore, a number of instruments used in creativity research are designed to measure constructs such as divergent thinking and primary-process thinking, which may only represent a narrow range of abilities related to creativity. All of these factors serve to compound the measurement problem that faces creativity researchers.

Investigators tend to select instruments for use in their studies that reflect their own theoretical perspective on creativity. At times, this tendency may lead to the selection of redundant measures. For instance, two of the three instruments that K. S. Bowers and van der Meulen (1971) administered to their subjects were measures of primary-process thinking. As a result, their battery represented only a narrow portion of the spectrum of creativity measures available to them.

Other researchers have effectively addressed the issue of redundant measures at the expense of replicability. For example, Perry et al. (1973) administered a comprehensive battery of creativity instruments that required nearly 3 hours of their subjects' time to complete. Moreover, one of the instruments selected by these investigators—the Kit of Reference Tests for Cognitive Factors (French, Ekstrom, & Price, 1963)—is so cumbersome and unfamiliar a measure that it has failed to appear in any other creativity studies in the hypnosis literature during the past 18 years.

The only creativity instruments that appear consistently in the research discussed here are the verbal and figural subtests of the TTCT. Although the presence of these instruments in many of the studies should facilitate comparison of the findings obtained in these studies, this benefit has been largely negated by the lack of consistency in administration of the TTCT. As we have seen, some investigators used a shortened version of the subtests. In some cases, the TTCT was given only to male subjects, and in others it was given only to females. One study used only high hypnotizable subjects.

The most radical departure from standardized administration procedures for the TTCT was undertaken by Gur and Reyher (1976). These authors modified the procedures in order to conceal the intellectual-task demands from their subjects. They reasoned that the standardized procedures were inadequate because "even a hypnotized subject is likely to become defensive and threatened when his creativity is being challenged and adopt his customary, problem-solving, task-oriented approach to tests" (p. 238).

Although the results of their study were not as convincing as they might have been, because none of the hypnotized subjects were given the TTCT with standardized instructions, Gur and Reyher (1976) did succeed in drawing attention to the notion that the administration of standardized creativity tests such as the TTCT may be inappropriate for use with hypnotized subjects. Their modification of the testing procedures for the TTCT encouraged subjects to use their imagination in formulating responses to the test questions and created a more comfortable, relaxed setting for the subjects, in contrast to the more stressful and demanding conditions normally associated with a standardized test-taking situation. In general, Gur and Reyher deviated from the standardized procedures in simple ways that seemed very reasonable. For example, allowing the subjects to respond orally to the TTCT tasks as opposed to requiring that they provide written responses is an effective way of minimizing the test-taking characteristics of the situation, and it also eliminates the distraction of having hypnotized subjects deal with writing implements and paper.

As reasonable as their modifications of the TTCT procedures may have been, Gur and Reyher received justified criticism from other investigators (see Ashton & McDonald, 1985) for deviating from the standardized testing procedures. By altering the procedures, they reduced the impact of their findings and made it difficult for other researchers to compare these findings to their own.

In selecting measures for use in their studies, researchers in this domain have tended to overlook the difference between "trait" and "state" measures. Tests of creative performance assess a single instance of creativity and thus may not be appropriate for use in research that examines the relationship of hypnosis and creativity at the level of personality. Problems arise when an individual's performance in a given context does not reflect the general tendencies of that individual. Even greater problems emerge, however, when personality measures are used in studies of hypnotic treatment conditions. The hypothesis in such studies should be that creative performance is enhanced in the context of hypnosis, not that hypnosis will have a lasting effect on the individual's personality. Trait measures such as the Barron–Welsh Revised Art Scale are inappropriate for this type of study.

Improving Measurement of Creativity in Hypnotic Settings

The methodological problems that have been described here have seriously impaired the study of the relationship between hypnosis and creativity. One problem that is of particular concern in our attempts to gain insight into the nature of this relationship is that none of the creativity instruments in existence is particularly appropriate for hypnosis research. In general, these instruments fail to meet the two criteria that are most critical to creativity research in a hypnotic setting: (1) nonreactivity and (2) ecological validity.

A "nonreactive" measure is one that can be obtained without affecting the subject's hypnotic experience. Most creativity instruments have a standard test format requiring written responses. Although some subjects may not be distracted by the administration of this type of instrument, it would be difficult to measure or control for the level of distraction induced by the instrument. A far more suitable alternative would be to minimize the possibility of distraction by designing a less intrusive format.

"Ecological validity" is a notion that is particularly relevant to state measures of creativity, which focus on creativity in a specific context as opposed to personality traits. The criticism of most creativity instruments is that the abilities they measure are distinct from the abilities that are responsible for creativity in a person's everyday environment (Weisberg, 1986). Creative expression in adults most commonly takes the form of storytelling. Even adults who no longer find the opportunity to engage in painting, dancing, or solving riddles still have the occasion to tell a bedtime story or tall tale. In hypnosis research, it is particularly important that a suggested activity be a part of the subject's everyday repertoire. There is no point in asking a hypnotized subject to carry out a task for which the subject has no aptitude or training. For instance, we would not ask a woman who does not dance to perform complex dance movements for us in the context of hypnosis. However, we might ask the same individual to imagine herself performing such dance movements, and then to describe the experience for us. In a hypnotic setting, it would be advantageous to find a creativity task that allows the subject to describe some imagined set of events, because such a task has a high probability of accessing a set of skills that the subject already has at his or her disposal.

At the University of Arizona, Kihlstrom and colleagues have been developing a measure of imaginative production that they believe has a high degree of ecological validity. "Imaginative production" is defined as the ability to generate novel and appropriate imagery in response to an open-ended storytelling task. The instrument consists of three imagery tasks, in which subjects are asked to experience and then describe (1) the features of an imagined place; (2) an interaction with imagined characters; and (3) a transformation into an imagined identity. Each task requires different levels of involvement in the imagined circumstances, thus offering subjects the opportunity for a wide range of response.

This measure of imaginative production was developed in part to reflect the importance of mental imagery in the experiences of hypnosis and creativity. Although measures exist for other types of skills related to imagery, such as imaginative involvement, fantasy proneness, and the control and vividness of imagery (for a review, see Sheehan, 1979a), there are virtually no measures that tap the more creative aspects of imagination (Khatena, 1987). Gur and Reyher (1976) tried to correct for this shortcoming by modifying the TTCT. As we have seen, this approach creates problems of generalizability. Instead, we propose that standardized assessment procedures such as our measure of imaginative production be developed that incorporate the types of innovations Gur and Reyher tried to bring to the TTCT. Such instruments should (1) be simple and quick to administer; (2) have a format that allows subjects to respond orally; and (3) encourage subjects to use their imaginations freely in formulating responses.

Relationship at the Level of Press

In an earlier section of the chapter, we have defined "press" as the interaction of individuals with their environment. There is support for the position that the situational variables giving rise to this interaction play a critical role for both hypnosis and creativity. In this section, we discuss the situational variables that have been linked to both processes, and we compare these variables.

Motivation and Creativity

In her work on creativity, Teresa Amabile has maintained the position that the individual's motivational orientation is strongly linked to creative performance, and that an environment that is conducive to an intrinsic motivational orientation will also facilitate creativity. Her research is guided by what she has termed the "intrinsic motivation" principle of creativity, which she states as follows: "People will be most creative when they feel motivated primarily by the interest, enjoyment, satisfaction, and challenge of the work itself—not by external pressures" (Hennessey & Amabile, 1988, p. 11).

A precursor of this principle is C. Rogers's (1954) notion of "conditions for creativity." He maintained that the most effective environments for promoting creativity are those characterized by elements of psychological safety and freedom from external evaluation. Research findings concerning the effects of rewards on creative task performance have provided a great deal of support for this position (for a review, see Hennessey & Amabile, 1988). The expectation of external evaluation or reward consistently diminishes creative performance on open-ended tasks for both children and adults.

Goal-Directed Behavior in Hypnosis

Social-psychological theorists have constructed a model that views hypnotic response as "scripted role enactment in which subjects modify responses strategically in terms of shifting role demands. . . . Hypnotic responses are regarded as goal-directed actions, and reports of involuntariness reflect context-generated interpretations of these goal-directed actions" (Lynn, Rhue, & Weekes, 1990, p. 170). According to this position, hypnotized subjects are actively controlling their responses in order to satisfy the role requirements of hypnotic suggestion.

Lynn and his associates view hypnotic behavior as creative problem solving in which subjects draw upon various cognitive strategies and abilities in order to achieve specific goals. These goals involve the experiencing of hypnotic events in order to fulfill implicit and explicit contextual demands. In Chapter 11 of this volume, Lynn and Sivec make the following claim: "The problem gestalt [in the hypnotic context] can be thought of as the constellation of attitudes about hypnosis, demand characteristics, and implicit and explicit expectations and performance standards" (p. 299).

Is Motivation Enough?

Amabile (1987) has convincingly argued that pressures to conform to goals that are extrinsic to a task serve to inhibit the individual's effectiveness in solving creative problems. This notion stands in direct contrast to Lynn's view of the hypnotized subject as a creative agent. If hypnotic behavior is directed by the "constellation" of demands and expectations that Lynn and his colleagues have described, then it seems unlikely that the context of hypnosis would be particularly conducive to creative behavior of any kind.

A more significant point, however, is that the effect sizes associated with manipulations of motivational orientation are vanishingly small (Amabile, 1987). The notion that the variable of motivation has limited predictive power should be self-evident. If a change in motivational orientation were sufficient to enhance creative performance, then creativity would be a rather commonplace experience. The mechanism by which creativity takes place is not well understood, but it is evident that the process involves much more than simple motivation.

Theoretical and Empirical Considerations for Future Work

Although there has been considerable speculation about the nature of creative thinking, the formal scientific study of creativity is a relatively recent development. J. P. Guilford, in a 1950 presidential address to the American Psychological Association, urged his colleagues to pursue this previously overlooked area of research; however, it was not until Guilford proposed his structure-of-intellect model in 1967, with its distinction between convergent and divergent thinking, that the systematic psychological study of creativity actually began to unfold. The earliest research on hypnosis and creativity dates from this time (e.g., P. G. Bowers, 1967).

It is evident that the best work in this field remains to be done. Although researchers have made some progress in understanding the nature of the relationship between hypnosis and creativity, their efforts have been hindered by the methodological problems that we have outlined in this chapter. The selection of appropriate creativity measures has proven to be a particularly challenging task for hypnosis researchers. There has been a tendency on the part of investigators in this field to confound state measures (of the creativity of particular products) with trait measures (of the creativity of particular people), and to overlook issues of ecological validity and reactivity in assessing the creativity of hypnotized subjects. In general, insufficient attention has been paid to the literature on creativity itself, particularly with respect to measurement issues.

In this chapter, we have attempted to demonstrate that many of the methodological problems besetting the study of hypnosis and creativity can be attributed to conceptual deficiencies. By introducing a simple organizational framework based on the principles governing creativity research in other domains, we have been able to identify specific limitations in the existing literature, as well as new directions that can be taken in this field.

Even if it is assumed that methodological obstacles can be overcome and that the relationship between hypnosis and creativity can be empirically established at some level, the theoretical implications of such findings will need to be explicated. What significance would there be in a finding that hypnotic susceptibility is correlated to personality measures of creativity, or that creative performance is enhanced in the hypnotic context? Of what benefit is it to the researcher to be able to establish that the experiences of hypnosis and of creativity have certain commonalities—that both may involve the suspension of the GRO or the effortless experiencing of ideas?

Empirical findings concerning the relationship between hypnosis and creativity could have enormous repercussions for existing theoretical viewpoints in the hypnosis literature. Of particular significance is the interaction of hypnosis and hypnotic susceptibility with the component processes of creativity. The experience of having a creative insight involves the following two events: (1) the generation of a new idea or image; and (2) the retrieval of this information into phenomenal awareness. Any condition, including hypnosis, that may favor the formation of such an insight must facilitate at least one of these events. Hypnosis theorists maintain a wide range of positions regarding not only the facilitation of creative insight in hypnosis, but also the mechanism by which such facilitation may occur. Here is a brief summary of these positions:

1. *No facilitation of creative insight takes place in hypnosis.* This position is advocated by some proponents of neodissociation theory, who suggest that incubation or consolidation activities may occur in a dissociated stream of consciousness, so that the individual remains unaware of cognitive processing taking place in the incubation stage. Because of this unawareness, the creative solution is experienced as coming to consciousness suddenly, in an unbidden manner. The experience of effortlessness associated with a creative insight is then illusory: Cognitive effort has been exerted, but the individual is not aware of this effort.

2. *Hypnosis facilitates the generation of new ideas or images.* This notion is consistent with psychoanalytic theory, as well as the model presented by P. G. Bowers in her work on effortlessness. In this model, restrictions in awareness increase the priming of associative networks outside of phenomenal awareness by reducing any interference on the part of conscious thought. The result of this process is that new associations are made, giving rise to creative insight.

Psychoanalytic theorists propose that the wellspring of creative insight is to be found in primary-process thinking—an imagistic mode of thought closely tied to primitive drives, and not constrained by reality concerns or formal logic. If, as Gill and Brenman (1959) and others have argued, hypnosis involves an adaptive regression or a regression in the service of the ego, then the resulting shift from secondary-process to primary-process thinking should allow new ideas and images to be generated.

3. *Hypnosis facilitates the retrieval of ideas and images into phenomenal awareness.* A number of cognitive processes related to memory, perception, learning, and problem solving take place outside of phenomenal awareness (see Kihlstrom , 1990). There is also a great deal of support for the

notion that imagination and fantasy provide a continuous backdrop to our unconscious thoughts (see P. G. Bowers & Bowers, 1979). Thus, it is conceivable that new ideas and images are being generated in a steady stream outside of awareness, but that only a small portion of this stream ever reaches awareness. Perhaps hypnosis contributes to creative insight by increasing the accessibility of some information processed outside of awareness.

The testing of competing hypotheses based on distinct theoretical perspectives could have a major impact on the ways in which both hypnosis and creativity are understood. But the types of logical inferences that we are describing cannot be made without the support of solid empirical work. At present, the most urgent need is for methodological consistency in the assessment of creativity. The selection of appropriate creativity measures is a critical first step in determining progress in this field.

As the quality of empirical work increases, we anticipate that researchers will begin to pursue questions of greater theoretical interest concerning the relationship of creativity and hypnosis. For instance, an entire research program could be developed in order to explore the interaction of hypnosis and hypnotizability with the various stages of the creative process. A number of intriguing questions emerge when we consider the nature of such an interaction: Does the initial representation of a problem differ in hypnosis, or in hypnotizable individuals, in comparison to controls? Are intuitions concerning the solubility of a problem stronger or more accurate? Does hypnosis, or hypnotizability, reduce incubation time? Is incubation outside of conscious awareness more effective than continued conscious efforts at problem solving? Do the insights produced in hypnosis differ qualitatively from those produced under other conditions? Research that addresses these questions goes directly to the heart of the processes underlying both hypnosis and creativity.

Acknowledgments

Preparation of this chapter, and research supporting the point of view expressed herein, was supported by a National Science Foundation Predoctoral Fellowship to Victor Shames, and by Grant No. MH-35856 from the National Institute of Mental Health to John F. Kihlstrom.

We wish to thank John F. Kihlstrom for contributing his time and ideas to this chapter. We also wish to acknowledge Teresa Woods for her assistance in gathering materials used in the chapter.

CHAPTER THIRTEEN

The Phenomenology of Hypnosis and the Experiential Analysis Technique

PETER W. SHEEHAN

The Nature of the Phenomenological Approach

A "phenomenological" perspective of hypnosis looks at personal experiences of hypnotic phenomena and attempts to describe them with as little bias or interpretation as possible (see Corsini, 1987, p. 482). The methodology that involves this way of looking at things maintains that personal experience, as reported by introspection, can be studied scientifically and is a genuine source of scientific data. In modern parlance, phenomenological data are typically regarded as subjective or private data, in comparison with objective or behavioral data. This kind of classification, however, should not be seen as negating the genuine validity of many verbal reports.

Adopting a phenomenological framework is a very useful means of exploring hypnotic phenomena. It enables us to look at processes, for example, in more detail than many other approaches afford, and it reveals the diversity and richness of hypnotic experience and behavior. The focus in such an approach is essentially on individual differences in response, the assumption being that there is wide heterogeneity in subjects' reactions to hypnotic suggestions. In each case, the whole person is viewed dynamically—not only as an organism with skills and abilities, but as a person in a social context. The approach incorporates a study of the nature of the person; in addition, however, it reaches out to take account of other important determinants of behavior and experience, such as the setting in which these occur, the relationship between the person and the hypnotist, the physical surroundings, and the person's specific attitudinal sets and expectancies.

Accounts of hypnosis that emphasize the person tend to focus on the hypnotic subject's ability to enter a state of hypnosis and to experience hypnotic phenomena. Such an emphasis often leads to a search for predispositions or personal cognitive propensities that define the meaning of the term "hypnotizability." Research of this kind typically centers on the study of imagination, absorption, attention, and dissociative capacity (see, e.g., Fromm & Kahn, 1990; Gruenewald, 1986). Trait-theoretical accounts of hypnosis, however, do not necessarily appeal to the phenomenology of hypnosis as a primary mode of explanation, although theoretical frameworks that utilize the concept of trait (e.g., E. R. Hilgard, 1965a, 1974; Orne, 1974; Shor, 1970, 1979) tend to highlight the state of hypnosis and emphasize the character of consciousness of a person when "under hypnosis." There are inventories that have been constructed specifically to measure the dispositional correlates of hypnotic consciousness (Kihlstrom, Register, Hoyt, Albright, Grigorian, Heindel, & Morrison, 1989) and to assess the patterning or structure of hypnotic consciousness (see Pekala & Kumar, 1989).

A complete understanding of hypnotic response is not possible, however, until a further range of important influences is taken into account. Especially significant among these are the contextual factors that shape hypnotic behavior and experience. These include the motivations and expectations of hypnotic subjects, including those emphasized strongly in the cognitive–behavioral theories of T. X. Barber (1979), Sarbin and Coe (1972), and most recently Spanos and Chaves (1989c).

With respect to assessment, the literature suggests that employing a variety of methods is the most useful approach to attempting to understand what is happening in the hypnotic setting. Assessment can be carried out either unilaterally by the hypnotist or experimenter, who interprets what is happening, or interactively by the hypnotist and subject, who discuss what has occurred. Phenomenological approaches (e.g., Sheehan, McConkey, & Cross, 1978; Shor, 1979) are interactive in character. Here, both participants explore the situation together in an unrestrained environment, in which the subject augments the data by contributing actively to an understanding of the hypnotic experience.

Despite the rich variety of theories and modes of assessment that are available to explain hypnotic events, most theorists make at least some appeal to the subjective experience of individuals under hypnosis in order to account for hypnotic happenings and occurrences. Indeed, whether the theoretical emphasis is on the subject's skills in hypnosis, expectancies, motivations, or states of consciousness, different theoretical frameworks tend to converge on the importance of understanding the internal cognitive processes at work when the subject responds to hypnotic suggestion. The essential character of the phenomenological approach is that it focuses explicitly on subjective experience and gives "experience" formal status in its model of explanation, in a way that other theoretical perspectives do not.

Some Historical Background

In the early 1960s, perhaps the most commonly employed indicator of a subject's depth of involvement in hypnosis was the ability of the subject to experience "difficult" (i.e., cognitive-delusory) hypnotic phenomena, such as hallucinations, posthypnotic responses, and amnesia. Attempts to gauge this ability were made through the construction of hierarchically-based behavioral scales (e.g., Friedlander & Sarbin, 1938; Shor & Orne, 1962; Weitzenhoffer & Hilgard, 1959) and a sampling of well-structured clinically oriented measures (e.g., O'Connell, Orne, & Shor, 1966). A related indicator of this involvement was "trance depth," which reflects how deeply a subject feels experientially that he or she is hypnotized (LeCron, 1953; O'Connell et al., 1966; Tart, 1979). Regardless of whether a measure was subjectively or behaviorally based, there was usually an underlying assumption in the construction of many of the early measures of hypnotic responsiveness that trance depth is unidimensional. Shor's three-factor theory, however, posited that it is not (Shor, 1962).

Significantly, Shor addressed the complexity of the hypnotic subject's involvement in hypnosis and formalized "experience" in terms of pre-scribed phenomenological methods. He viewed the measurement of the difficulty of items experienced and the level of the subjective experience of trance depth as distinct. Three factors were proposed as being responsible for the depth of trance: the generalized reality orientation of the subject, the nonconscious involvement of the subject in the hypnotic role, and the archaic involvement of the subject with the hypnotist. Shor's (1970) research also pointed to other important facets of the hypnotic situation, including drowsiness, relaxation, vividness of imagery, absorption, and access to the unconscious. Trance depth was seen as independent of these variables and characteristic of the phenomenological approach to hypno-sis. Formal status was afforded to individual differences in private experi-ence, not just in behavioral response. The nature of these differences was later explored intensively for heterohypnosis (Sheehan & McConkey, 1982) and for autohypnosis (Fromm & Kahn, 1990). McConkey and I developed the Experiential Analysis Technique (EAT), which is the primary focus of comment in this chapter. The emphasis of the EAT is on individual differ-ences in style of response; it draws strongly on the concept of "cognitive style" as a primary mediational construct in the explanation of hypnotic events.

Cognitive Styles

We (Sheehan & McConkey, 1982; Sheehan et al., 1978) first conceptualized three main styles of response: "concentrative," "independent," and "con-structive." These labels describe major strategies adopted by hypnotic subjects in responding to hypnotic suggestions and realizing positive hypnotic experiences. They are not claimed as exhaustive or independent categories, but appear to reflect discrete modes of cognitive processing that overlap with other styles researchers have identified elsewhere. These include for instance, the "imagic cognitive style" studied by Labelle, Laurence, Nadon, and Perry (1990), and the "detail" and "holistic" strategies studied by Crawford and Allen (1983). We feel, however, that our categories are made necessary by the need to handle the interface of reality and suggestion, and it seems instructive to define them here.

The "concentrative" or cooperative mode of cognizing is characterized by subjects' concentrating on the communications of the hypnotist and imagining a literal interpretation of the message communications. This style is illustrated by a subject's saying that he or she is trying to concentrate hard on what the hypnotist is saying and to experience what is suggested.

The "independent" mode of cognizing is characterized by subjects' interpreting the communications of the hypnotist in a manner that is meaningful to them. The subjects choose aspects of experience that they themselves consider appropriate to their situation, and respond in an individual or idiosyncratic fashion. This style is illustrated by a subject's saying that his or her arm is being lifted by a balloon (as suggested), but that the balloon has air pumped into it at irregular intervals and moves erratically, rather than regularly.

The "constructive" mode is characterized by subjects' considering the communications of the hypnotist from a position of preparedness to process incoming stimuli in a schematic way, so as to structure or reorganize events according to the hypnotist's suggestions. Subjects in this category appear to actively seek out ways to construct or synthesize the suggested experience; they appear to make an effort to plan to interpret reality and the demands of the suggestions so that they can nevertheless respond appropriately. This style is illustrated by a subject's saying that his or her arm is not being lifted by a balloon (as suggested), but is being lifted gently by someone standing next to the chair.

A subject may use one or more of these styles during the same hypnotic session, and to a considerable extent the choice of style varies with the task complexity and the nature of any conflict experienced in the hypnotic setting (Sheehan et al., 1978). There is evidence also (Bell, 1978) that some subjects who are high in susceptibility show greater flexibility in the use of cognitive styles than do low susceptible subjects, and there is clear evidence of meaningful individual differences in subjects' use of the "detail" and "holistic" strategies (see Crawford & Allen, 1983). It is important to recognize, in relation to the phenomenological model of hypnosis, that no one style typifies the response of hypnotic subjects to suggestion, and it is interesting to note that vastly different styles of response may be adopted by equally susceptible subjects. For example, some high susceptible subjects demonstrate a predominantly concentrative style, which is the least flexible of our three modes of processing, and the single-case studies of Connie and Susan reported by McConkey, Glisky, and Kihlstrom (1989) illustrate well the concentrative and constructive modes of response occurring among different hypnotic virtuosos.

In terms of a theoretical framework, cognitive style theory fits well overall with an interactional account of behavior and experience. A major assumption of this model is that hypnotic subjects are not passive responders. They actively cognize so as to fit their responses to the suggestions of the hypnotist, and frequently use problem-solving approaches to accomplish this goal. A second assumption is that the aptitudes and skills of the subject for hypnosis (in terms of imagery and other skills pertaining to hypnotizability) are important, but that their influence is modified substantially by the particular hypnotic situation or task that is presented (J. Jackson & Sheehan, 1986). Phenomenological evidence illustrates dramatically the operation of multiple streams of awareness in hypnotic subjects, and demonstrates marked differences in the ways that subjects process events while involved in hypnosis. Susceptible subjects clearly vary in the extent to which they may put a personal meaning or interpretation on the communication of the hypnotist, as well as in the degree to which they may manifest individuality or personal idiosyncrasy of response.

Specifically designed techniques of assessment are required to capture the multiple processes at work to account for this variability in response. The chapter turns now to describe the major types of techniques that have been used to investigate the phenomenological experience of hypnosis, and then focuses on the EAT in particular.

The Search for Meaningful Assessment

In 1979, Ronald Shor made an impassioned plea for research into hypnosis as a phenomenological experience, and the understanding of hypnosis as a complex subjective event. Experience was recognized by Shor as important and distinctive in its own right. Not unrelatedly, in the same year Nicholas Spanos and his associates (see Spanos & Chaves, 1989c) recorded "the danger of implicitly or explicitly assuming an equivalence between the treatments to which subjects are exposed and the nature of their experience" (Spanos, Radtke-Bodorik, Ferguson, & Jones, 1979, p. 290). More than 10 years later, Brian Fellows, in an analysis of content theories of hypnosis, concluded that "We are still very ignorant about how hypnotic procedures are perceived and what strategies are used to realize hypnotic phenomena" (Fellows, 1990, p. 89); the call here was for more basic, fine-grained research into the nature of hypnotic response and experience. When one surveys contemporary approaches to assessment in the literature, it seems that the major objectives of researchers are, on the one hand, to make the necessary detailed analysis of subjective experience, and, on the other, to do so by adopting methods that are as scientific and objective as possible.

Behavioral methods have obvious advantages in their appeal to publicly observable data, but they are limited in the extent to which they are able to focus on individual thoughts, images, and perceptions. The essential problems is that similar behavioral responses may occur for very different reasons. McConkey et al. (1989), for example, found very different styles for their two hypnotic subjects, who had equivalent susceptibility scores on two standard tests of hypnotizability. The subjects displayed essentially similar behavioral responses to the items; "despite this objective similarity, however, their post-experimental comments indicated that meaningful differences in subjective experience were [nevertheless] occurring" (p. 133).

Ultimately, appeal must be to verbal report. Verbal reports, however, are hazardous to interpret, and their alleged validity is frequently doubtful. On the one hand, Bates and Brigham (1990) point to the problem in their study of the Carleton Skills Training Program, when they suggest that verbal reports are as vulnerable to experimental demands as are objectively scored overt movements. On the other hand, when building in conditions designed to detect the influence of perceptions, attitudes, expectations, and motivations, the researcher has to be wary about losing the richness and variety of the very phenomena the experiment is designed to study. Furthermore, any undue emphasis on one type of factor may tend to conceal the presence of other influences.

When one is measuring subjective experience, the major challenge is to encourage and preserve the full range of responses that exist, while at the same time providing reliable and uncontaminated results. With these caveats in mind, there are some important questions that the phenomenological approach seems particularly well equipped to answer:

1. What distinguishes one individual's response from another's?
2. Is the hypnotic response simple or complex?
3. How does self-hypnosis (autohypnosis) relate to traditional hypnosis (heterohypnosis)?
4. What is the relevance of the interactions between subject aptitudes and the tasks being performed during hypnosis?
5. Are there distinct differences in patterns of responses to hypnotic tasks that exist among subjects with the same level of "hypnotizability"?
6. What personal attributes, or sets of attributes, correlate with traditional measures of hypnotic responsiveness?
7. How adequate are traditional measures of hypnotizability for assessing stylistic modes of response in the hypnotic setting?
8. What specific effects flow from variations in rapport between the hypnotist and the hypnotic subject?

9. What is the detailed character of the reported experiences of hypnotic phenomena, such as hallucinations, enhanced memory, amnesia, trance logic, and posthypnotic suggestions?
10. What outstanding negative or positive affect and associations are tied to personal memories uncovered during clinical hypnosis?

The Experiential Analysis Technique

The EAT seeks to address many of these questions. It allows for maximum flexibility in the reporting of data, and aims to encourage accuracy and honesty of response. Furthermore, it is as standardized and replicable as is commensurate with the nature of the data being collected. Attempts are made to reduce motivations that may be artifactually based on the hypnotic subject's relationship with the hypnotist. In addition, the data are analyzed in as objective a fashion as possible.

Some Antecedents of the Technique

Shor's Phenomenological Method

The method developed by Shor (1979) was an influential precursor to the EAT. Essentially, the method involves subjects' reporting retrospectively on their hypnotic experiences; these reports are then judged by a skilled examiner and rated according to specified criteria. The method aims at overcoming some of the problems inherent in the study of subjective experiences of hypnosis by attempting to elicit honest reports of experience and by rating these reports precisely.

Shor's original use of the method focused on the phenomenon of depth of hypnotic experience. But the method can equally well be applied to the study of a single hypnotic event, a number of hypnotic phenomena, self-hypnosis (see Fromm, Brown, Hurt, Oberlander, Boxer, & Pfeifer, 1981), or an entire hypnotic session. Specifically, the method assesses trance experience on eight distinct dimensions: trance, nonconscious involvement, archaic involvement, drowsiness, relaxation, vividness of imagery, absorption, and access to the unconscious. Judgments are based on the quality of experience, the main criterion being the degree of subjective conviction demonstrated by the hypnotic subject.

As argued earlier in this chapter, cognitive events during hypnosis are subtle and complex, and consequently are difficult to retrieve. Shor (1979) pointedly asserts that phenomenological data should not be used unless accurate recall has been established and is likely to remain. Thus his technique emphasizes the fact that special procedures are required to facilitate memory. The role of the examiner is seen as crucial to the outcomes of the technique. Shor asserts that the examiner must promote an atmosphere of open communication between himself or herself and the subject, who becomes a coinvestigator. The examiner is therefore a facilitator of immediate, accurate, and full response from the subject. Rapport with the subject is thus an essential condition for the technique to be applied correctly. At the same time, however, the examiner is seen as someone who should direct the flow of information by suitable questioning and should make judgments about the adequacy of each response.

The EAT, the development of which followed the construction of Shor's technique, shares with Shor's method its essential focus on the privacy of experience and on subjects as "investigators" of their own experience. Rather than emphasizing the multiple dimensions of hypnotic experience (judged in terms of processes such as imagery and dissociative capacity), however, the EAT focuses on the "reliving" of past events and on subjects' stylistic modes of cognitive processing. In doing so, it draws its origins from Kagan's method of Interpersonal Process Recall (IPR). I turn now to a brief consideration of this technique.

Interpersonal Process Recall

The procedures of the EAT are derived from the IPR method of Kagan, Krathwohl, and Miller (1963). This method in turn evolved from an observation that lecturers viewing video playbacks of their utterances often spontaneously reported many of the thoughts and concerns that had been going through their minds during these same events.

The IPR was developed as a learning tool for use in the counseling context, so that counselors in training could review and react to their contact with clients immediately after therapy sessions. An independent person, present at the review of each session, would inquire into the interaction between the counselor and client by stopping the tape and questioning the client about his or her underlying feelings and thoughts, thus facilitating and clarifying the information being recalled. Both clients and counselors benefited from this exercise. Evidence suggested, for example, that patients demonstrated greater insight into their experiences and showed increased ability to identify, label, and discuss the meaning of both their overt and their covert behavior; counselors learned more about the nature of their interactions with their clients (Kagan et al., 1963).

Prior to the establishment of the EAT in the literature (Sheehan et al., 1978), two studies acknowledged the use of the IPR in hypnosis. In the first of these, R. H. Woody, Krathwohl, Kagan, and Farquhar (1965) found that a combination of hypnosis and video technology both assisted and stimulated clients' recall in psychotherapy. In the second study, Hammer, Walker, and Diment (1978) specifically applied some of the IPR procedures to the study of hypnotic experience in an audiotape context. This study showed that the IPR technique was suited to detailing the subtleties of subjective hypnotic experience; it also demonstrated the availability of the data for more systematic analysis, thus highlighting the potential utility of Kagan's method for tapping the individual complexities of phenomenal events.

A Description of the Technique

In essence, the EAT consists of gathering the comments of hypnotic subjects about their hypnotic behavior and experience, as they view the video playback of their hypnotic sessions. The main stages of the process reflect the rationale of the method and are as follows (for more details, see Bell, 1978; Sheehan & McConkey, 1982; Sheehan et al., 1978):

1. The session between the hypnotist and the subject is videotaped.

2. The hypnotist introduces the subject to a second experimenter and leaves the test setting. The experimenter's role is primarily that of an independent inquirer who introduces the subject to the EAT session in a way that is designed to maximize the impact of the cues to recall. The instructions given by the inquirer at the beginning of the EAT session are prescribed as follows:

> In hypnosis research generally there is still wide interest in what actually does occur during hypnosis. In order to clarify what happened in your particular session, I am going to ask you to help us both by watching a videotape of things that happened during your hypnosis session.
>
> As [the hypnotist] told you at the beginning of the session, the hypnosis session has been videotaped, and we are going to play back that videotape now. Playing the videotape will provide for you a precise, detailed record of what happened and, therefore, you will probably find it easier to recall how you felt and what you thought, for instance, than you would if there were no playback of the videotape.
>
> Now, during your hypnotic session you probably felt and thought a lot of things that you didn't or weren't able to say aloud. Generally the mind works faster than the voice, for instance, and so there were probably times when you didn't have the time to say all you wanted. Perhaps also, you didn't want to tell some of the things to the hypnotist or else you might have just had some vague impressions or reactions or ideas that you weren't able to verbalize at the time. As you watch the videotape now, you'll find that these sorts of thoughts and feelings will come back to you. I want you to feel completely free to stop the videotape at any point and tell me about whatever it is that you are recalling. Anything at all that you recall, just stop the videotape right then and there and tell me about it, anything at all. It may be a little point that you remember or a bigger point that you wish to make. No matter how important you consider it to be, anytime you want to stop the videotape and comment is fine. All of your comments are important and valuable.
>
> It is important, though, that you stop the tape as soon as you want to comment on something. Don't wait till later but stop the videotape im-

mediately. It's a good idea to keep hold of this [stop–start switch] so that you can easily stop the playback. Okay, do you have any questions? Fine, if you're ready you can start the playback anytime you want. (Sheehan & McConkey, 1982, p. 84)[1]

3. The recording starts, and whenever the subject stops the tape, the inquirer records what the subject says. During the recording, the inquirer may attempt to solicit more information by using a set of standard probe questions relevant to the experience being studied. For a list of sample questions, see Table 13.1. Essentially, however, the objective is to let the subject (not the experimenter) reveal the nature of hypnotic experience.

4. The recorded data yielded by the EAT are analyzed for what they reveal about a subject's styles of response in hypnosis, and may be rated according to the particular concerns of the study conducted. Typically, also, multiple raters are used to index the reliability of the data.

Some Important Aspects of the Technique and the Role of the Inquirer

The EAT attempts in a number of ways to maintain independence from possible contaminating biases existing in the hypnotic testing. First, the inquirer and the hypnotist should be different people; the intent here is that the subject should not be constrained by the hypnotic relationship to react in a particular way during the playback session. Second, the inquirer typically should be unaware of the hypnotic performance of the subject, and so should have no preformed expectancies about the subject's hypnotic competencies. However, the video playback provides the inquirer with a literal and accurate record of what happened in the hypnotic session when he or she was not present. As in Shor's (1979) phenomenological method, the role of the inquirer is of critical importance to the success of the technique, although the nature of the role differs across the two methods. In the EAT, the inquirer specifically utilizes the skills of a nondirective counselor: paraphrasing, encouraging, and empathizing with the subject, and listening in a nonjudgmental fashion. The quality and quantity of subjective data derived from application of the method depend critically on a free and open atmosphere between the inquirer and hypnotic subject. If the rapport is poor, the response from the subject is likely to be inhibited, and the utility of the technique is thereby diminished.

In order to reduce the excessive influence of demand characteristics, the inquirer aims to provide subjects with minimal clues as to the nature of the information expected about the subjects' experiences. In practice, this means that questions used to probe for further information need to be appropriate to the content of the comments already made, rather than to the theoretical viewpoint or biases of the investigator. To this end, the

TABLE 13.1. Summary of EAT Inquiry Categories and Sample Questions

Inquiry categories	Sample questions
Cognitive	What were you thinking at the time? What thoughts were you having about the situation at that time? Were you consciously thinking about what was happening then? What was going on in your mind then?
Images	Were you having any fantasies at that moment? Were any pictures or images in your mind then? What was going on in your mind at that time? Did you imagine what the outcome might be?
Expectancies	What did you want to hear from the hypnotist? Were you expecting anything of the hypnotist at that point? What did you want to happen next? What were you expecting to happen next?
Image Presentation	How do you think you were coming across to the hypnotist? How did you want the hypnotist to see you at that point? What kind of image were you wanting to project? What message did you want to give the hypnotist?
Perceptions	How do you think the hypnotist was seeing you at that point? What did you think the hypnotist wanted at that point? How do you think the hypnotist felt about giving you this? Do you think your description of what took place would coincide with the hypnotist's?
Associations	What meaning did that have for you? Did this remind you of anything else you have experienced? Was this familiar to you? Did you connect that experience with anything in particular?
Sundry Feelings	How were you feeling about your involvement in the session at that point? What did you feel like doing? How were you feeling about your role as a subject at this point? What would you like to have said or done to the hypnotist at that point?
End of Session	What things did you learn from this recall session with the videotape? Did you like the "you" you saw on the screen? In retrospect, how do you think you felt about the hypnotist throughout the session? Were you satisfied with your behavior? Are there any parts you would like to see again? Did you enjoy talking about what you did in this way?

Note. Adapted from *Hypnosis and Experience: The Exploration of Phenomena and Process* (p. 86) by P. W. Sheehan and K. M. McConkey, 1982, Hillsdale, NJ: Erlbaum. Copyright 1982 by Lawrence Erlbaum Associates. Reprinted by permission of the publisher.

questions used are open-ended, brief, and tentative (see Table 13.1). Leading questions that may cue subjects as to what responses will satisfy the opinions of the inquirer are avoided.

In order to give the reader a feel for the technique and when it can be applied, the next section includes transcripts of parts of actual EAT sessions, taken from the literature. Examples illustrate both process and method in relation to the overall goal of the EAT, which is to clarify the meaning of hypnotic experiences.

The Technique in Use: Examples from the Literature

The examples chosen demonstrate how the EAT can be used to reveal a wide variety of aspects of hypnotic experience. Transcript segments have been selected that illustrate particularly interesting responses. It should be pointed out that the transcripts are not necessarily typical or atypical hypnotic records; rather, they uncover hitherto obscured or unreported aspects of hypnotic phenomena not generally highlighted in the literature. In all instances, subjects were watching videotapes of their own hypnotic sessions.

"Duality" during Age Regression

The concept of "duality" refers to the phenomenon of having simultaneous or alternating awareness of one's adult and childlike thoughts while experiencing age regression.

Laurence and Perry (1981), commenting on a study of the "hidden-observer" phenomenon in hypnosis (which includes duality in age regression), claim that "the verbal reports during the EAT inquiry convey the flavor of the differences between subjects reporting . . . duality in age regression, and the remaining subjects . . . whose regression was quasi-literal" (p. 338). "Quasi-literal" means, in this context, "as if literally" a child. The following examples of qualitative distinctions afforded by the EAT data (taken from Laurence & Perry, 1981, p. 338) are instructive about the likely processes underlying hypnotic responsiveness, and illustrate the major individual differences among hypnotic subjects themselves in their reaction to hypnotic age regression suggestions. The inquirer's questions are in parentheses.

Alternating Adult and Childlike Thinking

> The thing is . . . I was there, you know. It was as if I was there . . . but I wasn't very long: it came and went and it didn't stay. . . . I felt like I was . . . it

sort of felt like "What am I doing there?" and then the next thing I'm back there, and then "What am I doing here?" It felt like that. It felt like that I was looking at myself in a sense . . . something like you would do in a dream.

Quasi-Literal Experience

(Did you really feel you were 5 years old?) I had the feeling I was going with my mother. This is strange. I wasn't going to school yet so I felt 5½ on the verge of going for enrollment to school. (Did you have any sense of being adult at all?) I didn't have any sense of being an adult, no. (None at all?) None at all. (Not the slightest?) Not a fraction. No, nothing. (So you really felt you were 5 years old?) Yes.

Simultaneous Adult and Childlike Thinking

(Did you really feel you were 5 years old?) It was the same . . . it . . . especially when it came to writing my name again. I felt . . . you know, I was two people, one standing off looking at the other, and the other that was standing was saying, you idiot, you can write your name, why are you taking so long? Yet the one that's writing it is struggling away, to form these letters . . . can't. I'm trying the best I can.

Objective performance scales of hypnosis are not equipped to assess the fine-grained features of hypnotic responsiveness illustrated by these records. Hypnotic experience may illustrate either simultaneous or alternating states of consciousness, and both are distinct from quasi-literal experience. None, however, is necessarily more diagnostic of aptitude for hypnosis than another. We clearly need to know much more about stylistic features of experience if we are to properly assess the meaning of hypnotic performance.

Trance Logic

The next example is taken from Sheehan and McConkey (1982, pp. 142–144) and illustrates interesting features in the trance logic of a hypnotized subject. In this instance, the subject, who grew up in Germany, used German to the hypnotist, who was speaking in English. The example illustrates the subject's perception of the control of the hypnotist over the process, but also the use of questioning by the inquirer during an EAT session. The inquirer attempted to interact with the hypnotic subject to clarify the nature of her hypnotic experience. In this dialogue, "I" refers to the inquirer and "S" to the subject.

I: I noticed that you spoke in German to the hypnotist who was speaking in English. Do you have an explanation as to how that came about?

S: I could understand him all right. That was very natural.

I: It was natural for what [reason]?

S: That I could understand him. Like it's part, I don't know.

I: It is hard, I know. I can appreciate that. I suppose I'm just wondering whether you've got any thoughts on it at all.

S: No. I didn't think about it much. Put it that way.

I: Okay. You used the word "naturally." Are you able to say that it might have been natural that he would speak English and you would naturally understand [him]?

S: I think part of me was with him.

I: Okay. Can we just follow that for a little while? How was it that part of you was with him? In what sense was that?

S: The little girl who was there, who didn't like the teacher. It's very hard to explain. It was me and yet it was separate.

I: Right. And what's the part that was with the hypnotist?

S: Me.

I: What you're saying is that you could communicate with the hypnotist because part of you was with him.

S: It was really the hypnotist, who was sort of, well, really guiding. He was in control of this whole thing.

I: It seems to be a very difficult area for you.

S: Very difficult.

I: Yes.

S: It's very difficult to explain. It's almost as if I, well, part of me is there listening to him, but part of me is away from here. It was actually there all happening.

I: I find that really fascinating. Admittedly, we can't find explanations for all of it, but it happened.

S: Yes. Yes. [Starts tape.]

I: Good!

S: [Stops tape when hypnotist begins to count subject out of age-regressed situation. At this point, subject spontaneously interrupted the hypnotist.] I said it was snowing. I was still in the classroom while he was talking and I looked out of the window and snow was falling. And I thought it was such a pretty sight. And he said "You're going back," and I saw the snow and I thought "how beautiful it was" and I felt like saying, "Well, wait a minute. I just want to see the snow for a moment."

I: Just wait on because it's such a nice scene.

S: Mmm. I just wanted to watch that for a moment, and he was calling me back and I felt like saying, "Well, just a moment, you know!"

I: Just hang on a moment.

S: Yes. Yes.

I: Well, how come you didn't say that to him?

S: I was telling him that it was snowing.

I: Okay, but he didn't understand you.

S: Well, I guess at the time I thought he might.

I: How come he didn't pick up the fact that you were telling him that it was snowing?

S: Well, he didn't listen.

I: I mean if he's a sensitive sort of hypnotist he ought to have recognized that you said it was snowing [and] you'd like to stay there.

S: Well, maybe he was in a hurry. He tried to sort of, you know, rush things a little.

I: Yes. So, the fact you said to him, did he understand that?

S: Well, looking at it now, he probably didn't even understand what I was saying. But at the time, I certainly assumed that he'd understand what I'm saying.

I: Okay. So, at the time it seemed very correct that you should speak in the way that you did and that he ought to understand you.

S: Yes. Yes.

I: Okay. Looking back on it now, do you realize there's an explanation for what you've done?

S: Yes. It makes sense, now, but it didn't at the time.

I: Is that in perspective for you? Is there any conflict there?

S: No, not now.

I: Can you explain that for me?

S: At the time there was, you know, I was desperately trying to tell him that it was snowing and I'd just like to watch the snow for a moment. And he wouldn't listen to that, and he kept going, and eventually I thought, "Let it go," but now it makes sense. Obviously he couldn't understand what I was saying.

I: How did that affect you when you were actually saying to the hypnotist "it's snowing, it's snowing," and he didn't take any notice, or seem to take any notice?

S: You know, I just got a little bit tense because he didn't take notice of me.

I: Did you have any feelings about the fact that he didn't take notice of you?

S: Apart from feeling a little bit tense, and perhaps a little bit sad because I thought it was so beautiful. I hadn't seen snow for such a long time, you know, it was quite a novelty.

I: But you decided in the end to go with him?

S: I had no choice.

I: You had no choice. What makes you say that?

S: I guess he was, well, he was controlling the whole thing. He was telling me to, I don't know, he took me there and then he took me away from there. [Starts tape.]

I: Okay, good, fine.[2]

This example serves to illustrate a number of processes that underlie hypnotic experience. Duality, involuntariness, and seemingly paradoxical response interweave subtly with each other. The example illustrates the essential character of trance logic: The subject behaved (paradoxically) by talking in German as a small girl, while nevertheless clearly understanding the hypnotist, who spoke in English. The EAT data, however, reveal clearly that the subject herself (who was awake and reflecting on her experience) saw no incongruity at all in her hypnotic behavior. From her subjective point of view, her behavior was entirely predictable and logical. The data challenge current theoretical perspectives about trance logic. The incongruity we regularly theorize about, it seems, may reflect more the external observer's interpretation of what *seems* incongruous than any inherent process feature of the hypnotic experience itself.

Posthypnotic Amnesia

The examples that come next are from a study of posthypnotic amnesia (McConkey, Sheehan, & Cross, 1980, p. 104). While viewing videotapes of their behavior under hypnosis, a number of posthypnotically amnesic subjects commented spontaneously on the nature of their difficulties with recall, making distinctions that had not previously appeared in the literature. One subject said:

> All the words seem familiar, but I can't remember the sensations of it. . . . I sort of know these words, I think I've heard them before but it doesn't seem like me there . . . even when it happens, I have to believe it because it's there . . . but I can't sort of feel any of it . . . when I hear the voice I can sort of remember the words but I can't remember any of the sensations.

Another subject commented in a similar vein:

> I couldn't remember what had happened and when I saw it, it was just like new. . . . I remember [the hypnotist's] voice but I can't remember what happened . . . a couple of things came back to me but I couldn't remember the feeling as much as the movement . . . you know, I couldn't remember how I felt. . . . I couldn't really remember how I felt at the time, you know, my thoughts at the time.

The same distinction between behavioral and experiential memories was made by other amnesic subjects in different ways.

These amnesic subjects showed a consistent inability to recall ahead of the particular item they were viewing at any given time. Also, they seemed to need a particular cue to occur before they could remember the item presently being viewed. However, the amnesic subjects differed in the nature of their memories after viewing the videotape. Some indicated that they had knowledge of the events of the videotape, but could not access that knowledge. As one subject put it when commenting about her inability to recall the events of the videotape,

> It was just too much of an effort to remember anything. . . . I was trying to concentrate. . . . I know that I could have remembered if I really tried . . . it wasn't as if I'd forgotten it for good.

Reports of these kinds illustrate tangibly the multidimensional nature of amnesic experience. Forgetting in hypnosis is not simply the act of not remembering. Posthypnotically amnesic subjects may be conscious of remembering but may simply be unable to say so; they may forget and yet think they can remember (when they cannot); or they may fail mainly to make the effort to recall. The EAT data illustrate compellingly the multifactorial nature of hypnotic experience conceptualized long ago by Shor (1962), and highlight again the inadequacy of simple performance scales for tapping the inherently complex processes that underlie hypnotically suggested amnesic experience.

The next example focuses more on some of the procedural implications of the EAT, and relates them to a third phenomenon of hypnotic suggestion—the acceptance of false information suggested in hypnosis.

Pseudomemories: Using a Modification of the Technique

Laurence (1979) diverged from the standard EAT procedure of having the subject control the stopping of the videotape recorder. In this study, the recorder was stopped by the experimenter at predetermined points in order to obtain answers to a set of standard questions. This raises the possibility of subjects' being cued by the questions asked. Direction can be useful at times, however, and may serve the purposes of particular experimental designs. In order to guard against the subtle influence of demand characteristics on the judgments by raters of audiotaped data, tapes can be examined by independent raters who are unaware of the hypothesis of the experiment. Bryant and McConkey (1989a), for example, used this safeguard in their experiment on hypnotic blindness.

It is important, however, to sound a note of caution about the use of the more structured EAT viewing session. Laurence (1979) noted that much of the complexity of a hypnotized subject's experience is lost by structuring the inquiry session and limiting the analysis to questions concerning specific dimensions. Imposing structure on the inquiry session has a somewhat inhibiting influence on the degree to which subjects report their experiences; subjects generally restrict their comments in these circumstances to the material that the experimenter has indicated as being of interest. Thus there is a genuine danger of losing unanticipated pieces of information that may be relevant, as well as increased vulnerability to the influence of demand characteristics.

Recently, Labelle, Laurence, Nadon, and Perry (1990) investigated memory creation in hypnosis, using Laurence's modification of the EAT. They found that under appropriate conditions, personal attributes (e.g., absorption ability and facility for vivid imagery) predisposed people to confuse imagined noises suggested during hypnosis with reality. This led them to report "pseudomemories" as real memories. A crucial part of the investigation was to determine whether subjects really believed in the reality of the suggested noises or not. This was the point at which the researchers thought it appropriate to use a more structured version of the EAT. Preselected segments of videotaped material were presented to subjects and their comments were invited; the inquirer's task was to determine the validity of the pseudomemories.

A Clinical Application: The Hallucinatory Playback Version of the Technique

Salzman (1982) has devised another modification of the EAT for use in the clinical setting, where it can be adopted to aid recall in hypnotherapy. This version draws on the synthesizing or constructive aspects of subjects' fantasy. The indications are that this modification of the EAT can be clinically useful in facilitating vivid recall of therapy-related events. After termination of a hypnotherapy session, the client is subsequently put back into trance, with the prior suggestion that the client will watch a hallucinated (rather than real) playback of the events of the hypnotic session as it unfolds. The client is then requested to keep watching the scene and stop the imaginary recorder when he or she wants to comment; the hypnotist is told by the client when this is happening, and the hypnotist then listens to and records the client's comments. In this way, the posthypnotic context provides an opportunity for clients to distance themselves, so that preceding events can be replayed with some detachment.

There are advantages to this particular extension of the EAT for clinicians. It does not require the use of expensive equipment; it does not risk making clients anxious about the videotaping of very personal information; clients and therapists are not inhibited by the thought of a "hidden audience"; it does not involve the intrusion of a third party (the inquirer) into the therapeutic process; and, as noted above, it utilizes the positive, constructive aspects of clients' potential for fantasizing.

Other Applications

Table 13.2 lists some of the major uses of the EAT that have been published in the literature and the findings associated with these applications. The discussion now turns to considering other reporting techniques that have been used and evaluating them against the phenomenological model of hypnosis, as illustrated by the EAT.

Evaluation of Different Reporting Techniques

Phenomenological Inquiry and Convergence on Structure

By now there is considerable convergence in the literature on the significance and relevance of phenomenological inquiry, and this convergence stretches across the analysis of both heterohypnosis and autohypnosis. The Chicago paradigm (Fromm & Kahn, 1990), for example, offers an integrated methodology that challenges the assumption that the phenomena of autohypnosis are the same as those of heterohypnosis. The paradigm is oriented around analysis of the structure, content, and context of self-hypnosis, and derives its data from both qualitative and quantitative sources. Scoring categories, developed from the quantitative results of self-hypnosis questionnaires, are used in the analyses of diaries that provide the essential phenomenological data. In the development of the paradigm, subjects were required to keep diaries or journals following daily self-hypnosis sessions; these subjective reports of subjects were used as idiosyncratic data for full description and identification of the phenomena of self-hypnosis. The procedures are more structured than those of the EAT, but the methodology shares with the EAT and Shor's (1979) phenomenological method the use of introspective reports to help elucidate variations in experience. Its records, like those of other paradigms (including the EAT), typically illustrate high imaginative involvement, strong absorption, and at times strong emotion. Across techniques (see the discussion of the EAT examples, above), there are also substantial indications of the alteration of attentional processes. Shor's phenomenological method, Fromm and Kahn's diary methodology, and the EAT all involve procedures of assessment that yield, in a spontaneous way, conscious and unconscious material that can be related meaningfully to suggestions. Though autohypnosis and heterohypnosis are obviously not the same, the data nevertheless indicate substantial commonality with respect to the overall structure of hypnotic experience.

Common implications for process are also echoed in the application of the different techniques. The EAT, Shor's (1979) phenomenological method, and the Chicago paradigm (Fromm & Kahn, 1990) all clearly confirm, for example, the multidimensional nature of hypnotic experience.

TABLE 13.2. A Sampling of Applications of the EAT (Standard and Modified)

Reference	Topic	Major finding
	Standard EAT	
Sheehan, Statham, & Jamieson (1991b)	Factors affecting hypnotically involved pseudomemories	Pseudomemories influenced by both state (hypnosis) instruction and level of susceptibility for EAT (experience-derived scores).
Labelle, Laurence, Nadon, & Perry (1990)	Pseudomemories and imagic thinking	Pseudomemories created in high susceptibles only
Bryant & McConkey (1989a,b)	Hypnotic blindness	Blindness not due to demand characteristics; attribution supported false beliefs confirming hypnotic experiences
Sheehan & Statham (1989)	Pseudomemories and their acceptance	Interaction between trait and context factors in accepting pseudomemories
McCann & Sheehan (1987)	Breaching of pseudomemory under hypnosis	Original memory reversibly linked to pseudomemory
J. Jackson & Sheehan (1986)	Individual differences, imaging, and hypnotic susceptibility	Low and high susceptibles demonstrated intense imaginative involvement
Spanos, de Groot, Tiller, Weekes, & Bertrand (1985)	Trance logic, duality, and hidden-observer response	Cognitive activities underlying duality reports unrelated to hidden-observer responding
McConkey (1984)	Indirect suggestions	Individual variation in positive responses to indirect suggestion not a function of susceptibility
Sheehan (1982–1983)	Imaginative consciousness	High susceptibles showed more variation in cognitive strategies than low susceptibles
	Modified EAT	
Salzman (1982)	Clinical application (imaginary EAT, or IEAT) of EAT	IEAT of value in clinical cases for identifying anxiety-associated material
Nogrady, McConkey, Laurence, & Perry (1983)	Dissociation and duality in hypnosis studied in structured version of technique	Highly susceptible subjects were distinctive in their reports of multiple levels of awareness during hypnosis

There may be distinctive emphases in each (e.g., the EAT focuses on the relevance of styles of responding, whereas the Chicago paradigm emphasizes modes of ego functioning). But the evidence is strong across all of the techniques that hypnosis is not unidimensional in character and that the phenomena characterizing hypnotic responsiveness cannot be adequately tapped by objective, actuarial instruments of assessment alone.

Methodologies such as Shor's phenomenological method, the EAT, and the Chicago paradigm necessarily place strong emphasis on the relevance of hypnotic depth. There are alternative measures of depth, however (for a review of them, see Sheehan & McConkey, 1982). One is Field's (1965) Inventory Scale of Hypnotic Depth, in which subjects respond to 38 questions about various phenomena they may have experienced during the course of hypnosis. By virtue, however, of its emphasis on what people report generally about being hypnotized (Tart, 1979), this measure yields a rather more general assessment of trance experience than measures such as those reviewed in this chapter, which are characterized by a more specific assessment focus.

In any consideration of reporting procedures and techniques assessing subjective experience in the field of hypnosis, it is important to note that the literature encompasses a wide range of theoretical positions and research interests. It is not surprising, therefore, to find a wide variety of ways in which the subjective experience of hypnosis has been reported and discussed.

The most obvious distinction between methods of reporting subjective experience is the one between methods that emphasize the qualitative side of the experience and those that attempt to quantify experience. Open-ended techniques (e.g., Eiblmayr, 1987; Fromm & Kahn, 1990; Kihlstrom, Easton, & Shor, 1983) aim for a comprehensive survey of subjective experience. Experiments using more directive techniques, such as those that ask subjects to make specific response choices (e.g., Bartis & Zamansky, 1990; Pekala & Kumar, 1989; Schuyler & Coe, 1989), tend to focus on finding or testing for relationships between specific variables, subjective responsiveness being one of those investigated.

Let us consider first the emphasis on qualitative data. Experiments in this area have found that a major factor determining the quality of data produced is the degree of attention paid to controlling the influences that shape or distort the reporting context. A major influence in this respect is the rapport between hypnotist and subject.

Rapport

Evidence indicates that the subject has special motivations to please the hypnotist during a hypnotic session (Sheehan, 1971b, 1980), and rapport effects may clearly affect the reporting of subjective experience. One precaution against the occurrence of unwanted effects is to ensure that the hypnotist does not gather the data on which the assessment of experience rests. Another is to remove the hypnotist from the hypnosis session. This second option is obviously only available for autohypnosis rather than heterohypnosis studies; it was used in the landmark studies of Fromm and Kahn (1990) on self-hypnosis.

A particular rapport effect that may be operating in the response setting may arise from the data collector's actively fostering a cooperative and empathic relationship with the subject, in order to enhance both the quality and quantity of information. Rapport influences of this kind will increase the chances of the subject's responding in accord with the demand characteristics (Orne, 1969) of the overall experimental (or clinical) situation. In these instances, it becomes necessary to adopt procedures to take account of subjects' possible guessing of the biases of the experimenter and/or hypotheses of the experiment. The data collector may provide an obvious (though misleading) experimental rationale for the session, or may find an effective way of structuring the session to allow for the operation of demand characteristics. Experimenters have differing preferences for dealing with this type of influence and sometimes use a combination of methods. They may, for example, disguise the true aims of the experiment, and/or test for possible demand characteristic effects by including a pseudocontrol group that is strongly motivated to respond for nonexperimental reasons. The logic behind this latter strategy is well documented elsewhere (Orne, 1979a).

A number of procedures are available to tap the important dimension of rapport. One such measure is the Archaic Involvement Measure (AIM; M. R. Nash & Spinler, 1989). This test uses items derived from Shor's (1962) theoretical propositions and focuses on transference-like experiences among hypnotic subjects. The measure is positively correlated with behavioral responsiveness across the spectrum of hypnotizability, and scores on the test measure relevant aspects of hypnotic experience among high hypnotizable subjects.

Another important effect of rapport is the phenomenon of "countering" (Sheehan, 1971b, 1980), a process that M. R. Nash and Spinler (1989) argue may be related to subjects' performance on the AIM. Countering is a subject's responding in accord with the wishes of the hypnotist when social influences to respond otherwise are also present in the situation. For example, when subjects are faced during hypnosis with conflict between a nonhypnotic expectancy of how to behave and the hypnotist's apparent suggestion of how to behave, the subjects may ignore their preconception and "counter" the learned response, in order to respond in accord with the perceived wishes of the hypnotist. There are two intriguing findings in the data that relate to this phenomenon. The first is that counterers display a constructive (i.e., active and idiosyncratic) style of cognizing, which enables them to make personal sense of the conflicting demands by preserving the integrity of each (see "Cognitive Styles," above).

The second finding is that counterers, even though they demonstrate a higher degree of involvement with the hypnotist, fail reliably to score as highly on standard tests of susceptibility (e.g., the Stanford Hypnotic Susceptibility Scale, Form C) as subjects who do not counter (Sheehan, 1980). This second finding points to differential effects of rapport on subjects that are not explicable in terms of level of hypnotic susceptibility or simple willingness to comply with anticipated, obvious suggestions. Techniques like the EAT, which are sensitively attuned to detect the personal commitment of subjects to the hypnotist, are needed to detect subtle processes of this kind. It is difficult to see that techniques stressing objective, quantifiable responses, to the exclusion of subjective assessment, can be at all adequate for this task. Essentially, the "experience of the relationship" is what must be tapped to obtain a proper measure of rapport.

Properties of Qualitative and Quantitative Assessment

Another aspect of preserving the benefits of qualitative data is that the coding or categorizing of such data must be made as replicable as possible. For example, Lynn, Nash, Rhue, Frauman and Stanley (1983) scored essays obtained according to methods described by Spanos and Bodorik (1977), by using certain categories of sensation and summed sensation words to achieve specific scores. The use of raters who were unaware of the hypotheses of the experiment helped to guarantee consistency and to guard against ratings' being contaminated by experimenter bias.

A particular problem exists in regard to subjective data that are collected retrospectively (i.e., after the hypnotic session). Whole series of hypnotic events are typically experienced in the testing of hypnotic susceptibility, and the opportunity for distorted recall of what happened "after the event" is thus extensive. The special advantage of the EAT is that viewing the video recording refreshes the subject's memory, and so facilitates accurate recall of the physical events that actually occurred. A context is thus established for sensitively studying or assessing accompanying subjective events. Memories, however, may be available but still significantly distorted by subsequent or preceding events. Perry and Laurence (1980), for example, noticed that estimates of hypnotic depth are not necessarily spontaneous, but are "pegged" to the success or failure of responses to preceding hypnotic tasks. Kahn, Fromm, Lombard, and Sossi (1989), in a study of hypnotic depth, also pointed out that ratings of trance depth may influence subsequent ratings. The effects of subsequent responding is likely to be reduced by viewing a tape of the proceedings, as in the EAT, but effects of preceding tasks may still occur.

One further major advantage of qualitative methods is that they can be used to distinguish at times between groups when there is no apparent behavioral difference in response. In their study of hypnotic blindness, for example, Bryant and McConkey (1989a) found no significant differences in behavioral response among subjects. When subjects were separated into two groups on the basis of their reports of subjective experience, however, differences emerged. Analysis then showed that the speed of responding differed significantly between these two groups.

I turn now to those reporting techniques that emphasize the need to quantify responses. A number of relevant issues are highlighted in the literature. The first relates to the choice of type of scale to be used for the subject's report. P. G. Bowers, Laurence, and Hart (1988) point out the inadequacies of some forced-choice scales in which the options that are available to subjects do not cover the range of possible responses. Subjects, perceiving that they are obliged to use one or other of the options that are available to them (despite their irrelevance to what has been experienced), may use the scales in idiosyncratic ways that are potentially misleading (P. G. Bowers et al., 1988). These investigators opt for using a choice scale with an appropriate range of descriptor options. They prefer this to adopting Likert-type bipolar scales or numerical ratings, on the grounds that using descriptors provides more differentiation of response. In addition, they recommend the EAT as a "solid base" for producing these descriptors (p. 347).

Results in the "either–or" format have to be treated with some caution, bcause they may mask important differences in individual responses. For example, "yes–no" reports and even Likert-type scale ratings of involuntariness can at times conceal legitimate responses and distort judgments made on the basis of the data obtained. It is difficult to see how a subject can indicate the complex nature of a response on a simple dichotomous scale or a unidimensional scale of extent of effect. More sensitive techniques such as the EAT seem necessary to assess the subtle variations in response that occur.

When there are behavioral–subjective response mismatches in data, or when results are puzzling, a more in-depth, qualitative approach is strongly indicated. Positive rating scales appear incapable of uncovering sufficient individual variability to further our understanding of the phenomena under investigation. For example, substantial gains in susceptibility to hypnosis have been demonstrated in the work of Spanos and his associates (e.g., Spanos & Flynn, 1989a), but not in all subjects of the same level of initial susceptibility. Making a more detailed study of the "intransigents" with a qualitative approach such as the EAT may add considerably to our understanding of the underlying processes at work.

Finally, in any consideration of what measures of experience are appropriate for what purposes, the importance of establishing reliability, validity, and standardization of the data must be acknowledged. Significantly, Kirsch, Council, and Wickless (1990) assert that ad hoc subjective scoring systems do not have the uniformity and rigor of standardization necessary for close interlaboratory comparisons. In this respect, it is relevant to note that data on the reliability and validity of the EAT have been collected and are reported elsewhere (Sheehan & McConkey, 1982).

Summary, Comment, and Conclusions

The position of this chapter is that an understanding of what a hypnotized person perceives is fundamentally important to our explanation of hypnotic experience and events. As Tart (1979) argues, a significant internal experience is not reliably reflected in overt behavior. Experience cannot simply be observed objectively; it may not be reported spontaneously by the experiencer; and it may not even be elicited through ordinary forms of interaction. Frequently, it needs to be judiciously sought, and its meaning to the hypnotized person discovered, through appropriate techniques of assessment. Meaning to the participant is at the root of the phenomenological approach, and as Fromm (1975b) has argued elsewhere, study of the phenomenology of hypnosis is an idea whose time has come. Phenomenology is no longer a forbidding and risky province (Fromm et al., 1981; see also L. S. Johnson, 1981). It is central to our understanding of psychology (E. R. Hilgard, 1977c).

What phenomenological research has shown over the last decade is that hypnotic experience is both multifaceted and complex. It has given us a view of the hypnotic subject as a person who participates actively in the hypnotic process, who is susceptible to the influence of motivations and expectations, and who employs a variety of cognitive strategies so as to manage and respond to multiple levels of communication received in the hypnotic setting. Standard techniques of assessment, especially those emphasizing the primacy of behavioral data and those offering structured choices, are not equipped to reveal the full meaning of hypnotic responsiveness.

A major problem in phenomenological research is that, since the precise nature of underlying hypnotic experience is not well understood, the instruments routinely available to us to assess subjective experience are frequently not sensitive to the task of illustrating genuine individual variation in response. If an instrument of assessment assumes a unidimensional underlying process when there are multiple dimensions operating, then that instrument will produce equivalent ratings for very different experiences, and thus will be deficient in measuring overall experience. Measurement of trance depth poses just such a problem, and measurement of hypnotic experience in its full complexity even more so.

The EAT was designed with the specific purpose of revealing the full complexity of hypnosis. It assumes the primacy of experience and is based on the phenomenological model of hypnosis, which emphasizes what is perceived rather than what is real. It is a rich and sensitive instrument of assessment, and a very useful tool for analyzing the meaning of hypnosis. Stressing style as opposed to competency of response, it is sensitively attuned to measuring variability in response both within and across subjects responding to suggestion in the hypnotic setting. Although it is limited by the absence of rigor that characterizes more objective modes of assessment, it nevertheless carries specific advantages that can enrich our understanding of hypnosis.

Acknowledgments

I wish to thank Rosemary Robertson and Patricia Truesdale for their help in the preparation of this chapter. Research for the chapter was supported in part by a grant from the Australian Research Council.

Notes

1. The instructions are reprinted from *Hypnosis and Experienced: The Exploration of Phenomena and Process* (p. 84) by P. W. Sheehan and K. M. McConkey, 1982, Hillsdale, NJ: Erlbaum. Copyright 1982 by Lawrence Erlbaum Associates. Reprinted by permission of the publisher.

2. The dialogue is reprinted from *Hypnosis and Experience: The Exploration of Phenomena and Process* (pp. 142–144) by P. W. Sheehan and K. M. McConkey, 1982, Hillsdale, NJ: Erlbaum. Copyright 1982 by Lawrence Erlbaum Associates. Reprinted by permission of the publisher.

CHAPTER FOURTEEN

Self-Hypnosis, Personality, and the Experiential Method

STEPHEN KAHN
ERIKA FROMM

The study of self-hypnosis (SH) is a new way to explore the phenomena of the general field of hypnosis. It also creates a new perspective for viewing the different facets of personality and the unfolding of the self.[1] Although SH has been utilized in clinical practice for many years, no systematic exploration of its phenomena was undertaken until the 1970s. In 1972, our research group—Erika Fromm and her colleagues—began investigating SH at the University of Chicago. The research, which came to be known as the "Chicago paradigm" (L. S. Johnson, 1981), not only represented an experimental foray into a little-studied area; it also utilized a methodology that has yielded some very promising results. With this approach, referred to here as the "experiential method," clear and powerful relationships between personality and different aspects of SH have emerged. Parts of the self that can unfold and develop in the practice of SH have been identified.

The research conducted at Chicago over almost two decades began by examining the basic SH experience, first in its own right, and then later as compared to hypnotist-present hypnosis. As the research progressed, the methodology became more refined, and the study expanded to include richer details of the SH experience as well as the involvement of personality and the self. Through this refinement and expansion, a picture of the kind of individual who is more talented in SH and the aspects of trance allowing the self to unfold has emerged with greater clarity.

The Experiential Method and the Definition of Self-Hypnosis

Hypnosis has been defined as an altered state of consciousness in which absorption in internal experience becomes more profound while perceptions of the external environment are diminished or changed (D. P.

Brown & Fromm, 1986, pp. 3–4). These authors outline some of the changes that are characteristically involved: increased memory and imagery; dissociation; the deployment of different modes of attention; a more tranquil state of mind and body; perceived involuntarism; incongruous (trance) logic; and time distortion. These features are common to the experiences of heterohypnosis (HH) and SH. But how is SH conceived of as distinct from HH? The method of assessing these states—the experiential method—can shed some light on the differences.

In our research, we used two types of experiential approaches. The first is based on subjects' own retrospective assessment of their experiences. The second involves a deeper level of analysis, which enlists subjects as scientific collaborators in understanding their experience and in delineating its underlying structure and dimensions. We used both of these approaches to study SH. Ronald Shor (1979) outlined the experiential method for measuring hypnotic phenomena more systematically, and called the two approaches the "subjective approach" and the "phenomenological approach," respectively.

Utilizing this method meant establishing a different perspective and proceeding from a different set of assumptions with respect to the definition of SH. "Self-initiated SH" was defined as hypnotic experiences in the absence of a hypnotist that originate with and are generated by the subject. Rather than simply mimicking the procedure and technique of the hypnotist, the individual is encouraged to induce, manage, and direct his or her own trance. This version of SH should give greater freedom to the individual and permit the exploration of the inner experience of the person.

This experiential approach represented a break from the more traditional line of research in hypnosis. Ruch (1975) and L. S. Johnson (L. S. Johnson & Weight, 1976; L. S. Johnson, Dawson, Clark, & Sikorsky, 1983) have defined SH as hypnotic experiences induced and maintained through the subject's giving himself or herself the suggestions—suggestions, however, that are prescribed by the hypnotist. The hypnotist may or may not be present when the subject gives the suggestions. Ruch's and Johnson's experiments have focused more on the specific *behaviors* that are readily observed and assessed. Defining SH in this manner makes it less likely that differences will be found between SH and standard hypnosis. Our group, on the other hand, has defined SH in a way that allows subjects to maximize their individual experiences. The next section examines definitions of hypnosis and SH by organizing them according to how much of the self is involved in the experience.

Hypnosis and the Involvement of Self

The definition of hypnosis and therefore of SH is based on the assumptions about reality that are made and the perspective that is taken. The culture in which one lives provides the basic template of experience by consensually validating a set of assumptions for framing reality. Attending to certain aspects of reality enhances or creates one kind of experience, while attending to different aspects of the same reality can create a completely different kind of experience. Although Western culture now validates hypnosis as a legitimate phenomenon, each individual's experience of hypnosis can be very different. Within our culture, some individuals consider hypnosis to involve a total loss of both consciousness and control. Control is given over to the hypnotist, whose capabilities and skills cause or at the very least facilitate the subject's response. At the opposite end of the spectrum, hypnosis is conceived of as an active rather than a passive or purely receptive state, in which an individual can creatively shape his or her own response.

Particularly since the end of World War II, changes in the way hypnosis has been viewed have occurred. Both hypnotists and subjects have been influenced by these changes. Up until this time, hypnosis meant that the hypnotist took an authoritarian stance toward the subject, with style, content, wording, and intonation reflecting this stance. The subject as well as the hypnotist maintained this perspective. The subject believed that hypnosis meant somehow surrendering his or her will and even consciousness to the hypnotist. However, with the evolution of a more permissive approach, hypnotists began to view themselves as collaborators in or facilitators of the hypnotic experience. Many hypnotists now see themselves as providing direction and enhancement for the subjects' own capability, and the subjects as the repositories of the necessary talent for the hypnotic experience. The various beliefs about hypnosis today run the entire gamut from viewing it as a more passive state to seeing it as an ego-active or ego-receptive state, with the majority of those practicing it taking the latter viewpoint.

Thus, the differences in beliefs about hypnosis generate differences in the experience. In speaking of hypnosis, it may be more helpful to speak of different *kinds* of experience a subject may undergo. Hypnosis is characterized by different levels of involvement of the self (the subject) and the other (the hypnotist). At one end of the spectrum, hypnosis is controlled and directed by the hypnotist. At the other end, the phenomenon is qualitatively different; the self initiates and directs the process. (See Figure 14.1.) It is useful to view *all* hypnosis, both HH and SH, as falling along this continuum of initiation. The kind of hypnosis that emerges is predicated upon who directs the experience. Needless to say, both ends of the spectrum share the aspects of hypnosis as an altered state of consciousness that have been outlined above.

At either end of this continuum, neither the self (the subject) nor the other (the hypnotist) entirely predominates. When the hypnotist is the one who is primarily directing the experience, the self—although less salient— is never entirely absent. At the opposite end of the spectrum, where the self is initiating and directing the hypnosis, some aspects of the other are there, too, structuring the experience. In the former instance, where the

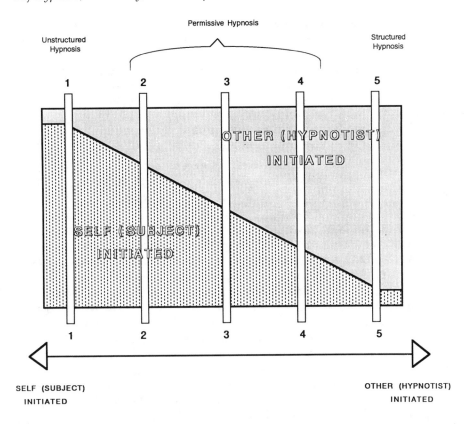

FIGURE 14.1. Continuum of self (subject) and other (hypnotist) involvement in hypnosis. Adapted from *Self-Hypnosis: The Chicago Paradigm* (p. 221) by E. Fromm and S. Kahn, 1990, New York: Guilford Press. Copyright 1990 by The Guilford Press. Adapted by permission.

hypnotist predominates, the self still colors the experience, even when the individual believes that his or her will and consciousness have been given over to a forceful and authoritarian other. The concept of the "hidden observer" suggests that the self remains on another level. In addition, the fantasies or images suggested by the hypnotist are imbued to a degree by the self with its own idiosyncratic aspects.

When the self predominates, the experience cannot be *entirely* initiated by the subject, because the subject's beliefs and expectations have been shaped and colored not only by the culture in which he or she lives, but by exposure to various kinds of hypnosis. Even with spontaneously occurring hypnosis, where the trance is entirely self-initiated, the individual's construction and comprehension of what has occurred are based on culturally shared definitions. If the cultural basis of the experience were absent, this might be the purest form of self-initiated hypnosis. However, it would be difficult for the individual to construe what has happened, and even more difficult to describe it to others.

There are two points to be made about the continuum depicted in Figure 14.1. First, just as depth fluctuates during trance, so too do the relative amounts of the self versus the other that are involved. At any point during trance, one can locate the kind of experience along the continuum. The fluctuations of self versus other can be small; they can cluster at one position along the continuum. However, they do not remain static. For example, a permissive hypnotist can utilize silence during trance to enhance the subject's private thoughts, fantasies, and suggestions. But a hypnotist who suggests and directs may move the experience more toward the hypnotist-initiated end of the spectrum.

Second, this continuum is *not* based on the presence or absence of the hypnotist. We have been able to show that an individual can achieve a deep state of hypnosis in the absence of a hypnotist (Fromm & Kahn, 1990). The question is what *kind* of hypnosis is achieved. That is, is it more "other-initiated" (Point 5 in Figure 14.1) or more "self-initiated" (Point 1)? At Point 5 on the spectrum, with the hypnotist present, the structure provided can be used to create an experience that adheres closely to what the hypnotist is suggesting. In the absence of structure, an individual can create an experience based on direction provided by the self (Point 1). But hypnosis with the hypnotist absent is not necessarily to be found at Point 1 and the more traditional kind of hypnosis (even with the hypnotist present) at Point 5, although it is certainly more likely. Some subjects can engage in self-directed experiences despite the intrusive presence of an authoritarian hypnotist. And other subjects, without a hypnotist, can vividly imagine the presence of one and can create a very rigidly defined and constricted experience based on suggestions and responses enacted "as if" hypnotist and structure were very much present.

How is the hypnotic experience different at the two ends of the spectrum? Over almost two decades, our research group endeavored to isolate and describe the differences in the hypnotic experience at each end of the spectrum. We defined the kind of hypnosis at Point 5 (other-initiated) as HH, and the kind of hypnosis at Point 1 (self-initiated) as SH. Thus, SH was considered to be hypnosis engendered by both self-directed suggestions and self-directed responses. The investigation focused on the *experiential* aspects of SH rather than the behavioral ones. The subjects in these studies were given a standard set of instructions for "laboratory-defined hypnosis," but were encouraged to use these only as a point of departure for exploring SH. This gave freer rein to the self and opened up the possibility for all to experience SH at Point 1 on the spectrum. The differences that emerged between these two forms of hypnosis and the evolution of the approach to examining them are outlined in the next section.

Experiential Research

The research conducted by our group (Fromm & Kahn, 1990) over nearly 20 years fell into three distinct phases. Although each successive phase explored the phenomena of SH more systematically and fully, the results of all three were comparable. The first phase involved conceptualization and preliminary or pilot studies spanning the years from 1972 to 1975. In the second phase, extensive questionnaires based on ideas that had been gleaned from the results of the pilot studies were created, administered, and analyzed. In these questionnaires, the subjects were asked to judge retrospectively how much or how little of various phenomena they had experienced during SH. This phase represented the subjective approach discussed above; it lasted from 1975 until 1981 (Fromm, Brown, Hurt, Oberlander, Boxer, & Pfeifer, 1981). The third phase, spanning the years 1982 to 1990, focused on the analysis of SH experiences as chronicled in daily diary entries. Through analyzing the diary entries each subject had to make immediately after each SH session, we isolated patterns and themes and examined the process of the immediate experience. This analysis represented the phenomenological approach. In order to give readers a full idea of the research and the method, we now outline the specifics of the approach.

Phase I, 1972–1975

During the pilot phase, two separate studies were performed. In the first, 36 male and female students at the University of Chicago were given hypnotic experiences at each end of the spectrum—one with the hypnotist present and directing the subject, and the other without the hypnotist. Each session lasted 90 minutes. To assess individual experience, an unstructured interview took place after the two trances. The second study, performed about a year later, attempted to broaden the experience on the SH end of the spectrum. Three male and three female subjects[2] were given three standard hypnosis experiences. For the next 4 weeks, they induced SH each day and chronicled their SH experiences in daily journal entries. A number of results emerged from these preliminary studies. First, in SH, the ego seemed to be subdivided to an even greater extent than in standard hypnosis. While in HH, the ego appeared to divide into an observing and an experiencing part; in SH another part was added—the "director." This directing and suggesting self seemed to become prominent in SH.

Second, we found that imagery appeared to be even more important in SH than in HH. Both vivid, reality-oriented imagery and primary-process, highly fantastic imagery (both of which came to be included later in our Imagery Production variable) were at the heart of the SH experience, even more so than in standard hypnosis. Third, the variable of Ego

Receptivity (Deikman, 1971) turned out to be a prominent feature of SH. Ego Receptivity is a mode of consciousness in which unconscious and preconscious material is allowed to emerge into awareness as the ego temporarily relinquishes deliberate control of internal experience, critical judgment, and goal-directed activity. Fourth, only the highly hypnotizable subjects were able to discriminate clearly between the two hypnotic states, HH and SH.

Finally, there were findings suggesting the influence of personality on the experience of SH: Some subjects, though clearly highly hypnotizable by someone else (as shown on the Stanford Hypnotic Susceptibility Scales given to all), could not attain more than very light SH states. These findings set the stage for the study of the effects of personality on SH in the next two phases.

Phase II, 1976–1981

During Phase II, findings from Phase I generated working hypotheses that could be explored more fully and tested in detail.

Sample Selection

Fifty-eight highly hypnotizable subjects were selected from an original group of 425 volunteers on the basis of (1) high hypnotizability and (2) freedom from psychopathology. The subjects who scored 9 or better on the Harvard Group Scale of Hypnotic Susceptibility (HGSHS:A; Shor & Orne, 1962) and on the Stanford Hypnotic Susceptibility Scale, Form C (SHSS:C; Weitzenhoffer & Hilgard, 1962) were administered the Rorschach (Rorschach, 1954) to screen out those with more or less serious emotional disorders. The 58 normal, highly susceptible individuals were chosen for participation in the SH experimental study because the pilot studies had indicated that these subjects would be the most capable of making distinctions and discriminations among the various kinds of hypnotic states. In addition, responding positively to a standard HH procedure seemed to help some subjects in inducing SH. Of the 58 highly hypnotizable subjects, a total of 30 volunteers, 17 males and 13 females, formed the final sample. The remaining 28 either dropped out during the 4 weeks of daily SH practice or did not complete the questionnaires.

Procedure

In addition to the Rorschach, the HGSHS:A, and the SHSS:C, subjects were administered the following measures before the experimental SH sessions began: the Stanford Profile Scale of Hypnotic Susceptibility, Form I (Weitzenhoffer & Hilgard, 1967); the Minnesota Multiphasic Personality Inventory (MMPI; Dahlstrom, Welsh, & Dahlstrom, 1972, 1975; Hathaway & McKinley, 1967); D. N. Jackson's (1974) Personality Research Form (PRF); and the Personality Orientation Inventory (POI; Shostrom, 1972). Having been given three measures of susceptibility, each subject had become familiar with standardly defined laboratory HH.

During the 4 weeks of the experiment, subjects practiced SH alone in a stimulus-free room in our laboratory for 1 hour daily. At the end of this hour, they detailed the contents of their SH experiences in a daily journal entry. The descriptions of the SH sessions in these journals served as the raw data for rating the level of Imagery Production, Absorption/ Fascination, and Ego Receptivity. Subjects were told to monitor their SH Trance Depth with a slightly revised version of Tart's (1979) Extended North Carolina Scale (ENCS) three times per SH session, recording these data in their journals. Midway through the 4-week period, the Stanford Profile Scale of Hypnotic Susceptibility, Form II (Weitzenhoffer & Hilgard, 1967), was given; Form I, which was given before the experiment began, was readministered at the end of the experiment. In addition, at the end of the 4 weeks, each subject completed three questionnaires detailing their experiences over the month. These extensive surveys were designed to assess many facets of SH. The first examined the SH experiences in and of themselves without reference to another mode. The second survey compared SH to standard HH, and the third examined SH over time (4 weeks).

In order to minimize experimenter effects, little monitoring of the subjects was done during the 4-week period. During a short checkup telephone call at the end of weeks 1 and 3, and a few minutes with one of the experimenters after week 2, no suggestions were given as to what was expected in the journals. Throughout the month-long experiment, therefore, the subjects' SH experiences were self-directed.

Sample Description

The final sample was comprised almost entirely of undergraduate or graduate students at the University of Chicago, most of whom were 17 to 26 years of age. The mean age of the sample was 25.18 with a standard deviation of 9.04. The oldest subject was 46. On the personality tests given before the SH experiments began, these subjects evidenced a strong theoretical orientation, a high level of curiosity, and a certain disregard for the opinions of others. The men seemed to be more flexible about their sex roles, while the women tended to adhere more to the traditional feminine role.

Results

Results can be divided into those characterizing the structure and those characterizing the content of the experience. In terms of the former, some aspects of trance, such as Absorption and the fading of the Generalized

Reality Orientation, provided the structure for both SH and standard HH. However, self-initiated SH characteristically also involved free-floating Attention, fluctuations in Trance Depth, and, most importantly, Ego Receptivity to stimuli arising from within the self. Ego Activity was present in SH and helped direct the process. Some subjects shifted back and forth between these two modes, and this seemed to heighten the experience. Attention was both expansive and focused, with concentrated Attention providing a backdrop for the experience.

The findings with regard to content were that vivid, idiosyncratic Imagery Production was again powerfully salient, with personal memories and adventures emerging with great frequency. Furthermore, although a number of subjects specifically attempted age regression in SH, most felt that they were more successful with age regression in the structured HH situation. Time distortion was a part of the SH experience as well as of HH. The results from the third questionnaire indicated that Ego Receptivity, Imagery Production, confidence in the ability to enter and maintain trance, and Trance Depth increased over time, while anxiety and doubt decreased. Although personality results were minimal, it was clear that spontaneity, openness, and a seeking attitude toward life led to more successful SH.

Phase III, 1981–1990

In Phase III, the constructs delineated in the first two phases were further explored. The diary entries were analyzed—quite a few years later than the questionnaires—by a different crew of raters. The ratings gleaned from the diaries allowed us to explore the results from the first two phases more completely. During this third period of analysis, the phenomenological approach was utilized. The subjects' experiences, as documented in their own words in the diaries they kept, became the basic units of analysis. The

TABLE 14.1. Intercorrelation of Personality Variables (Including Susceptibility) and SH Variables ($n = 30$; M $= 17$, F $= 13$)

	Ego Receptivity	SH Absorption/ Fascination	Imagery Production	Trance Depth	Composite SH
Outgoingness	.20	.18	.09	.23	.24
Impulsivity	.39*	.61***	.13	.16	.44*
POI Factor[a]	.48**	.59**	.23	.34*	.54**
Susceptibility	.44*	.30	.45*	.59**	.58**

Note. Adapted from *Self-Hypnosis: The Chicago Paradigm* (p. 178) by E. Fromm and S. Kahn, 1990, New York: Guilford Press. Copyright 1990 by The Guilford Press. Adapted by permission.

[a]The "POI Factor," derived from Shostrom's (1972) POI, measured Self-Actualization.

*$p \leq .05$. **$p \leq .01$. ***$p \leq .001$.

patterns of SH emerged with greater clarity and could then be related to personality factors from the PRF and the POI.

Each diary was meticulously examined and explored individually, without reference to the others, in order to determine what themes and patterns emerged for each subject. Part of the process was informed by Phase II. That is, some of the categories from analyses undertaken and the concepts explored in Phase II were subsequently utilized in Phase III; however, some new concepts also emerged. We then began coding the diaries for experiences commonly found during SH. A number of constructs had to be eliminated, since only a few subjects experienced them. Four constructs were coded, and the results are depicted in Table 14.1 and discussed below.[3]

Ego Activity and Ego Receptivity

The frequency and function of Ego Activity and Ego Receptivity and the alternations between them were clarified. Ego Activity occurred more frequently than Ego Receptivity and provided the structure for the unfolding of SH. Ego Receptivity allowed the facets of the self to emerge by providing the context that made it possible for them to "bubble up" from the unconscious. Although Ego Activity was actually found more frequently than Ego Receptivity in SH, Ego Receptivity seemed to be at the heart of the experience. The rhythm of alternation between the two was dictated by the needs of individuals. Subjects at times needed structure and guidance in the face of overwhelming affect, while at other times they could freely work through the emotions salient in their unconscious and preconscious lives.

One of the most important findings was that a specific cluster of personality traits influenced the experience (see Table 14.1). Independent persons who were at ease with themselves, and who were spontaneous and open to experience and to their own emotions, were able to allow more Ego Receptivity in SH. When Ego Activity predominated heavily over Ego Receptivity, the experience became dull and constricted. Only the rigid, nonspontaneous individuals tended to have this torpid type of SH trance.

Imagery Production

As in our earlier research, two kinds of imagery were found at the core of SH: reality-oriented imagery and primary-process imagery. These two variables, which were highly correlated, were merged into the variable called Imagery Production. This variable was the single most powerful variable in the SH cluster. Imagery Production and Ego Receptivity were highly correlated, but Imagery Production was the more powerful, in that it influenced Trance Depth beyond the influence of Ego Receptivity.

Personality characteristics were found to be influential, but primarily for the women in the sample. The results in Table 14.1 indicate a mild relationship when both sexes were taken together. The individuals with more immediate access to their impulses, who were more outgoing and more self-actualized, were able to experience more profound and vivid imagery in SH.

Trance Depth

Trance Depth could be accurately and effectively assessed with the ENCS. Trance Depth could be predicted by a number of other variables and seemed to indicate the overall quality of the experience. However, it turned out to be a less central variable than either Ego Receptivity or Imagery Production. Personality characteristics seemed to be less powerfully related to Trance Depth, though the different aspects of personality were correlated with it in much the same way as they were with Imagery Production. Trance Depth in SH was predicted by spontaneity, outgoingness, and self-actualization.

Absorption/Fascination

We measured how engrossed and involved the subjects became *during* trance (i.e., an *in vivo* assessment); we called this variable SH Absorption/Fascination. The trait of absorption (Tellegen & Atkinson, 1974) was related to our variable assessed *in vivo*, but there were some clear differences. Absorption/Fascination represented a specialized feature of SH and occurred less frequently than other aspects of SH. Not every SH trance was completely absorbing and filled with wonderment. When the SH trance was heightened to the extent of absorbed fascination, the influence of personality characteristics became the most profound. Again, the individuals who were self-actualized, and who readily and without fear could let themselves experience their own impulses, were the ones who found themselves absorbed and easily fascinated in SH.

Relationship of Personality to Overall Self-Hypnosis

The personality variable of Self-Actualization was clearly important in affecting the overall SH experience (measured by the Composite SH variable). However, Outgoingness was less important to overall SH, while being more internally attuned to one's impulse life (Impulsivity) became more crucial. As might be suspected, HH susceptibility had the strongest correlation with SH. If we consider susceptibility as a trait—more specifically, as a capability for engaging in HH—then it would be likely that this trait would enhance SH or would contribute to both SH and HH. However, it may also be the case that method variance contributed to the strength of the correlation. That is, the ability to engage in HH was measured by the hypnotist's scoring of specific hypnotic tasks *in vivo*. All the SH measures were based on reports in the diaries of *in vivo* occurrences. It is likely that these two kinds of *in vivo* measures would be more highly correlated with each other and would correlate less strongly with a paper-and-pencil measure (the POI or PRF).

In summary, the kind of person who enjoyed and could produce quite powerful SH experiences in this study was sensitive to and accepting of his or her impulse life, was self-actualized, and also demonstrated the ability to engage in HH.

Differential Relationship of Personality to Self-Hypnosis

Did the specific personality variables (including susceptibility) affect the various aspects of SH differentially? Susceptibility seemed more crucial to Trance Depth than to the other aspects of SH, although the correlations with Ego Receptivity and with Imagery Production were strong. Susceptibility thus was influential not only for structure and content, but even more so for the indicator of the overall experience, Trance Depth. The remaining personality traits that correlated with the Composite SH variable—Impulsivity and Self-Actualization—were correlated highly ($r = .66$, $p \le .001$). Thus it was not surprising that they followed the same pattern with respect to the four subfactors of SH. What was surprising was that the pattern differed from that of the susceptibility correlations. Whereas susceptibility seemed to have the strongest relationship to Trance Depth, Self-Actualization and Impulsivity most influenced the structural variables, particularly SH Absorption/Fascination. Susceptibility had no significant relationship to SH Absorption/Fascination. Thus, the capacity for HH was related to the ability to engage in SH and to have a successful experience. We believe that a general capacity to engage in an altered state is what underlies the ability to engage in either SH or HH. However, when it comes to a specific type of very involving experience, only those individuals who are more spontaneous and self-actualized and who are more attuned to their impulse life seem to become deeply absorbed in their SH trances.

Finally, the four SH variables were summarized into one composite measure, as noted above. This measure was then correlated with the combined personality variables (including susceptibility). A very strong relationship ($r = .57$, $p = .003$) between the personality measures and the Composite SH variable emerged.

In previous research on hypnosis, very few correlations between hypnosis variables and personality traits were found. Why was the correlation here so strong? Examining the ways in which this line of research departed from that of others may shed some light on this question.

One of the most important disjunctions with past research was the methodology. First, the SH experience was assessed via the experiential method, which enabled us to tap into its richer variations. The observable or behavioral aspects of SH were considered less important. Second, it was self-*initiated* hypnosis that was the focus of investigation, not the self-directed execution of hypnotist-initiated tasks. This gave more latitude and discretion to each individual, allowing the experiences to be more influenced by personal style. Finally, the assessment of the various aspects of SH was more rigorous and exacting than the assessment of general hypnotizability. The separate phenomena of SH (Ego Receptivity, Imagery Production, Trance Depth, Absorption/Fascination, etc.) were coded separately by two objective judges. Furthermore, a great many data points were summarized to yield the single measures of each of the SH phenomena. These data points were collected over a period of time. This wide-range, longitudinal data gathering is clearly very different from the usual type (a single judge rating a few instances of hypnotic behavior at one point in time). Thus, all of these factors contributed to increasing the accuracy of the measures.

In summary, the three phases of the research represented an ongoing refinement in the experiential method, with each successive phase rounding out and validating the work of the preceding phase. Phase I observations gleaned from descriptions of the process in semistructured interviews informed Phase II sample selection, procedure, and the questions selected for the three surveys. Phase III delineated the concepts further and devised a new experiential method of gleaning data (from the diaries). This method was grounded in the subjects' own version of the experience, and the constructs that emerged were based on this phenomenology. Thus, the research has established convergent validity (Campbell & Fiske, 1959) for the phenomena of self-initiated SH.

Future Research

The research we have described was exploratory. Future research in the area can undertake to test more specific hypotheses, but needs to be broader or to create further refinements in three areas: the sample, standards of comparison, and combination of approaches.

Sample Considerations

The small size of our sample was clearly appropriate for exploratory research. However, with only 30 subjects, statistical inference and generalizability were limited. Future research should be conducted on larger samples.

Three other aspects of the sample need to be closely scrutinized. First, our final sample included only those subjects who were highly hypnotizable, since these individuals seemed better able to discriminate between SH and HH. Our sample was also found to differ from the norm on several personality variables. It may have been the high level of curiosity coupled with low concern for social stereotypes that allowed our subjects to spend 1 hour daily in SH for 4 weeks, without compensation. Thus, future samples need to be more randomly selected in terms of both hypnotizability and motivational variables.

Second, sex differences need to be closely monitored and explored fully. In our research, sex differences emerged in the two variables at the heart of SH, Ego Receptivity and Imagery Production; furthermore, different personality characteristics influenced imagery for men and women. It will be imperative in all future research on SH to examine gender differences.

Finally, the historical context in which the experiment was conducted may have unduly influenced our subjects. These individuals had experienced the idealism, the social ferment, and the desire for large-scale change that characterized the 1960s. Consequently, our subjects may have been uniquely interested in hypnosis and the inner workings of the mind. Perhaps today, with such interests and attitudes less in vogue, the findings may differ.

Standards of Comparison

Although our research compared SH with HH, there was no comparison of both of these to the phenomena of the waking state. In future research, the occurrence, frequency, and quality of the factors we found to be characteristics of SH need to be studied in the waking state, for the purpose of establishing a baseline for comparison of the phenomena in SH.

Combination of Approaches

Our research utilized the experiential approach by analyzing retrospective questionnaires (the subjective approach) and by rating and analyzing ongoing accounts of the subjects' experience (the phenomenological approach). However, observable and operationally defined behaviors need to be analyzed (the behavioral approach) as well, to provide convergent assessment of the phenomenon of SH. This assessment can further clarify the limits of SH, the distinctions between SH and standard HH, and the influence of personality characteristics on the hypnotic experience.

Summary

Our research has shown that SH is a "many-splendored thing" that cannot be fully assessed and understood entirely by means of behavioral measures. The phenomenological approach for investigating SH has proved to be a viable and productive strategy for understanding the phenomena of self-initiated SH and for finding the personality characteristics of people who could easily and profitably engage in this activity. Important differences between self-initiated SH and hypnosis induced by another person have emerged, particularly in the area of Ego Receptivity. Ego Receptivity is at the heart of the SH experience. It allows the facets of the self to emerge and facilitates the bubbling up of conscious and preconscious material. The other important factors in SH are an increase in Imagery Production (which includes both primary-process imagery and reality-oriented imagery) and Absorption/Fascination. They all, in turn, contribute to Trance Depth in SH.

In addition, we have found that certain personality characteristics enable a person to go into deep SH trances. The spontaneous, self-actualized individual who is open to accepting his or her internal impulses is more likely to attain a rich SH experience than the rigid individual who has little fantasy and cannot "let go."

We hope that future research into the varieties of hypnotic experience will build on these explorations in personality and SH and will further refine the experiential method.

Notes

1. In this chapter, the word "self" is used to refer simply to the individual. It is not equivalent to the technical term "self" as used in psychoanalytic self psychology (see, e.g., Kohut, 1971).

2. These six subjects were chosen because they previously, out of their own curiosity, had meditated a great deal and had experimented with marijuana and other psychedelic drugs (as did so many students in the 1960s and 1970s). They also had taken two hypnosis courses taught by Fromm at the University of Chicago, in which they had proven to be not only excellent subjects but also keen self-observers, deeply interested in the scientific investigation of the phenomena of altered states of consciousness.

3. Some subjects were removed because of missing data or extreme scores.

CHAPTER FIFTEEN

The Effects of Hypnotic Procedures on Remembering: The Experimental Findings and Their Implications for Forensic Hypnosis

KEVIN M. McCONKEY

We must now plunge into the midst of the experimental phenomena of the hypnotic trance itself. A large and important group of these concern memory. One of the most remarkable of the latter is the alleged capacity of subjects in the hypnotic trance to recall events which are completely lost to the ordinary waking memory.—HULL (1933/1968, p. 105)

Although the focus of this chapter is on selected contemporary research on hypnosis and memory, it is useful to appreciate the experimental approaches and findings that existed earlier in this century. The eighth experiment in Hull's (1933/1968) landmark program of research on hypnosis concerned the impact of hypnosis on memory. In this experiment, Huse (1930) asked subjects to learn paired associates of a nonsense figure and a nonsense syllable. She found that hypnosis was not of any benefit to subjects' recall 1 day after they had learned these associates. These early negative findings notwithstanding, the impact of hypnosis on recently learned or observed material has been a major focus of research in recent years.

In other early research, Prince (1914), in his work on the unconscious, undertook a series of single-case studies in which subjects were asked to recall letters that they had written in the past and that were still available for comparison. He found that some, but not all, of these subjects could recall verbatim sections of these letters during hypnosis, whereas they could not achieve that degree of recall during the waking state. To test the impact of hypnosis on recall of remote material, Stalnaker and Riddle

(1932) asked subjects to recall the words of prose or verse (e.g., Longfellow's "The Village Blacksmith") that they had learned at least 1 year earlier. These researchers asked the subjects to recall this material both during hypnosis and during the waking state a total of eight times on different days. When the number of words that subjects recalled across these tests were summed, every subject showed greater recall during hypnosis than during the waking state. Although this finding appeared to support the notion that hypnosis increased recall for remote material, the qualitative observations made by Stalnaker and Riddle (1932) are critical in understanding the nature of this finding. Specifically, these authors observed that during hypnosis, the subjects tended to reconstruct or fabricate material when they were unable to recall the prose or verse in detail. That is, the subjects filled in the gaps in their remembering with plausible material. The degree to which hypnosis may lead subjects to fabricate or confabulate material during hypnosis has been a major focus of modern research.

Besides the core studies of Huse (1930) and Stalnaker and Riddle (1932), there is an important early study by R. W. White, Fox, and Harris (1940), who investigated the impact of hypnosis on recall for paired associates of nonsense material and for meaningful poetry and pictures. Their findings indicated that hypnosis did not benefit the recall of the nonsense material, but did benefit the recall of the meaningful material. R. W. White et al. (1940) interpreted this differential effect as occurring because nonsense material "allows little scope for the reconstructive activity which [is] characteristic of remembering" (p. 102), whereas meaningful material allows this type of "creative imagination" (p. 102), which leads to greater remembering.

The basic finding of R. W. White et al. (1940) has been observed in some studies but not in others. For instance, Dhanens and Lundy (1975) found that high hypnotizable subjects who received hypnosis together with motivating instructions improved their recall of contextual, but not nonsense, material. In a more sophisticated study by Cooper and London (1973), however, no such finding occurred. Cooper and London (1973) used high and low hypnotizable subjects in hypnotic and waking conditions in different orders of testing, and assessed their recall of meaningful material 2 weeks after learning. Although the recall of subjects was better on the second testing, this occurred whether hypnosis was involved or not; that is, the repeated testing itself led to increased recall. This selective summary of experimental studies conducted up to the mid-1970s sets the stage for the change in the level and sophistication of the research activity on the topic of hypnosis and memory since then.

This summary also sets the stage for the main issues that have been the focus of contemporary research, and that are discussed in this chapter. The focus of this chapter is on the experimental analysis of the effects of hypnosis on remembering, and the chapter has little to say directly about the practical use of hypnosis to enhance memory in the clinical or forensic setting. This is not because there is nothing to say, but because the issues surrounding the practical use of hypnosis have been discussed in several other sources (e.g., Laurence & Perry, 1988; Pettinati, 1988; Scheflin & Shapiro, 1989). It is useful, however, to provide a brief comment on the general context of the research that has been conducted on hypnosis and memory in recent years.

The Context of Contemporary Research on Hypnosis and Memory

Hypnosis and memory are areas of research that interact in a number of ways. This chapter focuses on the use of hypnosis to enhance or improve memory for witnessed events. Before I turn to consider that use of hypnosis, it is appropriate to comment briefly about some of the other ways in which hypnosis has been used in an attempt to influence memory. For example, the use of hypnosis to interfere with memory, in the sense of creating a functional amnesia, has been a major focus of research interest that has provided important information about the nature of hypnosis and memory (e.g., F. J. Evans, 1988). Also, the use of hypnosis to alter memory in a way that allows the possible exploration of aspects of psychopathology and emotional experience has been a focus of work that has provided insights into the interaction of mood and memory in particular (e.g., Friswell & McConkey, 1989). Finally, the use of hypnosis in the therapeutic setting to explore the nature and meaning of the rememberings of distressed individuals has pointed to important aspects of the nature of consciousness and personal experience in a way that provides fertile ground for research (e.g., Frankel, 1988).

Laying these interfaces between hypnosis and memory aside, this chapter focuses on the substantial degree of interest in and research conducted on the use of hypnosis to enhance memory since the mid-1970s. The theoretical, empirical, clinical, and legal controversy surrounding this influence of hypnosis on memory has had a substantial impact on the field of hypnosis. It is important to underscore that the influence of hypnosis on memory has been a major preoccupation of hypnosis researchers and practitioners in recent years. Most of the major hypnosis research laboratories throughout the world have conducted empirical work on hypnosis and memory in the last decade or so. The issues that have been investigated in these laboratories have been shaped by a variety of motivations, and have been determined by both scientific and practical concerns. To understand the laboratory research that has been conducted and that is reviewed selectively in this chapter, it is important to understand the general social context of work on hypnosis and memory.

Thus, it is appropriate to provide a summary listing of the major contemporary sources to which readers should turn for an understanding of the historical, clinical, and legal aspects of hypnosis and memory. The area that has become known as "forensic hypnosis" has given rise to several books (e.g., Laurence & Perry, 1988; Pettinati, 1988; Scheflin & Shapiro, 1989) and book chapters (e.g., Orne, Soskis, Dinges, & Orne, 1984; Sheehan & McConkey, in press; Wagstaff, 1989); a brief comment on some of the most recent books is provided. Laurence and Perry (1988) have given a historical and integrative analysis of the issues surrounding hypnosis, will, and memory, highlighting the route that hypnosis researchers and practitioners have followed to arrive at the current debate about forensic hypnosis. This book is an essential source for those wanting to understand fully the factors that have shaped the current state of empirical approaches to hypnosis and memory. In an equally timely volume, Pettinati (1988) has brought together a range of material on hypnosis and memory from various commentators. In the core section of that volume, Orne, Whitehouse, Dinges, and Orne (1988) provide a major statement on the issues involved in the forensic and clinical implications of using hypnosis in an attempt to enhance memory, and emphasize that "the same attributes of hypnosis that make it a useful adjunct to psychotherapy also create the greatest obstacles to its use in the forensic domain" (p. 55). This message can be seen also in the examination of applied uses and abuses of hypnotic age regression provided by Perry, Laurence, D'Eon, and Tallant (1988). In this analysis, these authors stress that an individual's experience of age regression is typically a combination of fact and fantasy. Consistent with the creative remembering referred to by R. W. White et al. (1940), the constructive and reconstructive processes of memory and the influences of hypnosis on those processes are recurring themes in much of the current literature on hypnosis and memory.

As can be inferred from my comments so far, there has been a burst of research on hypnosis and memory since the mid-1970s. Reflecting this activity, the *International Journal of Clinical and Experimental Hypnosis* has published two special issues on hypnosis and memory (October 1979 and October 1990); various review articles have appeared in a wide variety of journals (e.g., B. L. Diamond, 1980; Krass, Kinoshita, & McConkey, 1988; Mingay, 1987; Orne, 1979b; Perry & Laurence, 1983b; Pinizzotto, 1989; Relinger, 1984; M. C. Smith, 1983; Wagstaff, 1984); and the Council on Scientific Affairs of the American Medical Association (1985) has produced a major statement on the scientific basis of refreshing memory with hypnosis. Kihlstrom (1985a) summarized the major laboratory studies conducted in this area of activity up to that time, and concluded that "it seems difficult to maintain the position that hypnosis yields meaningful increases in memory" (p. 395). That is an essential conclusion of most studies that have been conducted since then, and it is a conclusion of this chapter.

Besides the historical roots of research on hypnosis and memory, and the scientific and professional context of contemporary research, it is important to understand both the general public's and many experts' perceptions and attitudes about the impact of hypnosis on memory. Individuals who agree to be hypnotized to enhance their memory most likely share the beliefs about hypnosis that are prevalent in the community generally. These beliefs have been investigated in several studies; the findings have shown that most people believe that hypnosis can make individuals remember information they cannot remember normally (Labelle, Lamarche, & Laurence, 1990; McConkey, 1986; McConkey & Jupp, 1985, 1986; L. Wilson, Greene, & Loftus, 1986).

Despite this general finding, some anomalies in the survey data indicate that a degree of skepticism may exist about the impact of hypnosis on memory, and that this skepticism has not been tapped fully by the survey methods that have been used. For instance, in one study (McConkey & Jupp, 1985), the respondents said that they would put less rather than more faith in the memory of people who have been hypnotized. Similarly, L. Wilson et al. (1986) reported that twice as many respondents indicated that they would put less rather than more faith in the testimony of someone who had been hypnotized; however, almost a third of the respondents said that they would put the same amount of faith in both hypnotic and nonhypnotic testimony. More recently, however, Labelle, Lamarche, and Laurence (1990) reported that the majority of individuals surveyed said that they would give more credibility to the testimony of someone who had been hypnotized than of someone who had not been hypnotized. Although most people generally believe that hypnosis enhances memory, at least some of those people express skepticism about the weight that they would give to those enhanced memories if they were presented as testimony in court.

This finding raises the question of how people would react to hypnotic testimony if they were in the role of jurors. In an investigation of this issue, Greene, Wilson, and Loftus (1989) used a jury simulation technique to study the effect of hypnotically refreshed testimony from a witness upon the decision making of jurors. The findings of these researchers indicated that the jurors viewed the hypnotic testimony with a degree of skepticism, and did not give it the status that they would give testimony based on the witness's immediate recollection of the events in question. Interestingly, and somewhat paradoxically, the jurors' exposure to hypnotically influenced testimony shaped the way in which they considered other evidence presented in the trial. Specifically, the calling of a previously hypnotized witness by the prosecution made the jurors more skeptical of the testimony of the other witnesses who were called by the prosecution. In a study that also used a jury simulation technique, Spanos, Gwynn, and Terrade (1989) investigated the effects on jurors' decision making of the testimony of experts who made either favorable or unfavorable comments about the hypnotically elicited testimony given by a rape victim. The findings of this study were complicated by the fact that the jurors tended to think that the defendant was not guilty even before they were exposed to the testimony of the experts; however, the findings essentially indicated that the jury verdict was not influenced by the conflicting testimony of the experts.

Spanos, Gwynn, and Terrade's (1989) interesting use of mock experts raises the question of whether experts who are willing to testify in actual cases agree about the impact of hypnosis on memory. Besides the inferences that can be drawn from the literature to answer this question (e.g., Orne, 1979b; B. L. Diamond, 1980), some empirical findings are available from the survey conducted by Kassin, Ellsworth, and Smith (1989). In this survey, experts on eyewitness memory were asked (among other questions) to judge the reliability of one statement concerning hypnotic retrieval (viz., "Hypnosis does not facilitate the retrieval of an eyewitness's memory") and another statement concerning hypnotic suggestibility (viz., "Hypnosis increases suggestibility to leading and misleading questions"). Whereas 40% of respondents placed some degree of reliability in the hypnotic retrieval statement, 33% believed that the relevant research findings were inconclusive; whereas 67% of the respondents placed some degree of reliability in the hypnotic suggestibility statement, 19% believed that the relevant research findings were inconclusive. In parallel with these findings, 52% of the respondents considered the hypnotic retrieval statement reliable enough to present as testimony in court, and 69% considered the hypnotic suggestibility statement reliable enough to make in that setting. Although these data can be criticized on a number of grounds (e.g., the adequacy of the sample of 63 respondents), the important point is that many experts felt capable of giving sworn testimony about the effects of hypnosis on eyewitness testimony, but disagreed about the extent to which firm statements about hypnotic retrieval and hypnotic suggestibility could be made on the basis of research on the hypnotic enhancement of memory. As will be seen in the remainder of this chapter, the experimental findings conflict almost as sharply as the views of these experts. This conflict, however, is probably more attributable to the procedural differences in the experimental approaches than to any substantive variation in the processes under investigation.

An Evaluative Summary of Experimental Approaches and Findings

With this broad background, the chapter turns now to an evaluative summary of selected experimental approaches and findings concerning the effects of hypnotic procedures on remembering. The studies that are discussed here have been selected to illustrate points of either convergence or divergence in the literature, and this chapter is not intended to be comprehensive in its coverage of the studies that have been conducted. Moreover, the focus is on studies that have been conducted in the last decade or so, and readers are referred elsewhere for reviews of the studies published earlier than that (e.g., see Pettinati, 1988; M. C. Smith, 1983).

In recent years, experimental research into the effects of hypnotic procedures on remembering has focused on three basic questions: (1) whether hypnosis increases remembering above and beyond that occurring in the normal waking state; (2) whether hypnosis leads subjects to become more vulnerable than they are in waking procedures to the distortions that occur in memory; and (3) whether hypnosis can lead to the intentional creation of false memories beyond that which might occur under waking conditions. These three issues—hypnotic hypermnesia, hypnotic distortions in memory, and hypnotic pseudomemory—are considered in turn. As will be seen, hypnotic procedures can be said to have potentially positive and negative effects on memory. Moreover, the varying findings that have been reported in the literature appear to have as much to do with the experimental methods used as they do with the phenomena being investigated. This is an important point to underscore. In work on hypnosis and memory (as in any area of research activity), the assumptions made, the methods of investigation used, and the findings obtained are intertwined in a way that needs to be recognized explicitly.

Hypnotic Hypermnesia

Hypermnesia can be said to occur when the repeated testing of memory leads to an increased degree of recall or recognition (for a review of hypermnesia in normal waking memory, see Payne, 1987). The hypermnesia paradigm of repeated testing has been used in several studies that have involved hypnosis. In the first major study of this sort, Dywan and Bowers (1983; see also Dywan, 1988) asked high and low hypnotizable subjects to recall, by giving written responses, pictures that they had been shown earlier. The recall of subjects was tested in this way three times immediately after they had viewed the pictures, once a day at home for a week, and then three times again in the laboratory in either hypnotic or motivated waking conditions. The findings of Dywan and Bowers (1983) indicated that the hypnotic procedures led to an increase in the number of both correct and incorrect items that subjects reported, and that this was especially the case for high hypnotizable subjects. Using similar stimuli, my colleagues and I (Nogrady, McConkey, & Perry, 1985) asked high and low hypnotizable subjects in either hypnotic, imagination, or waking conditions to recall repeatedly the names of line drawings of common objects or animals (e.g., spoon, kangaroo) that they had seen earlier. The basic findings indicated that the hypnotic procedures did not enhance the recall of subjects beyond that which occurred during the repeated waking attempts. However, the hypnotic procedures did lead high hypnotizable subjects to generate more incorrect material that they were confident was correct; that is, these subjects reported more "confident errors" (Nogrady et al., 1985).

In a further study, another colleague and I (McConkey & Kinoshita, 1988) gave high and low hypnotizable subjects repeated tests in either hypnotic or waking conditions to recall pictures that they had seen either 1 day or 1 week earlier. In contrast with the earlier findings (Nogrady et al., 1985), the results indicated that hypnotic procedures were associated with increased recall by subjects; specifically, in this study the subjects in the hypnotic condition reported more correct material. As in the Nogrady et al. (1985) study, however, the hypnotic procedures were also associated with an increased level of confidence by subjects in their recall, and high hypnotizable subjects who were tested in the hypnotic condition displayed the largest number of confident errors. Taken together, these studies indicate that recall can improve under some conditions when special procedures are used (i.e., hypermnesia can occur), but that the use of hypnotic procedures may or may not add to that improvement. Moreover, when hypnotic procedures do add to that improvement, this may be at the cost of increased error or excessive confidence being associated with the incorrect material.

The precise reason for this inconsistent state is not clear, and the various findings may be products as much of the methods of investigation as of the phenomenon being investigated. A study by Register and Kihlstrom (1987), for instance, also used a hypermnesia paradigm to investigate the effect of hypnosis on recall of pictures and words. They found that no increases in either accurate or inaccurate recollection were associated with the hypnotic procedures. Somewhat similarly, McKelvie and Pullara (1988) investigated the effects of hypnosis and level of processing on subjects' repeated recall of line drawings, and found that hypnosis had no general enhancement effect on recall. The combined effects of hypnosis and motivating instructions did have a facilitative effect on the recall of meaningful information in a study by DePiano and Salzberg (1981); the level of subjects' emotional arousal was not relevant, however. Crawford and Allen (1983) employed a task that involved detecting differences between successively presented picture pairs in which one member of the pairs was altered slightly. Across four experiments, these authors observed that hypnotizable rather than unhypnotizable subjects showed better performance on this visual discrimination task when it occurred in hypnosis rather than waking conditions. This finding suggests that visual memory can be enhanced during hypnosis for hypnotizable subjects at least.

Shields and Knox (1986) asked high hypnotizable subjects in hypnotic and waking conditions, and low hypnotizable subjects in a simulating condition, to perform deep- and shallow-processing tasks on a series of words; they then gave the subjects suggestions for increased memory and tested them on recall and recognition tasks. The findings indicated that hypnotic procedures enhanced the recall and recognition of verbal material that was processed at a deep level by subjects. Notably, this apparent hypnotic hypermnesia effect was not accompanied by an increase in the inaccurate recollections of subjects. This type of finding was also seen in a study by Stager and Lundy (1985). In this study, high and low hypnotizable subjects in either a hypnotic or a waking condition were shown a short movie, and were asked a series of questions about that movie immediately and again 1 week later. On the testing a week later, the high hypnotizable subjects in the hypnotic condition increased their accurate recall without showing an accompanying increase in inaccurate recall.

This finding was not confirmed, however, in a partial replication conducted by Lytle and Lundy (1988). In this second study, high and low hypnotizable subjects in hypnotic and waking conditions were given both free-recall and multiple-choice questions about the movie that they had seen 1 week earlier. Unlike Stager and Lundy (1985), Lytle and Lundy (1988) found that the high hypnotizable subjects in the hypnotic condition did not increase their accurate recall. High hypnotizable subjects in both the hypnotic and waking conditions, however, did show an increase in memory on the multiple-choice questions. Moreover, these subjects also showed an increase in their inaccurate recall on the free-recall questions. Lytle and Lundy (1988) explained these findings, and the difference between these and the Stager and Lundy (1985) results, in terms of a possible shift in the response criterion that was being used by the subjects in the hypnotic condition. Specifically, these authors argued that when the subjects were told that their memory would increase and that the material would come easily to mind, they gave answers to the free-recall and multiple-choice questions with a high degree of confidence. When the correct answer was available (i.e., in the multiple-choice questions), the high hypnotizable subjects were able to increase their correct responses. But when the correct answer was not available (i.e., in the free-recall questions), the high hypnotizable subjects increased their incorrect responses.

The possibility of a shift in response criterion as the basis for any apparent effect of hypnotic hypermnesia has been argued by Klatzky and Erdelyi (1985). They have contended on both conceptual and methodological grounds that hypnotic hypermnesia can be demonstrated only if the increase in correct recall occurs under conditions that prevent variation in the report criterion operating during the hypnotic and nonhypnotic tests of recall. One such condition is the use of a forced-recall procedure that requires subjects to provide a fixed number of responses on each recall attempt (e.g., Dywan & Bowers, 1983). This procedure is said to prevent variation in report criterion by requiring the same output from subjects on all tests of memory.

The importance of this methodological approach has been demonstrated by Whitehouse, Dinges, Orne, and Orne (1988) in their partial replication of the Stager and Lundy (1985) study. The movie, recall questions, and other procedures of Stager and Lundy (1985) were used by Whitehouse et al. (1988) to test high and low hypnotizable subjects in hypnotic and waking conditions. The major difference between the two studies was these authors' use of the forced-recall procedure that required subjects to provide an answer to every question. The findings indicated that no difference occurred in the level of accurate recall of subjects in the hypnotic and waking conditions. However, hypnotic procedures were associated with an increase in the confidence that subjects associated with the responses that they indicated were "guesses" on the initial waking-recall test. In interpreting their findings, Whitehouse et al. (1988) concluded that "the critical point is that because hypnosis yields information that otherwise would be withheld from the memory report, the process is one of facilitation of report tendency rather than an enhanced accessibility to stored memories" (p. 294).

The notion that hypnotic procedures may activate a process leading subjects to report material that they might not report otherwise is consistent with several other findings. For instance, Grabowski, Roese, and Thomas (1991) showed subjects a videotaped enactment of a crime, and tested the recall of high, medium, and low hypnotizable subjects in hypnotic and waking conditions. Although the subjects' recall scores were greater in the hypnotic than in the waking condition, this difference was not apparent when these scores were corrected for the subjects' increased rate of responding. This appears to indicate that a shift in report criterion was in effect here. Moreover, the subjects who were given the expectation that hypnosis would be used on the second recall test showed greater overall recall than did the subjects who were not given this expectation; again, however, this difference was not apparent when these scores were corrected for the subjects' rate of responding. Thus, this also appears to indicate that a shift in report criterion may occur if subjects are simply given the expectation that their recall will be tested again with hypnotic procedures.

One implication of the possible shift in report criterion concerns the confidence that subjects associate with their recall, whether that recall is accurate or inaccurate. Our studies (McConkey & Kinoshita, 1988; Nogrady et al., 1985) found that high hypnotizable subjects who were tested in hypnosis were distinctive in their production of confident errors. Given this, it is useful to look more closely at the issue of confidence and to determine the pattern of findings in other studies (see also Krass et al.,

1988). Wagstaff (1982), for instance, presented photographs of faces to subjects and 1 week later asked them to choose the previously seen face from an array of photographs. Subjects in the hypnotic condition were given the suggestion that they would clearly remember the previously seen photograph. Wagstaff's (1982) findings indicated that although hypnotic and waking subjects did not differ in the accuracy of their correct identifications, the hypnotic subjects made more incorrect identifications that they were sure were correct. That is, the hypnotic procedures led to a greater number of errors in recognition that the subjects were confident were correct. Although this finding is consistent with our results (McConkey & Kinoshita, 1988; Nogrady et al., 1985), it is not consistent with those of Mingay (1986), Gregg and Mingay (1987), and Yuille and McEwan (1985).

In his use of an incidental memory task to assess the effect of hypnosis on memory and confidence, Mingay (1986) found that hypnotic and waking subjects did not differ in terms of the accuracy of their memories or the confidence that they associated with their memories. In assessing the impact of hypnosis on memory for faces, Gregg and Mingay (1987) tested subjects in either a hypnotic or a waking condition and gave them very limited suggestions for the enhancement of their memory. The findings of Gregg and Mingay (1987) indicated that the hypnotic and waking subjects did not differ in terms of the number of accurate items recollected or the number of errors made. Yuille and McEwan (1985) assessed confidence in a lineup recognition task and found that the correlation between confidence and accuracy was positive and reliable across hypnotic, relaxation, and waking conditions. Because Yuille and McEwan (1985) did not report a breakdown of confidence ratings for the incorrect recognition responses that were given by subjects, however, it is not clear whether the hypnotic subjects may have displayed a greater number of confident errors. The variations in findings across these studies may be explained in terms of the different degrees of demand that appear to have been placed on subjects to display confidence in their recall or recognition. Importantly, across the studies that have used similar procedures, the findings have indicated that hypnotic procedures are associated with the generation of confident errors, especially for high hypnotizable subjects who are required to make repeated recall attempts (McConkey & Kinoshita, 1988; Nogrady et al., 1985).

In summary, experimental findings have indicated that hypnotic procedures may lead individuals to generate and report more material as memory than they would if hypnosis were not involved. The extent to which this occurs, however, seems to depend in part on the nature of the to-be-remembered material and on the nature of subjects' level of processing of that material. Moreover, the specific procedures that are used to test memory in the experimental studies may influence the extent to which hypnosis appears to have beneficial effects over various types of nonhypnotic procedures. Most importantly, perhaps, the experimental findings have indicated that hypnotic procedures may lead individuals to be inappropriately confident in the accuracy of their memory reports, and that this can occur when either accuracy or confidence is influenced by the hypnotic procedures. Given the constructive and reconstructive nature of memory generally, it is understandable that hypnotic procedures (or indeed any procedures intended to enhance memory) may lead subjects to report additional material in a way that allows them to integrate that material into their memory reports in a confident manner. The information that is remembered during hypnosis is typically reported in a context of implicitly and explicitly communicated acceptance of its accuracy (McConkey, 1988); because of this, it is not surprising that individuals who are exposed to hypnotic procedures have a tendency to display a degree of confidence in the remembered material that is not meaningfully associated with the accuracy of that material.

Hypnotic Distortions in Memory

The confidence associated with accurate and inaccurate recall and recognition has also been a salient issue in the studies that have investigated the degree to which hypnosis increases distortions in memory when misleading information is provided to subjects. For instance, W. H. Putnam (1979) showed hypnotizable subjects a videotape of a car–bicycle accident, and then questioned them in either a hypnotic or a waking condition either immediately or after 1 day. Subjects in the hypnotic condition were told that it would be possible to see the accident just as they had seen it the first time, and that they would be able to slow down or zoom in on the details of what they were seeing (i.e., the "television technique"). Both leading questions (i.e., ones implying a specific answer) and nonleading questions were asked by the experimenter, and the subjects rated how confident they were of their answers. The findings indicated that more errors were made in response to the leading questions by subjects in the hypnotic than in the waking condition. However, no appreciable difference occurred between the confidence ratings of subjects in the hypnotic and waking conditions. Thus, the hypnotic procedures were associated with a decrease in the accuracy, but not the confidence, of subjects' responses to the leading questions.

Similarly, Zelig and Beidleman (1981) showed hypnotizable subjects a segment of a stress-provoking film, and then questioned them in either a hypnotic or a waking condition. As in the W. H. Putnam (1979) study, subjects in the hypnotic condition were instructed to use the television technique; both leading and nonleading questions were asked by the experimenter; and the subjects rated how confident they were of their answers. The subjects in the hypnotic condition made more errors in response to the leading questions than did the subjects in the waking condition. Again, however, no appreciable difference occurred between the confidence ratings of subjects in the hypnotic and waking conditions. For both W. H. Putnam (1979) and Zelig and Beidleman (1981), then, even though the hypnotic subjects made more errors than did the waking subjects, the hypnotic and waking subjects were similarly confident of the accuracy of their answers.

G. S. Sanders and Simmons (1983) showed subjects a videotape of a pickpocket stealing a wallet, and 1 week later questioned them in either a hypnotic or a waking condition. In a subsequent lineup recognition task (in which the subjects were shown a videotape of a lineup), the memory distortion of subjects was evaluated by presenting a "leading target" individual who had not been in the original incident but who wore the same distinctive jacket as the pickpocket. On a structured-recall task, both leading and nonleading questions were asked, and subjects indicated in which of their responses they had enough confidence to testify about in court. The findings indicated that hypnotic subjects were more likely to respond on the basis of the misleading information in the lineup recognition task. On the structured-recall task, the hypnotic subjects were more likely than were the waking subjects to respond in accord with the leading questions. The proportion of subjects who were willing to testify in court about their responses did not differ between the hypnotic and waking conditions for either the lineup recognition task or the structured-recall task. Importantly, however, on the items in the structured-recall task that the subjects were willing to testify about, the hypnotic subjects were significantly less accurate than were the waking subjects. Thus, G. S. Sanders and Simmons (1983) observed that the use of hypnotic procedures was associated with a decrease in the accuracy of memory in response to leading questions. Despite this reduction in accuracy, however, the confidence that hypnotic subjects placed in their memories did not decrease. This finding is consistent with those of W. H. Putnam (1979) and Zelig and Beidleman (1981), and points to one way in which hypnosis may influence the relationship between accuracy and confidence.

Contrary to these findings, however, Yuille and McEwan (1985) reported that the responses of subjects to leading questions did not differ across hypnotic and nonhypnotic conditions. They employed both a lineup (photo identification) recognition task and a structured-recall task that included both leading and nonleading questions. In this study, highly hypnotizable subjects were shown a videotape of a bank robbery, and 1 week later they were questioned in either a hypnotic, a relaxation, or a waking condition; the subjects were told to use either the television technique or a guided-memory technique. Because of the differences between this study and the other studies, it is not clear what accounts for the discrepant results. One explanation relates to the different proportions of leading to nonleading questions across the studies. Specifically, this proportion was lower in Yuille and McEwan (1985) than in either W. H. Putnam (1979), Zelig and Beidleman (1981), or G. S. Sanders and Simmons (1983). Yuille and McEwan (1985) argued that if there were a large proportion of leading questions, then subjects might become aware of the inconsistency between the misinformation embedded in the questions and their memory, and come to doubt their memory. From this perspective, the discrepant findings can be understood as follows: Subjects in the hypnotic rather then the waking condition may have been more likely to accept misinformation when they became aware of the inconsistency, because of the large proportion of leading questions.

Perhaps the simplest explanation of the discrepant findings, however, is that the leading questions used by Yuille and McEwan (1985) simply were not effective in leading the subjects. This notion is supported by the finding that the rate of incorrect responses to leading questions in their study was not higher than the rate of incorrect responses to nonleading questions about similar information. As Sheehan and Tilden (1983) have pointed out, responses to questions involving misleading information depend critically on the stimulus features concerned. Thus, it is possible that Yuille and McEwan (1985) did not observe an effect of hypnosis on responses to leading questions because the questions did not lead subjects in the intended way. If this were the case, then Yuille and McEwan's (1985) findings cannot be said to provide evidence against the notion that hypnosis is associated with an increase in positive responses to leading questions.

Sheehan and his associates examined the effect of hypnosis on memory in a program of research (for a review, see Sheehan, 1988) that employed the paradigm developed by Loftus (e.g., Loftus, 1979). This paradigm involves subjects' being tested for their memory of a previously witnessed event. As part of the testing, the experimenter introduces false information about the event. Subjects are then retested on recall and/or recognition tasks, and the focus is on whether the introduced misinformation is reported as memory by the subjects. In the studies by Sheehan and his associates, high and low hypnotizable subjects were shown a slide series that depicted an apparent wallet-snatching event, and the misinformation was presented either before (Sheehan & Tilden, 1983, 1984, 1986) or during (Sheehan & Grigg, 1985; Sheehan, Grigg, & McCann, 1984; Sheehan & Statham, 1989) hypnosis. Three of the studies (Sheehan & Grigg, 1985; Sheehan & Tilden, 1984; Sheehan et al., 1984) tested subjects according to the procedures of the real–simulating model of hypnosis (Orne, 1959). This model compares the performance of subjects high (real) and low (simulating) in hypnotizability; the latter are instructed to simulate hypnosis in front of a hypnotist who does not know which subjects are responding genuinely and which subjects are faking. The responses of simulating subjects are considered to index the potential impact of demand characteristics on the responses of real subjects. The studies by Sheehan and his associates indexed memory performance through both recall and recognition tasks, as noted above, and subjects were asked to rate their confidence.

Across the studies, two major patterns of findings can be said to have emerged. When the misinformation was given before hypnosis, the extent to which subjects incorporated the misinformation into their memory reports was not influenced by either hypnosis or hypnotizability (Sheehan & Tilden, 1983, 1986), and was similar across both real and simulating conditions (Sheehan & Tilden, 1984). In contrast, when the misinformation was given during hypnosis, the misinformation effect was greater for high than for low hypnotizable subjects in hypnosis (Sheehan & Grigg, 1985), and for real than for simulating subjects (Sheehan et al., 1984). The findings concerning confidence essentially mirrored those concerning the accuracy of subjects' memory. Neither hypnosis nor hypnotizability was seen to influence the confidence ratings that were associated with the acceptance of misinformation introduced before hypnosis, and real and simulating subjects were similarly confident about their responses. In contrast, when the misinformation was given during hypnosis, real subjects were appreciably more confident than were simulating subjects. Thus, the extent to which hypnosis is associated with an increase in the incorporation of misleading information into memory may be based on demand characteristics when the information is presented before hypnosis, but not when the misinformation is given during hypnosis.

As Sheehan and Statham (1989) have pointed out, however, the situation concerning the hypnotic distortion of memory is not straightforward. Rather, hypnotic distortions in memory are highly variable in their extent, depend on the hypnotizability of the individuals involved, and depend also on the general context of memory testing and on whether the distorting influences occur during hypnosis or in the waking state. The essential message from these studies is that many factors interact to shape the nature of the memory reports of subjects, and the use of hypnotic procedures is just one of those factors; on some occasions hypnosis may be a major factor, and on other occasions it may not.

Although the distorting effects of hypnosis may be real, they are also inconsistent. Register and Kihlstrom (1988), for instance, induced memory errors through the use of misleading questions during hypnosis. The subjects were given a short story, and their free recall was tested. Four days later, the subjects were given a number of free-recall tests, and were interrogated during hypnosis with either misleading or objective questions for the story details. The subjects gave more incorrect information on the final waking free-recall test as a result of the misleading information that was given during the hypnotic interrogation process. That is, although hypnosis essentially did not enhance the accuracy of subjects' memory, it was associated with a greater degree of acceptance and incorporation of misleading information for both hypnotizable and unhypnotizable subjects. As Register and Kihlstrom (1988) pointed out, hypnotic subjects in their study did not show improvements in memory and were susceptible to the effects of misleading questions.

In summary, the hypnotic distortion of memory is a phenomenon that is highly variable, and its occurrence appears to be dependent upon the procedures used in the laboratory setting. The type of hypnotic procedures used, the hypnotizability of subjects, the nature of the leading and misleading questions, the timing of the introduction of those questions, and the way in which memory is tested have all been shown to play a role in determining the nature and extent of hypnotic distortions in memory. Although the precise impact of procedural differences needs to be understood in greater detail, the laboratory studies on this aspect of hypnosis and memory point to the extent to which hypnotic subjects will accept subtle changes in their memory and will incorporate those changes into their beliefs about the accuracy of their memory.

Hypnotic Pseudomemory

Giving misleading information to subjects can be extended to the giving of subtle suggestion to alter memory, and a distinct body of research exists on the phenomenon of hypnotic pseudomemory. Many anecdotal reports, in fact, have pointed to the apparent ease with which memory can be changed intentionally through hypnotic suggestion, and to the apparent strength of the person's confidence in this hypnotically created false memory (e.g., see Laurence & Perry, 1988). Hypnotic pseudomemory can be said to occur when a hypnotized individual accepts a suggestion for information that is false and subsequently reports that false information as veridical memory after being awakened from hypnosis. Laurence and Perry (1983; see also Laurence, Nadon, Nogrady, & Perry, 1986) adapted the procedure of Orne (1979b) in the first experimental study of this phenomenon. They hypnotically age-regressed high hypnotizable subjects to a night of the previous week, and suggested to them that they were woken by noises on that night. After being awakened from hypnosis, the subjects were asked by another experimenter about the events of that night. Laurence and Perry (1983) reported that most of the subjects who accepted the suggestion in the first place displayed pseudomemory by indicating in the waking state that they had been woken by noises on that night. Moreover, even when these subjects were told that the hypnotist had suggested the noises to them, almost half of the subjects maintained that the noises had occurred on the actual night, even though they had not mentioned any noises when they were originally asked about that night. As has been well documented (e.g., M. R. Nash, 1987; M. R. Nash, Drake, Wiley, Khalsa, & Lynn, 1986), hypnotic age regression in no way implies an accurate reliving of a specific event, and it is highly unlikely that the noises did actually occur on the night in question.

This original study, and a number that followed it, focused on the responses of subjects in conditions that involved hypnotic but not nonhypnotic procedures (Labelle, Laurence, Nadon, & Perry, 1990; Laurence & Perry, 1983; Lynn, Milano, & Weekes, 1991; McCann & Sheehan, 1988; Spanos & McLean, 1986). As a colleague and I (McConkey and Kinoshita, 1986) have argued, however, these studies do not allow any strong inferences to be drawn about the relevance of the use of hypnotic versus nonhypnotic procedures to the creation of pseudomemory. Studies that have tested subjects in both hypnotic and nonhypnotic procedures have yielded quite divergent results. Spanos, Gwynn, Comer, Baltruweit, and de Groh (1989), for instance, showed high and low hypnotizable subjects a videotape of a simulated armed robbery, and 1 week later showed them a simulated newscast of a suspect's arrest. One week after that, the subjects were questioned about the offender in either a hypnotic or a nonhypnotic condition. A similar number of subjects in the hypnotic and nonhypnotic conditions misattributed characteristics of the suspect to the offender. In similar fashion, my colleagues and I (Barnier & McConkey, in press; McConkey, Labelle, Bibb, & Bryant, 1990) suggested false memories to high and low hypnotizable subjects in either a hypnotic or a nonhypnotic condition, and reported that a similar number of hypnotic and waking subjects gave a pseudomemory response on the standard test of recall. Moreover, Lynn, Weekes, and Milano (1989) used Orne's (1959) real–simulating paradigm of hypnosis and found that the pseudomemory responses of real (hypnotic) and simulating (nonhypnotic) subjects were similar.

A quite different set of findings has been reported by Sheehan and his associates (Sheehan, Statham, & Jamieson, 1991a,b; Sheehan, Statham, Jamieson, & Ferguson, 1991). These investigators conducted various studies in which they suggested pseudomemories to high, medium, and low hypnotizable subjects in hypnosis and waking conditions. They found that more hypnotic than nonhypnotic subjects reported the false memories on memory tests that were given either immediately after (Sheehan et al., 1991b) or 2 weeks after (Sheehan et al., 1991a) the pseudomemories had been suggested. Moreover, they observed that high hypnotizable subjects in the hypnotic condition were the subjects most likely to report the false memories (Sheehan et al., 1991b; Sheehan, Statham, Jamieson, & Ferguson, 1991). Because of the arguments that can be made at a theoretical level about the possible impact of hypnosis on the creation of false memories (e.g., see Laurence & Perry, 1988; Orne et al., 1988), and the conflict that exists in the findings of recent studies (e.g., Barnier & McConkey, in press; McConkey et al., 1990; Sheehan et al., 1991a,b), the precise role played by hypnotic procedures in the creation of false memories cannot be specified with precision at this point.

If hypnotic procedures do have an appreciable influence on pseu-domemory creation and maintenance, then this influence should be seen in high rather than low hypnotizable subjects. Because of this, several studies have focused on high hypnotizable subjects (e.g., Laurence & Perry, 1983; McCann & Sheehan, 1988; Spanos & McLean, 1986) and other studies have examined the demand characteristics that may influence the behavior of high hypnotizable subjects (Lynn, Weeks, & Milano, 1989). The studies that have tested high, medium, and/or low hypnotizable subjects have highlighted the relevance of hypnotizability to the creation of false memories. For instance, Labelle, Laurence, et al. (1990) suggested a false memory to high, medium, and low hypnotizable subjects in a hypnot-ic condition, and found that the high and medium, but not the low, hypnotizable subjects displayed a pseudomemory. Spanos, Gwynn, Com-er, et al. (1989) found that across hypnotic and nonhypnotic conditions, high hypnotizable subjects misattributed characteristics of a suspect to the offender during interrogation more often than did low hypnotizable sub-jects. Our studies (Barnier & McConkey, in press; McConkey et al., 1990) both found that more high than low hypnotizable subjects in the hypnotic and nonhypnotic conditions accepted the suggestion for false memory, and reported the false memory when tested by an independent experimen-ter under standard conditions of memory testing. Sheehan et al. (1991a,b) and Sheehan, Statham, Jamieson, and Ferguson (1991) observed that more high than medium or low hypnotizable subjects reported suggested pseudomemories in both hypnotic and nonhypnotic conditions. Given the consistency of these findings, it is clear that hypnotizability is relevant to the acceptance and reporting of suggested memories, whether or not hypnotic procedures are involved. Like studies of hypnotic hypermnesia and hypnotic distortion of memory, studies of hypnotic pseudomemory point to the relationship of hypnotizability to memory performance, es-pecially to the errors that occur in that memory performance.

A number of recent studies of hypnotic pseudomemory have ex-amined the role played by the general context of the memory test in determining whether or not subjects show a pseudomemory response. The impact of general contextual cues in this way is especially important to understand, since Lynn, Weekes, and Milano's (1989) use of the real–simulating paradigm has indicated that an explanation of pseudomemory responding on the basis of demand characteristics cannot be ruled out. Spanos and McLean (1986) also showed that pseudomemory responding can be influenced by the communication features of the social setting of the memory test, and concluded that hypnotic pseudomemory reflected a bias in subjects' reporting rather than an alteration in their memory. In a further study, Spanos, Gwynn, Comer, et al. (1989) found that when subjects were cross-examined in an attempt to break down their memory reports that misattributed characteristics of a suspect to the offender, a similar number of subjects who had given those reports in a hypnotic or a nonhypnotic condition rejected them. That is, the hypnotic procedures that had been used did not protect subjects, as it were, from the effects of cross-examination in a different context of memory testing.

The role of contextual cues has been investigated also in studies by McCann and Sheehan (1988) and Sheehan, Statham, Jamieson, and Ferguson (1991). These authors showed that pseudomemory responding can be influenced by the similarity of the contexts in which the false memory suggestion is given and the memory of subjects is tested, by the verifiability of the suggested false memory, and by the salience of that memory. The relevance of these variables underscores the importance of the perceived link between the false memory suggestion and the memory test in determining whether or not subjects give a pseudomemory response. The exploration of this link is seen in our work (Barnier & McConkey, in press; McConkey et al., 1990). We (McConkey et al., 1990) tested subjects' pseudomemory first when they were with the experimenter who gave them the suggestion, a second and third time when they were with a second experimenter, and a fourth time when they were contacted away from the laboratory by a third experimenter. The pseudomemory responses of subjects did not differ across the memory tests in the laboratory setting, but they declined appreciably when the subjects were contacted away from the laboratory.

In a further study, we (Barnier & McConkey, in press) tested the memory of subjects first when they were with one experimenter and a second and third time when they were with a second experimenter. On the third and final memory test, this second experimenter adopted an informal approach and told subjects that the suggested events might or might not have been depicted in the slide series of a purse snatching that they had seen earlier. Most of the subjects who had shown a pseudomemory response changed their reports. That is, the shift in the context of the memory test (from formal to informal) resulted in a substantial decrease in the pseudomemory responding of subjects. This type of finding raises the question of the degree to which the memory of subjects is changed by the procedures, the extent to which they are altering their reports to accord with the perceived experimental demands, or the degree to which the suggestion is operating in something of the way of a posthypnotic suggestion that wears off over time or across situations. These issues have not been resolved to date, although it does seem to be the case that there may not be anything particularly hypnotic about hypnotic pseudomemory.

In recent years, studies of hypnotic pseudomemory have moved from suggesting one false memory to subjects (Labelle, Laurence, et al., 1990; Laurence & Perry, 1983; Lynn, Weekes, & Milano, 1989; McConkey et al., 1990; Spanos & McLean, 1986) to suggesting more than one false memory (Barnier & McConkey, in press; McCann & Sheehan, 1988; Lynn, Milano, & Weeks, 1991; Sheehan et al., 1991a,b; Sheehan, Statham, Jamieson, & Ferguson, 1991; Spanos, Gwynn, Comer, et al., 1989). In various studies, McCann and Sheehan (1988), Sheehan et al. (1991a,b), and Sheehan, Statham, Jamieson, and Ferguson (1991) showed subjects a videotape of a simulated bank robbery and gave subjects false suggestions about the robber's swearing, wearing a mask, and entering from a particular direction. They found that the pseudomemory responding of subjects was associated differentially with the three false suggestions, and explained this in terms of the salience of the suggested events. Spanos, Gwynn, Comer, et al. (1989) focused on eight characteristics of a suspect and an offender that differed, and found that most subjects misattributed some of the characteristics of the suspect to the offender; that is, different patterns emerged for different subjects.

In quite distinct research, Lynn, Milano, and Weeks (1991) gave subtle suggestions concerning an event that did occur (pencils dropping) as well as an event that did not occur (a telephone ringing) during a previous session. They found that the subjects were incorrect or unsure of the event that did occur as often as they were of the event that did not occur. That is, these authors observed faulty memory for both a "suggested" real event and a suggested false event. In a similar vein, we (Barnier & McConkey, in press) also used a suggested real event (moustache on robber) in conjunction with two suggested false events (scarf on robber; flowers dropped by victim). We observed that both high and low hypnotizable subjects' reports of the false memories and the actual memory were influenced by the social context of the memory test. In this sense, the subjects' memory of the false events was no more or less fixed than was their memory of the real event. The findings of these two studies highlight the importance of not assuming that "actual" memories cannot be influenced in the same way that "false" memories can. Many processes are at work in shaping the memory of subjects and the way in which that memory is reported, and it is wrong to assume that variation in memory is necessarily a function of hypnotic procedures.

In summary, it appears that hypnotizability is the most important factor in the acceptance of a false memory suggestion, and that hypnotizability may interact with the use of hypnotic procedures. The context of memory testing, however, exerts a major influence on subjects' memory reports, and when the link between the false memory suggestion and the memory test is weakened, a decrease in pseudomemory responding can be seen to occur. Although this suggests that social-psychological factors play a major role in hypnotic pseudomemory, it is important to underscore that highly hypnotizable subjects—especially those tested under hypnotic procedures in at least some studies—are much more likely to respond to a pseudomemory suggestion and to display a false memory.

Concluding Comments

The experimental findings on hypnotic hypermnesia, hypnotic distortions in memory, and hypnotic pseudomemory indicate that hypnotic procedures have potentially positive and negative effects on memory. Put simply, sometimes hypnosis appears to have a positive effect and sometimes it appears to have a negative effect on the memory performance of subjects. One problem with this situation, of course, is that it is very difficult to predict when hypnosis will have positive and when it will have negative effects. The burst of research since the mid-1970s has not helped greatly in this regard. The procedures of the experiments vary so widely in this area that there have been very few replicated (positive or negative) findings. Some work has been programmatic, however, and that work has provided important information on the major parameters determining the effects of hypnotic procedures on memory. Nevertheless, an essential conclusion is that too much work on hypnosis and memory has told us too little about the basic processes that are involved. Perhaps this is because there are no sound theoretical reasons to expect that hypnosis will enhance normal waking memory.

Hypermnesia occurs, distortions in memory occur, and pseudomemory occurs—but the introduction of hypnosis does not reliably lead to more of any of these phenomena occurring. Nevertheless, some researchers have been too eager to attribute to "hypnosis" improvements in and errors of memory that perhaps would have been more correctly attributed to the variation normally occuring in memory. Analyses of the experimental findings on hypnosis and memory have more often than not ended in dire warnings about the negative effects or in proselytizing claims about the positive effects of hypnosis on memory. Overstatement of either kind is not a reasonable conclusion, however. Rather, it is time for the researchers who continue to be interested in this area to recognize more obviously that rhetoric and simple manipulation of parameters have both played too great a role in shaping experimental research; it is time now for more careful theorizing and methods of inquiry to be used in the laboratory.

It is time also to try to bring experimental and quasi-experimental methods of inquiry into field research on forensic hypnosis. The inferences that can be drawn from laboratory research and applied to the forensic use of hypnosis are limited in various ways (see M. C. Smith, 1983; Wagstaff, 1984), and there is a need for well-conducted field studies; very few such studies exist in the literature. Yuille and Kim (1987) reported a field study of selected cases in which hypnosis had been used in police investigations. Their analysis of the material in the case records indicated that hypnosis was found to substantially increase the amount of information that the witnesses provided, and that this increase occurred without any loss in the accuracy of the information. This contrasts markedly with many experimental findings. Moreover, as Yuille and Kim (1987) pointed out, the hypnotic procedures included instructions to use a number of normal memory aids (e.g., imagery, context reinstatement), and thus the apparent increase in recall may have been as much a function of these nonhypnotic aspects of the procedures as they were of the hypnotic aspects. From this perspective, many of the anecdotal reports about the effects of hypnosis on memory in the forensic setting may simply have been misattributions of those (positive or negative) effects to hypnosis, when perhaps they should have been correctly attributed to any of a number of nonhypnotic aspects of the memory enhancement procedure. This is not to deny the substantial weight that such a misattribution can carry; indeed, the use of hypnosis to influence memory has led to a number of individuals' becoming victims of misinformation and misuse of hypnosis.

In pointing to the research directions that the area of hypnosis and memory needs to take, Pettinati (1988) has argued for more field research, more clinical research, more systematic case compilation, greater examination of hypnotic versus nonhypnotic interrogation techniques, and greater examination of individual differences in remembering. There is little doubt that research will proceed in these and other relevant directions. Such research is needed to help correct some of the forensic excesses that will probably continue to occur, albeit (let us hope) at a lesser level than that of the last decade or so. The essential message that contemporary experimental findings carry, and will probably continue to carry, is that there is a need for a cautious approach and a critical evaluation of the effects of hypnotic procedures on remembering. Many of the effects may be more apparent than real; those that are real may be highly variable.

Given these findings from experimental research on the effects of hypnotic procedures on remembering, we can ask whether it is worth using hypnosis to enhance the memory of witnesses of crime in the forensic setting. Given the complexity of the scientific findings, the professional and ethical issues, and the legal concerns that surround forensic hypnosis (see McConkey & Sheehan, in press; Sheehan & McConkey, in press), the answer would have to be "no" in most instances. If a decision is made nevertheless to proceed with the use of hypnosis, it should be understood clearly that the experimental findings provide no guarantee that any benefits (e.g., increased accurate recall) will be obtained through its use, and that some costs (e.g., inaccurate recall, inappropriate confidence) may well be incurred through its use. This is the strongest inference that should be drawn from the experimental findings by those who are considering using forensic hypnosis. Given this, a balanced evaluation of the potential costs and benefits of the effects of hypnosis on memory should limit the use of forensic hypnosis in any substantial way.

Acknowledgments

The preparation of this chapter was supported in part by a grant from the Australian Research Council and the Criminology Research Council of Australia. I am grateful to Amanda Barnier for her assistance during the preparation of this chapter.

CHAPTER SIXTEEN

Clinical Hypnosis Research since 1986

DANIEL P. BROWN

In *Hypnotherapy and Hypnoanalysis* (D. P. Brown & Fromm, 1986) and *Hypnosis and Behavioral Medicine* (D. P. Brown & Fromm, 1987), Erika Fromm and I discussed the clinical literature on the use of hypnosis in psychodynamic treatment and behavioral medicine before 1986. This chapter reviews the developments and findings on clinical hypnosis research in the years since then, as a way to update our understanding of new developments in the application of clinical hypnosis.

Behavioral Medicine

Pain

It is generally accepted that hypnosis offers an advantage in the treatment of pain and that successful outcome of pain control is related to hypnotizability (D. P. Brown & Fromm, 1987; Wadden & Anderton, 1982). This favorable view of hypnosis for pain control was derived primarily from experimental rather than clinical studies of pain control. There have been few well-designed clinical trials demonstrating the effects of hypnosis in the treatment of clinical pain syndromes.

The clinical studies on pain control in the past several years have yielded inconsistent results. Freeman, MacCaulay, Eve, Chamberlain, and Bhat (1986) conducted a clinical trial comparing self-hypnosis to a control procedure for reducing pain associated with labor in childbirth. A total of 65 subjects were randomly assigned either to a hypnotic or a nonhypnotic condition. All subjects attended weekly prenatal classes after the 32nd week of gestation. In addition to the prenatal classes, hypnotic subjects

427

were given suggestions for relaxation and transfer of analgesia from one hand to the abdominal area. There were no significant differences in the amount of pain relief, but women in the hypnotic condition reported greater satisfaction with the labor experience.

Spinhoven and Linssen (1989) reported changes in 45 patients with low back pain who participated in a group program consisting of a psychoeducational approach to their pain, and who also received training in self-hypnosis. Patients reported significant favorable posttreatment changes: reduction in the use of pain medication and increased activity level. There was no reported change in pain intensity. The relative contribution of the psychoeducational approach and hypnosis was unclear. Since no external control group was used, it was difficult to know whether hypnosis contributed anything unique to the results, or whether the positive changes were due to nonspecific treatment effects. Like the Freeman et al. (1986) study, this study failed to demonstrate a unique contribution of hypnosis to pain relief, although a number of other favorable subjective changes were reported.

In a third study, Edelson and Fitzpatrick (1989) compared the relative efficacy of cognitive–behavioral and hypnotic treatment of chronic pain. A total of 20 chronic pain subjects were assigned (nonrandomly) to one of three treatment conditions: hypnotherapy or cognitive–behavioral treatment, and a control condition (in which patients talked about their pain experience). The cognitive–behavioral treatment consisted of modifying negative self-statements regarding pain experience, and reinterpretation of pain as numbness. Hypnotic treatment consisted of the same treatment as the cognitive–behavioral treatment, following a standard hypnotic induction. Each group received four 1-hour treatment sessions over a 2-week period. Both treatment groups showed significant changes, whereas there were none in the control group. Subjects in the cognitive–behavioral group had reduced pain ratings on the McGill Pain Questionnaire and increased levels of daily activity as reported in the Fordyce Activity Log. Subjects in the hypnosis group showed reduction in pain ratings, but no change in activity level. Because the cognitive–behavioral and hypnotic induction group showed similar pain reduction ratings, the hypnotic induction failed to offer any therapeutic advantage. In addition, it failed to increase significantly the likelihood that patients would normalize daily activity in the face of pain.

Taken as a unit, these studies imply that hypnosis may be useful in altering a variety of subjective experiences associated with acute and chronic clinical pain, but not necessarily in altering the pain experience per se. However, failure to demonstrate a positive treatment effect on pain experience could be attributable to various methodological weaknesses of each study or to a narrow approach to hypnotic pain control. Some evidence exists that effective pain control is contingent on the type of pain coping strategy utilized, and especially on matching the specific hypnotically suggested coping strategy to the coping resources of the individual pain patient (D. P. Brown & Fromm, 1987). None of the three studies discussed above attempted to control for the type of hypnotic pain coping strategy used. Furthermore, none of the studies adequately addressed the issue of hypnotizability and its association with outcome; nor did they control for a variety of nonspecific factors that could have explained the outcome.

More convincing findings come from the programmatic work of A. F. Barabasz and M. Barabasz (1989; see also Barabasz & Barabasz, Chapter 7, this volume) in well-designed studies on restricted environmental stimulation therapy (REST) and its enhancing effects on hypnotizability and pain control. The Barabaszs had demonstrated in their previous work (Barabasz & Barabasz, 1989) that the use of REST temporarily enhanced hypnotizability in experimental subjects. A. F. Barabasz (1982) further documented that use of the REST methodology enhanced hypnotizability, and in turn offered an opportunity to teach low hypnotizable subjects more effective strategies for pain control. The 1989 investigation tested whether this effect might also obtain for chronic pain patients. A total of 20 subjects were assigned to either a treatment or a control condition. Subjects in the treatment condition received 6 hours of REST; those in the control group did not. Subjects in the REST condition were also divided into two groups: one with a high situational demand, favoring increase of hypnotizability following the experience; and another with a low situational demand, in which the experimental hypotheses were intentionally disguised. The Stanford Hypnotic Susceptibility Scale, Form C (Weitzenhoffer & Hilgard, 1962), an ischemic pain test, and a posthypnotic suggestion for pain relief were given before and after the REST. A significant increase in hypnotizability was found in the experimental but not in the control condition. Significant decreases in pain scores were also found in the experimental but not control condition. There were no differences in the high and low demand groups, which suggests that the results were more a function of hypnotizability than of task motivation. Although this study clearly shows the relative contribution of hypnotizability to pain control in a clinical population of pain patients, it must be remembered that patients reported a decrease in response to ischemic pain (an experimental measure). Measures of chronic pain were not the focus of the study. The study also suffers from a lack of follow-up. Nevertheless, the study is valuable in that it attempts to differentiate between nonspecific treatment effects and hypnotic effects in the control of pain in the clinical population.

Overall, it is clear that better-designed studies controlling for hypnotizability, situational demands, and type of pain coping strategy utilized are needed, if we are to be able to draw more definitive conclusions about the efficacy of hypnosis with *clinical* pain populations.

Headache

Research on hypnotherapy for headaches since 1986 has not significantly advanced our previous understanding of the clinical efficacy of hypnosis with headaches. According to a previous review (D. P. Brown & Fromm, 1987), the effectiveness of behavioral medicine interventions with headaches ranges from 40% to 90%, and that of hypnotic interventions ranges from 35% to 65%. Comparative studies of hypnotherapy and other behavioral medicine techniques have yielded equivocal results. We stated (D. P. Brown & Fromm, 1987) that the failure to achieve better outcomes is largely attributable to the fact that most studies have favored unidimensional over multidimensional treatment protocols.

P. Davidson (1987) reported a 70% improvement in 10 migraine patients with H. Spiegel and D. Spiegel's unidimensional hypnotherapy approach. The patients showed a significant decrease in the severity and frequency of their headaches after four treatment sessions. No control group was used, and no follow-up data were given. In a better-designed clinical trial, van Dyck, Zitman, Linssen, and Spinhoven (1991) randomly assigned 55 tension headache patients to autogenic training or future-oriented hypnotic imagery, combined with suggestions to enhance coping and to decrease headache pain and frequency over time. Patients in both groups received a total of four treatment sessions. No external control group was used. The results of both treatment groups were equivocal, and the data of all treatment groups were pooled for analysis. Significant pre–post differences were then found: Ratings of headache intensity, medication use, and associated depressive and anxiety symptoms decreased. Pain reduction was correlated significantly with hypnotizability across groups, as measured by the Stanford Hypnotic Clinical Scale (Morgan & Hilgard, 1978–1979a), and also with a subjective rating of depth of relaxation and involvement in imagery. In this study, the positive treatment outcome seemed to be related more to hypnotizability than to the type of treatment.

In a well-designed study, Olness, MacDonald, and Uden (1987) compared the relative efficacy of self-hypnosis to the use of propranolol and to placebo treatment in children from ages 6 to 12 suffering from classic migraines. A total of 28 patients were randomly assigned to one of three treatment conditions in a 3-month by 3-month crossover design: propranolol in one group and placebo in another for 3 months, and then vice versa for 3 months, after a 1-month baseline period prior to either. After the initial 7 months, all children were taught self-hypnosis for 3 months. Self-hypnosis included suggestions for relaxation, pleasant imagery, and pain control. Self-hypnosis emphasized self-regulation. A significant reduction in the frequency of headaches was found only after self-hypnosis treatment. No changes were reported in the subjective ratings of headache severity or in objective ratings of headache duration. Self-hypnosis was superior to the pharmacological intervention. Unfortunately, the relationship of treatment outcome to hypnotizability was not studied.

Although it is clear that hypnosis and self-hypnosis offer some advantage, a definitive clinical study remains to be done. It is unclear why headache frequency and not severity was affected in one study (Olness et al., 1987) and headache severity in another (van Dyck et al., 1991). More careful attention needs to be paid to the type of suggestions given, in the context of multimodal treatment that includes relaxation and suggestions for pain control as well as for muscular and vascular control. Moreover, whether a formal hypnotic induction adds to the overall treatment gain has not yet been firmly established.

Asthma

The prevailing view is that hypnosis is generally effective in the treatment of asthma (D. P. Brown & Fromm, 1987; Wadden & Anderton, 1982). Early controlled clinical studies comparing hypnosis to various control conditions (Maher-Loughnan, McDonald, Mason, & Fry, 1962) described positive treatment effects primarily in terms of subjective effects (e.g., decreased wheezing) and behavioral indices (e.g., decreased use of bronchial dilators). Clinical trials that utilized objective measures of pulmonary functioning reported largely negative results (Edwards, 1960). Thus, although hypnosis may offer *some* advantage in the treatment of asthma, it remains to be established whether or not hypnotic interventions can alter the physiological basis of the illness—namely, bronchial spasm and tissue inflammation.

Two recent studies have attempted to determine the impact on hypnosis on objective measures of airways flow, in addition to the subjective and behavioral outcome measures. Morrison (1988) studied 16 asthmatic patients over a 1-year course of hypnotherapy. Hypnotic relaxation, direct suggestions to alter breathing rate, and ego-strengthening suggestions were given. Each patient also practiced self-hypnosis daily for 5 to 15 minutes. Subjects served as their own controls. After 1 year, a number of objective changes were noted: The number of admissions to the hospital and the duration of stay in the hospital had diminished, and a reduction or total cessation in steroid use had occurred in 14 to 16 patients. Although improvements in peak flow after hypnotherapy were reported for most subjects, these changes in airways flow were highly variable and not always reproducible. The hypnotic suggestions, however, were shown to directly affect the rate and volume of breathing. Morrison alludes to the fact that the inconsistency in the peak flow results may have been related to compliance. The lack of a comparison control group, and the fact that all patients shared the same physician, make it hard to conclude whether the beneficial effects were results of hypnotherapy, transference, or other nonspecific treatment factors.

A randomized controlled clinical trial conducted by Ewer and Stewart (1986) allows us to draw more definitive conclusions about the efficacy of hypnosis with asthmatics. Hypnotizability was assessed with the Stanford Hypnotic Clinical Scale (Morgan & Hilgard, 1978–1979a). A total of 39 patients were divided into high and low hypnotizable groups and then randomly assigned to either a treatment or a control condition. Hypnotic interventions included suggestions for relaxation, ego strengthening, guided imagery, self-hypnosis, and symptom challenge. Dependent measures included subjective measures of symptom evaluation; behavioral measures of medication use; and subjective sensitivity ratings and objective measures of peak flow and airways response after a methacholine challenge. High hypnotizable subjects in the treatment group showed significant changes in pulmonary functioning (forced vital capacity and peak expiratory flow), as well as objective decreases in bronchial hyperactivity as measured by the methacholine challenge test. Low hypnotizable subjects in the treatment group and high hypnotizable subjects in the control group showed decreased subjective but not objective sensitivity during the methacholine challenge test. High hypnotizable subjects in the treatment group also had significant reductions in the subjective evaluation of symptoms, such as wheezing, inhibition of activity, and use of medication, relative to low hypnotizable and no-treatment control subjects.

This well-designed study clearly demonstrates that hypnosis affects more than a patient's subjective evaluation of his or her asthmatic condition. Hypnotic intervention directly affects physiological processes; it reduces the hyperresponsiveness of the airways and improves airways flow in highly hypnotizable patients. Thus, this study lends further strong support to the conclusion reached earlier by Wadden and Anderton (1982) that hypnotizability is positively related to the outcome with asthmatics when hypnotherapy is used. A more recent study of nonhypnotic relaxation therapy with asthma (Murphy, Lehrer, Karlin, Swartzman, Hochron, & McCann, 1989) reached similar conclusions: When a nonhypnotic behavioral intervention was used, a significant change in the response to the methacholine challenge test was correlated with hypnotizability.

Gastrointestinal Disorders

In *Hypnosis and Behavioral Medicine*, we (D. P. Brown & Fromm, 1987) wrote that "the treatment of gastro-intestinal disorders with hypnosis has not yet evolved substantially compared with, say, hypnotic treatment of pain and other physiological disorders. Few detailed and proven treatment protocols are available" (p. 117). Whorwell, Prior, and Faragher (1984) undertook the first controlled study comparing the effectiveness of hypnosis, psychotherapy, and placebo treatment for irritable bowel syndrome (IBS). Only the hypnotherapeutic treatment proved effective. More recent research from this clinical research group has convincingly demonstrated the advantage of hypnosis in the treatment of gastrointestinal disorders, such as IBS and duodenal ulcer. In the original study, IBS patients were randomly assigned to one of three treatment conditions: hypnosis, supportive psychotherapy, and placebo treatment. Hypnotic interventions, called "gut-directed hypnotherapy," focused on direct suggestions for relaxation and ego strengthening. Only the patients in the hypnotic group showed significant treatment gains at a 3-month follow-up. The weakness of the study was that it lacked an extended follow-up.

A subsequent study, designed to correct these limitations, reported follow-up data on the 15 original IBS patients previously reported to be successfully treated with hypnosis (Whorwell, Prior, & Colgan, 1987). The later study also contributed another 35 IBS patients treated with hypnosis to the overall data pool. Only 2 patients out of the total sample of 50 patients experienced a single relapse episode of the IBS at the 18-month follow-up. Some attempt was made to identify patient characteristics that predicted the outcome. The success rate with classical cases of IBS (meeting all diagnostic criteria) was 95%, whereas the success rate of atypical cases associated with a wide spectrum of associated symptoms of psychopathology was between 40% and 60%. Age was a factor, in that the success rate was 100% in IBS patients under 50 and only 25% in patients over 50 years of age.

Further evidence for the efficacy of hypnosis of IBS has been given by Harvey, Hinton, Gunary, and Barry (1989). A total of 33 patients with refractory IBS were treated with hypnosis in four 40-minute sessions over a 7-week interval. Twenty of the patients showed improvement at a 3-month follow-up. Although this study lacks the rigor of an adequate experimental design, the results are entirely consistent with the positive results of the original Whorwell et al. (1984) well-designed study. A major finding in the Harvey et al. (1989) study was that group hypnotic treatment (with up to eight patients) was as effective as individual hypnotherapy.

In more recent work, Prior, Colgan, and Whorwell (1990) have focused on psychological mechanisms by which hypnosis works with IBS. Physiological studies were conducted on patients treated with hypnotherapy, who were compared with a no-treatment control group. Thirteen of the 15 hypnotherapy patients, but no control patients, showed significant decreases in symptoms such as abdominal pain, distension, and disturbance in bowel habit. A significant decrease in rectal sensitivity, but not in rectal motor activity as measured by anorectal manometry techniques, was found in diarrhea-predominant IBS patients. The authors concluded that one mechanism by which gut-directed hypnotherapy works is to desensitize IBS patients to the discomforting visceral sensations associated with IBS.

Since the pioneering study by Whorwell et al. (1984) on IBS, other studies have investigated essentially the same treatment strategy with duodenal ulcers. Tosi, Judah, and Murphy (1989) reported on a 3 × 4 multifactorial repeated-measures design consisting of pretreatment, posttreatment, and follow-up testing of 25 patients in one of four conditions: rational stage-directed hypnotherapy, cognitive restructuring, hypnosis only, and a nontreatment control. Hypnosis, consisting of cognitive restructuring of self-defeating beliefs and associated behaviors, contributed to a significant decrease in symptoms and associated beliefs. Colgan, Faragher, and Whorwell (1988) also conducted a trial with 30 patients with rapidly relapsing duodenal ulcers, who were matched and randomly assigned to a hypnotherapy or a control condition. After successful treatment of the duodenal ulcers with ranitidine, the drug was discontinued for 10 weeks. During this interval, the patients in the hypnotherapy group received seven hypnotherapy sessions and were given an audiotape for daily self-hypnosis. The control group was seen by clinicians for the same amount of time but did not receive hypnotherapy. One year after discontinuance of ranitidine, 100% of the control patients, but only 53% of the hypnotherapy patients, had relapsed.

Taken as a whole, this group of studies suggests that hypnotherapy can be effective in the treatment of certain types of gastrointestinal disorders. The effectiveness, in my opinion, is dependent on the type of hypnotherapy utilized. The hypnotic interventions used in most of these studies primarily involve ego-strengthening suggestions, a type of hypnotic cognitive therapy. It is well established that there is a strong association between negative cognitions, notably worry, and IBS symptoms (Latimer, 1983). Direct hypnotic suggestions to increase psychological well-being or to restructure cognitions may be particularly well matched to this patient population's unique characteristics. In addition to altering visceral sensitivity, gut-directed hypnotherapy may serve as a hypnotic cognitive therapy that alleviates negative cognitions, which otherwise serve to exacerbate (and may even predispose patients to) IBS symptoms.

Skin Disorders

Although it is generally believed that hypnosis is effective in the treatment of a wide variety of skin diseases (D. P. Brown & Fromm, 1987, Scott, 1960), there have been relatively few controlled clinical trials using hypnosis in the treatment of skin disorders. However, numerous clinical cases have been reported anecdotally in the literature. The research study most often cited is based on only six subjects. Sinclair-Gieben and Chalmers (1959) treated six patients with bilateral warts. Direct hypnotic suggestions and graded posthypnotic suggestions were given that the warts would disappear, but only on one side of the body; they did. Surman, Gottlieb,

An important study that has appeared in recent years on insomnia is that of Stanton (1989a). He conducted a controlled clinical study with 45 subjects matched on their baseline sleep onset latency, and then randomly assigned them to one of three treatment conditions: hypnotherapy, stimulus control, and placebo treatment. The placebo control entailed imagining neutral presleep images. Each group was given four weekly 30-minute treatment sessions. Hypnosis consisted of hypnotic imagery to go to a special place and ego-strengthening suggestions for subjects to let go of their problems. Demand characteristics were controlled by using counterdemand instructions in which subjects were told that improvement in their sleep condition would not occur until their fourth treatment session. Sleep onset latency at the end of the third treatment session was used as the primary outcome measure for the counterdemand condition, and sleep onset latency at the end of the fourth session was used for the demand condition. A significant reduction of sleep onset latency was found only in the hypnotherapy group: Subjects in this treatment group were able to reduce their baseline sleep onset latency by over 50% by the end of the second treatment session. Since no differences were observed between the counterdemand and the demand conditions, Stanton concluded that the positive treatment effect was attributable to hypnosis, and not to demand characteristics or other nonspecific treatment factors.

The Stanton (1989a) study adds further evidence to the view that hypnosis offers a unique advantage to the short-term treatment of insomnia, at least when nightly sleep onset latency is taken as an outcome measure. Since the Stanton study, unlike the Borkovec and Fowles (1973) study, demonstrated the superiority of hypnosis over behavioral treatment, one possible interpretation of the difference is that the two studies entailed different types of hypnotic suggestion. In addition to suggestions of hypnotic relaxation, Stanton's subjects were given ego-strengthening suggestions to "let go of their problems." Once again, this hypnocognitive approach may be particularly well matched to insomniacs, who suffer from a condition of "cognitive hyperactivity" (Borkovec, 1982).

Psychoneuroimmunology

A rapidly growing area in behavioral medicine is psychoneuroimmunology (D. P. Brown & Fromm, 1987). Unfortunately, controlled clinical studies of hypnotherapy with patients with immune-related illnesses have lagged behind studies of nonhypnotic interventions. Following the pioneering work of Black and his associates (Black, 1963; Black, Humphrey, & Niven, 1963) on the effects of direct hypnotic suggestions on allergic response, several studies have appeared since 1986 on hypnosis and immediate and delayed immunosensitivity. Locke, Ransil, Covino, Toczydlowski, Lohse,

Dvorak, Arndt, and Frankel (1987) failed to demonstrate a significant effect of direct hypnotic suggestions on delayed immunosensitivity in 12 highly hypnotizable subjects as compared to 30 low-hypnotizability controls. Suggestions to either enhance or suppress the size of the allergic skin response or the degree of cellular infiltration failed to produce any significant treatment effect.

Zachariae, Bjerring, and Arendt-Nielsen (1989) did find a significant effect on both immediate and delayed immunosensitivity, using direct hypnotic suggestions and guided imagery. Direct hypnotic suggestions were effective in reducing the flair but not the wheal reaction to immediate immunosensitivity to a histamine prick test. Hypnotic guided imagery was effective in significantly modifying the size of the flair and induration in response to delayed immunosensitivity to tuberculin antigen (Mantoux test). Laser doppler flowmetry and ultrasonic measures of skin thickness were used to demonstrate significant changes in regional blood flow and cellular infiltration following hypnosis. The discrepancies between the two studies with respect to the effects of hypnosis on delayed immunosensitivity may have resulted from the different types of hypnotic suggestions given.

Another important clinical study has recently appeared. Haanen, Hoenderdos, Romunde, Hop, Mallee, Terwiel, and Hekster (1991) studied the effects of hypnotherapy on patients with refractory fibromyalgia. A total of 40 patients were randomly assigned to 12 weeks of either hypnotherapy or physical therapy. Hypnotherapy consisted of hypnotic relaxation, suggestions to alter sensory perceptions (especially pain perception), and ego-strengthening suggestions. Patients were also given a 30-minute audiotape to use for daily self-hypnosis. Patients in the physical therapy group practiced progressive muscle relaxation and received massage therapy. Patients in the hypnotherapy group had significantly less pain, fatigue upon awakening, and sleep disturbance than those in the physical therapy group. They also reported significantly less overall discomfort, fewer symptoms, and less use of medications. These effects were still observable at a 3-month follow-up. Objective measures were taken of the number of tender points within the musculature; they were not significantly reduced after either treatment. The authors conclude that hypnotherapy may be useful in alleviating the subjective distress associated with fibromyalgia, but does not necessarily lead to a biological effect. The lack of an external control group, a comparison of treatments with and without hypnotic induction, a comparison of demand and nondemand treatment suggestions, or a measure of hypnotizability makes it impossible to ascertain whether hypnosis per se contributed significantly to the reported positive treatment factor.

The most interesting and potentially important study on hypnosis and psychoneuroimmunology to appear recently is a long-term prospective study of survival rate in women with breast cancer (D. Spiegel, Bloom,

Kraemer, & Gottheil, 1989). A total of 86 women with metastasized breast cancer were randomly assigned to either a treatment or a control group. The control group received routine oncological care. In addition, the treatment group received 1½ hours of weekly supportive group therapy and self-hypnosis for pain control. Follow-up was done every 4 months for the first year. No differences in survival rate were apparent 1 year after treatment. At a 10-year follow-up, only three patients were alive; however, the survival rate for those patients in the group therapy/self-hypnosis group ($\bar{X}$ = 36.6 months) was double that in the control group ($\bar{X}$ = 18.9 months). This is one of the few prospective studies available. Since the difference in survival rate was highly significant ($p < .0001$), the study has generated considerable interest in the past few years. It is quite clear that psychosocial interventions significantly affect survival rate in terminal breast cancer patients, yet it is unclear what worked. Was it the group support? Was it the fact that patients had a context to express feelings? Was it the self-hypnosis? Or was it something else? Research is currently being done to ascertain whether or not self-hypnosis contributed to the positive outcome.

Chronic Illness

Another growing area within behavioral medicine is the use of psychosocial interventions as an adjunct to the treatment of chronic illness (D. P. Brown & Fromm, 1987). Although hypnosis has not been used extensively in this area, a few interesting and promising exploratory studies have appeared in the past several years. Ratner, Gross, Casas, and Castells (1990) studied the effects of hypnotherapy on compliance with regular insulin injections among adolescent insulin-dependent diabetics. A small sample size was used—only seven patients, each serving as his or her own control. A 6-month documented history of noncompliance with diet, insulin injections, and blood/urine testing served as the baseline measure of noncompliance. Blood hemoglobin and fasting blood sugar levels were used as indices of control over hyperglycemia. Hypnotic suggestion emphasized self-regulation of the disease. Patients also visualized and reinforced treatment goals during self-hypnosis twice daily. A significant drop in fasting blood sugar and hemoglobin levels occurred over three hypnotic sessions as compared to the pretreatment levels. Despite the small sample size, the results suggest that hypnosis and self-hypnosis hold some promise in improving compliance with medical regimens in the treatment of certain chronic illnesses such as diabetes.

In another study, Swirsky-Sacchetti and Margolis (1986) studied the effects of self-hypnosis on hemophilia. A total of 30 hemophiliacs were randomly assigned to self-hypnotic treatment or to a waiting-list control group. The self-hypnosis group received a 6-week training program in

provements in both nausea and vomiting were reported in the majority of patients.

Hockenberry-Eaton and Cotanch (1989) studied the effects of hypnotherapy on perceived self-confidence in children undergoing chemotherapy for the treatment of cancer. Twenty-two children were randomly assigned to a self-hypnosis treatment group and a group receiving standard medical care. Self-hypnosis practice emphasized increased control and mastery. Relative to the control children, the children in the self-hypnosis group had significant increases in five of six dimensions of perceived self-confidence. Both groups showed increases in social and academic confidence after treatment.

Wall and Womack (1989) studied the effects of hypnosis on distress associated with bone marrow aspiration and lumbar puncture in pediatric oncology patients. A total of 20 subjects were randomly assigned to an hypnotic treatment condition or a cognitive strategy condition. Subjects in both groups received instructions in coping strategies designed to distance the children psychologically from uncomfortable medical procedures. Subjects in the hypnosis group were also given a hypnotic induction. Both groups showed significant decreases in pain but not anxiety. Hypnotizability did not correlate with pain reduction.

It appears from these studies that hypnotic interventions hold some promise in reducing subjective distress, enhancing psychological well-being, increasing recovery rate, and decreasing associated symptoms in patients undergoing uncomfortable medical and surgical procedures. However, much more work needs to be done with carefully controlled, randomized, blind clinical trials designed to discriminate among the differential effects of hypnotizability, hypnotic induction, situational demands, and type of hypnotic suggestions before definitive conclusions can be drawn as to the relative efficacy of hypnotic interventions as an adjunct to such procedures.

A few studies have also appeared in which hypnosis has been used with obstetrical and gynecological patients. Omer, Friedlander, and Palti (1986) and Omer (1987) investigated the effects of hypnotic relaxation as an adjunct to pharmacotherapy with 39 pregnant women hospitalized for premature labor contractions. Another 74 women in the control group received pharmacological treatment alone. Hypnotic suggestions focused on relaxation, increased control over bodily processes (including uterine contractions), and future time orientation to completion of the pregnancy at full term. Patients in the hypnosis group were also given audiotapes for daily self-hypnosis practice. The rate of pregnancy prolongation and mean weight of the infants were both significantly higher in the hypnosis group than in the medication control group. This study suffers from a number of methodological flaws—for example, nonrandom assignments to conditions, unmatched demographic and medical variables across groups, greater treatment time and therapist contact in the treatment group, and failure to assess hypnotizability. Thus, it is impossible to say whether hypnosis contributed to the significant treatment effects. The preliminary findings are important enough, however, to merit carefully designed controlled clinical trials on the effects of hypnosis in delaying premature labor.

In another study, Venn (1986) compared the efficacy of hypnosis to the Lamaze method for childbirth. A total of 122 women self-selected for one of three treatment groups: Lamaze classes alone ($n = 8$), hypnosis alone ($n = 17$), or Lamaze plus hypnosis ($n = 25$). Subjects who volunteered were given the Stanford Hypnotic Clinical Scale (Morgan & Hilgard, 1978–1979a) (only a small portion of the subjects in the groups volunteered to take the hypnotizability test). Group hypnosis training included suggestions for pain control, age progression through the birth experience, and posthypnotic suggestions to re-enter hypnosis at the appropriate time during labor and delivery. There were no significant differences between treatment groups in self-ratings or nurses' ratings of pain experience or well-being during labor, use of medication, or duration of labor. Hypnotizability was moderately correlated with subjective reports of less pain and discomfort during delivery, but only in the Lamaze group in which sufficient subjects took the hypnotizability scale. Although Venn concludes that there may be "functional similarities between hypnosis and Lamaze" (1986, p. 79), the failure to assign women randomly to the treatment conditions makes it difficult to distinguish between self-selection and treatment effects.

Health-Risk and Addictive Behaviors

Traditionally, clinical studies on hypnosis and smoking have been poorly designed. Moreover, the wide variety of hypnotic treatment strategies utilized has led to marked variations in treatment outcomes, which make it difficult to draw conclusions (D. P. Brown & Fromm, 1987). In an authoritative review of the literature, Wadden and Anderton (1982) concluded that hypnosis is not a uniquely effective strategy for smoking cessation or weight reduction. In response to this quite negative conclusion, we (D. P. Brown & Fromm, 1987) stated that the largely inconsistent and often poor maintenance rate at long-term follow-up intervals is more a problem with often ill-conceived hypnotic strategies to stop smoking or lose weight than with hypnosis per se. Within the field of behavioral medicine, there has been a distinct shift toward multimodal or broad-spectrum treatment approaches and also toward maintenance or relapse prevention strategies for weight loss and smoking cessation in particular, as well as for addictive behaviors in general (D. P. Brown & Fromm, 1987; Marlatt & Gordon, 1985). Nevertheless, by the time of the publication of *Hypnosis and Behavioral Medicine* (D. P. Brown & Fromm, 1987), few controlled clinical trials using primarily mulitmodal or relapse prevention approaches to hypnosis and weight reduction or smoking cessation had appeared in the literature. Multimodal strategies include interventions designed to address a number of dimensions of complex addictive behaviors: increasing motivation; facilitating coping; encouraging self-management of the habit per se; providing alternatives to the manner in which the habit is used in the service of affect regulation; altering negative cognitions and self-images that reinforce the addiction; decreasing negative social influences; and attenuating withdrawal states and risk situations for relapse.

The research literature on hypnosis and smoking and weight loss in the last several years can be grouped into three categories: (1) comparative efficacy studies; (2) multimodal hypnotic interventions; and (3) single-session hypnotic interventions. Consistent with our earlier conclusions (D. P. Brown & Fromm, 1987), results of the multimodal studies merit serious consideration.

The comparative efficacy studies have generally failed to show an advantage of hypnotic interventions over other methods. Hyman, Stanley, Burrows, and Horne (1986) compared hypnosis to focused smoking and to attention placebo and waiting list control conditions in 60 subjects. Smoking rates were not significantly different at the 3- and 6-month follow-ups. Frank, Umlauf, Wonderlich, and Ashkanazi (1986) compared different types of hypnotic treatments: two hypnotic sessions, four hypnotic sessions plus a booster; or two hypnotic sessions plus two behavioral sessions with a booster. A group hypnotic treatment protocol was used to enhance motivation and to facilitate coping strategies to quit smoking. There were no significant differences across treatments in the number of cigarettes smoked. A total of 31% of all subjects were abstinent at the end of treatment, and 20% at the 6-month follow-up. Success was negatively correlated with scores on the Creative Imagination Scale. Considering that most smoking interventions show recidivism to a baseline maintenance of about 20% by the second year after treatment, the results of these comparative efficacy studies are not impressive.

The results of multimodal interventions, in which hypnosis is integrated into a broad-spectrum treatment protocol, are more promising. T. B. Jeffrey, Jeffrey, Greuling, and Gentry (1985) developed a five-session treatment protocol, which included behavioral management of the habit, cognitive interventions, hypnotic relaxation, hypnotic reinforcement of the commitment to stop smoking, suggestions for smoking cessation, ego strengthening, and hypnotic control of craving to smoke. A total of 35 subjects in the group treatment sessions were compared to 30 waiting-list control subjects. Significantly more subjects in the multimodal hypnosis treatment group were abstinent than in the control group. A total of 63% in the hypnosis group were abstinent at the end of the treatment, and 31% maintained abstinence at a 3-month follow-up.

In a subsequent study, L. K. Jeffrey and Jeffrey (1988) added another dimension to this treatment; they called it "exclusion therapy." All smokers were required to maintain abstinence for 48 hours just prior to the treatment. A total of 120 subjects were randomly assigned to the hypnotic treatment condition, half of them with and half of them without a pretreatment abstinence condition. There were no significant differences between the treatment conditions. The abstinence rate in both groups was 59% at the end of treatment and 37% at the 3-month follow-up point. Unfortunately, the 1988 study lacked a control group, and no measures of hypnotizability were used in the earlier study. Nevertheless, compared to the predicted baseline recividism rate of 20%, multimodal hypnotic protocols may offer a distinct advantage to smoking cessation; still, a 3-month follow-up is too short to permit conclusions to be drawn about the efficacy of multimodal treatment.

The efficacy of multimodal hypnotherapy for weight loss has also been investigated (Cochrane & Friesen, 1986). A total of 60 obese women (>20% overweight) were randomly assigned to one of three conditions: group hypnosis; group hypnosis plus self-hypnosis; and a control group. Hypnosis in both treatment conditions included a group hypnotic induction, group suggestions to enhance motivation, ego strengthening, and facilitation of patients' decision making about weight treatment goals. Individualized hypnotic suggestions helped each patient identify unconscious factors related to weight loss. Patients in the treatment groups attended two weekly 3-hour sessions over a month. Whereas patients in the control group did not lose weight, patients in both treatments groups had a significant mean weight loss of 7–8 pounds at the end of the treatment and of about 17 pounds at a 6-month follow-up. Various measures of patient characteristics were included in the study. These included measures of suggestibility, imagery absorption, self-concept, family-of-origin conflict, age of onset of obesity, educational level, and socioeconomic status. None of these variables were significantly related to weight loss. Cochrane and Friesen concluded that hypnotherapy is a useful treatment for weight reduction. The addition of self-hypnosis did not add anything to the positive treatment outcome. The mean weight loss of 17 pounds at the 6-month follow-up is consistent with the expected weight loss from behaviorally oriented interventions (D. P. Brown & Fromm, 1987), although at least a 2-year follow-up interval is usually required in the weight loss field before clear conclusions can be reached (Stunkard, 1977).

The other popular approach to smoking and hypnosis entails a single-session treatment. Neufeld and Lynn (1988) reported their findings on a 2-hour single-session multimodal hypnotic protocol. The treatment manual included hypnotic suggestions to increase motivation, to induce relaxation, to alter self-image by visualizing the self as a nonsmoker, to identify risk situations and enhance coping strategies to prevent relapse, and to enhance the health benefits from smoking cessation. Abstinence rates were 26% at a 3-month follow-up and 19% at a 6-month follow-up. A study with more promising results was conducted by Williams and Hall (1988). A total of 60 subjects were assigned to a single-session hypnotic treatment, a placebo condition, or a non-treatment control condition. Subjects in the hypnotic condition received primarily hypnotic cognitive therapy, adapted from H. Spiegel (1970) and Stanton (1978). Subjects in the treatment group were significantly more abstinent (60%) than the controls (40%) following treatment. About 45% of the subjects maintained their abstinence at a 48-month follow-up.

A. F. Barabasz, Baer, Sheehan, and Barabasz (1986) studied a variety of treatment variables in 307 patients who utilized group hypnotic treatment for smoking cessation. The primary intervention was a single-session hypnotic approach. A number of subgroups were used, each of which varied the length of the session, the use of additional sessions, the use of posttreatment booster sessions, and the use of adjunctive sessions with REST. Some subgroups were led by interns and some by experienced psychologists. The primary hypnotic intervention employed H. Spiegel's (1970) approach to maintaining commitment to health. Abstinence rates at various follow-up points varied considerably, from 4% to 47%. The highest abstinence rates were found when experienced clinicians were used, when patients were given more treatment contact, and when REST (see Barabasz & Barabasz, Chapter 7, this volume) was used as an adjunct to hypnotherapy (the 47% abstinence rate was achieved at a 20-month follow-up in the hypnosis plus REST condition). In contrast to the previous negative conclusions of Wadden and Anderton (1982), hypnotizability was correlated significantly with the treatment outcome of this study.

The studies discussed above suggest that single-session treatment is worth considering as a brief cost-effective approach to smoking cessation. To the extent that tentative conclusions can be drawn, despite the various methodological weaknesses in the studies, it appears that unidimensional treatment emphasizing primarily hypnocognitive interventions (H. Spiegel, 1970; Stanton, 1978) yield better results than multimodal approaches (Neufeld & Lynn, 1988) in single-session hypnotic treatment. It may be that multimodal protocols are too complex for patients to grasp in a single session. Moreover, positive treatment outcomes may depend more on hypnotizability in single-session treatment than is the case over a number of sessions, where a variety of nonhypnotic variables may effect treatment outcome. At any rate, the A. F. Barabasz et al. (1986) paper is valuable in helping us to appreciate the complex number of variables that must be addressed if significant progress is to be made in the use of hypnosis for weight reduction and smoking cessation.

Psychiatric Conditions

Very few controlled clinical trials of hypnotherapy for psychiatric conditions have appeared in recent years. Several studies are worth noting, although each suffers from methodological limitations. Der and Lewington (1990) used a single-subject design to study the effects of hypnotherapy on panic attacks. After a 2-week baseline period, the subject was treated with hypnotherapy for 13 weeks. The hypnotic method was largely cognitive—an integration of hypnotically enhanced self-control strategies and rational–emotive therapy. According to the subject's reports and responses to objective symptom inventories, there was a reduction in anxiety-related symptoms. Although this study provides more data than an anecdotal case report, it is hard to make treatment generalizations from a single case.

Clarke and Reynolds (1991) conducted an outcome study on hypnotherapy and bruxism with eight patients. Hypnotic suggestions emphasized enhanced awareness of and control over masseter muscle activity. Nightly electromyographic (EMG) measurements of masseter activity served as the outcome measure, along with subjective ratings of pain. Relative to baseline measurements taken before treatment began, the bruxers showed a significant decrease in EMG activity and subjective reports of pain. Treatment gains were maintained up to 36 months. Griffiths (1989) investigated the outcome of hypnobehavioral therapy with 12 bulimia nervosa patients. Treatment consisted of 4 weeks of behavioral therapy followed by 4 weeks of hypnotherapy. Hypnotic suggestions emphasized enhanced self-control and mastery. Significant reductions in bingeing and vomiting were observed after treatment and at a 9-month follow-up. However, the lack of control groups or a crossover design between the behavioral and hypnotherapy treatment makes it difficult to assess the relative contribution of hypnosis to the positive treatment outcome.

One very important large-scale controlled outcome study was conducted on patients in The Netherlands with a diagnosis of posttraumatic stress disorder (Brom, Kleber, & Defares, 1989). The study included 112 patients who had been victims of violent crimes, had lost someone close to murder or suicide, or had suffered a serious traffic accident. Patients typically scored very high on the Impact of Events Scale (Horowitz, Wilner, & Alvarez, 1979), which measures intrusion and avoidance symptoms in response to traumatization. All patients were randomly assigned to one of four conditions: (1) desensitization therapy, in which subjects were presented with traumatic scenes from a hierarchy while in a relaxed state; (2) hypnobehavioral therapy, in which patients learned to cope better with traumatic imagery while in trance; (3) brief psychodynamic therapy, emphasizing resolution of conflicts triggered by the traumatic experience; and (4) a waiting-list control. All treatment was conducted by therapists

patients with chronic urticaria (Shertzer & Lookingbill, 1987), and proneness to nausea and vomiting during pregnancy (Apfel, Kelley, & Frankel, 1986). Although it is tempting to speculate about some underlying mechanism by which normal hypnotic ability is transmuted into psychopathology, notably psychophysiological and dissociative disorders, some caution is necessary. Most of these studies in question simply demonstrate a correlation between hpnotizability and psychopathology, and a correlation does not imply a causal relationship.

Current and Future Trends

An examination of the clinical research on hypnotherapy in the past several years makes it clear that the preponderance of controlled clinical research during that period was done in the domains of behavioral medicine in particular and medicine in general. *Hypnosis and Behavioral Medicine* (D. P. Brown & Fromm, 1987) was written with the intent of inviting a greater integration of the respective fields of hypnotherapy and behavioral medicine. It is encouraging to see the increased application of hypnosis in the field of behavioral medicine, and even more encouraging to see the number of clinical research studies appearing the literature that document the efficacy of hypnosis in the treatment (or adjunctive treatment) of psychophysiological and medical illnesses. Data are accumulating that enable us to carefully evaluate the efficacy of hypnosis in treating pain, headache, asthma, gastrointestinal disorders, skin disorders, immune diseases, and insomnia, as well as in facilitating adjustment to noxious medical procedures and chronic illnesses. The main contributions of hypnosis to clinical outcome lie in positive subjective effects (decreased distress and increased well-being) and in behavioral changes (symptom reduction, a decrease in the use of medication and the frequency of medical visits). Whether or not hypnosis can alter the underlying pathophysiology of psychophysiological disorders and chronic illnesses remains largely untested, though there are interesting suggestive findings with respect to asthma, hemiparesis, premature labor, and metastatic breast cancer.

With respect to habit disorders, the efficacy of hypnosis is not firmly established. The percentages of hypnotized patients who stop smoking or lose weight, and who maintain the treatment gains for reasonable follow-up intervals of 1 to 2 years, vary considerably across clinical research reports; as a result, it is impossible to say whether or not hypnosis consistently adds anything unique to the treatment outcome. Instead of attempting to demonstrate the efficacy of hypnosis in the treatment of health-risk behaviors, a more promising research strategy in recent years has been to identify the numerous complex variables relevant to treatment outcome. These include patient and therapist characteristics, the nature of the therapeutic interaction, and the context of the treatment and the intervention used (which in this case includes the nature of the hypnotic induction and the specific hypnotic suggestions given). A. F. Barabasz et al.'s (1986) follow-up study on smoking cessation and Cochrane and Friesen's (1986) study on weight control at least move in the direction of identifying a range of relevant variables, in addition to investigating the relative efficacy of hypnotherapy with health risk behaviors. Certainly much more work needs to be done in this area.

The main surprise in reviewing hypnotherapy research since 1986 is the absence of controlled clinical trials of hypnotherapy with psychiatric disorders. The one important exception is the study by Brom et al. (1989) on posttraumatic stress disorder. Then again, judging from the rapid proliferation of clinical literature on posttraumatic stress disorder in the past decade, it is just as surprising that only *one* reasonably well-designed controlled clinical outcome study has appeared in the literature. Several anecdotal reports have appeared regarding multiple personality disorder patients who were successfully treated with hypnosis (Coons, 1986; Kluft, 1985; Ross, Norton, & Fraser, 1989; Ross, Norton, & Wozney, 1989). However, controlled clinical trials using hypnosis as the primary intervention with such patients have not yet appeared. In contrast, about 40 clinical reports (mostly anecdotal) on hypnosis and dissociative disorders have appeared in the hypnosis journals or in the journal *Dissociation* since 1986. Although there appears to be tremendous interest in the use of hypnosis in the treatment of posttraumatic stress and dissociative disorders, the field simply has not evolved enough to generate a foundation of solid clinical outcome studies. Yet the paper by Brom et al. (1989) is indeed a very promising beginning. It is all the more puzzling, then, that controlled studies of hypnotherapy in more established areas of psychiatric treatment (e.g., anxiety, phobias, conversion disorders, grief reactions, and habit disorders) have been virtually nonexistent in recent years.

Neglected Areas

This reflection on the areas of hynotherapy research that have developed in the past several years makes it easier to see the blind spots in such research. First, considering the enormous amount of research conducted on drug efficacy in this country, it is amazing that there has been virtually no research on the interaction of hypnosis and drug-induced states. It is likely that many patients treated with hypnosis take medication for their main complaint and/or other conditions. But we know virtually nothing about how various medications affect hypnotic responsiveness, or how hypnosis may potentiate or attenuate drug effects. It is well established that set and setting greatly affect drug experiences (Tart, 1969). Likewise, the types of cognitive tasks carried out in hypnosis and situational variables significantly affect hypnotic responsiveness. Therefore, research on the interaction of drug effects, hypnotic suggestions, expectation effects, and contextual variables would be quite useful.

With respect to psychiatric conditions, there has been far too little work on hypnosis with affective disorders. Since cognitive therapy has made significant contributions to the treatment of depression (Burns, 1980), it is surprising to see so few studies on hypnocognitive therapy and depression. It would be useful to see research on the applications of Hartland's (1965) ego-strengthening suggestions or Stanton's (1989b) rational–emotive hypnotherapy in *controlled* clinical studies with depressive patients. Moreover, the use of hypnosis with bipolar patients is controversial. There are arguments for (Feinstein & Morgan, 1986) and against (D. P. Brown & Fromm, 1986) its use. These clinical arguments need to be backed up by research.

Another rapidly developing area of clinical hypnosis is the hypnoanalytic treatment of severely disturbed patients—that is, schizophrenic, borderline, and narcissistic patients. A number of important clinical papers and books on the theory and practice of hypnoanalysis with such patients have appeared in the literature (E. L. Baker, 1981, 1987, 1990; Fromm, 1984; D. P. Brown, 1985; D. P. Brown & Fromm, 1986; Copeland, 1986; Sands, 1986; Hodge, 1988). Although claims have been made about the efficacy of hypnosis in the treatment of certain severely disturbed patients, virtually no clinical research studies have examined these claims. Priority should be given to outcome studies for potentially useful treatments with the chronically mentally ill.

Another "hot" clinical area is the treatment of alcoholism and other substance abuse. Since our (D. P. Brown & Fromm, 1987) review of the hypnotherapy literature in this area, only a few anecdotal case reports have been published (Orman, 1991; Stanton, 1987); no controlled outcome studies on hypnotherapy with substance abuse have appeared. If this field is to address current social and clinical problems, much more work is needed in this area.

Finally, it is quite rare to find a reference in the clinical hypnosis literature to the use of hypnosis with patients from ethnic minority groups. Since 1986, one clinical article has described the use of hypnosis with Hispanic burn patients (Dobkin de Rios & Friedman, 1987). In another article, Richeport (1988) argues that it is important to understand cultural differences in framing hypnotic treatment. With the exception of these two articles, no other references to the concerns of ethnic minorities could be found in the clinical hypnosis literature surveyed, and certainly no controlled clinical studies have been conducted on hypnotherapy with ethnic minority populations.

A Shift toward Integrative Hypnotherapy

In the past several years, a number of authors have clearly articulated the theoretical foundations that guide their use of hypnosis in psychotherapy. Some (D. P. Brown & Fromm, 1986; Lavoie, 1990; Watkins, 1986) have presented consistent theoretical explanations of the psychodynamic theories underlying their approaches to hypnotherapy and hypnoanalysis. Others (D. P. Brown & Fromm, 1987; E. L. Baker, 1990; Copeland, (1986) have detailed the essential features of a structural/developmental psychoanalytic theory as it applies to the hypnoanalytic treatment of the severely disturbed psychiatric patient. Several clinicians have articulated the essential features of their behavioral (D. P. Brown & Fromm, 1987; Spinhoven, 1987) and cognitive–behavioral (Stanton, 1989a,b; Okhowat, 1985) approaches to hypnotherapy. Still other clinicians have attempted to integrate family systems theory and hypnotherapy (Brink, 1986–1987; Lind, 1989; Somer, 1990).

In my opinion, the best clinicians mature beyond identification with a particular theoretical position and are able to move flexibly across diverse theoretical perspectives to select the theory and related treatment approach, or combination of approaches, that best matches a given patient's needs. When the data of the individual case are used to guide the selection of a treatment from among diverse possibilities, the selection process is by no means haphazard or eclectic, but systematic and intregative. As I see it, integrative psychotherapy is probably the wave of the future as we come to understand which treatments are best matched to which conditions. In anticipation of this trend, more studies are necessary in which the outcome of hypnotherapy conducted from diverse theoretical perspectives is compared with respect to selected patient populations. For example, this chapter has reported a number of positive outcome studies in which hypnocognitive therapy was matched to specific patient populations whose illnesses had a high cognitive load (notably patients with IBS and insomnia). In an ideal sense, criteria may be developed to guide clinical treatment planning, so that we know which particular approach to hypnotherapy is best suited to a particular syndrome or personality type.

Design Strategy

There are four types of clinical research designs, intended to meet different goals. Clinical efficacy studies are designed to answer these questions: Does a particular treatment work? Is it effective? Comparative efficacy studies are designed to compare the relative efficacy of two or more treatment approaches: For example, is hypnotherapy more effective than progressive muscle relaxation or a cognitive–behavioral approach to the treatment of insomnia? Multimodal studies compare the relative contribution of a number of combined treatment strategies to the overall variance of the clinical outcome. A sample question here is as follows: How much do motivational enhancement, hypnotic relaxation, behavioral habit management, hypnocognitive therapy, and relapse prevention strategies each contribute to the overall treatment outcome, when these combined strategies are used for smoking cessation? Finally, individualized designs allow the individual patient to select and/or tailor hypnotic imagery and suggestions within the overall treatment frame. The question here is this: Are individual treatment protocols more or less effective than standardized treatment protocols? In the field of behavioral medicine, the majority of the studies have been comparative efficacy studies, with a more recent shift toward more sophisticated multimodal and individualized designs (D. P. Brown & Fromm, 1987). In the area of psychotherapy research in general, a number of internally consistent treatment manuals are appearing; the components of these treatments can be added or subtracted as a means of assessing the relative contribution of each component to the overall outcome (Beutler & Clarkin, 1991).

The hypnotherapy studies reviewed here follow the same trend as do other studies of behavioral medicine and psychotherapy outcome. Newer research areas (e.g., treatment of eczema or duodenal ulcer) are primarily represented by clinical efficacy studies. A number of comparative efficacy studies have emerged, in which hypnosis and (typically) behavioral or cognitive–behavioral treatments have been compared. There are, however, still very few multimodal and individualized treatment designs represented in the studies reviewed. Because a trend toward integrative psychotherapy, along with the development of clearly articulated treatment manuals, is anticipated, more multimodal and individualized designs are warranted.

The Standard of Research Design

In reflecting on the clinical hypnosis research over the past several years, I find it encouraging to see an increase both in the number of clinical studies and in the number of well-designed controlled clinical studies, in contrast to poorly designed post hoc comparisons of nonrandomized groups (Beutler, Crago, & Machado, 1991). The standard of hypnotic research has been raised somewhat by the well-designed studies that have appeared. By "well-designed," I mean studies that use appropriately matched control groups along with experimental groups; that randomize assignment into these groups; that conduct the treatment in a blind way, wherever possible; and that also control for situational demands (e.g., through the use of placebo controls, simulator controls, counterdemand suggestions, etc.). Such ideal designs, although easy to carry out in experimental settings with normal subjects, are much harder to implement with clinic patients. The fact that a number of the studies reviewed here move in the direction of meeting most of these criteria is encouraging and suggests that a clear standard of hypnotherapy research is evolving.

Nevertheless, even the best of these studies fall far short of the ideal. The evolving standard of psychotherapy outcome research addresses the complex interaction of different important variables: (1) specific treatment; (2) therapist qualities; (3) patient characteristics; (4) specific problem area; and (5) nature of the setting (Beutler & Clarkin, 1991). Psychotherapy process research has also emphasized the importance of understanding the therapist–patient relationship (Beutler et al., 1991). Within the wider context of psychotherapy research, it is too simple to ask the hypnotherapy outcome question, "Does hypnosis work in treating certain symptoms?" (D. P. Brown & Fromm, 1987, p. 57). Clinical outcome studies of hypnotherapy must control for at least six specific types of variables: (1) treatment variables (the approach to hypnosis, the style of hypnosis used, the nature and wording of suggestions given); (2) hypnotherapist variables (the level of experience of the hypnotherapist, the characteristics of the hypnotherapist); (3) the characteristics of the given patient population; (4) the nature of the presenting problem; (5) the nature of the setting (the context of the treatment, and the expectational and situational demands inherent in that context); and (6) the quality of the hypnotherapeutic relationship.

If there is one major flaw in most of these outcome studies, I believe that it is the recurrent failure to control for the type of hypnotic suggestions utilized in each type of clinical trial. Unfortunately, it is still quite rare to see a research report that includes the entire wording of the hypnotic protocol used in the treatment. This curious omission merits some explanation. In part, it can be attributed to the greater emphasis on studying hypnotherapy outcome than on hypnotherapy process. Within the wider context of psychotherapy research, the evolving standard is likely to be a integration of process and outcome research (Beutler et al., 1991). Thus, I anticipate that more emphasis will be given to the hypnotherapy process in the future by investigators studying hypnotherapy outcome. Since there is much we do not know about the process of hypnotherapy, it may be advisable to follow the general recommendation of L. Horwitz and his associates for psychotherapy process research—namely, that future research engage in hypothesis finding about therapy process as much as in hypothesis testing about therapy outcome (L. Horwitz, Allen, Colson, Frieswyk, Gabbard, Coyne, & Newsom, 1991).

ful use of language and individualized strategy are of the utmost importance in the process and for the outcome of hypnotherapy. Future hypnotherapy research should strive to integrate process and outcome perspectives, as is already the trend in other psychotherapy research. Through utilizing both the construct of hypnotizability and the specificity theory of hypnotic responsivity in clinical hypnotherapy research, we may strengthen the scientific base on which the art of clinical hypnosis is built.

CHAPTER SEVENTEEN

The Measurement of Hypnotic Ability

CAMPBELL PERRY
ROBERT NADON
JENNIFER BUTTON

Attempts to measure the ability to experience hypnosis first began within the context of 19th-century clinical practice (Perry & Laurence, 1980). Braid (1855/1970), for example, proposed a tripartite classification in terms of three "stages" or degrees of hypnotic depth, which he labeled "slight hypnosis," "deep hypnosis," and "hypnotic coma." The first of these referred to what is experienced by approximately 90% of the population. At that time, given the close parallel drawn between hypnosis and nocturnal sleep, a degree of lethargy was most commonly reported (as opposed to the more frequent current experience of relaxation). At the same time, the person in "slight hypnosis," then as now, had no subsequent loss of memory. The subsequent two "stages" involved different forms of posthypnotic amnesia: "Deep hypnosis" involved being able to remember the events of a particular hypnotic session only in a subsequent one, whereas "hypnotic coma" represented a permanent amnesia for what was experienced in a particular hypnosis session.

These last two amnesias are rarely if ever seen today, mainly because current investigators see posthypnotic amnesia as a suggested phenomenon rather than as "spontaneous." By contrast, the amnesias of a century and a half ago appear to have been the products of shared implicit views held by both hypnotic practitioners and hypnotized patients about the manner in which hypnotic response manifests itself; the belief of both patients and therapists that "spontaneous" amnesia was to be expected most likely led to its occurrence in those patients possessing the abilities of the highly hypnotizable. Viewed in this manner, such amnesias offer striking instances of how the demand characteristics (Orne, 1959) of history markedly influenced the behavior observed in hypnosis at these earlier times.

A review of the literature reveals that many clinicians subsequent to Braid attempted to further categorize degrees of responsivity to hypnosis; Bernheim (1886/1889) proposed nine such categories, each defined in terms of behavioral responses that were thought to have subjective accompaniments. Interestingly, Bernheim's taxonomy of hypnotic responsivity bears a close resemblance to that of one of the current standardized measuring instruments of hypnotic ability (see Perry & Laurence, 1980, for a review of this literature).

The current situation is for the most part markedly different in all but one major respect. A certain degree of standardization in the measurement of what is now called "hypnotic responsivity" (used in this chapter as synonymous with "hypnotic susceptibility," "hypnotizability," and "hypnotic ability") has been achieved as the result of work beginning in the late 1950s, which led to the development of the Stanford scales (Weitzenhoffer & Hilgard, 1959, 1962, 1967). Despite this degree of standardization, the past three decades have also witnessed a proliferation of measuring instruments based variously upon such considerations as an investigator's theoretical position about the nature of hypnosis, the perceived differential exigencies of clinical and laboratory hypnosis, and various beliefs about which hypnotic items best tap the hypnotized person's experience of hypnosis.

The present chapter seeks to explore some current issues in the measurement of hypnotic ability in the light of current diversity in measuring instruments. It focuses upon the four measures[1] most commonly utilized in the current practice of both laboratory and clinical hypnosis.

The Problem in Current Perspective

More than 30 years have elapsed since Weitzenhoffer and Hilgard (1959) introduced the first viable measures of hypnotizability into the field. The Stanford Hypnotic Susceptibility Scale, Forms A and B (SHSS:A and SHSS:B) were parallel forms of a 12-item measuring instrument, each taking approximately 1 hour to administer, and each comprised of individual items of progressively greater difficulty. Methods for evaluating hypnotic susceptibility already existed at this time; for various reasons, however, their properties as measurement devices were less than optimal (see E. R. Hilgard, 1965a, for a review). With the demonstration of the SHSS:A and SHSS:B's measurement properties, the field appeared finally to be moving towards having a uniform yardstick, against which experimental studies from different investigators could be gauged.

This impression was reinforced soon afterward with the introduction of the Stanford Hypnotic Susceptibility Scale, Form C (SHSS:C), also authored by Weitzenhoffer and Hilgard (1962). Like the earlier two forms, it consisted of 12 items of progressively greater difficulty and required approximately 1 hour to administer. The SHSS:C differed from its earlier counterparts in possessing greater "top"; that is, it contained not merely items of progressively greater difficulty (in common with the SHSS:A and SHSS:B), but, overall, a greater proportion of more difficult cognitive items. The earlier impression, and indeed hope, of a standard "tape measure" for the evaluation of hypnotizability appeared even closer to fruition.

This growing trend continued with Shor and Orne's (1962) construction of a group version of the SHSS:A, which they called the Harvard Group Scale of Hypnotic Susceptibility, Form A (HGSHS:A). More is said about the rationale of this scale subsequently; for the present, it is sufficient to indicate that its implementation permitted group administration to samples of up to 20 subjects simultaneously. This saving of time, however, was not the sole or even the primary rationale for the development of the HGSHS:A, although some investigators have since utilized it primary for this reason. The problems resulting from this exclusive utilization of the HGSHS:A are likewise discussed in a later section. One major result of this successful development of HGSHS:A as a group administered scale is that nowadays its forerunners (SHSS:A and SHSS:B) are rarely utilized, at least by laboratory researchers.

In the following years, there was a proliferation of shorter scales of measurement. One of these, the Barber Suggestibility Scale (BSS), was first reported in a study performed by T. X. Barber and Glass (1962). The BSS consisted of eight items, and was reported as taking from 10 to 12 minutes to administer and score. Norms and psychometric properties were published subsequently (T. X. Barber, 1965). Barber's main rationale for developing this scale was that, in his view, the earlier scales were "intertwined with the administration of a hypnotic induction procedure and predicated upon the presumed presence of 'trance' "; this meant, from Barber's perspective, that they were "not conducive to experimental manipulation of independent variables prior to assessment of response" (T. X. Barber, 1965, p. 810).

At the time when he wrote this rationale, Barber was deeply interested in the related questions of whether hypnosis permitted transcendence of basic capacities. He was also interested in the question of whether the term "hypnosis" was expendable. He developed this view as a result of a large number of studies he performed during this period; these usually indicated that performance in a hypnosis condition could not be distinguished from performance in what he called a "task motivation" condition.[2] He did not, however, provide any rationale for introducing so brief an induction procedure—one that took only 20% of the time it takes to administer the HGSHS:A and SHSS:C, and that consisted of several fewer items.

Like the SHSS:A and SHSS:B, the BSS came subsequently to be abandoned in favor of a group-administered scale. The Carleton University Responsiveness to Suggestion Scale (CURSS) was first reported in three simultaneously published papers in the early 1980s (Spanos, Radtke, Hodgins, Stam, & Bertrand, 1983; Spanos, Radtke, Hodgins, Bertrand, Stam, & Dubreuil, 1983; Spanos, Radtke, Hodgins, Bertrand, Stam, & Moretti, 1983). Spanos, the first author of all three papers, performed much of his early work with Barber; not surprisingly, he shares many (though not all) of the theoretical beliefs of his former coinvestigator. Consequently, the CURSS, like the BSS, is a relatively short measuring instrument; it consists of a 5-minute induction period followed by seven items, each of which takes 50 seconds to administer (approximately 6 minutes in all). In addition, four different indices of susceptibility (to be discussed later) take an additional several minutes for the subject to self-score, so that in all, the CURSS appears to take approximately 25 to 30 minutes to administer and score.[3]

Although all of the aforementioned brief measures of hypnotic ability were developed in the experimental, laboratory context, clinicians were becoming interested at this time in obtaining measures of hypnotizability from patients. As opposed to the experimental interest in sampling a wide band of experiences a person may have in hypnosis (thus implying longer measures in terms of time), the clinical interest was in developing brief estimates of hypnotic responsivity, in order to determine a person's suitability for therapy in which hypnosis was utilized as a part of the treatment program.

A pioneer of this trend was H. Spiegel (1972), who first introduced the Hypnotic Induction Profile (HIP) to the field. The HIP is not quite like any other measure of hypnotic responsivity, and in its early days at least, it generated a considerable degree of controversy. The details of the procedure are discussed later; the main point is that it sought to obtain an estimate of what was referred to as "clinically usable hypnotizability." More recently, performance on the HIP has been characterized as "a statement of the relationship between a person's potential for trance and his ability to experience it and maintain it" (H. Spiegel & Spiegel, 1978, p. 41)—a perspective not found in any other measurement approach to hypnotic ability.

The present chapter focuses on these four measures of hypnotizability—namely, the longer measures as exemplified by the HGSHS:A and SHSS:C, and the briefer CURSS and HIP. Each of these measures is first described, and the data that exist on their interrelationships are then presented. Specifically, this chapter addresses the question of the degree to which these four scales provide equivalent measures; that is, do they measure the same individuals in a consistent manner? An allied question concerns whether they are equally successful in identifying highly hypnotizable individuals. It should be emphasized that the answers to these questions are imperfect ones; the analysis, however, highlights the problems with which present-day and future hypnosis researchers will need to grapple.

Longer Measures of Hypnotic Ability

As indicated earlier, of measures that are still currently in frequent usage, the HGSHS:A and the SHSS:C are the most commonly employed measures of hypnotizability. This is particularly so in the laboratory; indeed, their administration length (approximately 1 hour each) has led some clinical investigators to reject them on the grounds of feasibility. This is based upon the belief that a clinician has too pressing a set of time commitments to be realistically able to perform so extensive and detailed a measuring procedure (M. J. Diamond, 1989; E. L. Rossi, 1989). Other clinicians report hesitating to utilize the SHSS:C (though they quite often incorporate the SHSS:A and SHSS:B into their practice) because it includes some challenge items; here the legitimate concern is that failure on such items will translate into therapeutic failure (E. Fromm, personal communication to C. Perry, September 24, 1991). Too few clinical professionals have commented on these issues, however, for us to be able to evaluate this issue of excessive time constraints.

Accordingly, the present discussion must perforce be restricted to laboratory uses of the HGSHS:A and SHSS:C. Even a cursory examination of the laboratory literature on these two instruments reveals a considerable cleavage among experimental researchers in the usage of these instruments; the split is between those who utilize the HGSHS:A as a sole measure of hypnotizability, as opposed to those who like to administer the HGSHS:A first, followed by the more cognitively demanding SHSS:C. In the following sections, each is separately evaluated, following which they are compared.

The Harvard Group Scale of Hypnotic Susceptibilty, Form A

The HGSHS:A may well be the most widely used measuring instrument in the field of hypnosis. As indicated earlier, it was adapted from the SHSS:A by Shor and Orne (1962), consists of 12 items, and takes approximately 1 hour to administer. Its most valuable characteristic is that it is group-administered by audiocassette; it thus provides substantial savings of time, in that a group of up to 20 individuals can be tested simultaneously within the space of 1 hour.[4] As indicated earlier, however, there were other, more compelling reasons than the saving of time that led to the decision to construct an audiotaped, group-administered, standardized measure of hypnotizability.

The HGSHS:A was intended as a preliminary screening device, designed to serve as a nonthreatening initial estimate of hypnotic responsivity. This was a major consideration in the decision to record it on audiocassette; Shor and Orne (1962) believed that such a procedure conveyed the implicit message that hypnosis is a sufficiently benign procedure to be induced in groups via mechanical means. Less well known is the fact that the person who narrated the induction for the recording was the late Lee Dumas, who for many years was a nightclub entertainer in the Boston area. His only connection with the field (although it is almost certain to have been an important one) was that he himself was highly responsive to hypnosis; he thus had an understanding of the subjective alterations that hypnosis can activate (L. Dumas, 1964).

Over a span of almost 30 years, the HGSHS:A has been evaluated extensively for its properties as a measuring instrument. During this period, normative studies have been performed at Harvard University (Shor & Orne, 1963); the University of California at Berkeley (Coe, 1964); the University of Queensland, Australia (Sheehan & McConkey, 1979); and Concordia University, Montréal, Canada (Laurence & Perry, 1982). More recently, German (Bongartz, 1985) and Spanish (Lamas, del Valle-Inclan, Blanco, & Diaz, 1989) norms have been constructed. Thus, it is possible to evaluate the measuring properties of the HGSHS:A both over time and across several different cultures.

There are numerous ways of performing such an evaluation. One preferred way is to compare the item difficulties of the 12 HGSHS:A items across different samples—that is, the percentage of individuals passing each item, where the smaller the percentage of passing, the greater the difficulty of the item. All six normative studies have reported these pass percentages for each item; they are presented in Table 17.1. Discrepancies in the item difficulties of the six normative groups are apparent. To begin with, when the difficulties of the amnesia suggestion are compared across samples, only the Canadian sample (19%) approaches the general estimate of its occurrence within the general population. The figure usually is put at 10–15% of all individuals. For the remaining five samples, the difficulty of amnesia ranges from 33% to 52%. Much the same is found for posthypnotic suggestion, which is thought to be an even more difficult item than posthypnotic amnesia; here, the range of pass percentages is from 15% to 36%.

Additional cross-comparison is difficult, since the Australian and Canadian sample used the standard audiotaped version recorded by Dumas; the German and Spanish versions were audiotaped translations; and the Boston and Berkeley samples were administered orally by an experimenter. Thus, discrepancies might be the result of any of a number of factors: differences in language,[5] in culture, in method of presentation, and in the degree to which the subjects were prepared for hypnosis. On this last point, it should be noted that the Canadian sample was given a 2-hour lecture on hypnosis; this was designed to allay any fears, misconceptions, and misgivings that subjects might have about hypnosis. A part of this procedure involved answering questions that subjects had about hypnosis. Furthermore, the administration of the HGSHS:A was

TABLE 17.1. Item Difficulty: Percentages of Subjects Passing Each Item of the HGSHS:A in Six Normative Samples

Item	Spain 1989 (n = 220)	Germany 1985 (n = 374)	Canada 1982 (n = 535)	Australia 1979 (n = 1,944)	Berkeley 1964 (n = 168)	Boston 1963 (n = 132)
1. Head falling	73	73	65	61	68	86
2. Eye closure	64	73	63	57	56	74
3. Hand lowering	60	83	66	71	71	89
4. Arm immobil- ization	58	52	47	36	35	48
5. Finger lock	67	57	50	53	52	67
6. Arm rigidity	69	52	47	41	48	57
7. Hands moving	79	74	64	71	77	86
8. Verbal inhibi- tion	74	49	43	42	44	50
9. Hallucination	29	47	23	25	33	39
10. Eye catalepsy	59	47	36	38	39	56
11. Posthypnotic suggestion	29	31	15	17	34	36
12. Amnesia	52	36	19	33	35	48
Mean % pass per item	59	56	45	45	49	61

part of a laboratory exercise; the students were told that they were not obliged to undergo the hypnotic procedure, but they were expected to write a laboratory report. Very few students actually missed the hypnosis testing on the HGSHS:A; this sampling procedure, however, may mean that the Canadian sample is not typical of what is obtained by more traditional volunteer recruitment procedures.

Another set of problems is posed by the data presented in Table 17.1: Not merely do item difficulties fluctuate by sample, but samples differ in terms of the percentage of persons passing items overall. Clearly, a method by which these discrepancies can be evaluated is needed. There is no ideal solution to this problem, but, a rough assessment of the issue is possible. It can be argued that regardless of these sample differences (and whatever their origin may be) if the HGSHS:A is truly a robust measuring instrument, the item difficulties in each sample relative to the others should be fairly similar. That is, head falling should be a fairly simple item in all six samples, and amnesia and posthypnotic suggestion should be relatively difficult. Thus, one can rank-order the item difficulties in each of the samples and intercorrelate them. Furthermore, since (with a few ex-

TABLE 17.2. Intercorrelations of HGSHS:A Item Difficulties in Six Samples, and Their Correlations with the Order of Presentation of Items

	1.	2.	3.	4.	5.	6.	7.
1. Spain	—	.65	.66	.79	.79	.70	.47
2. Germany		—	.99	.94	.91	.92	.84
3. Canada			—	.94	.91	.94	.88
4. Australia				—	.98	.97	.71
5. Berkeley					—	.97	.67
6. Boston						—	.72
7. Order of presentation							—

ceptions) the items of HGSHS:A were ordered in terms of item difficulty (from least to most difficult), performance of these six samples should correlate at least moderately with order of item presentation. The results of this analysis are set out in Table 17.2.

There are several striking features of this analysis. To begin with, there is remarkably high correlation of the item difficulties of the German, Canadian, Australian, Boston, and Berkeley samples; all are greater than .90. This suggests strongly that the HGSHS:A is not greatly affected by language and cultural differences; even for the Spanish sample, the correlations, though lower, are all still statistically significant. Furthermore, this analysis indicates that the HGSHS:A is relatively stable over time since, the Boston and Berkeley samples were tested in the early 1960s, and the Australian, Spanish, German, and Canadian samples were tested from 15 to 25 years after the Berkeley sample. Finally, it is of some interest that there are relatively high correlations between most of the HGSHS:A samples and the order of presentation of items. Only the Spanish sample fails to correlate significantly with order of presentation of items, which was the same for all samples. Again, on this criterion, the HGSHS:A can be said to consist of items of progressively greater difficulty,[6] and it can be concluded overall that the HGSHS:A is relatively unaffected by sociocultural factors. The fact, however, that there are variations in outcomes on individual items suggests one important conclusion: In general, the investigator who relies upon the HGSHS:A as a sole measure for determining hypnotizability categorizations may have many errors of classification in his or her data. We return to this point following our discussion of other measures of hypnotic responsivity.

The Stanford Hypnotic Susceptibility Scale, Form C

In 1962, Weitzenhoffer and Hilgard introduced the SHSS:C. As indicated earlier, it was designed to have more "top" to it through the utilization of more cognitive items of greater difficulty. Although some easy items are presented initially, such as hand lowering and hand separation, the remaining 10 items are difficult; the range of pass percentages has been reported to be from 9% to 48%. Like the HGSHS:A, the SHSS:C is still in widespread use, and has become (as will be seen when other measures are presented) the touchstone against which new measures of hypnotizability are evaluated.

Some investigators have modified certain items of the SHSS:C for various reasons. In research at Concordia University, for instance, the anosmia-to-ammonia item has been removed and replaced by a posthypnotic suggestion that the subject will stand up when a cue is given. The reason for this is that it is difficult to standardize the anosmia item; the instruction is to hold a bottle of ammonia (of unspecified strength) 3 inches from the subject's nose, in order to test the suggestion that the sense of smell has been lost. Invariably, if the experimenter suspects that this sense has not been lost, he or she will hold the ammonia further away from the nose so as to avoid a coughing fit. Furthermore, the replacement of anosmia by a posthypnotic suggestion is helpful in confirming the subject's response to this item on the HGSHS:A.

In addition, the age regression instructions to re-experience grades 5 and 2 has been replaced by a suggestion to regress to the age of 5 years old. This alteration was made in the hope of eliciting more childlike behavior. The scoring, has also been modified to assess the degree to which the subject experiences a "reliving" of the suggested age.[7] Furthermore, all references during the initial relaxation induction period to hypnosis as being akin to sleep have been removed, since it is now well established that the electroencephalographic (EEG) pattern of hypnosis is not in any way similar to the four stages of sleep that have been identified via EEG (see F. J. Evans, 1979, for a review). These are relatively minor changes; their effect upon cross-comparison of hypnotizability categories by other investigators using the SHSS:C is likely to be minimal.

The norms for the SHSS:C were originally obtained for 203 subjects (Weitzenhoffer & E. Hilgard, 1962), and subsequently boosted to 307 subjects because of some irregularity in the earlier sample. These are presented in Table 17.3. Before we comment upon these normative data, we should state that not all investigators have followed E. R. Hilgard's (1965) recommendation for classifying subjects into a fourfold categorization ("very high," "high," "medium," and "low"). Some use a very "soft" criterion of treating scores of from 8 to 12 as high, and from 0 to 4 as low, with the remaining scores (from 5 to 7) being classified as medium. Others are more severe, classifying scores from 9 to 12 as high and from 0 to 2 as low. Then again, there are studies that classify highly susceptible subjects as individuals who pass the SHSS:C amnesia criterion and most of its other 11 items. This classification is based upon the assumption that posthypnotic amnesia is associated with the classical somnambulism that has been

TABLE 17.3. Norms for the SHSS:C ($n = 307$)

General level	Raw score	Number of cases	Percentage of cases
Very high	12	7	2
	11	8	3
High	10	19	6
	9	15	5
	8	30	10
Medium	7	29	9
	6	29	9
	5	33	11
Low	4	24	8
	3	33	11
	2	48	16
	1	22	7
	0	10	3

Mean = 5.19; standard deviation = 3.09.

Note. From *Hypnotic Susceptibility* (p. 236) by E. R. Hilgard, 1965, New York: Harcourt, Brace & World. Copyright 1965 by Harcourt, Brace & World. Reprinted by permission.

described for more than 200 years in the historical literature of hypnosis (Laurence & Perry, 1988). This may appear at first glance to defeat the purpose of cross-comparison with other studies, but, as will be seen, it need not.

The distribution of the SHSS:C is multimodal (see E. R. Hilgard, 1965a, p. 237), with modes appearing at the scores of 2, 5, 8, and 10. This might suggest an empirical basis for classifying subjects scoring from 10 to 12 as high, from 8 to 9 as high medium, from 5 to 7 as medium, and from 0 to 4 as low. This is a matter of preference; the main point to be drawn from the normative data is that the distribution of hypnotizability within a college population (and there is only slight reason to think that students are unrepresentative of the general population) is anything but normal—as is so commonly reported.

An inspection of the item difficulties of the SHSS:C reveals that it is, as its constructors intended, an ascending scale in which (with one exception) the items begin with very easy ones and rapidly become progressively more difficult. These are presented in Table 17.4, along with the correlations of each item with total score (minus the particular item) and retest reliabilities. This table indicates that only the amnesia item of SHSS:C is aligned out of its order of presentation. This item difficulty is, however, higher than the commonly believed figure of 10–15%, which traditionally has been taken as the percentage of hypnotically amnesic subjects. The

TABLE 17.4. Item Difficulty, Correlation of Item with Total Score, and Estimated Reliability of Individual Items for the SHSS:C

Item	Percent passing ($n = 203$)	Correlation with total score minus this item (biserial r's) ($n = 203$)	Retest reliability coefficients (tetrachoric r's)
1. Hand lowering	92	.60	.77 ($n = 307$)
2. Moving hands apart	88	.49	.65 ($n = 307$)
3. Mosquito hallucination	48	.80	.76 ($n = 307$)
4. Taste hallucination	46	.75	.60 ($n = 35$)
5. Arm rigidity	45	.76	.67 ($n = 307$)
6. Dream	44	.57	.63 ($n = 58$)
7. Age regression	43	.68	.69 ($n = 58$)
8. Arm immobilization	36	.81	.60 ($n = 307$)
12. Amnesia	27	.85	.74 ($n = 307$)
9. Anosmia to ammonia	19	.65	.65 ($n = 58$)
10. Hallucinated voice	9	.63	.70 (estimated)
11. Negative hallucination	9	.87	.60 ($n = 35$)

Note. From *Hypnotic Susceptibility* (p. 238) by E. R. Hilgard, 1965, New York: Harcourt, Brace & World. Copyright 1965 by Harcourt, Brace & World. Reprinted by permission.

range of correlations between each item and total score minus that item is from .49 to .87, and the Kuder–Richardson total scale reliability index (see Note 6) was reported by E. R. Hilgard (1965a, p. 237) as .85. Furthermore, he reported the correlation between the SHSS:A and SHSS:C as .72; this is lower than the correlation between the SHSS:A and SHSS:B because of the addition of new and more difficult items. Since the SHSS:A and SHSS:B have been superseded by the HGSHS:A, however, it is of interest to examine the degree to which the group scale is related to the SHSS:C.

Relationship between the HGSHS:A and SHSS:C

In a recent paper examining the relationship between the HGSHS:A and SHSS:C, Register and Kihlstrom (1986) noted that there are many merits to relying on the HGSHS:A alone to assess hypnotizability. They stated that

> the group-administered, tape recorded format insures that unhypnotizable and hypnotizable subjects are treated alike by the hypnotist; and the procedure permits the easy accumulation of large amounts of data. Several studies of unselected samples, however, show that HGSHS:A correlates only about $r = .60$ with SHSS:C (Bentler & Roberts, 1963; Coe, 1964; [F. J.] Evans & Schmeidler, 1966). (pp. 85–86)

Using some earlier unpublished data from samples of 112 and of 107 subjects, Register and Kihlstrom (1986) confirmed these earlier findings; the correlations within the two separate samples between the two scales were .60 and .57 respectively. More troubling, though, was the finding that when the two samples were pooled, only 36% of subjects scoring in the highest range on the HGSHS:A (11–12) continued to perform comparably on the SHSS:C.

Register and Kihlstrom proceeded to seek replication of this finding. A sample of 96 subjects was tested on both scales; again, the correlation of .62 was similar to that of the first study they had reported, and again, only 33% of subjects scoring in the highest range on the HGSHS: A maintained this performance on the SHSS:C. Given this uniformity of results for the two studies, we feel that pooling the two studies is justified; the results are presented in Table 17.5. This table indicates that of the 315 subjects, 148 (47%) were categorized identically on the HGSHS:A and SHSS:C. The greatest agreement on the two scales was in the low hypnotizable category; of 92 subjects scoring in this category on the HGSHS:A, 65 of them (71%) were classified as low in hypnotizability on the SHSS:C. For the remaining three categories, the corresponding figures were, respectively, 29% (medium), 46% (medium high), and 34% (high). An alternative analysis reveals that of these 315 subjects, only 47% of them performed identically on the two scales; 30% scored lower on the SHSS:C, and 23% scored higher on it. As already seen, most of this effect can be attributed to the fact that

TABLE 17.5. Joint Distribution of Hypnotizability as Classified by the HGSHS:A and SHSS:C ($n = 215$)

HGSHS:A classification	SHSS:C classification								Total
	Low (0–4)		Medium (5–7)		High (8–10)		Virtuoso (11–12)		
	n	%	n	%	n	%	n	%	
Low (0–4)	65	71	17	18	10	11	0	0	92
		60		22		11		0	
Medium (5–7)	36	39	27	29	24	26	5	5	92
		33		34		25		15	
Medium high (8–10)	7	7	29	30	44	46	16	17	96
		6		37		46		48	
Very high (11–12)	0	0	6	17	17	49	12	34	35
		0		8		18		36	
Total	108		79		95		33		315

Note. The data are condensed from Tables 1 and 2 (pp. 86 and 89) of Register and Kihlstrom (1986).

low hypnotizability tends to be the category best measured (in terms of consistency) by the two scales.

These data speak eloquently to the issue of testing for hypnotizability with the HGSHS:A only. Almost half of the time, a subject's score on the HGSHS:A leads to a different classification from that obtained with the SHSS:C. Partly, this is a matter of the HGSHS:A's having little "top" of difficult cognitive items. Allied to this is the fact that the HGSHS:A provides the great majority of subjects with their first experience of hypnosis; it is reasonable to think that some HGSHS:A scores will reflect compliance to suggestions, while others will be the result of subjects' "holding back" until they have assured themselves that they are in a safe and protected situation.

Briefer Measures of Hypnotizability

Following the publication of the Stanford scales between 1959 and 1962, and of the HGSHS:A during the same period, there was a development that was to have profound consequences for measurement in the field of hypnosis. For various reasons, many investigators, both experimental and clinical, felt that it was important to save as much time as possible in the evaluation of a subject's or a patient's degree of hypnotizability.

In the present chapter, two brief measures are discussed. As already indicated, the first brief experimental measure of hypnotizability was the BSS of T. X. Barber (1965); throughout the 1960s and 1970s, it was utilized extensively by proponents of the social psychological position. It disappeared almost without a trace during the 1980s, partly because Barber's interests became more clinical in nature, and also because of the development of an alternative measuring instrument within this group of investigators, the CURSS of Spanos and colleagues.

The first report of a clinical measure of hypnotizability was a paper by H. Spiegel (1972), in which he reported the result of relating an "eye roll" test to a privately published measure (H. Spiegel & Bridger, 1970), the HIP. In the 1972 paper, Spiegel stated that the eyeroll takes 5 seconds to administer, while the HIP was reported as taking an additional 5–10 minutes. Subsequently, the eye roll sign became a part of the HIP (see H. Spiegel & Spiegel, 1978; D. B. Stern, Spiegel, & Nee, 1978–1979); overall performance on the HIP was described as measuring "clinically usable hypnotic capacity" (D. B. Stern et al., 1978–1979), which may be different from "hypnotizability" as it is measured in the laboratory. This conceptualization of hypnotic ability in terms of a practical criterion appears to put the HIP at some variance with more conventional formulations of hypnotizability; as will be seen, though, it is still possible to evaluate this particular measuring instrument against more orthodox measures.

As indicated earlier, other brief measures have been developed during the period under review, but for one reason or another these have been little utilized or else abandoned by their own constructors. Accordingly, the present analysis focuses upon the HIP and the CURSS.

The Hypnotic Induction Profile

A particularly impressive feature of the HIP is that from the very start, H. Spiegel (1972) sought to buttress his clinical observations with empirical data; the initial report relating eye roll to hypnotic susceptibility was based upon a sample of 2,000 consecutive cases seen between October 1968 and June 1970. In this initial paper, the impressive claim was made that hypnotizability could be accurately estimated in three patients out of four, simply on the basis of what a clinical patient did when looking upwards while closing the eyelids. On the basis of subsequent work with the HIP, the eyeroll has come to be seen by its constructor (soon to be joined by his son, David) as but one component of the overall profile.

The procedure has been described in considerable detail by H. Spiegel and Spiegel (1978). The eye roll consists of four components. Initially, in what is termed the "up-gaze," the subject is asked to turn the eyes upwards as far as he or she can. The amount of sclera (white of the eye) between the iris and the lower lid is rated on a 5-point scale from 0 to 4, with higher scores indicating a greater amount of sclera showing. This is not scored nowadays, since it was found to have only a small correlation with the remainder of the scale (H. Spiegel & Spiegel, 1978, p. 52).

In the second phase of the eye roll procedure, characterized as "roll," the subject is asked to close the eyes slowly while maintaining the up-gaze. Like the up-gaze, the roll is a measure of the amount of visible sclera between the lower border of the iris and the lower eyelid; it is scored on the same 5-point scale as that used for the up-gaze. Occasionally, during the first and/or second phase of the eye roll procedure, both eyes may veer inward simultaneously, thus causing a squint. This is scored also, this time on a 3-point rating scale, but only when it occurs simultaneously in both eyes.

Finally, what is called the "eye roll sign" is scored. It consists of adding together the roll and squint scores. For example, a roll score of 1 and a squint score of 1 yields an eye roll sign score of 2. No attempt is made to distinguish a score of 2 that is obtained in this manner from a score of 2 based upon a score of 2 without a squint. It is difficult to evaluate this procedure, given that elsewhere it has been noted that "ER [eye roll] was a serendipitous observation. Why ER is a meaningful measure is not clear" (D. B. Stern et al., 1978–1979, p. 110). Nevertheless, it should not be dismissed out of hand; for example, Faria (1819) reported a comparable index of hypnotizability when he observed that *époptes* (his term for highly hypnotizable subjects) often show a rapid, sustained fluttering of the eyelashes when the eyes are slightly shut.

Rather, the issue needs to be more thoroughly researched; in particular, a comment by H. Spiegel and Spiegel (1978) requires careful attention. They noted that "accurately rating eye-roll signs takes a great deal of practice. You may not feel confident in judging them until you have seen fifty to a hundred" (p. 55). This suggests that a certain amount of subjectivity may be buried in the procedure; given variations in the shape and size of eyes, both in absolute terms and relative to facial dimensions, this would not be surprising. Now that videotape technology is within the reach of even moderately funded research laboratories, empirical evaluation of this possible subjectivity in judging the eye roll component of the HIP is possible. It may be no greater than it is for other established hypnotizability measures. A study of a small sample of 39 male volunteers (Sheehan, Latta, Regina, & Smith, 1979), however, has provided the only data on this issue thus far. Sheehan et al. concluded that "the role of the rater was not influential; and that the pattern of intercorrelations among component scores on HIP was somewhat similar to that previously reported for patients" (p. 109) by H. Spiegel and his colleagues.

Following the procedure used to determine the eye roll sign, an additional procedure is used to derive the remaining HIP score. It involves a suggestion of arm levitation (i.e., that the hand and arm feel so light and weightless they will float effortlessly to an upright position, as if the hand were a balloon). From this single item, a number of measures are obtained. These are posthypnosis subjective ratings of "tingle" (the feeling of "tingling" or "pins and needles" during levitation), "dissociation" (the degree of connectedness between the hand and wrist of the levitated arm, and those of the control arm), "signaled arm levitation" (LEV; the number of reinforcements, and the time taken for the arm levitation to occur), "control differential" (CD; a measure of subjective difference in the degree of control experienced in the levitated arm and the control arm), and "cutoff" (an index of the subject's ability to terminate hypnosis immediately when dehypnotiztion is suggested). In addition, scores for "amnesia" (an optional measure of whether the subject recalls the cutoff instruction) and "float" (a measure of the degree of overall buoyancy the subject remembers having experienced in hypnosis) are obtained.

One measure of particular interest that is obtained from a summation of some of these scores is for "induction" (IND). It consists of a summation of the scores for dissociation, LEV, CD, cutoff, and float. The IND score is the one that has most commonly been utilized in the comparison of the HIP with other measures of hypnotizability.

The specifics of these measures, including the rating scales employed, are presented elsewhere by (H. Spiegel & Spiegel, (1978). The interested reader is referred to this source for the additional details; the present purpose is simply to furnish sufficient information to make the following section on the comparison of HIP with other measures comprehensible.

Comparison of the HIP with Other Measures

Experimental Studies

During the 1970s the HIP justifiably attracted considerable interest among both clinicians and experimental researchers, both for its brevity and for its unorthodox manner of measuring hypnotizability. Accordingly, studies were performed at both M. T. Orne's laboratory in Philadelphia and E. R. Hilgard's laboratory at Stanford to compare the eye roll sign and HIP with the more traditional HGSHS:A and SHSS:C measures. The results of these studies were reported in a single paper (Orne, Hilgard, Spiegel, Spiegel, Crawford, Evans, Orne, & Frischholz, 1979); they are summarized briefly here.

The Philadelphia sample involved 87 paid volunteers who had participated in studies at this laboratory during the course of the previous 1 to 10 years. They had been extensively evaluated for hypnotizability (on such measures as the HGSHS:A or the SHSS:A and SHSS:C) prior to their participation in the study, and had "demonstrated a consistent response to hypnosis over time" (Orne et al., 1979, p. 89) to the extent of having attained a stable measure of plateau hypnotizability.[8] The HIP was administered by H. Spiegel, who was presented to subjects as "a distinguished visiting professor and an authority on hypnosis participating in an important collaborative effort" (Orne et al., 1979, p. 90). It was hoped that this procedure would facilitate rapport with the subject volunteers, while approximating the expectancies that a private patient would have about an eminent clinician.

By contrast, the Stanford study was performed with 58 paid volunteers, and the HIP was administered in advance of the traditional (SHSS:A and SHSS:C) measures.[9] The HIP data were collected by D. Spiegel, and no attempt was made, as at Philadelphia, to mimic the atmosphere of a private clinical practice by representing him as an authority in the field of hypnosis.

For the eye roll sign, low correlations (ranging from .10 to .18) were found at both Philadelphia and Stanford when it was related to the Stanford scales. For the IND score of HIP, a statistically significant relationship was found at Philadelphia, but not at Stanford, between it and the SHSS:A and SHSS:C. When the 2 samples were combined, however, the relationships found at Philadelphia continued to hold. Perhaps the most representative of these values is the correlation of .34 ($p < .001$) that was obtained when the two samples were combined, and scores on both of the traditional measures are combined and averaged; a moderate relationship can be inferred.

Orne et al. (1979) presented a wealth of other analyses; most do not touch on the issues under examination here and are not discussed. One finding of interest, however, is provided in Table 5 of Orne et al. (1979, p. 94). This table presented IND cross-comparisons with the SHSS:A and SHSS:C separately for the Philadelphia and Stanford samples. The data for the two samples have been pooled to form Table 17.6, even though it is recognized that there were almost twice as many subjects posting low IND scores at Stanford as at Philadelphia, χ^2 (1) = 3.93, $p < .05$. Two things can be seen from this table. At both Philadelphia and Stanford, all subjects who obtained high hypnotizability scores (11–12) on the Stanford scales also scored in the same way on the IND score of the HIP. On this measure, however, 82% of subjects at Philadelphia tested by H. Spiegel and 67% of subjects at Stanford tested by D. Spiegel obtained high IND scores (6.25–10) on the HIP. This result is difficult to interpret; Stanford scores were presented in four categories (11–12, 8–10, 5–7, 0–4), whereas performance on the HIP was dichotomized (0–6.25, 6.25–10). Thus the finding may have been influenced by the different scoring categorizations employed for the respective measures (see Tukey, 1986, for a discussion of this issue).

In addition, E. R. Hilgard (1978–1979) has maintained that "there is little justification for asserting that the IND is successful in selecting poor hypnotic responders" (p. 80). He based this conclusion on the data provided by the Stanford sample, which indicated that "of those scoring between 0 and 6, the low end of the IND, . . . 32% scored 8–10 on SHSS:A and 29% that high on SHSS:C" (p. 80). At that point in time, he appears not

TABLE 17.6. Cross-Comparison of IND Scores on the HIP with SHSS:A and SHSS:C Scores for the Combined Philadelphia and Stanford Samples

	SHSS:A		SHSS:C	
	IND: Low (0–6.25)	IND: High (6.25–10)	IND: Low (0–6.25)	IND: High (6.25–10)
11–12	0	17	0	18
8–10	11	37	7	39
5–7	8	37	10	28
0–4	16	19	18	25
Total	35	110	35	110

Note. Adapted from "The Relation between the Hypnotic Induction Profile and the Stanford Hypnotic Susecptibility Scales, Forms A and C" (Table 5, p. 94) by M. T. Orne, E. R. Hilgard, H. Spiegel, D. Spiegel, H. J. Crawford, F. J. Evans, E. C. Orne, and E. J. Frischholz, 1979, *International Journal of Clinical and Experimental Hypnosis, 27,* 85–102. Copyright 1979 by *International Journal of Clinical and Experimental Hypnosis.* Adapted by permission.

to have had the Philadelphia data available to him. Inspection of the combined data of Table 17.6 indicates that 11 of 35 low IND scorers (31%) scored from 8–10 on the SHSS:A, as opposed to 7 of 35 low IND scorers (20%) on the SHSS:C. This figure, however, needs to be compared with the data of Register and Kihlstrom (1986); 10 subjects scoring low on the HGSHS:A (11%) scored from 8 to 10 on the SHSS:C (see Table 17.5).

It appears, though, that the HIP is more generous in assigning higher hypnotizability scores than is the SHSS:C, since 110 of 145 subjects (76%) scored at the higher end of the HIP. In addition, although there is no significant difference between the number of subjects variously assigned high and low scores on the two scales for the SHSS:A, χ^2 (1) = 3.80, $p >$ .05, the difference is highly significant for the SHSS:C, χ^2 (1) = 9.83, $p <$ .01. This may be because most of the IND score is based upon performance on the very easy item of arm levitation, which has an item difficulty of about 90%. It could, however, just as easily be an artifact of the IND's and SHSS:C's different scoring criteria for very high, high, medium, and low hypnotizability. In particular, and in hindsight, dichotomizing the HIP distribution may not have been in the best interests of its cross-comparison.

A subsequent study (Frischholz, Tryon, Velios, Fisher, Maruffi, & Spiegel, 1980) compared the performance of 63 subjects on the HIP and SHSS:C, which were administered in counterbalanced order. Here, the relationship was stronger; the IND score of HIP correlated .63 with SHSS:C, and when "depth" ratings derived from the two scales were compared, the correlation was found to be .78. This suggests, a higher degree of equivalence between the IND measure of the HIP and the SHSS:C. It suggests also that the HIP may be an alternative to the HGSHS:A as an initial estimate of hypnotic ability, given that both measures correlate about .60 with the SHSS:C. Again, however, it should be noted that both the HGSHS:A and SHSS:C sample a broad band of responses in hypnosis, whereas the HIP is reliant upon the easy item of arm levitation. Unfortunately, Frischholz et al. (1980) did not present a table comparable to those of Orne et al. (1979) and of Register and Kihlstrom (1986), indicating the extent to which these two measures locate subjects of different degrees of hypnotizability.

Studies Involving Clinical Populations

An alternative method of evaluating a measuring instrument is to compare it with others for its ability to differentiate various clinical populations. The finding of moderate to good correlations between the HIP and the Stanford scales (depending upon the study cited) does not, in itself, invalidate the HIP as a measuring instrument; since it is rare to obtain a perfect test–retest reliability for any measuring instrument in psychology, a certain amount of error is to be expected. On this particular point, data reported by Pettinati and her associates (Pettinati, Horne, & Staats, 1985; Pettinati, Kogan, Evans, Wade, Horne, & Staats, 1990) are invaluable.[10]

In an initial study on this issue, Pettinati et al. (1985) administered the HIP and HGSHS:A in counterbalanced order, followed by the SHSS:C as a third measure, to 86 female patients. Of these, 65 had been diagnosed as having anorexia nervosa, and 21 had diagnoses of bulimia. Of the 65 anorexics, 19 were "abstainers" (individuals who lose weight only by strict dieting and exercise), while the remaining 46 were "purgers" (patients who use purging—typically self-induced vomiting and laxative abuse—to lose weight). Hypnotizability data on the three measures are presented in Table 17.7.

It can be seen from this table that on all three scales bulimics were more hypnotizable than purgers, who in turn were more hypnotizable than abstainers. This is reassuring; it suggests that the three measures were providing comparable differentiations. They differed, though, in terms of the level of statistical significance with which they distinguished the three samples; the effect was most pronounced for the SHSS:C, where the high level of statistical significance may have been attributable to the SHSS:C's being overall a more exacting and difficult scale, and/or to its always having been the third testing instrument (as a result of the previous two experiences of hypnosis with the HGSHS:A and HIP, subjects may have been approaching plateau). On the other hand, the HIP differentiated the three patient groups at the .05 level, whereas the effect was a nonsignificant trend for the HGSHS:A. These data suggest that the SHSS:C is the instrument of preference for differentiating clinical groups; the possibility of an order effect, however, must temper this interpretation.

A subsequent study (Pettinati et al., 1990) compared six groups of subjects, five of which consisted of various clinical populations. These were patients diagnosed variously as having anorexia nervosa ($n = 19$), schizophrenic disorders ($n = 28$), major depression ($n = 20$), substance use disorders ($n = 23$), and bulimia ($n = 23$). A sample of normal college

TABLE 17.7. Hypnotizability of Anorexic Subgroups (Abstainers and Purgers) and Bulimic Patients

| | Mean score (SD) | | | | |
| | Anorexia | | | | |
Scale	Abstain ($n = 19$)	Purge ($n = 46$)	Bulimia	F	p
HIP	4.66 (3.2)	4.93 (3.2)	7.13 (2.4)	4.58	<.05
HGSHS:A	6.11 (2.7)	7.11 (2.7)	8.05 (2.3)	2.74	<.10
SHSS:C	5.00 (2.3)	6.13 (2.6)	7.71 (1.7)	6.97	<.01

Note. From "Hypnotizability in Patients with Anorexia Nervosa and Bulimia" (Table 3, p. 1015) by H. M. Pettinati, R. L. Horne, and J. S. Staats, 1985, *Archives of General Psychiatry, 42,* 1014–1016. Copyright 1985 by the American Medical Association. Reprinted by permission.

students ($n = 58$) taken from the published data of Orne et al. (1979) was used as a comparison group, since these subjects had all been tested with the HIP and SHSS:C (and, unlike the patient groups, had been brought very close to plateau by the use of other measures of hypnotizability). In this study, the HIP was administered first, and the SHSS:C from 2 to 3 weeks later. Since the six groups differed significantly in age, both mean hypnotizability scores and age-adjusted mean hypnotizability scores were presented and analyzed. The results, however, were highly similar for observed and age-adjusted means; accordingly, the latter are presented in Table 17.8. The table indicates that both the HIP and the SHSS:C differentiated the six groups, though this time—in a reversal of the finding of the earlier study, and despite the possible advantage that may have ensued from the SHSS:C's being administered second—the effect was more pronounced statistically for the HIP. Of interest, also, is that on both scales (as in the earlier study), bulimics were significantly more hypnotizable than anorexics.

The Carleton University Responsiveness to Suggestion Scale

The final measure of hypnotizability to be reviewed in this chapter is the CURSS, which, despite the unfortunate connotations of its acronym, has many positive features as a measuring instrument. It consists of seven items: two ideomotor items (arm levitation, arms moving apart), two motor challenge items (arm catalepsy, arm immobility), and three cognitive suggestions (auditory hallucination, visual hallucination, and amnesia for all preceding events). Although item difficulties have not been published (except in the form of a figure, thus making them difficult to calculate precisely), these seven items would appear to sample the range of hypnotic items quite well. Each item takes approximately 50 seconds to administer (approximately 6 minutes in all for the seven items), and is preceded by a 5-minute hypnotic induction procedure. The CURSS can be administered either individually or in groups by means of an audiocassette, and, as with the HGSHS:A, items are self-scored by subjects on a number of subscales described below.

Like the induction procedure of the BSS, which preceded the CURSS, the induction procedure of the CURSS can be replaced by the task-motivational instructions of T. X. Barber (1969). As indicated earlier, these types of instructions can be especially relevant when research questions such as whether normal capacities can be transcended via hypnosis, or whether an effect is due to hypnosis or of enhanced motivation, are being addressed. In addition, a number of different scores can be derived from the CURSS. These are as follows:

1. *Objective score* (CURSS:O), which is simply the number of items to which subjects make an appropriate overt response; that is, they respond

TABLE 17.8. Adjusted Scores on Two Hypnotizability Scales for Patients in Five DSM-III Diagnostic Categories and for Normal Control Subjects

	Patient group					Normal college students ($n = 58$)	F	p
Scale	Anorexia nervosa ($n = 19$)	Schizophrenic disorders ($n = 28$)	Major depression ($n = 20$)	Substance use disorder ($n = 23$)	Bulimia ($n = 23$)			
HIP	4.23_a	$4.98_{a,b}$	$6.00_{b,c,d}$	7.57_e	$6.72_{c,d,e}$	$6.51_{d,e}$	5.5	<.001
SHSS:C	4.92_f	$5.83_{f,g}$	$7.28_{g,h}$	$7.31_{h,i}$	7.48_h	$6.08_{f,g,i}$	3.3	<.01

Note. Same subscript means a nonsignificant difference between two means. From "Hypnotizability of Psychiatric Inpatients According to Two Different Scales" (Table 1, p. 72) by H. M. Pettinati, L. G. Kogan, F. J. Evans, J. H. Wade, R. L. Horne, and J. S. Staats, 1990, *American Journal of Psychiatry, 147,* 69–75. Copyright 1990 by the American Psychiatric Association. Reprinted by permission.

overtly in a manner consistent with passing the item behaviorally. Scores range from 0 to 7.

2. *Subjective score* (CURSS:S), which indicates the degree to which subjects report experiencing an item in the manner suggested. For each item, subjects are required to indicate on a 4-point scale whether they experienced each item "not at all" (score = 0) or "a great deal" (score = 3). Thus CURSS:S scores range from 0 to 21.

3. *Objective Involuntariness score* (CURSS:OI), which indicates the degree to which subjects objectively pass a suggestion *and* experience their response as occurring involuntarily. The involuntariness is scored on the same 4-point scale as that used for the CURSS:S, though no points are awarded for a failed response to an item that the subject rates as involuntary to some degree. Once again, CURSS:OI scores range from 0 to 21.

4. *Voluntary Cooperation score* (CURSS:VC), which appears to be a measure of compliance. It is described as reflecting "the number of suggestions that were passed by overt criteria, but did not have their execution rated as at least moderately involuntary" (moderately involuntary = a score of 2) (Spanos, Radtke, Hodgins, Bertrand, Stam, & Dubreuil, 1983, p. 556).

It should be noted that all of these scores are rating-scale formalizations of open-ended questions typically asked by the experimenter following the administration of the SHSS:C. Classically, a response reflecting the subjective alterations occurring in hypnosis includes the following: The subject responds to the suggestion behaviorally (O), reports an alteration in subjective experience (S), reports that it was accompanied with a feeling of involuntariness (OI),[11] and does not simply exhibit compliance (VC). Although there is much merit in seeking to systematize and objectify these subjective components of hypnotic response through these scores (as opposed to relying upon the experimenter to ask such questions systematically during the posthypnosis period), it appears from reports of research utilizing the CURSS that such corrective factors are not taken into account in determining that a subject is highly responsive to hypnosis.

A typical statement of how high hypnotizability is determined for the purpose of being included in a study comes from Spanos and Katsanis (1989); they report of a study involving five groups of highly hypnotizable subjects:

> Fifty Carleton University undergraduates (ages 18–30) who in previous testing had obtained high scores (5–7) on the objective dimension of the Carleton University Responsivity to Suggestion Scale (CURSS:O: Spanos, Radtke, Hodgins, Stam, & Bertrand, 1983) volunteered to participate in a study on suggestion and pain. (p. 184)

A footnote adds:

> Along with objective responding, the CURSS also assesses subjective [responding] (CURSS:S) and the extent to which objective responses are rated as feeling involuntary (CURSS:OI scores). Separate ANOVAS indicated no significant differences between treatments on any CURSS dimensions (all $ps < .1$). (p. 184)

This indicates that no attempt was made to "correct" CURSS:O scores by reference to S, OI, and VC scores. It means that some individuals identified as highly hypnotizable on the CURSS:O may not have had an appropriate subjective experience of hypnosis, and/or may not have experienced the items passed as having an involuntary component; furthermore, they may have been scored as compliant on the VC measure, though this particular measure was not apparently obtained in this particular study. Regardless of one's theoretical orientation, these would appear to be important data.

Since Spanos and Katsanis (1989) ran five groups of 10 subjects each, we do not know the proportion of subjects who fulfilled optimal conditions for high hypnotic susceptibility—only that there were equivalent proportions of subjects per group who had CURSS:S and CURSS:OI scores that were consistent with their objective scores. It is clear that further attention to this point is needed. Moreover, a ready empirical solution to the problem is available: All that is required is to compare outcomes of studies utilizing "corrected" and "uncorrected" CURSS:O scores. Differences in findings would provide an argument for taking dissonant S, OI, and VC scores into consideration.

There is one final way in which the CURSS differs from the HGSHS:A, SHSS:C, and HIP. The HGSHS:A and SHSS:C are predicated upon the assumption that hypnotic responsivity reflects subjects' abilities; hence the instructions represent responsivity to hypnosis as both a willingness to cooperate and an ability to experience subjective alterations. The HIP appears, to be based upon similar assumptions, as can be seen from the various components of the IND score discussed earlier. By contrast, subjects who receive the CURSS are told only that "Your ability to be hypnotized depends entirely on your willingness to cooperate" (Spanos, 1983, p. 1). There have been no comparisons of the CURSS and HIP; differences in performance between the CURSS and the HGSHS:A or SHSS:C may be the result of the different manners in which responsivity to hypnosis is represented. That is, representing hypnotic responsivity as a "willingness to cooperate," as opposed to representing it as this same willingness *and* an ability to experience subjective alterations, may often result in quite different outcomes—especially as it appears that O scores are not "corrected" by S, OI, and VC performances.

Comparison of the CURSS:O with the HGSHS:A and SHSS:C

Since the practice is to screen subjects in terms of their performance on the CURSS:O, "uncorrected" for subjective, involuntariness, and compliance reports, it is legitimate to compare CURSS:O scores with scores on the HGSHS:A and SHSS:C. A preliminary caution is required, however. In all but one study (Spanos, Lush, Smith, & de Groh, 1986), Spanos and his colleagues did not report how they represented the CURSS:O, HGSHS:A, and SHSS:C to subjects. Here we may wonder whether CURSS:O was represented as involving a willingness to cooperate, and the other scales as involving both this willingness and an ability to experience subjective alterations. A report by Spanos, Radtke, Hodgins, Bertrand, Stam, and Moretti (1983) indicated a correlation of .62 between CURSS:O and HGSHS:A performances for a sample of 107 subjects, and a correlation of .65 between CURSS:O and SHSS:C performances in a second sample of 102 subjects. Given that the HGSHS:A and SHSS:C correlate with each another at about the level of .60, as we have already seen, it is unusual to find that the CURSS:O correlates almost as well with a relatively easy scale as it does with one that is relatively difficult. No attempt was made by Spanos and colleagues to account for this apparent paradox, and it is possible that they did (and still do) not see it as such. It may, however, be the result of how hypnosis was represented to subjects when the different scales were employed.

Spanos, Radtke, Hodgins, Bertrand, Stam, and Moretti (1983) presented no data comparing hypnotizability categorizations for the CURSS:O and HGSHS:A. However, following Register and Kihlstrom (1986), they performed an analysis comparing CURSS:O, CURSS:S, CURSS:OI, and CURSS: VC performances with SHSS:C performance. In the interests of brevity, Table 17.9 presents this comparison only for the CURSS:O and SHSS:C. It should be noted that in this study the CURSS:O was first administered, followed by the SHSS:C within an interval of 2–4 weeks. If the same analysis as that employed for Register and Kihlstrom's (1986) comparison of the HGSHS:A and SHSS:C is applied, it can be seen that 66 subjects (65%) were categorized identically across hypnotizability categories (i.e., were highs, mediums, and lows on both testing occasions). In addition, 21 subjects (20%) performed better on the SHSS:C than on the CURSS:O, and 15 subjects (15%) performed worse on the SHSS:C. Most interestingly, the CURSS:O and SHSS:C showed quite good agreement in identifying lows (69% and 79%) and highs (75% and 64%); their greatest divergence was in the identification of medium hypnotizables (43% and 38%).

A similar picture emerged when the CURSS:O and a modified (10-item) version of the SHSS:C were administered to 108 student volunteers in counterbalanced order (Spanos, Salas, Menary, & Brett, 1986). The data are presented in Table 17.10. It can be seen that 71 of the 108 subjects

TABLE 17.9. Frequencies and Percentages of Subjects Classified as High, Medium, and Low in Hypnotizability on the CURSS:O and SHSS:C

	SHSS:C score						
	Low (0–4)		Medium (5–7)		High (8–12)		
CURSS:O	n	%	n	%	n	%	Total
Low	38	69	11	20	6	11	55
		79		42		21	
Medium	9	39	10	43	4	17	23
		19		38		14	
High	1	4	5	21	18	75	24
		2		19		64	
Total	48		26		28		102

Note. From "The Carleton University Responsiveness to Suggestion Scale: Relationship with Other Measures of Hypnotic Susceptibility, Expectancies, and Absorption" (Table 8, p. 731) by N. P. Spanos, H. L. Radtke, D. C. Hodgins, L. D. Bertrand, H. J. Stam, and P. Moretti, 1983, *Psychological Reports, 53,* 723–734. Copyright 1983 by *Psychological Reports.* Reprinted by permission.

(66%—almost the same proportion as that found in the previous study) were classified in the same way by both the CURSS:O and SHSS:C. Since the two scales were administered in counterbalanced order, nothing can be inferred from the finding that 22 of the 108 subjects (20%) performed better on the modified SHSS:C, and 15 of them (14%) performed worse. Once again, though, there was better agreement between the two scales for lows (69% and 77%) and highs (71% and 59%) than for the medium subjects (58% and 51%). As in the earlier study, most of the subjects classified as mediums on the CURSS:O were classified as lows on the SHSS:C.

Some Longitudinal Data

From the foregoing analyses, it is clear that multiple measures of hypnotizability yield similar, but not identical, classifications of subjects as high, medium, or low in hypnotizability. A recent longitudinal study (Piccione, Hilgard, & Zimbardo, 1989) of the SHSS:A as used in 1960, 1970, and 1985 indicates, however, that a similar problem exists even when the same measuring instrument is employed across a quarter of a century. The Piccione et al. (1989) paper followed an earlier report (Morgan, Johnson & Hilgard, 1974) comparing performance on the SHSS:A across an average of 10 years between 1960 and 1970. In this earlier study, a correlation of .60 was found for the total sample of 85 subjects tested on the two occasions. From scatterplots provided in this report, it was possible to calculate the stability of performance on the two occasions. Of the 85 subjects, 51 of

TABLE 17.10. Frequencies and Percentages of Subjects Classified as High, Medium, and Low in Hypnotizability on the CURSS:O and a Modified, 10-Item SHSS:C Administered in Counterbalanced Order

	Modified SHSS:C/O[a]						
	Low (0–4)		Medium (5–7)		High (8–10)		
CURSS:O	n	%	n	%	n	%	Total
Low (0–2)	42	69	15	25	4	7	61
		77		41		24	
Medium (3–4)	11	33	19	58	3	9	33
		20		51		18	
High (5–7)	1	7	3	21	10	71	14
		2		9		59	
Total	54		37		17		108

Note. From "Comparison of Overt and Subjective Responses to the Carleton University Responsiveness to Suggestion Scale and the Stanford Hypnotic Susceptibility Scale under Conditions of Group Administration" (Table 4) by N. P. Spanos, J. Salas, E. P. Menary, and P. J. Brett, 1986, Psychological Reports, 58, 847–856. Copyright 1986 by Psychological Reports. Reprinted by permission.
[a] A 10-item modification of SHSS:C scored objectively (O).

them (60%) performed identically on the two testings, 17 (20%) scored higher in 1970 than in 1960, and the remaining 17 (20%) scored lower.

Over the 25-year period from 1960 to 1985 (Piccione et al., 1989), the sample was reduced to 50 subjects. Of the 50, 31 subjects (62%) were categorized identically on the two occasions, 6 (12%) showed decrements in performance, and 13 (26%) performed better in 1985 than they had in 1960. An examination of retest correlations revealed that for the 10-year period 1960–1970, $r = .64$; for the 15-year period 1970–1985, $r = .82$; and for the entire 25-year period, $r = .71$.

Although these data are consistent with the long-held belief that hypnotizability is a stable characteristic of the individual, it is clear that more attention needs to be paid to the issue of measurement. To the extent that careful measurement is essential for experimental and clinical research, the results of this chapter's analysis of the main scales currently in use suggests that the certain procedures need to be adopted in the future. These are discussed in the following section.

Discussion

The most telling finding that emerges from the present analysis is that any study relying upon a single measure of hypnotizability is likely to misrepresent a sample's performance on this variable. The degree to which this may occur depends upon which single measure is used. From Register and Kihlstrom's (1986) data comparing performance on the HGSHS:A and SHSS:C (which are relatively "easy" and "difficult" scales, respectively), a mere 47% of subjects performed identically upon the two measures, whereas 23% performed better on the SHSS:C and 30% performed worse. This suggests strongly that exclusive reliance upon the HGSHS:A as a sole measure of hypnotic ability is likely to yield misleading results, at least on some occasions. At the same time, the conclusion may need to be tempered by the fact that, as indicated earlier, different investigators tend to use different cutoff points in determining their hypnotizability classifications.

In addition, two studies by Spanos and his associates (Spanos, Radtke, Hodgins, Bertrand, Stam, & Moretti, 1983; Spanos, Salas, Menary, & Brett, 1986) found almost identical patterns of a relationship between CURSS:O and SHSS:C scores: 65% and 66% of subjects performed identically on the two occasions, 20% of subjects in both studies had better performances on the SHSS:C, and approximately 15% performed worse. The lack of an analysis comparing the HIP and SHSS:C does not permit any conclusion, though the finding of a moderate but statistically significant correlation between these two measures in one study (Orne et al., 1979) and a more robust one in another (Frischholz et al., 1980) suggests that it may not be prudent to utilize the HIP as a single experimental measure.

A general lack of research over the last 30 years into the measurement properties of these various scales, however, prevents firm conclusions from being drawn. Although it is clear that the discrepancy between HGSHS:A and SHSS:C performance is mainly, but not entirely, a matter of overall item difficulty, other discrepancies noted throughout this chapter are not as easily explained. For example, there is the question of whether there would be greater correspondence between CURSS:O and SHSS:C scores were the former to be "corrected" by S, OI, and VC scores. Furthermore, would this correspondence be increased if subjective, involuntariness, and compliance scores were obtained systematically on the SHSS:C? Again, there is the question posed by the finding that the CURSS:O correlates equally well with the "easier" HGSHS:A and the "more difficult" SHSS:C. This may be a question of how the scales (and thus hypnosis) are represented to subjects, though the finding of Spanos, Lush, Smith, and de Groh (1986) suggests that this is not the case.

Alternatively, the CURSS may be tapping into a dimension that is partially measured by the HGSHS:A and partially by the SHSS:C. This, though theoretically possible, appears improbable, given the almost identical relationship found between the CURSS and SHSS:C in two separate studies (Spanos, Radtke, Hodgins, Bertrand, Stam, & Moretti, 1983; Spanos, Salas, Menary, & Brett, 1986). Clearly, these are questions that call for further examination, with particular reference to the issue of the degree to which scales tap compliance as opposed to subjects' abilities (see Tellegen, 1978–1979).

There is also the question of whether "clinically usable hypnotic capacity," which is thought to underlie performance on the HIP, is in some manner different from laboratory conceptualizations of hypnotizability as an ability of the individual. Some clinical investigators have argued that if an individual has some degree of hypnotizability, however slight, he or she can be treated successfully by a hypnotic procedure. If this is what proponents of the HIP mean by "clinically usable capacity," there is probably no real disagreement. Furthermore, the scoring procedure utilized by the HIP is intuitively appealing; it is eminently sensible to suppose that the more experiences such as dissociation, arm levitation, control differential, cutoff, and float a person reports having, the more hypnotizable that person is. On the other hand, the use of the "easy" item of arm levitation as the core performance element of the HIP may mean that some degree of imprecision in measurement is unavoidable. This may not matter in the clinical setting; it is likely to matter a good deal when the issue is an experimental one.

Given the data on plateau susceptibility, which suggest that many individuals do not reach their optimal degree of hypnotizability in one session, it would appear that an investigator who takes at least two measures of hypnotic ability is likely to be on firmer ground in terms of the reproducibility of findings by other, independent investigators. This conclusion is strongly reinforced by the longitudinal study of Piccione et al. (1989); although developmental considerations may temper this conclusion, the reliance on a single measure of hypnotizability, even on the same subjects over time, may produce a degree of measurement error. It should be added, though, that measurement error may at times be confounded with "true" change.

At the same time, we acknowledge that it is not always possible to obtain multiple measures of hypnotizability. In one case (John, Hollander, & Perry, 1983), a sample of snake and spider phobics became unexpectedly available, and constraints were such that only the HGSHS:A could be administered, though this was performed individually rather than in groups. At that time, however, four different studies of the relationship between hypnotizability and phobia had been conducted, and three of them had found a relationship between these two variables. Thus, the decision to obtain a single hypnotizability measure appeared justifiable, given what was then known. The problem, of course, is that even three studies that are in agreement can be in error. The majority of subsequent published studies on this issue have likewise favored the hypothesized link between hypnotizability and phobia; although this lessens the possibility that the majority of studies are in error, it still does not exclude it entirely.

It is clear that current understanding of the measurement issue surrounding hypnotic ability is not as complete as is often believed by investigators in the field. The issues that have been raised in this chapter cannot be resolved by fiat; rather, some patient and careful research is required before investigators can determine the degree to which single-measure studies of hypnotic ability really provide accurate estimates of this characteristic of the individual. Such data are of value in their own right; more importantly, an empirical resolution to the issues raised in this chapter could help to reduce the often acrimonious disagreements that occur when different investigators, utilizing different measuring instruments, obtain different findings on the same question. This in itself would help to civilize the already quite civilized field of hypnosis—perhaps beyond recognition, by current standards.

Acknowledgments

This chapter was prepared while Campbell Perry was in receipt of Natural Sciences and Engineering Research (NSERC) of Canada Grant No. A6361, and shared a grant from Fonds pour la Formation des Chercheurs et l'Aide à la Recherche (FCAR) de Québec (Principal Investigator: Jean-Roch Laurence); Perry was also supported by an Internal Research Grant from Concordia University. Robert Nadon was supported partially by Social Sciences and Humanities Research Council (SSHRC) of Canada Research Fellowship Grant No. 455-90-0072, and by SSHRC Grant No. 410-91-0737. All of these sources are acknowledged gratefully for their assistance.

Notes

1. A number of scales have been constructed over the last three decades and are not considered here. As will be indicated later in the text, the Stanford Hypnotic Susceptibility Scales, Forms A and B (SHSS:A and SHSS:B; Weitzenhoffer & Hilgard, 1959) are not considered here because they have been superseded by the Harvard Group Scale of Hypnotic Susceptibility, Form A (HGSHS:A; Shor & Orne, 1962). Likewise, the Barber Suggestibility Scale (BSS; T. X. Barber, 1965) has been replaced by the Carleton University Responsiveness to Suggestion Scale (CURSS; Spanos, Radtke, Hodgins, Stam, & Bertrand, 1983; Spanos, Radtke, Hodgins, Bertrand, Stam, & Dubreuil, 1983; Spanos, Radtke, Hodgins, Bertrand, Stam, & Moretti, 1983) and is not discussed for the same reason. A number of other measuring instruments are not discussed for other reasons. The Stanford Profile Scales of Hypnotic Susceptibility, Forms I and II (Weitzenhoffer & Hilgard, (1967) were devised as extensions of the earlier Stanford measures, by providing additional test data on subjects who had scored very highly on the SHSS:C. It may be a sad commentary on the present state of research on hypnotizability that they have rarely been utilized. They are available, however, for future researchers who may pose more complex hypotheses about the nature of high hypnotizability. Similarly, the Stanford Clinical Hypnotic Scale in separate forms for adults and children (Morgan and Hilgard (1978–1979a,b) is essentially a five-item version of the SHSS:C; it likewise has been little utilized. The Diagnostic Rating Procedure (DRP; O'Connell, Orne, & Shor, 1966) is one of the more interesting attempts to provide a

brief but flexible clinical measure of hypnotizability. It consists of four items; one is ideomotor, one is a challenge suggestion, another involves a hallucinatory response, and a final item involves amnesia and posthypnotic response. It is unlike any other measuring instrument of hypnotizability, in that the operator is free to choose the item content of the four test suggestions utilized. The DRP has not been promoted by M. T. Orne, mainly because he did not want it to stand in the way of the adoption of the Stanford scales. Finally, there are "special-purpose" scales such as the Stanford Hypnotic Arm Levitation Induction and Test (E. R. Hilgard, Crawford, & Wert, 1979), and the "tailored" SHSS:C (E. R. Hilgard, Crawford, Bowers, & Kihlstrom, 1979). These also have been utilized rarely.

2. Barber's "task motivation" instructions were designed to partial out the effects of extraneous motivational variables that might facilitate responses to hypnosis. Subjects are typically told that other individuals perform well on similar imaginal tasks; that they are expected to cooperate and try to the best of their ability to perform the designated task; that they will perform optimally if they try very hard; and that if they do not try hard, the experiment will fail, and the experimenter will be made to look foolish. See Sheehan and Perry (1976) for a detailed analysis of these task motivation procedures.

3. These are estimates, since Spanos and his colleagues rarely report the time taken to administer the CURSS; given that students tend to vary in the time spent in filling out questionnaires, between 25 and 30 minutes appears to be a realistic estimate.

4. Occasionally, there are reports of use of the of HGSHS:A with groups as large as 500 students in a large lecture hall. The savings in time are considerable with this procedure; however, an experimenter is in a much better position to cater to the individual needs of a small sample than to those of so large a group.

5. In this connection, Bongartz (1985) reported that "in German, the term 'hypnotized' is strongly associated with the idea that an individual no longer has free will . . . 'to become hypnotized' [was] translated as . . . 'to reach a hypnotic state'" (p. 132). In a similar vein, Lamas et al. (1989) reported that in an initial sample of 133 students, 82% of them passed the amnesia item by recalling 3 or fewer of the 12 HGSHS:A items; these authors felt that the wording of the amnesia recall instructions may have been ambiguous. Even after instruction was changed, 45% of a subsequent sample of 70 subjects passed the amnesia item (still much higher than most of the other samples in Table 17.1). In their final normative sample of 220 subjects, the item difficulty for amnesia was 52%. Interestingly, for Shor and Orne's (1963) normative sample, the item pass percentage for amnesia was 48%. Very little can be inferred from such data; howerver, they highlight the problem(s) of cross-cultural comparison. The discrepancies across the amnesia item for the six samples could variously reflect an idiosyncratic instruction from the hypnotist, idiosyncratic perceptions of the amnesia instructions by some of the samples, prior exposure to accurate information about hypnosis (in the case of the Montréal group), and/or cultural similarities and differences. In addition, none of these studies evaluated reversal of amnesia in determining performance on the amnesia item.

6. Another method of evaluating the measuring characteristics of scales is to calculate the Kuder–Richardson total scale reliability index (KR20) for the six sam-

ples. KR20 seeks to evaluate the homogeneity of a test by providing a measure of the degree of consistency of subjects' responses. An example provided by Anastasi (1968) may help clarify what is at issue here. She writes:

> If one test includes only multiplication items, while another comprises addition, subtraction, multiplication, and division items, the former test will probably show more inter-item consistency than the latter. In the latter, more heterogeneous test, one subject may perform better in subtraction than in any of the other arithmetic operations; another subject may score relatively well on the division items, but more poorly in addition, subtraction, and multiplication, and so on. (p. 84)

In terms of these criteria, the Canadian (KR20 = .84), Australian (KR20 = .76), Berkeley (KR20 = .77), and Boston (KR20 = .80) samples all strongly suggest homogeneity for the HGSHS:A; the Spanish (KR20 =.68) and German (KR20 = .62) samples imply it less strongly. What this appears to mean within the present context is that items of the HGSHS:A are arranged in relative order of difficulty, so that all persons who score 5 on it do so by passing the first five items, as opposed, for example, to passing items 1, 4, 7, 9 and 12. This substantiates in part the impression gained from Table 17.2, where it can be seen that only the Spanish sample's pattern of item difficulties fails to correlate with order of presentation of items. As indicated earlier, there is no way of knowing why this should be so.

7. The original SHSS:C criterion of a change in handwriting is no longer accepted by current investigators as evidence of age regression. For one thing, it is easily simulated; for another, some subjects report feeling the suggested age without showing any change in handwriting. Furthermore, it has been shown (Orne, 1951), that the handwriting and drawings of age-regressed adults, though appearing to be childlike, invariably show an adult overlay. Citing the noted child psychologist Karen Machover, who evaluated the drawings of a group of regressed adults, Orne described such productions as "sophisticated oversimplification."

8. "Plateau hypnotizability" is a term introduced by Shor, Orne, and O'Connell (1962); it refers to the fact that many subjects do not reach optimal or "plateau" level of hypnotizability at their first experience of hypnosis. Such factors as fear of being controlled by the hypnotist, inability to "let go," or fear of having an unpleasant experience may mean that some subjects may participate in several sessions before reaching a point of maximal response; after this point has been reached, there will be little improvement in their overall performance.

9. At Philadelphia, subjects were tested initially on either the SHSS:A or the HGSHS:A, whereas at Stanford all initial testing was on the SHSS:A. These data were pooled for the Philadelphia sample, given the evidence of comparability of the two measures. In the text, for reasons of simplicity, this first testing is referred to as involving the SHSS:A. Apart from this minor discrepancy, all subjects at both locations were tested on the SHSS:C and HIP.

10. An additional report by Pettinati and Wade (1986) discusses additional data obtained by Pettinati et al. (1985). These do not bear on the questions under examination.

11. The issue of involuntariness appears to be more complex than Spanos and his colleagues represent it to be. Some responses to hypnosis involve both effort in the attempt to experience a suggested effect, and a feeling that once this attempt

was made, the effect occurred involuntarily. For instance, subjects will sometimes report effortfulness in experiencing a suggestion to age-regress to 5 years old, and of being able to have the experience only when they ceased trying (see P. G. Bowers, 1986, and Perry & Laurence, 1986, for discussions of this point).

References

Acosta, E., & Crawford, H. J. (1985). Iconic memory and hypnotizability: Processing speed, skill or strategy differences? *International Journal of Clinical and Experimental Hypnosis, 33,* 236–245.

Adams, J. L. (1974). *Conceptual blockbusting.* Palo Alto, CA: Stanford Alumni Association.

Ader, R., Felton, D., & Cohen, N. (1990). Interactions between the brain and the immune system. *Annual Review of Pharmacology and Toxicology, 30,* 561–602.

Akpinar, S., Ulett, G. A., & Itil, T. M. (1971). Hypnotizability predicted by computer-analyzed EEG pattern. *Biological Psychiatry, 3,* 387–392.

Alman, B. M., & Carney, R. E. (1980). Consequences of direct and indirect suggestions on success of posthypnotic behavior. *American Journal of Clinical Hypnosis, 23,* 112–118.

Amabile, T. M. (1984). Social environments that kill creativity. In S. S. Grysskiewicz, J. T. Shields, & S. J. Sensabaugh (Eds.), *Blueprint for innovation* (pp. 1–18). Greensboro, NC: Center for Creative Leadership.

Amabile, T. M. (1987). The motivation to be creative. In S. G. Isaksen (Ed.), *Frontiers of creativity research* (pp. 223–254). Buffalo, NY: Bearly Limited.

Amadeo, M., & Yanovski, A. (1975). Evoked potentials and selective attention in subjects capable of hypnotic analgesia. *International Journal of Clinical and Experimental Hypnosis, 23,* 200–210.

American Psychiatric Association. (1980). *Diagnostic and statistical manual of mental disorders* (3rd ed.). Washington, DC: Author.

American Psychiatric Association (1987). *Diagnostic and statistical manual of mental disorders* (3rd ed., rev.). Washington, DC: Author.

Anastasi, A. (1968). *Psychological testing* (3rd ed.). New York: Macmillan.

Andersen, M. S. (1985). Hypnotizability as a factor in the hypnotic treatment of obesity. *International Journal of Clinical and Experimental Hypnosis, 33,* 150–159.

Andreassi, J. L., Balinsky, B., Gallichio, J. A., De Simone, H. H., & Mellers, B. W. (1976). Hypnotic suggestion of stimulus change and visual cortical evoked potential. *Perceptual and Motor Skills, 42,* 371–378.

Andresen, B., Stemmler, G., Thom, E., & Irrgang, E. (1984). Methodological conditions of congruent factors: A comparison of EEG frequency between hemispheres. *Multivariate Behavioral Research, 19,* 3–32.

Apfel, R. J., Kelley, S. F., & Frankel, F. H. (1986). The role of hypnotizability in the pathogenesis and treatment of nausea and vomiting of pregnancy. *Journal of Psychosomatic Obstetrics and Gynaecology, 5,* 179–186.

Arendt, N. L., Zachariae, R., & Bjerring, P. (1990). Quantitative evaluation of hypnotically suggested hyperaesthesia and analgesia by painful laser stimulation. *Pain, 42,* 243–251.

Arnold, M. B. (1946). On the mechanism of suggestion and hypnosis. *Journal of Abnormal and Social Psychology, 41,* 107–128.

Arnolds, D. E. A. T., Lopes Da Silva, F. H., Aitink, J. W., Kamp, A., & Boeijinga, P. (1980). The spectral properties of hippocampal EEG related to behaviour in man. *Electroencephalography and Clinical Neurophysiology, 50,* 324–328.

Ås, A. (1962). Non-hypnotic experiences related to hypnotizability in male and female college students. *Scandinavian Journal of Psychology, 2,* 112–121.

Ås, A. (1963). Hypnotizability as a function of non-hypnotic experiences. *Journal of Abnormal and Social Psychology, 66,* 142–150.

Ås, A., O'Hara, J. W., & Munger, M. P. (1962). The measurement of subjective experiences presumably related to hypnotic susceptibility. *Scandinavian Journal of Psychology, 3,* 47–64.

Ashton, M. A., & McDonald, R. D. (1985). Effects of hypnosis on verbal and non-verbal creativity. *International Journal of Clinical and Experimental Hypnosis, 33,* 15–26.

Atkinson, R. C., & Shiffrin, R. M. (1971). The control of short-term memory. *Scientific American, 224,* 82–90.

Atkinson, R. P. (1990, October). *Enhancement of visual perception: Influences of hypnotizability in waking and hypnotic conditions.* Paper presented at the annual meeting of the Society for Clinical and Experimental Hypnosis, Tucson, AZ.

Atkinson, R. P., & Crawford, H. P. (in press). Individual differences in afterimage duration: Relationships to hypnotic susceptibility and visuospatial skills. *American Journal of Psychology.*

Atwood, G. (1971). An experimental study of visual regression. *Cognitive Psychology, 2,* 290–299.

Baer, L., Carey, R., & Meminger, S. (1986). Hypnosis for smoking: A clinical follow–up. *International Journal of Psychosomatics, 33*(3), 13–16.

Bakan, P., & Svorad, D. (1969). Resting EEG alpha and asymmetry of reflective lateral eye movements. *Nature, 223,* 975–976.

Baker, E. L. (1981) An hypnotherapeutic approach to enhance object relatedness in psychotic patients. *International Journal of Clinical and Experimental Hypnosis, 124,* 136–147.

Baker, E. L. (1987). The state of the art of clinical hypnosis. *International Journal of Clinical and Experimental Hypnosis, 35,* 203–214.

Baker, E. L. (1990). Hypnoanalysis for structural pathology: Impairments of self-representation and capacity for object involvement. In M. L. Fass & D. Brown (Eds.), *Creative mastery in hypnosis and hypnoanalysis: A festschrift for Erika Fromm* (pp. 279–286). Hillsdale, NJ: Erlbaum.

Baker, E. L., & Copeland, D. R. (1978). *Hypnotic susceptibility of psychotic patients: A comparison of schizophrenics and psychotic depressives,* Unpublished manuscript, Research Institute of Mental Sciences, Houston, TX.

Baker, R. A. (1990). *They call it hypnosis.* Buffalo, NY: Prometheus Books.

Baker, S. R., & Boas, D. (1983). The partial reformulation of a traumatic memory of a dental phobia during trance: A case study. *International Journal of Clinical and Experimental Hypnosis, 31,* 14–18.

Balint, M. (1968). *The basic fault: Therapeutic aspects of regression.* London: Tavistock.

Balthazard, C. G. (1990). *The hypnosis scales: Still some fundamental unresolved issues after 100 years.* Unpublished manuscript, Peat Marwick Stevenson & Kellogg, Toronto.

Balthazard, C. G., & Woody, E. Z. (1985). The "stuff" of hypnotic performance: A review of psychometric approaches. *Psychological Bulletin, 98,* 283–296.

Balthazard, C. G., & Woody, E. Z. (1989). Bimodality, dimensionality, and the notion of hypnotic types. *International Journal of Clinical and Experimental Hypnosis, 37,* 70–89.

Balthazard, C. G., & Woody, E. Z. (1992). The spectral analysis of hypnotic performance with respect to "absorption." *International Journal of Clinical and Experimental Hypnosis, 40,* 21–43.

Bandler, R., & Grinder, J. (1975). *Patterns of the hypnotic techniques of Milton H. Erickson, M.D.* (Vol. 1). Cupertino, CA: Meta Publications.

Bandura, A. (1982). Self-efficacy mechanism in human agency. *American Psychologist, 37,* 122–147.

Banquet, J. P. (1973). Spectral analysis of the EEG in meditation. *Electroencephalography and Clinical Neurophysiology, 35,* 143–151.

Bányai, E. I., & Hilgard, E. R. (1976). A comparison of active–alert hypnotic induction with traditional relaxation induction. *Journal of Abnormal Psychology, 85,* 218–224.

Bányai, E. I., Mészáros, I., & Csokay, L. (1985). Interaction between hypnotist and subject: A social psychophysiological approach (preliminary report). In D. Waxman, P. C. Misra, M. Gibson, & M. A. Baker (Eds.), *Modern trends in hypnosis* (pp. 97–108). New York: Plenum Press.

Barabasz, A. F. (1976). Treatment of sleep disturbances in mildly depressed patients by hypnosis and cerebral electrotherapy. *American Journal of Clinical Hypnosis, 19,* 120–122.

Barabasz, A. F. (1980a). EEG alpha, skin conductance and hypnotizability in Antarctica. *International Journal of Clinical and Experimental Hypnosis, 28,* 63–74.

Barabasz, A. F. (1980b). Effects of hypnosis and perceptual deprivation on vigilance in a simulated radar target–detection task. *Perceptual and Motor Skills, 50,* 19–24.

Barabasz, A. F. (1982). Restricted environmental stimulation and the enhancement of hypnotizability: Pain, EEG alpha, skin conductance and temperature responses. *International Journal of Clinical and Experimental Hypnosis, 30,* 147–166.

Barabasz, A. F. (1983). EEG alpha–hypnotizability correlations are not simple covariates of subject self-selection. *Biological Psychology, 17,* 169–172.

Barabasz, A. F. (1990a). A review of Antarctic behavioral research. In A. Harrison, Y. Clearwater, & C. McKay (Eds.), *The human experience in Antarctica: Applications to life in space* (pp. 201–208). New York: Springer-Verlag.

Barabasz, A. F. (1990b). Eingeschranke stimulation durch die Umwelt ruft spontane Hypnose fur die Schmerrzkontrolle beim cold pressor test hervor. *Experimentelle und Klinishe Hypnose, 4*(2), 95–105.

Barabasz, A. F. (1990c). Flotation restricted environmental stimulation elicits spontaneous hypnosis. In R. Van Dyck, A.J. Spinhoven, W. Vander Does, Y. R. Van Rood, & W. DeMoor (Eds.), *Hypnosis: Current theory, research and practice* (pp. 113–119). Amsterdam: Free University Press.

Barabasz, A. F. (1990d, July). *Effects of sensory deprivation on EEG theta and skin conductance.* Paper presented at the 5th International Congress of Psychophysiology, Budapest.

Barabasz, A. F., Baer, L., Sheehan, D. V., & Barabasz, M. (1986). A three year clinical follow-up of hypnosis and restricted environmental stimulation therapy for smoking. *International Journal of Clinical and Experimental Hypnosis, 34,* 169–181.

Barabasz, A. F., & Barabasz, M. (1985). Effects of restricted environmental stimulation: Skin conductance, EEG alpha and temperature responses. *Environment and Behavior, 17,* 239–253.

Barabasz, A. F., & Barabasz, M. (1989). Effects of restricted environmental stimulation: Enhancement of hypnotizability for experimental and chronic pain control. *International Journal of Clinical and Experimental Hypnosis, 37,* 217–231.

Barabasz, A. F., & Barabasz, M. (1990). [Subject types: Fifty experiments, one thousand subjects.] Unpublished data.

Barabasz, A. F., & Barabasz, M. (1992). *Suggestibility and mentations in flotation restricted environmental stimulation: Differences between high and low hypnotizable subjects.* Manuscript submitted for publication.

Barabasz, A. F., Barabasz, M., Dyer, R., & Rather, N. (1992). Effects of chamber REST, flotation REST and relaxation on transient mood state. In A. Barabasz & M. Barabasz (Eds.), *Clinical and experimental restricted environmental stimulation: New developments and perspectives* (pp. 113–120). New York: Springer-Verlag.

Barabasz, A. F., & Gregson, R. A. M. (1979). Antarctic wintering-over, suggestion and transient olfactory stimulation: EEG evoked potential electrodermal responses. *Journal of Biological Psychology, 9,* 285–295.

Barabasz, A. F., & Lonsdale, C. (1983). Effects of hypnosis on P300 olfactory evoked potential amplitudes. *Journal of Abnormal Psychology, 92,* 520–523.

Barabasz, A. F., & McGeorge, C. M. (1978). Biofeedback, mediated biofeedback and hypnosis in peripheral vasodilation training. *American Journal of Clinical Hypnosis, 21,* 23–37.

Barabasz, A. F., & Sheehan, D. V. (1983). [Lack of sequelae: Clinical hypnosis with 600 patients.] Unpublished data.

Barabasz, A. F., & Tellegen, A. (1992). *Absorption–hypnotizability correlations are not simple covariates of experimental context.* Manuscript in preparation.

Barabasz, M. (1987). Trichotillomania: A new treatment. *International Journal of Clinical and Experimental Hypnosis, 16,* 169–181.

Barabasz, M. (1991). Hypnotizability in bulimia. *International Journal of Eating Disorders, 10,* 117–120.

Barabasz, M., & Barabasz, A. F. (1987). Controlling experimental and situational demand variables in restricted environmental stimulation research. In J. W. Turner, Jr., & T. H. Fine (Eds.), *Second International Conference on Restricted Environmental Stimulation* (pp. 110–121). Toledo, OH: IRIS.

Barabasz, M., Barabasz, A. F., & Dyer, R. (1990). *Effects of restricted environmental stimulation therapy (REST) on alcohol consumption.* Paper presented at the 98th Annual Convention of the American Psychological Association, Boston.

Barabasz, M., Barabasz, A. F., & O'Neill, M. (1991). Effects of experimental context, demand characteristics and situational cues. *Perceptual and Motor Skills, 73,* 83–92.

Barabasz, M., & Spiegel, D. (1989). Hypnotizability and weight loss in obese subjects. *International Journal of Eating Disorders, 8,* 335–341.

Barber, J. (1977). Rapid induction analgesia: A clinical report. *American Journal of Clinical Hypnosis, 19,* 138–149.

Barber, J. (1980). Hypnosis and the unhypnotizable. *American Journal of Clinical Hypnosis, 23,* 4–9.

Barber, J., & Mayer, D. J. (1977). Evaluation of the efficacy and neural mechanism of a hypnotic analgesia procedure in experimental and clinical dental pain. *Pain, 4,* 41–48.

Barber, T. X. (1961). Physiological effects of "hypnosis." *Psychological Bulletin, 58,* 390–419.

Barber, T. X. (1962). Toward a theory of "hypnotic" behavior: The "hypnotically induced dream." *Journal of Nervous and Mental Disease, 135,* 206–221.

Barber, T. X. (1963). The effects of "hypnosis" on pain: A critical review of experimental and clinical findings. *Psychosomatic Medicine, 25,* 303–333.

Barber, T. X. (1964). Hypnotizability, suggestibility and personality: V. A critical review of research findings. *Psychological Reports, 14* (Monograph Suppl. 13), 299–320.

Barber, T. X. (1965). Measuring "hypnotic-like" suggestibility with and without "hypnotic induction": Psychometric properties, norms, and variables influencing response to the Barber Suggestibility Scale (BSS). *Psychological Reports, 16* (Monograph Suppl. 3), 809–844.

Barber, T. X. (1969). *Hypnosis: A scientific approach.* New York: Van Nostrand Reinhold.

Barber, T. X. (1970). *LSD, marihuana, yoga, and hyponosis.* New York: Aldine.

Barber, T. X. (1979). Suggested ("hypnotic") behavior: The trance paradigm versus an alternative paradigm. In E. Fromm & R. E. Shor (Eds.), *Hypnosis: Developments in research and new perspectives* (2nd ed., pp. 217–271). New York: Aldine.

Barber, T. X. (1984). Changing "unchangeable" bodily processes by (hypnotic) suggestions: A new look at hypnosis, cognitions, imagining, and the mind–body problem. In A. A. Sheikh (Ed.), *Imagination and healing* (pp. 69–128). New York: Baywood.

Barber, T. X. (1985). Hypnosuggestive procedures as catalysts for psychotherapy. In S. J. Lynn & J. P. Garske (Eds.), *Contemporary psychotherapies: Models and methods.* (pp. 334–376). Columbus, OH: Charles E. Merrill.

Barber, T. X., & Calverley, D. C. (1964a). Empirical evidence for a theory of "hypnotic" behavior: Effects of pretest instructions on response to primary suggestions. *Psychological Record, 14,* 457–467.

Barber, T. X. & Calverley, D. C. (1964b). Experimental studies in hypnotic behavior: Suggested deafness evaluated by delayed auditory feedback. *British Journal of Psychology, 55,* 439–446.

Barber, T. X., & Calverley, D. S. (1964c). The definition of the situation as a variable affecting "hypnotic–like" suggestibility. *Journal of Clinical Psychology, 20,* 438–440.

Barber, T. X., & Calverley, D. S. (1964d). Toward a theory of hypnotic behavior: Effects on suggestibility of defining the situation as hypnosis and defining response to suggestions as easy. *Journal of Abnormal and Social Psychology, 68,* 585–592.

Barber, T. X., & Calverley, D. S. (1964e). An experimental study of "hypnotic" (auditory and visual) hallucinations. *Journal of Abnormal Psychology, 68,* 13–20.

Barber, T. X., & Calverley, D. S. (1964f). Comparative effects of "hypnotic-like" suggestibility of recorded and spoken suggestions. *Journal of Consulting Psychology, 28,* 384.

Barber, T. X., & Calverley, D. S. (1965a). Empirical evidence for a theory of "hypnotic" behavior: Effects on suggestibility of five variables typically included in hypnotic induction procedures. *Journal of Consulting Psychology, 29,* 98–107.

Barber, T. X., & Calverley, D. S. (1965b). Empirical evidence for a theory of "hypnotic" behavior: The suggestibility enhancing effects of motivational suggestions, relaxation–sleep suggestions, and suggestions that the S will be effectively hypnotized. *Journal of Personality, 33,* 256–270.

Barber, T. X., & Calverley, D. S. (1966). Toward a theory of "hypnotic" behavior: Experimental analysis of suggested amnesia. *Journal of Abnormal Psychology, 71,* 95–106. Aldine.

Barber, T. X., & Glass, L. B. (1962). Significant factors in hypnotic behavior. *Journal of Abnormal and Social Psychology, 64,* 222–228.

Barber, T. X., & Hahn, K. W. (1962). Physiological and subjective responses to pain producing stimulation under hypnotically/suggested and waking-imagined "analgesia." *Journal of Abnormal and Social Psychology, 65,* 411–418.

Barber, T. X., Karacan, I., & Calverley, D. S. (1964). "Hypnotizability" and suggestibility in chronic schizophrenia. *Archives of General Psychiatry, 11,* 439–451.

Barber, T. X., Spanos, N. P., & Chaves, J. F. (1974). *Hypnosis, imagination and human potentialities.* Elmsford, NY: Pergamon Press.

Barber, T. X., & Wilson, S. C. (1977). Hypnosis, suggestions, and altered states of consciousness: Experimental evaluation of the new cognitive–behavioral theory and the traditional trance-state theory of "hypnosis." In W. E. Edmonston (Ed.), *Conceptual and investigative approaches to hypnosis and hypnotic phenomena. Annals of the New York Academy of Sciences, 296,* 34–47.

Barber, T. X. & Wilson, S. C. (1978). The Barber Suggestibility Scale and the Creative Imagination Scale: Experimental and clinical applications, *American Journal of Clinical Hypnosis, 21,* 84–108.

Barlow, D. H., Hayes, S. C., & Nelson, R. O. (1984). *The scientist practitioner.* Elmsford, NY: Pergamon Press.

Barnier, A. J., & McConkey, K. M. (in press). Reports of real and false memories: The relevance of hypnosis, hypnotizability, and test context. *Journal of Abnormal Psychology.*

Barrett, D. (1979). The hypnotic dream: Its relation to nocturnal dreams and waking fantasies. *Journal of Abnormal Psychology, 88,* 584–591.

Barrios, M. V., & Singer, J. L. (1981–1982). The treatment of creative blocks: A comparison of waking imagery, hypnotic dream, and rational discussion techniques. *Imagination, Cognition, and Personality, 1,* 89–109.

Barron, F. (1965). Creativity. In T. Newcomb (Ed.), *New directions in psychology II* (pp. 1–134). New York: Holt, Rinehart & Winston.

Barron, F. & Harrington, D. M. (1981). Creativity, intelligence, personality. *Annual Review of Psychology, 32,* 349–376.

Barry, H., Jr., MacKinnon, D. W., & Murray, H. A. (1930). Studies in personality: A. Hypnotizability as a personality trait and its typological relations. *Human Biology, 3,* 1–36.

Bartis, S. P., & Zamansky, H. S. (1986). Dissociation in hypnotic amnesia. *American Journal of Clinical Hypnosis, 29,* 103–108.

Bartis, S. P., & Zamansky, H. S. (1990). Cognitive strategies in hypnosis: Toward resolving the hypnotic conflict. *International Journal of Clinical and Experimental Hypnosis, 38,* 168–182.

Bartlett, F. C. (1932). *Remembering.* Cambridge, England: Cambridge University Press.

Bates, B. L. (1990). Compliance and the Carleton Skills Training Program. *British Journal of Experimental and Clinical Hypnosis, 7,* 159–164.

Bates, B. L. & Brigham, T. A. (1990). Modifying hypnotizability with the Carleton Skills Training Program: A partial replication and analysis of components. *International Journal of Clinical and Experimental Hypnosis, 38,* 183–195.

Bates, B. L., Miller, R. J., Cross, H. J. & Brigham, T. A. (1988). Modifying hypnotic suggestibility with the Carleton Skills Training Program. *Journal of Personality and Social Psychology, 55,* 120–127.

Bauer, R. M., & Craighead, W. E. (1979). Psychological responses to the imagination of fearful and neutral situations: The effects of imagery instructions. *Behavior Therapy, 10,* 389–403.

Baum, D., & Lynn, S. J. (1981). Hypnotic susceptibility level and reading involvement. *International Journal of Clinical and Experimental Hypnosis, 29,* 366–374.

Beahrs, J. O., Harris, D. R., & Hilgard, E. R. (1970). Failure to alter skin inflammation by hypnotic suggestion in five subjects with normal skin reactivity. *Psychosomatic Medicine, 32,* 627–631.

Beaumont, J. G., Young, A. W., & McManus, I. C. (1984). Hemisphericity: A critical review. *Cognitive Neuropsychology, 1,* 191–212.

Beck, E. C., & Barolin, G. S. (1965). The effect of hypnotic suggestion on evoked potentials. *Journal of Nervous and Mental Disease, 140,* 154–161.

Beck, E. C., Dustman, R. E., & Beier, E. C. (1966). Hypnotic suggestions and visually evoked potentials. *Electroencephalography and Clinical Neurophysiology, 20,* 397–400.

Beckmann, J. (1987). Metaprocesses and the regulation of behavior. In F. Halisch & J. Kuhl (Eds.), *Motivation, intention and volition* (pp. 371–386). Berlin: Springer-Verlag.

Belicki, K., & Belicki, D. (1986). Predisposition for nightmares: A study of hypnotic ability, vividness of imagery, and absorption. *Journal of Clinical Psychology, 42,* 714–718.

Belicki, K., & Bowers, P. G. (1982). The role of demand characteristics and hypnotic ability in dream change following a presleep instruction. *Journal of Abnormal Psychology, 91,* 426–432.

Bell, G. (1978). *A phenomenological study of hypnosis using the Experiential Analysis Technique.* Unpublished honors thesis, University of Queensland, Brisbane, Queensland, Australia.

Bem, D. J. (1967). Self-perception: An alternative interpretation of cognitive dissonance phenomena. *Psychological Review, 74,* 183–200.

Bennett, H. L., Benson, D. R., & Kuiken, D. A. (1986). Preoperative instructions for decreased bleeding during spine surgery. *Anesthesiology, 65,* A245.

Bentler, P. M., & Roberts, M. R. (1963) Hypnotic susceptibility assessed in large groups. *International Journal of Clinical and Experimental Hypnosis, 11,* 93–97.

Bernheim, H. (1884). *De la suggestion dans l'état hypnotique et dans l'état de veille.* Paris: Octave Doin.

Bernheim, H. (1886). *De la suggestion et de ses applications à la thérapeutique*. Paris: Octave Doin.

Bernheim, H. (1887). *Suggestive therapeutics: A treatise on the nature and uses of hypnotism* (C. A. Herter, Trans.). Westport, CT: Associated Booksellers. (Original work published 1886)

Bernheim, H. (1889). *Suggestive therapeutics: A treatise on the nature and uses of hypnotism* (C. A. Herter, Trans.). New York: G. P. Putnam's Sons. (Original work published 1886)

Bernheim, H. (1971). *Automatisme et suggestion*. Paris: Librarie Felix Alcan. (Original work published 1884)

Bernstein, E. M., & Putnam, F. W. (1986). Development, reliability, and validity of a dissociation scale. *Journal of Nervous and Mental Disease, 174*, 727–735.

Bertrand, A. J. F. (1823). *Traité du somnambulisme et des différentes modifications qu'il présente*. Paris: J. G. Dentu.

Bertrand, L. D., & Spanos, N. P. (1984–1985). The organization of recall during hypnotic suggestions for complete and selective amnesia. *Imagination, Cognition and Personality, 4*, 249–261.

Bertrand, L. D., Spanos, N. P., & Parkinson, B. (1983). Test of the dissipation hypothesis of hypnotic amnesia. *Psychological Reports, 52*, 667–671.

Bertrand, L. D., Stam, H. J., & Radtke, H. L. (1990). *The Carleton Skills Training Package for modifying hypnotic susceptibility: A replication and extension*. Unpublished manuscript, University of Calgary.

Besemer, S. I., & O'Quin, K. (1987). Creative product analysis: Testing a model by developing a judging instrument. In S. G. Isaksen (Ed.), *Frontiers of creativity research* (pp. 341–357). Buffalo, NY: Bearly Limited.

Beutler, L. E. (1979). Toward specific psychological therapies for specific conditions. *Journal of Consulting and Clinical Psychology, 47*, 882–897.

Beutler, L. E., & Clarkin, J. (1991). Future research directions. In L. E. Beutler & M. Crago (Eds.), *Psychotherapy research* (pp. 329–334). Washington, DC: American Psychological Association Press.

Beutler, L. E., Crago, M., & Machado, P. P. P. (1991). The status of programmatic research. In L. E. Beutler & M. Crago (Eds.), *Psychotherapy research* (pp. 325–328). Washington, DC: American Psychological Association.

Binet, A. (1896). *On double consciousness*. (2nd ed.). Chicago: Open Court.

Binet, A., & Féré, C. (1888). *Animal magnetism*. New York: Appleton.

Bion, W. R. (1977). *Seven servants*. New York: Jason Aronson.

Birkett, D. A. (1982). Warts and their management. *The Practitioner, 226*, 1251–1254.

Bishay, E. G., & Lee, C. (1984). Studies of the effects of hypnoanesthesia on regional blood flow by transcutaneous oxygen monitoring. *American Journal of Clincal Hypnosis, 27*, 64–69.

Bishay, E. G., Stevens, G., & Lee, C. (1984). Hypnotic control of upper gastrointestinal hemmorrhage: A case report. *American Journal of Clinical Hypnosis, 27*, 22–25.

Bitter, E. J. (1975). An empirical investigation of the relationship between hypnosis and transference (Doctoral dissertation, University of Montana, 1974). *Dissertation Abstracts International, 35*(10), 5099B.

Black, S. (1963). Inhibition of immediate-type hypersensitivity response by direct suggestion under hypnosis. *British Medical Journal, vi*, 925–929.

Black, S., Humphrey, J. H. & Niven, J. S. F. (1963). Inhibition of Mantoux reaction by direct suggestion under hypnosis. *British Medical Journal, i,* 1649–1652.

Blankfield, R.P. (1991). Suggestion, relaxation, and hypnosis as adjuncts in the care of surgery patients: A review of the literature. *American Journal of Clinical Hypnosis, 33*(3), 172–187.

Blatt, T., Dixon, M., & Laurence, J.-R. (1990, October). *Differential acquisition of automatic responses among high and low hypnotizable subjects.* Paper presented at the annual meeting of the Society for Clinical and Experimental Hypnosis, Tucson, AZ.

Bliss, E. L. (1984a). Spontaneous self–hypnosis in multiple personality disorder. *Psychiatric Clinics of North America, 7,* 135–148.

Bliss, E. L. (1984b). A symptom profile of patients with multiple personalities, including MMPI results. *Journal of Nervous and Mental Disease, 172,* 197–202.

Bliss, E. L. (1986). *Multiple personality, allied disorders and hypnosis.* New York: Oxford University Press.

Block, J. (1965). *The challenge of response sets.* New York: Appleton-Century-Crofts.

Blum, G. S., & Barbour, J. S. (1979). Selective inattention to anxiety-linked stimuli. *Journal of Experimental Psychology: General, 108,* 182–224.

Blum, G. S., Geiwitz, P. J., & Stewart, C. G. (1967). Cognitive arousal: The evolution of a model. *Journal of Personality and Social Psychology, 5,* 138–151.

Blum, G. S., & Nash, J. (1981). Posthypnotic attentuation of a visual illusion as reflected in perceptual reports and cortical event-related potentials. *Academic Psychology Bulletin, 3,* 251–271.

Blum, G. S., Porter, M. L., & Geiwitz, P. J. (1978). Temporal parameters of negative visual hallucination. *International Journal of Clinical and Experimental Hypnosis, 26,* 30–44.

Bogen, J. E. (1973). The other side of the brain: An appositional mind. In R. Ornstein (Ed.), *The nature of human consciousness* (pp. 101–125). San Francisco: W. H. Freeman.

Boneau, C. A. (1990). Psychological literacy: A first approximation. *American Psychologist, 45,* 891–900.

Bongartz, W. (1985). German norms for the Harvard Group Scale of Hypnotic Susceptibility: Form A. *International Journal of Clinical and Experimental Hypnosis, 33,* 131–139.

Bonke, B., Schmitz, P. I. M., Verhage, F., & Zwaveling, A. (1986). Clinical study of so-called unconscious perception during general anaesthesia. *British Journal of Anaesthesia, 58,* 957–964.

Borenstein, M., & Cohen, J. (1988). *Statistical power analysis: A computer program.* Hillsdale, NJ: Erlbaum.

Borkovec, T. D. (1982). Insomnia. *Journal of Consulting and Clinical Psychology, 50,* 880–895.

Borkovec, T. D., & Fowles, D. C. (1973). Controlled investigation of the effects of progressive and hypnotic relaxation on insomnia. *Journal of Abnormal Psychology, 82,* 153–158.

Botto, R. W., Fisher, S., & Soucy, G. P. (1977). The effect of a good and a poor model on hypnotic susceptibility in a low demand situation. *International Journal of Clinical and Experimental Hypnosis, 25,* 175–183.

Boucher, R. C., & Hilgard, E. R. (1962). Volunteer bias in hypnotic experimentation. *American Journal of Clinical Hypnosis, 5,* 49–51.

Bower, G. H. (1975). Cognitive psychology: An introduction. In W. K. Estes (Ed.), *Handbook of learning and cognitive processes* (Vol. 1, pp. 25–80). Hillsdale, NJ: Erlbaum.

Bowers, K. S. (1966). Hypnotic behavior: The differentiation of trance and demand characteristic variables. *Journal of Abnormal Psychology, 71,* 42–51.

Bowers, K. S. (1967). The effects of demands for honesty on reports of visual and auditory hallucinations. *International Journal of Clinical and Experimental Hypnosis, 15,* 31–36.

Bowers, K. S. (1968). Hypnosis and creativity. *International Journal of Clinical and Experimental Hypnosis, 16,* 38–52.

Bowers, K. S. (1971). Sex and susceptibility as moderator variables in the relationship of creativity and hypnotic susceptibility. *Journal of Abnormal Psychology, 78,* 93–100.

Bowers, K. S. (1973a). Hypnosis, attribution, and demand characteristics. *International Journal of Clinical and Experimental Hypnosis, 21,* 226–238.

Bowers, K. S. (1973b). Situationism in psychology. *Psychological Review, 80,* 307–336.

Bowers, K. S. (1976). *Hypnosis for the seriously curious.* Monterey, CA: Brooks/Cole.

Bowers, K. S. (1979). Time distortion and hypnotic ability: Underestimating the duration of hypnosis. *Journal of Abnormal Psychology, 88,* 435–439.

Bowers, K. S. (1981). Do the Stanford scales tap the "classic suggestion effect"? *International Journal of Clinical and Experimental Hypnosis, 29,* 42–53.

Bowers, K. S. (1983). *Hypnosis for the seriously curious.* New York: Norton. (Original work published 1976)

Bowers, K. S. (1984a). On being unconsciously influenced and informed. In K. S. Bowers & D. Meichenbaum (Eds.), *The unconscious reconsidered* (pp. 227–272). New York: Wiley.

Bowers, K. S. (1984b). Hypnosis. In N. S. Endler & J. M. Hunt (Eds.), *Personality and the behavioral disorders* (2nd ed., Vol. 1, pp. 439–475). New York: Wiley.

Bowers, K. S. (1987a). Revisioning the unconscious. *Canadian Psychology, 28,* 93–104.

Bowers, K. S. (1987b). Response to commentaries. *Canadian Psychology, 28,* 124–132.

Bowers, K. S. (1990). Unconscious influences and hypnosis. In J. L. Singer (Ed.), *Repression and dissociation: Implications for personality theory, psychopathology, and health* (pp. 143–178). Chicago: University of Chicago Press.

Bowers, K. S. (1991a). Dissociation in hypnosis and multiple personality disorder. *International Journal of Clinical and Experimental Hypnosis, 39,*155–176.

Bowers, K. S. (1991b, October 18). *Dissociative control, imagination, and the phenomenology of dissociation.* Invited paper presented at the Dissociation Workshop for the Mind–Body Network, Palo Alto, CA.

Bowers, K. S., & Brenneman, H. A. (1979). Hypnosis and the perception of time. *International Journal of Clinical and Experimental Hypnosis, 27,* 29–41.

Bowers, K. S., & Brenneman, H. A. (1981). Hypnotic dissociation, dichotic listening, and active versus passive modes of attention. *Journal of Abnormal Psychology, 90,* 55–67.

Bowers, K. S., & Davidson, T. M. (1991). A neodissociative critique of Spanos's social-psychological model of hypnosis. In S. J. Lynn & J. W. Rhue (Eds.), *Theories of hypnosis: Current models and perspectives* (pp. 105–143). New York: Guilford Press.

Bowers, K. S., & Kelly, P. (1979). Stress, disease, psychotherapy, and hypnosis. *Journal of Abnormal Psychology, 88,* 490–505.

Bowers, K. S., Regehr, G., Balthazard, C. G., & Parker, K. (1990). Intuition in the context of discovery. *Cognitive Psychology, 22,* 72–110.

Bowers, K. S., & van der Meulen, S. J. (1970). Effect of hypnotic susceptibility on creativity test performance. *Journal of Personality and Social Psychology, 14,* 247–256.

Bowers, P. G. (1967). Effect of hypnosis and suggestions of reduced defensiveness on creativity test performance. *Journal of Personality, 35,* 311–322.

Bowers, P. G. (1978). Hypnotizability, creativity and the role of effortless experiencing. *International Journal of Clinical and Experimental Hypnosis, 26,* 184–202.

Bowers, P. G. (1979). Hypnosis and creativity: The search for the missing link. *Journal of Abnormal Psychology, 88,* 564–572.

Bowers, P. G. (1982). The classic suggestion effect: Relationship with scales of hypnotizability, effortless experiencing, and imagery vividness. *International Journal of Clinical and Experimental Hypnosis, 30,* 270–279.

Bowers, P. G. (1982–1983). On not trying so hard: Effortless experiencing and its correlates. *Imagination, Cognition and Personality, 2,* 3–13.

Bowers, P. G. (1986). Understanding reports of nonvolition. *Behavioral and Brain Sciences, 9,* 469–471.

Bowers, P. G., & Bowers, K. S. (1979). Hypnosis and creativity: A theoretical and empirical rapprochement. In E. Fromm & R. E. Shor (Eds.), *Hypnosis: Developments in research and new perspectives* (2nd ed., pp. 351–379). New York: Aldine.

Bowers, P. G., Laurence, J.-R., & Hart, D. (1988). The experience of hypnotic suggestions. *International Journal of Clinical and Experimental Hypnosis, 36,* 336–349.

Braid, J. (1843). *Neurypnology, or the rationale of nervous sleep considered in relation with animal magnetism, illustrated by numerous cases of its successful application in the relief and cure of disease.* London: John Churchill.

Braid, J. (1970). The physiology of fascination and the critics criticized. In M. M. Tinterow (Ed.), *Foundations of hypnosis: From Mesmer to Freud* (pp. 365–389). Springfield, IL: Charles C Thomas. (Original work published 1855)

Braid, J. (1960). *Braid on hypnotism: The beginnings of modern hypnosis* (rev. ed. of *Neurypnology,* A. E. Waite, Ed.). New York: Julian. (Original work published 1843)

Braun, B. G., & Sachs, R. G. (1985). The development of multiple personality disorder: Predisposing, precipitating, and perpetuating factors. In R. P. Kluft (Ed.), *Childhood antecedents of multiple personality* (pp. 37–64). Washington, DC: American Psychiatric Press.

Brentar, J., & Lynn, S. J. (1989). Negative effects and hypnosis: A critical examination. *British Journal of Experimental and Clinical Hypnosis, 6,* 75–84.

Breuer, J., & Freud, S. (1955). Studies on hysteria: I. On physical mechanisms of hysterical phenomena: Preliminary communication. In J. Strachey (Ed. and Trans.), *The standard edition of the complete psychological works of Sigmund Freud* (Vol. 2, pp. 1–181). London: Hogarth Press.

Brink, N. E. (1986–1987). Three stages of hypno–family therapy for psychosomatic problems. *Imagination, Cognition and Personality, 6,* 263–270.

Brom, D., Kleber, R. J., & Defares, P. B. (1989). Brief psychotherapy for posttraumatic stress disorders, *Journal of Consulting and Clinical Psychology, 57*(5), 607–612.

Brown, D. P. (1985). Hypnosis as an adjunct to the psychotherapy of the severely disturbed patient: An affective development approach. *International Journal of Clinical and Experimental Hypnosis, 33,* 281–301.

Brown, D. P. (1990). Erika Fromm: An intellectual history. In M. L. Fass & D. P. Brown (Eds.), *Creative mastery in hypnosis and hypnoanalysis: A festschrift for Erika Fromm* (pp. 3–29). Hillsdale, NJ: Erlbaum.

Brown, D. P., & Fromm, E. (1986). *Hypnotherapy and hypnoanalysis.* Hillsdale, NJ: Erlbaum.

Brown, D. P., & Fromm, E. (1987). *Hypnosis and behavioral medicine.* Hillsdale, NJ: Erlbaum.

Brown, S. W. (1984). Retrospective duration judgements of a hypnotic time interval. In J. Gibbon & L. Allan (Eds.), *Timing and time perception. Annals of the New York Academy of Sciences, 423,* 583–584.

Bruder, G. E. (1991). Dichotic listening: New developments and applications in clinical research. In R. A. Zappulla, F. F. LeFever, J. Jaeger, & R. Bilder (Eds.), *Windows on the brain: Neuropsychology's technological frontiers. Annals of the New York Academy of Sciences, 620,* 217–232.

Bryant, R. A., & McConkey, K. M. (1989a). Hypnotic blindness: A behavioral and experiential analysis. *Journal of Abnormal Psychology, 98,* 71–77.

Bryant, R. A., & McConkey, K. M. (1989b). Hypnotic blindness, awareness and attribution. *Journal of Abnormal Psychology, 98,* 443–447.

Bryant, R. A., & McConkey, K. M. (1989c). Hypnotic emotions and physical sensations: A real–simulating analysis. *International Journal of Clinical and Experimental Hypnosis, 37,* 305–319.

Buckner, L. G., & Coe, W. C. (1977). Imaginative skill, wording of suggestions, and hypnotic susceptibility. *International Journal of Clinical and Experimental Hypnosis, 25,* 27–35.

Burnett, C. T. (1925). Splitting the mind. *Psychological Monographs, 34*(No. 2).

Burns, A., & Hammer, G. (1970, October). *Hypnotizability and amenability to social influence.* Paper presented at the meeting of the Society for Clinical and Experimental Hypnosis, Philadelphia.

Burns, D.D. (1980). *Feeling good: The new mood therapy.* New York: Signet.

Busse, T. V., & Mansfield, R. S. (1980). Theories of the creative process: A review and a perspective. *Journal of Creative Behavior, 14,* 91–103.

Cameron, N., & Rychlak, J. F. (1980). *Personality development and psychopathology: A dynamic approach.* Boston: Houghton Mifflin.

Campbell, D. T. (1957). Factors relevant to the validity of experiments in social settings. *Psychological Bulletin, 54,* 297–312.

Campbell, D. T., & Fiske, D. W. (1959). Convergent and discriminant validation by the multitrait–multimethod matrix. *Psychological Bulletin, 56,* 81–105.

Carlson, E. B., & Putnam, F. W. (1988, August). *Further validation of the Dissociative Experiences Scale.* Paper presented at the meeting of the American Psychological Association, New Orleans.

Carlson, E. B., & Putnam, F. W. (1989). Research on dissociation and hypnotizability: Are there two pathways to hypnotizability? *Dissociation, 2,* 32–38.

Carroll, L. [Dodgson, C. L.] (1989). Sylvie and Bruno concluded. In *The complete works of Lewis Carroll*. London: Nonesuch Press. (Original work published 1893)

Cass, W. A. (1941). An experimental investigation of the dissociation hypothesis utilizing a posthypnotic technique (Abstract). *Psychological Bulletin, 38,* 744.

Ceci, S. J., Peters, D., & Plotkin, J. (1985). Regulation of social science research. *American Psychologist, 40*(9), 994–1002.

Cermak, L. S., & Craik, F. I. M. (Eds.). (1979). *Levels of processing in human memory.* Hillsdale, NJ: Erlbaum.

Chapman, L. G., Goodell, H., & Wolff, H. G. (1959). Increased inflammatory reaction induced by central nervous system activity. *Transactions of the Association of American Physicians, 72,* 84–109.

Charcot, J. M. (1882). Sur les divers états nerveux déterminés par l'hypnotisation chez les hystériques. *Comptes Rendus Hebdomadaires des Séances de l'Académie des Sciences* [On different nervous states as they appear when hysterics are hypnotized. *Biweekly Accounts of the Meetings of the Academy of Sciences*], *94,* 403–405.

Charcot, J. M. (1889). *Clinical lectures on the diseases of the nervous system* (T. Savill, Trans.). London: New Sydenham Society.

Chaves, J. F. (1968). Hypnosis reconceptualized: An overview of Barber's theoretical and empirical work. *Psychological Reports, 22,* 587–608.

Chaves, J. F. (1989). Hypnotic control of clinical pain. In N. P. Spanos & J. F. Chaves (Eds.), *Hypnosis: The cognitive–behavioral perspective* (pp. 242–272). Buffalo, NY: Prometheus Books.

Chaves, J. F., & Barber, T. X. (1974). Cognitive strategies, experimenter modeling and expectation in the attenuation of pain. *Journal of Abnormal Psychology, 83,* 356–363.

Chaves, J. F., & Brown, J. F. (1987). Spontaneous coping strategies for pain. *Journal of Behavioral Medicine, 10,* 263–276.

Cheesman, J., & Merikle, P. M. (1986). Distinguishing conscious from unconscious perceptual processes. *Canadian Journal of Psychology, 40,* 343–367.

Chen, A. C. N., Dworkin, S. F., & Bloomquist, D. S. (1981). Cortical power spectrum analysis of hypnotic pain control in surgery. *International Journal of Neuroscience, 13,* 127–136.

Chertok, L. (Ed.). (1969). *Psychophysiological mechanisms of hypnosis.* New York: Springer.

Chiofalo, L., & Coe, W. C. (1982). A failure to support the relationships of selected traits and hypnotic responsiveness in drama students. *American Journal of Clinical Hypnosis, 24,* 200–203.

Chodoff, P. (1974). The diagnosis of hysteria: An overview. *American Journal of Psychiatry, 131,* 1073–1078.

Christensen, P. R., Merrifield, P. R., & Guilford, J. P. (1958). *Consequences: Manual of administration, scoring, and interpretation.* Beverly Hills, CA: Sheridan Supply.

Cikurel, K., & Gruzelier, J. H. (1990). The effect of an active–alert hypnosis induction on lateral asymmetry in haptic processing. *British Journal of Experimental and Clinical Hypnosis, 7,* 17–25.

Clarke, J. H., & Reynolds, P. J. (1991). Suggestive hypnotherapy for nocturnal bruxism: A pilot study. *American Journal of Clinical Hypnosis, 33*(4), 248–253.

Clynes, M., Kohn, M., & Lifshitz, K. (1964). Dynamics and spatial behavior of light evoked potentials, their modification under hypnosis, and on-line correlation in relation to rhythmic components. *Annals of the New York Academy of Sciences, 112,* 468–509.

Cochrane, G., & Friesen, J. (1986). Hypnotherapy in weight loss treatment. *Journal of Consulting and Clinical Psychology, 54,* 489–492.

Coe, W. C. (1964). Further norms on the Harvard Group Scale of Hypnotic Susceptibility, Form A. *International Journal of clinical and Experimental Hypnosis, 12,* 184–190.

Coe, W. C. (1978). The credibility of posthypnotic amnesia: A contextualist's view. *International Journal of Clinical and Experimental Hypnosis, 26,* 218–245.

Coe, W. C. (1989a). Posthypnotic amnesia: Theory and research. In N. P. Spanos & J. F. Chaves (Eds.), *Hypnosis: The cognitive–behavioral perspective* (pp. 110–148). Buffalo, NY: Prometheus Books.

Coe, W. C. (1989b). Hypnosis: The role of sociopolitical factors in a paradigm clash. In N. P. Spanos & J. F. Chaves (Eds.). *Hypnosis: The cognitive–behavioral perspective* (pp. 418–436). Buffalo, NY: Prometheus Books.

Coe, W.C., Allen, J.L., Krug, W.M., & Wirzmann, A.G. (1974). Goal-directed fantasy in hypnotic responsiveness: Skill, item wording, or both? *International Journal of Clinical and Experimental Hypnosis, 22,* 157–166.

Coe, W. C., Basden, B. H., Basden, D., Fikes, T., Gargano, G. J., & Webb, M. (1989). Directed forgetting and posthypnotic amnesia: Information processing and social contexts. *Journal of Personality and Social Psychology, 56,* 189–198.

Coe, W. C., Basden, B. H., Basden, D., & Graham, C. (1976). Posthypnotic amnesia: Suggestions of an active process in dissociative phenomena. *Journal of Abnormal Psychology, 85,* 455–458.

Coe, W. C., & Ryken, K. (1979). Hypnosis and risks to human subjects. *American Psychologist, 34,* 673–681.

Coe, W. C., St. Jean, R. L., & Burger, J. M. (1980). Hypnosis and the enhancement of visual imagery. *International Journal of Clinical and Experimental Hypnosis, 28,* 225–234.

Coe, W. C., & Sarbin, T. R. (1977). Hypnosis from the standpoint of a contextualist. *Annals of the New York Academy of Sciences, 296,* 2–13.

Coe, W. C., & Sarbin, T. R. (1991). Role theory: Hypnosis from a dramaturgical and narrational perspective. In S. J. Lynn & J. W. Rhue (Eds.), *Theories of hypnosis: Current models and perspectives* (pp. 303–323). New York: Guilford Press.

Coe, W. C., & Sluis, A. S. E. (1989). Increasing contextual pressures to breach posthypnotic amnesia. *Journal of Personality and Social Psychology, 57,* 885–894.

Coe, W. C., & Steen, P. (1981). Examining the relationship between believing one will respond to hypnotic suggestions and hypnotic responsiveness. *American Journal of Clinical Hypnosis, 24,* 22–32.

Coe, W. C., & Yashinski, E. (1985). Volitional experiences associated with breaching posthypnotic amnesia. *Journal of Personality and Social Psychology, 48,* 716–722.

Coffman, J. A., Mefferd, J., & Golden, C. J. (1981). Cerebellar atrophy in schizophrenia. *Lancet, i,* 666.

Cohen, J. (1977). *Statistical power analysis for the behavioral sciences* (rev. ed.). New York: Academic Press.

Cohen, J. (1988). *Statistical power analysis for the behavioral sciences* (2nd ed.). Hillsdale, NJ: Erlbaum.

Colgan, S. M., Faragher, E. B., & Whorwell, P. J. (1988). Controlled trial of hypnotherapy in relapse prevention of duodenal ulceration. *Lancet, i,* 1299–1300.

Collison, D. A. (1975). Which asthmatic patients should be treated by hypnotherapy? *Medical Journal of Australia, 1,* 776–781.

Comins, J., Fullam, F., & Barber, T. X. (1975). Effects of experimenter modeling, demands for honesty, and initial level of suggestibility on response to hypnotic suggestions. *Journal of Consulting and Clinical Psychology, 43,* 668–675.

Conn, L., & Mott, T. (1984). Plethysmographic demonstration of rapid vasodilation by direct suggestion: A case of Raynaud's Disease treated by hypnosis. *American Journal of Clincal Hypnosis, 26,* 166–170.

Coons, P. M. (1986). Treatment progress in 20 patients with multiple personality disorder. *Journal of Nervous and Mental Disease, 174*(12), 715–721.

Cooper, L. M., & London, P. (1973). Reactivation of memory by hypnosis and suggestion. *International Journal of Clinical and Experimental Hypnosis, 21,* 312–323.

Cooper, L. M., & London, P. (1976). Children's hypnotic susceptibility, personality, and EEG patterns. *International Journal of Clinical and Experimental Hypnosis, 24,* 140–148.

Copeland, D. R. (1986). The application of object relations theory to the hypnotherapy of developmental arrests: The borderline patient. *International Journal of Clinical and Experimental Hypnosis, 34,* 157–168.

Coppola, R. (1986). Issues in topographic analysis of EEG activity. In F. H. Duffy (Ed.), *Topographic mapping of brain electrical activity* (pp. 339–346). Boston: Butterworths.

Coppola, R., & Chassy, J. (1986). Subjects with low versus high frequency alpha rhythm reveal different topographic structure. *Electroencephalography and Clinical Neurophysiology, 63,* 41.

Corby, J. C., Crawford, H. J., Hink, R., Capell, B. S., & Roth, W. T. (1980, October). *EEG correlates of hypnosis and hypnotic susceptibility.* Paper presented at the annual meeting of the Society for Clinical and Experimental Hypnosis, Chicago.

Corby, J. C., Roth, W. T., Zarcone, V. P., & Kopell, B. S. (1978). Psychophysiological correlates of the practice of tantric yoga meditation. *Archives of General Psychiatry, 35,* 571–577.

Corsini, R. J. (Ed.). (1987). *Concise encyclopedia of psychology.* New York: Wiley.

Coulter, J. (1989). *Mind in action.* Atlantic Highlands, NJ: Humanities Press.

Council, J. R., & Huff, K. D. (1990). Hypnosis, fantasy activity, and reports of paranormal experiences in high, medium, and low fantasizers. *British Journal of Experimental and Clinical Hypnosis, 7,* 9–15.

Council, J. R., Kirsch, I., & Hafner, L. P. (1986). Expectancy versus absorption in the prediction of hypnotic responding. *Journal of Personality and Social Psychology, 50,* 182–189.

Council, J., Kirsch, I., Vickery, A. R., & Carlson, D. (1983). "Trance" vs. "skill" hypnotic inductions: The effects of credibility, expectancy, and experimenter modeling. *Journal of Consulting and Clinical Psychology, 51,* 432–440.

Council, J. R., Waters, C., Sanderson, S., & Svenby, P. (1991, August). Beyond hypnosis: Research on the generality of context effects. In M. R. Nash (Chair), *Context and cognition in hypnosis.* Symposium conducted at the meeting of the American Psychological Association, San Francisco.

Council on Scientific Affairs, American Medical Association. (1985). Scientific status of refreshing recollection by the use of hypnosis. *Journal of the American Medical Association, 253,* 1918–1923.

Crasilneck, H. B., & Hall, J. A. (1959). Physiological changes associated with hypnosis: A review of the literature since 1948. *International Journal of Clinical and Experimental Hypnosis, 7,* 950.

Crasilneck, H. B., McCranie, E. J., & Jenkins, M. T. (1956). Special indications for hypnosis as a method of anesthesia. *Journal of the American Medical Association, 162,* 1606–1608.

Crawford, H. J. (1978). *Relationship of hypnotic susceptibility to imagery vividness, absorption and daydreaming styles.* Paper presented at the annual meeting of the Western Psychological Association, San Francisco.

Crawford, H. J. (1981). Hypnotic susceptibility as related to gestalt closure tasks. *Journal of Personality and Social Psychology, 40,* 376–383.

Crawford, H. J. (1982a). Hypnotizability, daydreaming styles, imagery vividness, and absorption: A multidimensional study. *Journal of Personality and Social Psychology, 42,* 915–926.

Crawford, H. J. (1982b). Cognitive processing during hypnosis: Much unfinished business. *Research Communications in Psychology, Psychiatry and Behavior, 7,* 169–179.

Crawford, H. J. (1986). Imagery processing during hypnosis: Relationships to hypnotizability and cognitive strategies. In M. Wolpin, J. E. Shorr, & L. Krueger (Eds.), *Imagery: Recent practice and theory* (pp. 13–32). New York: Plenum.

Crawford, H. J. (1989). Cognitive and physiological flexibility: Multiple pathways to hypnotic responsiveness. In V. Ghorghui, P. Netter, H. Eysenck, & R. Rosenthal (Eds.), *Suggestion and suggestibility: Theory and research* (pp. 155–168). Berlin: Springer-Verlag.

Crawford, H. J. (1990a). Cognitive and psychophysiological correlates of hypnotic responsiveness and hypnosis. In M. L. Fass & D. P. Brown (Eds.), *Creative mastery in hypnosis and hypnoanalysis: A festschrift for Erika Fromm* (pp. 47–54). Hillsdale, NJ: Erlbaum.

Crawford, H. J. (1990b, July). *Cold pressor pain with and without suggested analgesia: EEG correlates as moderated by hypnotic susceptibility level.* Paper presented at the 5th International Congress of Psychophysiology, Budapest.

Crawford, H. J. (1991a). Cold pressor pain with and without suggested analgesia: EEG correlates as moderated by hypnotic susceptibility level. In J. Gruzelier et al. (Eds.), *Frontiers of psychophysiology.*

Crawford, H. J. (1991b, October). *The hypnotizable brain: Attentional and disattentional processes.* Presidential address delivered at the annual meeting of the Society for Clinical and Experimental Hypnosis, New Orleans.

Crawford, H. J. (1992). Psychophysiological comparisons of REST and hypnosis: Implications for future research. In A. F. Barabasz & M. Barabasz (Eds.),

Clinical and experimental restricted environmental stimulation: New developments and perspectives (pp. 175–186). New York: Springer-Verlag.

Crawford, H. J., & Allen, S. N. (1983). Enhanced visual memory during hypnosis as mediated by hypnotic responsiveness and cognitive strategies. *Journal of Experimental Psychology: General, 112,* 662–685.

Crawford, H. J., Allen, S. H., & Kiefner, M. G. (1983, October). *Effect of hypnosis on the retention of high- and low-imagery paired associates.* Paper presented at the annual meeting of the Society for Clinical and Experimental Hypnosis, Boston.

Crawford, H. J., & Barabasz, A. F. (in press). Phobias and intense fears: Facilitating their treatment with hypnosis. In J. W. Rhue, S. J. Lynn, & I. Kirsch (Eds.), *Handbook of clinical hypnosis.* Washington, DC: American Psychological Association.

Crawford, H. J., Brown, A., & Moon, C. (1991). *Sustained attentional abilities: Differences between low and high hypnotizables.* Manuscript submitted for publication.

Crawford, H. J., Clarke, S. N., Kitner-Triolo, M., & Olesko, B. (1989). *EEG correlates of emotions: Moderated by hypnosis and hypnotic level.* Paper presented at the annual meeting of the American Psychological Association, New Orleans.

Crawford, H. J., Crawford, K., & Koperski, B. J. (1983). Hypnosis and lateral cerebral function as assessed by dichotic listening. *Biological Psychiatry, 18,* 415–427.

Crawford, H. J., Gur, R., Skolnick, B., Gur, R., & Benson, D. (1986, July). *Regional cerebral blood flow and hypnosis: Differences between low and high hypnotizables.* Paper presented at the 3rd International Congress of Psychophysiology, Vienna.

Crawford, H. J., Hilgard, J. R., & Macdonald, H. (1982). Transient experiences following hypnotic testing and special termination procedures. *International Journal of Clinical and Experimental Hypnosis, 30,* 117–126.

Crawford, H. J., Kitner-Triolo, M., Clarke, S., & Brown, A. (1988 October). *EEG patterns accompanying induced happy and sad moods: Moderating effects of hypnosis and hypnotic responsiveness level.* Paper presented at the annual meeting of the Society for Clinical and Experimental Hypnosis, Asheville, NC.

Crawford, H. J., Macdonald, H., & Hilgard, E. R. (1979). Hypnotic deafness: A psychophysical study of responses to tone intensity as modified by hypnosis. *American Journal of Psychology, 92,* 193–214.

Crawford, H. J., & MacLeod-Morgan, C. (1986). *Right ear advantage of low and high hypnotizables in waking and hypnosis: Comparisons of passive and active alert inductions with focused and nonfocused attention instructions.* Unpublished manuscript.

Crawford, H. J., Mészáros, I., & Szabó, C. (1989). EEG activation of low and high hypnotizables during waking and hypnosis: Rest, math and imaginal tasks. In D. Waxman, D. Pedersen, I. Wilkie, & P. Mellett (Eds.), *Hypnosis: The 4th European Congress at Oxford* (pp. 76–85). London: Whurr.

Crawford, H. J., Nomura, K., & Slater, H. (1983). Spatial memory processing: Enhancement during hypnosis. In J. C. Shorr, J. Conella, G. Sobel, & T. Robin (Eds.), *Imagery: Theoretical aspects and applications* (pp. 209–216). New York: Plenum Press.

Crawford, H. J., Skolnick, B. E., Benson, D. M., Gur, R. E., & Gur, R. C. (1985,

August). *Regional cerebral blood flow in hypnosis and hypnotic analgesia.* Paper presented at the 10th International Congress of Hypnosis and Psychosomatic Medicine, Toronto.

Crawford, H. J., Wallace, B., Nomura, K., & Slater, H. (1986). Eidetic–like imagery in hypnosis: Rare but there. *American Journal of Psychology, 99,* 527–546.

Cross, W. P., & Spanos, N. P. (1988–1989). The effects of imagery vividness and receptivity on skill training induced enhancements in hypnotic susceptibility. *Imagination, Cognition and Personality, 8,* 89–103.

Crowne, D. P., Konow, A., Drake, K. J., & Pribram, K. H. (1972). Hippocampal electrical activity in the monkey during delayed alternation problems. *Electroencephalography and Clinical Neurophysiology, 33,* 567–577.

Crowne, D. P., & Marlowe, D. (1964). *The approval motive.* New York: Wiley.

Cunnington, B. R., & Torrance, E.P. (1965). *Sounds and images.* Boston: Ginn.

Dahlstrom, W. G., Welsh, G. S., & Dahlstrom, L. (1972). *An MMPI handbook: Vol. 1. Clinical interpretation.* Minneapolis: University of Minnesota Press.

Dahlstrom, W.G., Welsh, G.S., & Dahlstrom, L. (1975). *An MMPI handbook: Vol. 2. Research applications.* Minneapolis: University of Minnesota Press.

Darnton, R. (1968). *Mesmerism and the end of the enlightenment in France.* Cambridge, MA: Harvard University Press.

Darrow, C. W., Henry, C. E., Gill, M., Brenman, M., & Converse, M. (1950). Frontal–motor parallelism and motor–occipital in-phase activity in hypnosis, drowsiness and sleep. *Electroencephalography and Clinical Neurophysiology, 2,* 355.

Dave, R. (1979). Effects of hypnotically induced dreams on creative problem-solving. *Journal of Abnormal Psychology, 88,* 293–302.

Davidson, P. (1987) Hypnosis and migraine headache: Reporting a clinical series. *Australian Journal of Clinical and Experimental Hypnosis, 15,* 111–118.

Davidson, R. J., Chapman, J. P., Chapman, L. J., & Henriques, J. B. (1990). Asymmetrical brain electrical activity discriminates between psychometrically-matched verbal and spatial cognitive tasks. *Psychophysiology, 27,* 528–543.

Davidson, T. M., & Bowers, K. S. (1991). Selective hypnotic amnesia: Is it a successful attempt to forget or an unsuccessful attempt to remember? *Journal of Abnormal Psychology, 100,* 133–143.

Davis, G. A. (1971). Instruments useful in studying creative behavior and creative talent: Part II. Non-commercially available instruments. *Journal of Creative Behavior, 5,* 162–165.

Davis, S., Dawson, J. G., & Seay, B. (1978). Prediction of hypnotic susceptibility from imaginative involvement. *American Journal of Clinical Hypnosis, 20,* 194–198.

Deabler, H. L., Fidel, E., Dillenkoffer, R. L., & Elder, S. T. (1973). The use of relaxation and hypnosis in lowering blood pressure. *American Journal of Clinical Hypnosis, 16,* 75–83.

De Benedittis, G., & Carli, G. (1990). Psineurobiologia dell'ipnosi. In M. Tiengo (Ed.), *Seminari sul dolore* (pp. 59–116). Milan: Centro Studi sull'Analgesia, Università degli Studi di Milano.

De Benedittis, G., & Longostreui, G. P. (1988, July). *Cerebral blood flow changes in hypnosis: A single photon emission computerized tomography (SPECT) study.* Paper presented at the 4th Conference of the International Organization of Psychophysiology, Prague.

De Benedittis, G., Panerai, A. A., & Villamira, M. A. (1989). Effects of hypnotic analgesia and hypnotizability on experimental ischemic pain. *International Journal of Clinical and Experimental Hypnosis, 37*, 55–69.

De Benedittis, G., & Sironi, V. A. (1986). Deep cerebral electrical activity in man during hypnosis. *International Journal of Clinical and Experimental Hypnosis, 34*, 63–70.

De Benedittis, G., & Sironi, V. A. (1988). Arousal effects of electrical deep brain stimulation in hypnosis. *International Journal of Clinical and Experimental Hypnosis, 36*, 96–106.

DeBono, E. (1968). *The use of lateral thinking in the generation of new ideas.* New York: Basic Books.

Deckert, G. H., & West, L. J. (1963a). Hypnosis and experimental psychopathology. *American Journal of Clinical Hypnosis, 5*, 256–276.

Deckert, G.H., & West, L.J. (1963b). The problem of hypnotizability: A review. International Journal of Clinical and Experimental Hypnosis, 11, 205–235.

D'Eon, J. L. (1989). Hypnosis in the control of labor pains. In N. P. Spanos & J. F. Chaves (Eds.), *Hypnosis: The cognitive–behavioral perspective* (pp. 273–296). Buffalo, NY: Prometheus Books.

de Groh, M. (1989). Correlates of hypnotic susceptibility. In N. P. Spanos & J. F. Chaves (Eds.), *Hypnosis: The cognitive–behavioral perspective* (pp. 32–63). Buffalo, NY: Prometheus Books.

de Groot, H. P., & Gwynn, M. I. (1989). Trance logic, duality, and hidden observer responding. In N. P. Spanos & J. F. Chaves (Eds.), *Hypnosis: The cognitive–behavioral perspective* (pp. 187–205). Buffalo, NY: Prometheus Books.

de Groot, H. P., Gwynn, M. I., & Spanos, N. P. (1988). The effects of contextual information and gender on the prediction of hypnotic susceptibility. *Journal of Personality and Social Psychology, 54*, 1049–1053.

Deikman, A. J. (1963). Experimental meditation. *Journal of Nervous and Mental Disease, 136*, 329–343.

Deikman, A. J. (1971). Bimodal consciousness. *Archives of General Psychiatry, 25*, 481–489.

Dellas, M., & Gaier, E. L. (1970). Identification of creativity: The individual. *Psychological Bulletin, 73*, 55–73.

Delmonte, M. M. (1984). Meditation: Similarities with hypnoidal states and hypnosis. *International Journal of Psychosomatics, 31*, 24–34.

De Pascalis, V., & Imperiali, M. G. (1984). Personality, hypnotic susceptibility and EEG responses: Preliminary study. *Perceptual and Motor Skills, 59*, 371–378.

De Pascalis, V., Marucci, F. S., & Penna, P. M. (1989). 40-Hz EEG asymmetry during recall of emotional events in waking and hypnosis: Differences between low and high hypnotizables. *International Journal of Psychophysiology, 7*, 85–96.

De Pascalis, V., Marucci, F., Penna, P. M., & Pessa, E. (1987). Hemispheric activity of 40 Hz EEG during recall of emotional events: Differences between low and high hypnotizables. *International Journal of Psychophysiology, 5*, 167–180.

De Pascalis, V., & Palumbo, G. (1986). EEG alpha asymmetry: Task difficulty and hypnotizability. *Perceptual and Motor Skills, 62*, 139–150.

De Pascalis, V., & Penna, P. M. (1990). 40-Hz EEG activity during hypnotic induction and hypnotic testing. *International Journal of Clinical and Experimental Hypnosis, 38*, 125–138.

De Pascalis, V., Silveri, A., & Palumbo, G. (1988). EEG asymmetry during covert mental activity and its relationship with hypnotizability. *International Journal of Clinical and Experimental Hypnosis, 36,* 38–52.

DePiano, F. A., & Salzberg, H. C. (1979). Clinical applications of hypnosis to three psychosomatic disorders. *Psychological Bulletin, 86,* 1223–1235.

DePiano, F. A., & Salzberg, H. C. (1981). Hypnosis as an aid to recall of meaningful information presented under three types of arousal. *International Journal of Clinical and Experimental Hypnosis, 29,* 383–400.

Der, D., & Lewington, P. (1990). Rational self-directed hypnotherapy: A treatment for panic attacks. *American Journal of Clinical Hypnosis, 32*(3), 160–167.

Derman, D., & London, P. (1965). Correlates of hypnotic susceptibility. *Journal of Consulting Psychology, 29,* 537–545.

DeVoge, J. T., & Sachs, L. B. (1973). The modification of hypnotic susceptibility through imitative behavior. *International Journal of Clinical and Experimental Hypnosis, 21,* 70–77.

Dhanens, T. P., & Lundy, R. M. (1975). Hypnotic and waking suggestions and recall. *International Journal of Clinical and Experimental Hypnosis, 23,* 68–79.

Diamond, B. L. (1980). Inherent problems in the use of pretrial hypnosis on a prospective witness. *California Law Review, 68,* 313–349.

Diamond, M. J. (1972). The use of observationally presented information to modify hypnotic susceptibility. *Journal of Abnormal Psychology, 79,* 174–180.

Diamond, M. J. (1974). Modification of hypnotizability: A review. *Psychological Bulletin, 81,* 180–198.

Diamond, M. J. (1977). Hypnotizability is modifiable: An alternative approach. *International Journal of Clinical and Experimental Hypnosis, 25,* 147–166.

Diamond, M. J. (1989) Is hypnotherapy art or science? *American Journal of Clinical Hypnosis, 32,* 11–12.

Diamond, M. J., Gregory, J., Lenney, E., Steadman, C., & Talone, J. M. (1974). An alternative approach to personality correlates of hypnotizability: Hypnosis-specific mediational attitudes. *International Journal of Clinical and Experimental Hypnosis, 12,* 346–353.

Diamond, M. J., Steadman, C., Harada, D., & Rosenthal, J. (1975). The use of direct instructions to modify hypnotic performance: The effects of programmed learning procedures. *Journal of Abnormal Psychology, 84* 109–113.

Diamond, M. J., & Taft, R. (1975). The role played by ego permissiveness and imagery in hypnotic responsivity. *International Journal of Clinical and Experimental Hypnosis, 23,* 130–138.

Dierks, T., Mauer, K., & Zacher, A. (1989). Brain mapping of EEG in autogenic training (AT). *Psychiatry Research, 29,* 433–434.

Dillon, R. F., & Spanos, N. P. (1983). Proactive interference and the functional ablation hypothesis: More disconfirmatory data. *International Journal of Clinical and Experimental Hypnosis, 31,* 47–56.

Dimond, S. J. (1980). *Neuropsychology.* London: Butterworths.

Dixon, M., Brunet, A., & Laurence, J.-R. (1990). Hypnotizability and automaticity: Toward a parallel distributed processing model of hypnotic responding. *Journal of Abnormal Psychology, 99,* 336–343.

Dixon, M., Labelle, L., & Laurence, J.-R. (in press). A multivariate approach to the prediction of hypnotizability. *International Journal of Clinical and Experimental Hypnosis*

Dixon, M., & Laurence, J.-R. (1992). Hypnotic susceptibility and verbal automaticity: Automatic and strategic processing differences in the Stroop color naming task. *Journal of Abnormal Psychology, 101,* 344–347.

Dixon, N. F. (1981). *Preconscious processing.* New York: Wiley.

Dobkin de Rios, M., & Friedman, J. K. (1987). Hypnotherapy with Hispanic burn patients. *International Journal of Clinical and Experimental Hypnosis, 35,* 87–94.

Domangue, B. B., Margolis, C. G., Lieberman, D., & Kaji, H. (1985). Biochemical correlates of hypnoanalgesia in arthritic pain patients. *Journal of Clinical Psychiatry, 46,* 235–238.

Domino, G. (1970). Identification of potentially creative persons using the Adjective Check List. *Journal of Consulting and Clinical Psychology, 35,* 48–51.

Donaldson, S. K., & Westerman, M. A. (1986). Development of children's understanding of ambivalence and causal theories of emotions. *Developmental Psychology, 22,* 655–662.

Dragutinovich, S., & Sheehan, P. W. (1986). Hypnotic susceptibility and cortical modulation of stimulus intensity. *Australian Journal of Clinical and Experimental Hypnosis, 14,* 1–14.

Drake, S. D., Nash, M. R., & Cawood, G. N. (1990–1991). Imaginative involvement and hypnotic susceptibility: A re-examination of the relationship. *Imagination, Cognition and Personality, 10,* 141–155.

Dubreuil, D. L., Spanos, N. P., & Bertrand, L. D. (1982–1983). Does hypnotic amnesia dissipate with time? *Imagination, Cognition and Personality, 2,* 103–113.

Ducat, S. (1985). Science and psychoanalysis. *International Journal of Biosocial Research, 7,* 94–107.

Dudek, S. Z. (1980). Primary process ideation. In R. H. Woody (Ed.), *Encyclopedia of clinical assessment* (Vol. 1, pp. 520–539). San Francisco: Jossey-Bass.

Dumas, L. (1964). Subjective report of inadvertent hypnosis. *International Journal of Clinical and Experimental Hypnosis, 12,* 53–62.

Dumas, R. A. (1976). *Operant control of EEG alpha and hypnotizability.* Unpublished doctoral dissertation, Stanford University.

Dumas, R. A. (1977). EEG alpha–hypnotizability correlations: A review. *Psychophysiology, 14,* 431–438.

Dumas, R. A. (1980). Cognitive control in hypnosis and biofeedback. *International Journal of Clinical and Experimental Hypnosis, 28,* 53–62.

Dumas, R. A., & Spitzer, E. (1978). Influences of subject self-selection on the EEG alpha–hypnotizability correlation. *Psychophysiology, 15,* 606–608.

Durio, H. F. (1975). Mental imagery and creativity. *Journal of Creative Behavior, 9,* 233–244.

Durndell, A. J., & Wetherick, N. E. (1976). The relation of reported imagery to cognitive performance. *British Journal of Psychology, 67,* 501–506.

Dwyer, J. H. (1983). *Statistical models for the social and behavioral sciences.* New York: Oxford University Press.

Dynes, J. B. (1947). Objective method for distinguishing sleep from the hypnotic trance. *Neurological Psychiatry, 57,* 84–93.

Dywan, J. (1988). The imagery factor in hypnotic hypermnesia. *International Journal of Clinical and Experimental Hypnosis, 36,* 312–326.

Dywan, J., & Bowers, K. S. (1983). The use of hypnosis to enhance recall. *Science, 222,* 184–185.

Edelson, J. & Fitzpatrick, J. L. (1989). A comparison of cognitive–behavioral and hypnotic treatments of chronic pain, *Journal of Clinical Psychology, 45*(2), 316–323.

Edmonston, W. E., & Grotevant, W. R. (1975). Hypnosis and alpha density. *American Journal of Clinical Hypnosis, 17,* 221–232.

Edmonston, W. E., & Moscovitz, H. C. (1990). Hypnosis and lateralized brain functions. *International Journal of Clinical and Experimental Hypnosis, 38,* 70–84.

Edwards, G. (1960). Hypnotic treatment of asthma: Real and illusory results. *British Medical Journal, ii,* 492–497.

Eiblmayr, K. (1987). Trance logic and the circle-touch test. *Australian Journal of Clinical and Experimental Hypnosis, 15,* 133–145.

Eisen, M. (in press). A psychodynamic model of hypnosis. In J. W. Rhue, S. J. Lynn, & I. Kirsch (Eds.), *Handbook of clinical hypnosis.* Washington, DC: American Psychological Association.

Ekehammer, B. (1974). Interactionism in personality from a historical perspective. *Psychological Bulletin, 81,* 1026–1048.

Ellenberger, H. F. (1970). *The discovery of the unconscious: The history and evolution of dynamic psychiatry.* New York: Basic Books.

Elson, B. D., Hauri, P., & Cunis, D. (1977). Physiological changes in yoga meditation. *Psychophysiology, 14,* 52–57.

Engstrom, D. R., London, P., & Hart, T. (1970a). Hypnotic susceptibility increased by EEG alpha training. *Nature, 227,* 1261–1262.

Engstrom, D. R., London, P., & Hart, T. (1970b). EEG alpha feedback training and hypnotic susceptibility. *Proceedings of the 78th Annual Convention of the American Psychological Association, 5,* 837–838.

Epstein, S., & O'Brien, E. J. (1985). The person–situation debate in historical and current perspective. *Psychological Bulletin, 98,* 513–537.

Erdelyi, M. H. (1985). *Psychoanalysis: Freud's cognitive psychology.* New York: Freeman.

Erickson, M. H., & Erickson, E. (1944). Concerning the nature and character of post-hypnotic behavior. *Journal of General Psychology, 24,* 95–133.

Erickson, M. H., & Kubie, L. S. (1941). The successful treatment of a case of acute hysterical depression by a return under hypnosis to a critical phase of childhood. *Psychoanalytic Quarterly, 10,* 583–609.

Erickson, M. H., & Rossi, E. L. (1980). The February man: Facilitating new identity in hypnotherapy. In E. L. Rossi (Ed.), *The collected papers of Milton H. Erickson on hypnosis* (Vol. 4, pp. 525–542). New York: Irvington.

Erickson, M. H., Rossi, E. L., & Rossi, S. (1976). *Hypnotic realities.* New York: Irvington.

Ernest, C. H. (1977). Imagery ability and cognition: A critical review. *Journal of Mental Imagery, 2,* 181–216.

Evans, C., & Richardson, P. H. (1988). Improved recovery and reduced postoperative stay after therapeutic suggestions during general anaesthesia. *Lancet, ii,* 491–493.

Evans, F. J. (1963, August 23). *A factor analysis of hypnosis phenomena.* Paper presented at the 17th International Congress of Psychology, Washington, DC.

Evans, F. J. (1967). An experimental indirect technique for the induction of hypnosis. *International Journal of Clinical and Experimental Hypnosis, 15,* 72–85.

Evans, F. J. (1979). Hypnosis and sleep: Techniques for exploring cognitive activity during sleep. In E. Fromm & R. E. Shor (Eds.), *Hypnosis: Developments in research and new perspectives* (2nd ed., pp. 139–183). New York: Aldine.

Evans, F. J. (1983, October). *The hypnotizable subject: The hypnotizable patient.* Presidential address presented at the 35th Annual Meeting of the Society for Clinical and Experimental Hypnosis, Boston.

Evans, F. J. (1988). Posthypnotic amnesia: Dissociation of context and content. In H. M. Pettinati (Ed.), *Hypnosis and memory* (pp. 157–192). New York: Guilford Press.

Evans, F. J., & Kihlstrom, J. F. (1973). Posthypnotic amnesia as disrupted retrieval. *Journal of Abnormal Psychology, 82,* 317–323.

Evans, F. J., Kihlstrom, J. F., & Orne, E. C. (1973). Quantifying subjective reports during posthypnotic amnesia. *Proceedings of the 81st Annual Convention of the American Psychological Association, 8,* 1077–1078.

Evans, F. J., & Orne, M. T. (1965). Motivation, performance and hypnosis. *International Journal of Clinical and Experimental Hypnosis, 13*(2), 103–116.

Evans, F. J., & Schmeidler, D. (1966) Relationships between the Harvard Group Scale of Hypnotic Susceptibility and the Stanford Hypnotic Susceptibility Scale: Form C. *International Journal of Clinical and Experimental Hypnosis, 14,* 333–343.

Evans, F. J., & Thorn, W. A. (1966). Two types of posthypnotic amnesia: Recall amnesia and source amnesia. *International Journal of Clinical and Experimental Hypnosis, 14,* 162–179.

Evans, M. G. (1991). The problems of analyzing multiplicative components. *American Psychologist, 45,* 6–15.

Ewer, T. C., & Stewart, D. E. (1986). Improvement in bronchial hyper-responsiveness in patients with moderate asthma after treatment with a hypnotic technique. *British Medical Journal, i,* 1129–1132.

Ewin, D. M. (1986a). The effect of hypnosis and mental set on major surgery and burns. *Psychiatric Annals, 16,* 115–118.

Ewin, D. M. (1986b). Emergency room hypnosis for the burned patient. *American Journal of Clinical Hypnosis, 29,* 7–21.

Eysenck, H. J. (1947). *Dimensions of personality.* London: Routledge & Kegan Paul.

Eysenck, H. J., & Furneaux, W. D. (1945). Primary and secondary suggestibility: An experimental and statistical study. *Journal of Experimental Psychology, 35,* 485–503.

Fairbairn, W. R. D. (1952). Object relationships and dynamic structure. In W. R. D. Fairbairn, *An object-relations theory of the personality.* New York: Basic Books. (Original work published 1946)

Faria, J. C. da, Abbé. (1819). *De la cause du sommeil lucide: Ou Etude de la nature de l'homme.* Paris: Mme Horiac.

Faria, J. C. da, Abbé. (1906). *De la cause du sommeil lucide: Ou l'étude de la nature de l'homme* [*On the cause of lucid sleep: A study of the nature of man*] (2nd ed., D. G. Dalgado, Ed.). Paris: Henri Jouve. (Original work published 1819)

Farthing, G. W., Venturino, M., & Brown, S. W. (1983). Relationship between two different types of imagery vividness questionnaire items and three hypnotic susceptibility scale factors: A brief communication. *International Journal of Clinical and Experimental Hypnosis, 31,* 8–13.

Fass, M. L., & Brown, D. P. (Eds.). (1990). *Creative mastery in hypnosis and hypnoanalysis: A festschrift for Erika Fromm.* Hillsdale, NJ: Erlbaum.

Faw, V., Sellers, D. J., & Wilcox, W. W. (1968). Psychopathological effects of hypnosis. *International Journal of Clinical and Experimental Hypnosis, 16*, 26–37.

Feigl, H. (1958). The "mental" and the "physical." In H. Feigl, M. Scriven, & G. Maxwell (Eds.), *Minnesota studies in the philosophy of science* (Vol. 2, pp. 370–498). Minneapolis: University of Minnesota Press.

Feinstein, D., & Morgan, M. (1986). Hypnosis in regulating bipolar affective disorders. *American Journal of Clinical Hypnosis, 29*, 29–38.

Fellows, B. J. (1990). Current theories of hypnosis: A critical overview. *British Journal of Experimental and Clinical Hypnosis, 7*, 81–92.

Fellows, B. J., & Armstrong, V. (1977). An experimental investigation of the relationship between hypnotic susceptibility and reading involvement. *American Journal of Clinical Hypnosis, 20*, 101–105.

Fenwick, P. (1987). Meditation and the EEG. In M. A. West (Ed.), *The psychology of meditation* (pp. 104–117). Oxford: Clarendon Press.

Ferenczi, S. (1980). Introjection and transference. In E. Jones (Ed. and Trans.), *First contributions to psychoanalysis* (pp. 35–93). New York: Brunner/Mazel. (Original work published 1909)

Festinger, L. (1954). A theory of social comparison processes. *Human Relations, 7*, 117–140.

Field, P. B. (1965). An inventory scale of hypnotic depth. *International Journal of Clinical and Experimental Hypnosis, 13*, 238–249.

Finke, R. A., & Macdonald, H. (1978). Two personality measures relating hypnotic susceptibility to absorption. *International Journal of Clinical and Experimental Hypnosis, 26*, 178–183.

Flavell, J. (1985). *Cognitive development* (2nd ed.). Englewood Cliffs, NJ: Prentice-Hall.

Foenander, G., Burrows, G. D., Gerschman, J., & Horne, D. J. (1980). Phobic behavior hypnotic susceptibility. *Australian Journal of Clinical and Experimental Hypnosis, 8*, 41–46.

Forisha, B. (1980). *Patterns of creativity and mental imagery in men and women.* Paper presented at the annual meeting of the American Psychological Association, Montréal.

Forisha, B., & Nagy, J. (1979). *Creativity and imagery in men and women.* Unpublished manuscript, University of Michigan, Dearborn.

Frank, R. G., Umlauf, R. L., Wonderlich, S. A., & Ashkanazi, G. S. (1986). Hypnosis and behavioral treatment in a worksite smoking cessation program. *Addictive Behaviors, 2*, 59–62.

Frankel, F. H. (1976). *Hypnosis: Trance as a coping mechanism.* New York: Plenum Medical.

Frankel, F. H. (1974). Trance capacity and the genesis of phobic behavior. *Archives of General Psychiatry, 31*, 261–263.

Frankel, F. H. (1982). Hypnosis and hypnotizability scales: A reply. *International Journal of Clinical and Experimental Hypnosis, 30*(4) 377–392.

Frankel, F. H. (1988). The clinical use of hypnosis in aiding recall. In H. M. Pettinati (Ed.), *Hypnosis and memory* (pp. 247–265). New York: Guilford Press.

Frankel, F. H. (1990). Hypnotizability and dissociation. *American Journal of Psychiatry, 147*, 823–829.

Frankel, F. H., & Orne, M. T. (1976). Hypnotizability and phobic behavior. *Archives of General Psychiatry, 33*, 1259–1261.

Franklin, B., de Bory, G., Lavoisier, A. L., Bailly, J. S., Majault, Sallin, D'Arcet, J., Guillotin, J. I., & Leroy, J. B. (1784). *Rapport des Commissaires chargés par le Roy de l'examen du magnétisme animal.* Paris: Bibliothéque Royale.

Frauman, D. C., Lynn, S. J., Hardaway, R., & Molteni, A. (1984). Effect of subliminal symbiotic activation on hypnotic rapport and susceptibility. *Journal of Abnormal Psychology, 93,* 481–483.

Fredericks, L. E. (1967). The use of hypnosis in hemophilia. *American Journal of Clinical Hypnosis, 10,* 52–55.

Free, M. L., & Oei, T. P. S. (1989). Biological and psychological processes in the treatment and maintenance of depression. *Clinical Psychology Review, 9,* 653–688.

Freeman, R. M., MacCaulay, A. J., Eve, L., Chamberlain, G. V. P., & Bhat, A. V. (1986). Randomised trial of self hypnosis for analgesia in labour. *British Medical Journal, 292,* 657–658.

French, J. W., Ekstrom, R. B., & Price, L. A. (1963). *Manual for Kit of Reference Tests for Cognitive Factors.* Princeton, NJ: Educational Testing Service.

Freud, A. (1948). *The ego and the mechanisms of defense.* New York: International Universities Press. (Original work published 1926)

Freud, S. (1953). The interpretation of dreams. In J. Strachey (Ed. and Trans.), *The standard edition of the complete psychological works of Sigmund Freud* (Vol. 4, pp. 1–338; Vol. 5, pp. 339–621). London: Hogarth Press. (Original work published 1900)

Freud, S. (1955). Group psychology and the analysis of the ego. In J. Strachey (Ed. and Trans.), *The standard edition of the complete psychological works of Sigmund Freud* (Vol. 18, pp. 69–143). London: Hogarth Press. (Original work published 1921)

Freud, S. (1957). Thoughts for the times on war and death. In J. Strachey (Ed. and Trans.), *The standard edition of the complete psychological works of Sigmund Freud* (Vol. 14, pp. 275–300). London: Hogarth Press. (Original work published 1915)

Freud, S. (1957). A metapsychological supplement to the theory of dreams. In J. Strachey (Ed. and Trans.), *The standard edition of the complete psychological works of Sigmund Freud* (Vol. 14, pp. 222–235). London: Hogarth Press. (Original work published 1917)

Freud, S. (1959). Charcot. In E. Jones (Ed.), J. Riviere (Trans.), *Sigmund Freud: Collected papers* (Vol. 1, pp. 9–23). New York: Basic Books. (Original work published 1893)

Freud, S. (1960). Jokes and their relation to the unconscious. In J. Strachey (Ed. and Trans.), *The standard edition of the complete psychological works of Sigmund Freud* (Vol. 8, pp. 9–236). London: Hogarth Press. (Original work published 1905)

Freud, S. (1961). The ego and the id. In J. Strachey (Ed. and Trans.), *The standard edition of the complete psychological works of Sigmund Freud* (Vol. 19, pp. 3–66). London: Hogarth Press. (Original work published 1923)

Freud, S. (1963). Introductory lectures on psycho-analysis. In J. Strachey (Ed. and Trans.), *The standard edition of the complete psychological works of Sigmund Freud* (Vols. 15–16, pp. 9–463). London: Hogarth Press. (Original work published 1916–1917)

Freud, S. (1964). New introductory lectures on psycho-analysis. In J. Strachey (Ed. and Trans.), *The standard edition of the complete psychological works of Sigmund Freud* (Vol. 22, pp. 7–182). London: Hogarth Press. (Original work published 1933)

Freundlich, B., & Fisher, S. (1974). The role of body experience in hypnotic behavior. *International Journal of Clinical and Experimental Hypnosis, 22,* 68–83.

Fricton, J. R., & Roth, P. (1985). The effects of direct and indirect hypnotic suggestions for analgesia in high and low susceptible subjects. *American Journal of Clinical Hypnosis, 27,* 226–231.

Frid, M., & Singer, G. (1980). The effects of naloxene on human pain reactions during stress. In C. Peck & M. Wallace (Eds.), *Problems in pain: Proceedings of the first Australia–New Zealand Conference on Pain* (pp. 78–86). Elmsford, NY: Pergamon Press.

Friedland, M. R. (1976). *A comparison of three methods for inducing hypnosis* (Doctoral dissertation, University of Oregon). *Dissertation Abstracts International, 37,* 3071B–3072B. (University Microfilms No. 76-27, 643)

Friedlander, J. W., & Sarbin, T. R. (1938). The depth of hypnosis. *Journal of Abnormal and Social Psychology, 33,* 453–475.

Friedman, H., & Taub, H. A. (1978). A six-month follow-up of the use of hypnosis and biofeedback procedures in essential hypertension. *American Journal of Clinical Hypnosis, 20,* 184–188.

Friedman, H., & Taub, H. A. (1986). Hypnotizability and speed of visual information processing. *International Journal of Clinical and Experimental Hypnosis, 36,* 234–241.

Friedman, H., Taub, H. A., Sturr, J. F., & Monty, R. A. (1987). Visual information processing speed in hypnotized and nonhypnotized subjects. *Journal of General Psychology, 114,* 363–372.

Friedman, H., Taub, H. A., Sturr, J. F., & Monty, R. A. (1990). Hypnosis and hypnotizability in cognitive task performance. *British Journal of Experimental and Clinical Hypnosis, 7,* 103–107.

Frischholz, E. J. (1985a). Hypnotizability and psychosis: a meta-analytic review. In J. Fawcett (Chair), *Psychopathology and hypnotizability symposium.* Symposium conducted at the meeting of the American Psychiatric Association, Dallas, TX.

Frischholz, E. J. (1985b). The relationship among dissociation, hypnosis, and child abuse in the development of multiple personality. In R. P. Kluft (Ed.), *Childhood antecedents of multiple personality* (pp. 99–120). Washington, DC: American Psychiatric Press.

Frischholz, E. J., Spiegel, D., Spiegel, H., Balma, D. L., & Markell, C. S. (1982). Differential hypnotic responsivity of smokers, phobics, and chronic-pain control patients: A failure to confirm. *Journal of Abnormal Psychology, 91,* 269–272.

Frischholz, E. J., Spiegel, D., Spiegel, H., Lipman, L.S., & Bark, N. (1988). Psychopathology and hypnotizability. Unpublished manuscript.

Frischholz, E. J., Spiegel, D., Trentalange, M.J., & Spiegel, H. (1987). The Hypnotic Induction Profile and absorption. *American Journal of Clinical Hypnosis, 30,* 87–93.

Frischholz, E. J., Tryon, W. W., Vellios, A. T., Fisher, S., Maruffi, B. L., & Spiegel, H. (1980) The relationship between the Hypnotic Induction Profile and the Stanford Hypnotic Susceptibility Scale, Form C: A replication. *American Journal of Clinical Hypnosis, 22,* 185–196.

Friswell, R., & McConkey, K.M. (1989). Hypnotically induced mood. *Cognition and Emotion, 3,* 1–26.

Fromm, E. (1965a). Hypnoanalysis: Theory and two case excerpts. *Psychotherapy: Theory, Research and Practice, 2,* 127–133.

Fromm, E. (1965b). Awareness versus consciousness. *Psychological Reports, 16,* 711–712.

Fromm, E. (1972). Activity and passivity of the ego in hypnosis. *International Journal of Clinical and Experimental Hypnosis, 20,* 238–251.

Fromm, E. (1975a). Autohypnosis and heterohypnosis: Phenomenological similarities and differences. In L.-E. Unestahl (Ed.), *Hypnosis in the seventies* (pp. 24–28). Örebro, Sweden: Veje Förlag.

Fromm, E. (1975b). Self-hypnosis: A new area of research. *Psychotherapy: Theory, Research and Practice, 12,* 295–301.

Fromm, E. (1976). Altered states of consciousness and ego psychology. *Social Service Review, 50,* 557–569.

Fromm, E. (1977). An ego psychological theory of altered states of consciousness. *International Journal of Clinical and Experimental Hypnosis, 25,* 372–387.

Fromm, E. (1978–1979). Primary and secondary process in waking and in altered states of consciousness. *Journal of Altered States of Consciousness, 4,* 115–128.

Fromm, E. (1979). The nature of hypnosis and other altered states of consciousness: An ego-psychological theory. In E. Fromm & R. E. Shor (Eds.), *Hypnosis: Developments in research and new perspectives* (2nd ed., pp. 81–103). New York: Aldine.

Fromm, E. (1981). How to write a clinical paper: A brief communication. *International Journal of Clinical and Experimental Hypnosis, 29,* 5–9.

Fromm, E. (1984). Hypnoanalysis—with particular emphasis on the borderline patient. *Psychoanalytic Psychology, 1,* 61–76.

Fromm, E. (1987). Significant developments in clinical hypnosis during the past 25 years. *International Journal of Clinical and Experimental Hypnosis, 35,* 215–230.

Fromm, E. (1988). Self-hypnosis and the creative imagination. In I. Shafer (Ed.), *The incarnate imagination: Essays in theology, the arts and social sciences in honor of Andrew Greeley. A festschrift* (pp. 15–24). Bowling Green, OH: Popular Press.

Fromm, E., Brown, D. P., Hurt, S. W., Oberlander, J. Z., Boxer, A. M., & Pfeifer, G. (1981). The phenomena and characteristics of self-hypnosis. *International Journal of Clinical and Experimental Hypnosis, 29,* 189–246.

Fromm, E., & Gardner, G. G. (1979). Ego psychology and hypnoanalysis: An integration of theory and technique. *Bulletin of the Menninger Clinic, 43,* 413–423.

Fromm, E., & Hurt, S. W. (1980). Ego-psychological parameters of hypnosis and altered states of consciousness. In G. D. Burrows & L. Dennerstein (Eds.), *Handbook of hypnosis and psychosomatic medicine* (pp. 13–27). New York: Elsevier/North-Holland.

Fromm, E., & Kahn, S. (1990). *Self-hypnosis: The Chicago paradigm.* New York: Guilford Press.

Fromm, E., Lombard, L., Skinner, S. H., & Kahn, S. (1987–1988). The modes of the ego in self-hypnosis. *Imagination, Cognition and Personality, 7,* 335–349.

Fromm, E., Oberlander, M. I., & Gruenewald, D. (1970). Perceptual and cognitive processes in different states of consciousness: The waking state and hypnosis. *Journal of Projective Techniques and Personality Assessment, 34,* 375–387.

Fromm, E., & Shor, R. E. (Eds.). (1972). *Hypnosis: Research developments and perspectives.* Chicago: Aldine-Atherton.

Fromm, E., & Shor, R. E. (Eds.). (1979). *Hypnosis: Developments in research and new perspectives* (2nd ed.). New York: Aldine.

Frumkin, L. R., Ripley, H. S., & Cox, G. B. (1978). Changes in cerebral hemispheric lateralization with hypnosis. *Biological Psychiatry, 13,* 741–750.

Frumkin, L. R., Ripley, H. S. , & Cox, G. B. (1979). A dichotic index of laterality that scores linguistic errors. *Cortex, 15,* 687–691.

Futterman, A. D. (1990). *Experimentally-induced high and low arousal positive and negative mood states: Immunologic and autonomic nervous system responses.* Unpublished doctoral dissertation, University of California at Los Angeles.

Galbraith, G. C., Cooper, L. M., & London, P. (1972). Hypnotic susceptibility and the sensory evoked response. *Journal of Comparative and Physiological Psychology, 80,* 509–514.

Galbraith, G. C., London, P., Leibovitz, M. P., Cooper, L. M., & Hart, J. T. (1970). EEG and hypnotic susceptibility. *Journal of Comparative and Physiological Psychology, 72,* 125–131.

Galin, D. (1974). Implications for psychiatry of left and right cerebral specialization: A neurophysiological context for unconscious processes. *Archives of General Psychiatry, 31,* 572–583.

Gardner, R. W., Holzmann, P. S., Klein, G. S., Linton, H. P., & Spence, D. P. (1959). Cognitive control: A study of individual consistencies in cognitive behavior. *Psychological Issues, 1,* 1–186.

Gazzaniga, M. S. (1970). *The bisected brain.* New York: Appleton-Century-Crofts.

Gearan, P. (1990, August). Expectancy change as a mediator of hypnotizability enhancement. In I. Kirsch (Chair), *Hypnotizability and interpretational sets: Conflicting evidence.* Symposium conducted at the meeting of the American Psychological Association, Boston.

Geiselman, R. E., Fisher, R. P., MacKinnon, D. P., & Holland, H. L. (1985). Eyewitness memory enhancement in the police interview: Cognitive retrieval mnemonics versus hypnosis. *Journal of Applied Psychology, 70,* 401–412.

Geiselman, R. E., MacKinnon, D. P., Fishman, D. L., Jaenicke, C., Larner, B. R., Schoenberg, S., & Swartz, S. (1983). Mechanisms of hypnotic and nonhypnotic forgetting. *Journal of Experimental Psychology: Learning, Memory, and Cognition, 9,* 626–635.

Geiselman, R. E., & Machlovitz, H. (1987). Hypnosis memory recall: Implications for forensic use. *American Journal of Forensic Psychology, 1,* 37–47.

Geiser, D. S. (1989). Psychosocial influences on human immunity. *Clinical Psychology Review, 9,* 689–715.

Getzels, J. W. (1975). Creativity: Prospects and issues. In I. A. Taylor & J. W. Getzels (Eds.), *Perspectives in creativity.* Chicago: Aldine.

Gfeller, J. D., Lynn, S. J., & Pribble, W. E. (1987). Enhancing hypnotic susceptibility: Interpersonal and rapport factors. *Journal of Personality and Social Psychology, 52,* 586–595.

Gibbons, D. E. (1975). Hypnotic vs. hyperempiric induction procedures: An experimental comparison. *Journal of the American Society of Psychosomatic Dentistry and Medicine, 22,* 35–42.

Gibbons, D. E. (1976). Hypnotic vs. hyperempiric induction procedures: An experimental comparison. *Perceptual and Motor Skills, 42,* 834.

Gibson, H. B. (1985). Dreaming and hypnotic susceptibility: A pilot study. *Perceptual and Motor Skills, 60,* 387–394.

Gill, M. M. (1972). Hypnosis as an altered and regressed state. *International Journal of Clinical and Experimental Hypnosis, 20,* 224–237.

Gill, M. M., & Brenman, M. (1959). *Hypnosis and related states: Psychoanalytic studies in regression.* New York: International Universities Press.

Glass, L. B., & Barber, T. X. (1961). A note on hypnotic behavior, the definition of the situation, and the placebo effect. *Journal of Nervous and Mental Diseases, 132,* 539–541.

Glisky, M. L., Tataryn, D. J., Tobias, B. A., Kihlstrom, J. F., & McConkey, K. M. (1991). Absorption, openness to experience, and hypnotizability. *Journal of Personality and Social Psychology, 60,* 263–272.

Goebel, R. A., & Stewart, C. G. (1971). Effects of experimenter bias and induced subject expectancy on hypnotic susceptibility. *Journal of Personality and Social Psychology, 18,* 263–272.

Goffman, E. (1959). *The presentation of self in everyday life.* Garden City, NY: Doubleday.

Gold, S. R., & Reilly, J. P. (1985–1986). Daydreaming, current concerns, and personality. *Imagination, Cognition and Personality, 5,* 117–125.

Goldstein, A., & Hilgard, E. R. (1975). Lack of influence of the morphine antagonist naloxone on hypnotic analgesia. *Proceedings of the National Academy of Sciences USA, 72,* 2041–2043.

Gorassini, D. R., & Spanos, N. P. (1986). A social cognitive skills approach to the successful modification of hypnotic susceptibility. *Journal of Personality and Social Psychology, 50,* 1004–1012.

Gordon, M. C. (1973). Suggestibility of chronic schizophrenic and normal males matched for age. *International Journal of Clinical and Experimental Hypnosis, 21,* 284–288.

Gorton, B. E. (1962). Current problems of physiologic research in hypnosis. In G. H. Estabrooks (Ed.), *Hypnosis: Current problems.* New York: Harper & Row.

Gott, P. S., Hughes, E. C., & Whipple, K. (1984). Voluntary control of two lateralized conscious states: Validation by electrical and behavioral studies. *Neuropsychologia, 22,* 65–72.

Gough, H. G. (1979). A creative personality scale for the Adjective Check List. *Journal of Personality and Social Psychology, 37,* 1398–1405.

Gough, H. G., & Heilbrun, A. (1965). *The Adjective Check List manual.* Palo Alto, CA: Consulting Psychologists Press.

Grabowski, K. L., Roese, N. J., & Thomas, M. R. (1991). The role of expectancy in hypnotic hypermnesia: A brief communication. *International Journal of Clinical and Experimental Hypnosis, 34,* 193–197.

Graham, K. R. (1977). Perceptual processes and hypnosis: Support for a cognitive-state theory based on laterality. In W. E. Edmonston, Jr. (Ed.), *Conceptual and investigative approaches to hypnosis and hypnotic phenomena. Annals of the New York Academy of Sciences, 296,* 274–283.

Graham, K. R., & Patton, A. (1968). Retroactive inhibition, hypnosis and hypnotic amnesia. *International Journal of Clinical and Experimental Hypnosis, 16,* 68–74.

Graham, K. R., Wright, G. W., Toman, W. J., & Mark, C. R. (1975). Relaxation and hypnosis in the treatment of insomnia. *American Journal of Clinical Hypnosis, 18,* 39–42.

Greaves, G. B. (1980). Multiple personality: 165 years after Mary Reynolds. *Journal of Nervous and Mental Disease, 168,* 577–596.

Green, J. P., Kvaal, M. S., Lynn, S. J., Mare, M. S., & Sandberg, M. S. (1991). Dissociations, fantasy proneness, and hypnotizability: A test of context effects.

In E. J. Frischholz (Chair), *Dissociation and multiple personality: Research on artifacts and contextual moderators*. Symposium conducted at the meeting of the American Psychological Association, San Francisco.

Greene, E., Wilson, L., & Loftus, E. F. (1989). Impact of hypnotic testimony on the jury. *Law and Human Behavior, 13,* 61–78.

Greenwald, A. G., Pratkanis, A. R., Leippe, M. R., & Baumgardner, M. H. (1986). Under what conditions does theory obstruct research progress? *Psychological Review, 93,* 216–229.

Gregg, V. H., & Mingay, D. J. (1987). Influence of hypnosis on riskiness and discriminability in recognition memory for faces. *British Journal of Experimental and Clinical Hypnosis, 4,* 65–75.

Gregory, J., & Diamond, M. J. (1973). Increasing hypnotic susceptibility by means of positive expectancies and written instructions. *Journal of Abnormal Psychology, 82,* 363–367.

Griffiths, R. A. (1989). Hypnobehavioural treatment for bulimia nervosa: Preliminary findings, *Australian Journal of Clinical and Experimental Hypnosis, 17*(1), 79–87.

Grosz, H. J., & Zimmerman, J. (1965). Experimental analysis of hysterical blindness: A follow-up report and new experimental data. *Archives of General Psychiatry, 13,* 255–260.

Gruenewald, D. (1982). A psychoanalytic view of hypnosis. *American Journal of Clinical Hypnosis, 24,* 185–190.

Gruenewald, D. (1986). Dissociation: Appearance and meaning. *American Journal of Clinical Hypnosis, 29,* 116–122.

Gruenewald, D., Fromm, E., & Oberlander, M. I. (1972). Hypnosis and adaptive regression: An ego-psychological inquiry. In E. Fromm & R. E. Shor (Eds.), *Hypnosis: Research developments and perspectives* (pp. 495–509). Chicago: Aldine-Atherton.

Gruenewald, D., Fromm, E., & Oberlander, M. I. (1979). Hypnosis and adaptive regression: An ego-psychological inquiry. In E. Fromm & R. Shor (Eds.), *Hypnosis: Developments in research and new perspectives* (2nd ed., pp. 619–635). New York: Aldine.

Gruzelier, J. H. (1987). Individual differences in dynamic process asymmetries in the normal and pathological brain. In A. Glass (Ed.), *Individual differences in hemispheric specialization* (pp. 301–329). New York: Plenum.

Gruzelier, J. H. (1988). The neuropsychology of hypnosis. In M. Heap (Ed.), *Hypnosis: Current clinical, experimental and forensic practices* (pp. 68–76). London: Croom Helm.

Gruzelier, J. H. (1990). Neuropsychophysiological investigations of hypnosis: Cerebral laterality and beyond. In R. Van Dyck, P. H. Spinhoven, & A. J. W. Van Der Does (Eds.), *Hypnosis: Theory, research and clinical practice* (pp. 37–51). Amsterdam: Free University Press.

Gruzelier, J. H., Allison, J., & Conway, A. (1988). A psychophysiological differentiation between hypnotic behaviour and simulation. *International Journal of Psychophysiology, 6,* 331–338.

Gruzelier, J. H., & Brow, T. D. (1985). Psychophysiological evidence for a state theory of hypnosis and susceptibility. *Journal of Psychosomatic Research, 29,* 287–302.

Gruzelier, J., Brow, T. D., Perry, A., Rhonder, J., & Thomas, M. (1984). Hypnotic susceptibility: A lateral predisposition and altered cerebral asymmetry under hypnosis. *International Journal of Psychophysiology, 2,* 131–139.

Gruzelier, J. H., Eves, F. F., & Connolly, J. F. (1981). Habituation and phasic reactivity in the electrodermal system: Reciprocal hemispheric influences. *Physiological Psychology, 9,* 313–317.

Gruzelier, J. H., Hancock, J., & Maggs, R. (1991). EEG topography during word versus face recognition memory in high and low susceptibles in baseline and hypnosis. *International Journal of Psychophysiology, 11,* 36.

Gruzelier, J., Hancock, J., & Maggs, R. (in press). Susceptibility-related changes in recognition memory for words versus faces after instructions of hypnosis. *International Journal of Psychophysiology.*

Gruzelier, J. H., & Phelan, M. (1991). Stress induced reversal of a lexical divided visual-field asymmetry accompanied by retarded electrodermal habituation. *International Journal of Psychophysiology, 11,* 269–276.

Gruzelier, J. H., Thomas, M., Conway, A., Liddiard, D., Jutai, J., McCormack, K., Golds, J., Perry, A., Rhonder, J., & Brow, T. (1987). Involvement of the left hemisphere in hypnotic induction: Electrodermal, haptic, electrocortical and divided visual-field evidence. In B. Taneli, C. Perris, & B. Kemali (Eds.), *Advances in biological psychiatry: Vol. 16. Neurophysiological correlates of relaxation and psychopathology* (pp. 6–17). Basel: Karger.

Gruzelier, J. H., & Warren, K. (1992). *Neuropsychological evidence of left frontal inhibition with hypnosis.* Manuscript submitted for publication.

Guerra, G., Guantieri, G., & Tagliaro, F. (1985). Hypnosis and plasmatic beta-endorphins. In D. Waxman, P. C. Misra, M. Gibson, & M. A. Basker (Eds.), *Modern trends in hypnosis* (pp. 259–266). New York: Plenum.

Guerrero-Figueroa, R., & Heath, R. G. (1964). Evoked responses and changes during attentive factors in man. *Archives of Neurology, 10,* 74–84.

Guilford, J. P. (1950). Creativity. *American Psychologist, 5,* 444–454.

Guilford, J. P. (1959). Traits of creativity. In H.H. Anderson (Ed.), *Creativity and its cultivation: Addresses presented at the inter-disciplinary symposia on creativity, Michigan State University, East Lansing, Michigan* (pp. 142–161). New York: Harper.

Guilford, J. P. (1967). *The nature of human intelligence.* New York: McGraw-Hill.

Gur, R. C., & Gur, R. E. (1974). Handedness, sex and eyedness as moderating variables in the relation between hypnotic susceptibility and functional brain asymmetry. *Journal of Abnormal Psychology, 83,* 635–643.

Gur, R. C., & Reyher, J. (1976). Enhancement of creativity via free imagery and hypnosis. *American Journal of Clinical Hypnosis, 18,* 237–249.

Gustafson, R., & Kallmen, H. (1989). Alcohol effects on cognitive and personality style in women with special reference to primary and secondary process. *Alcoholism: Clinical and Experimental Research, 13,* 644–648.

Haanen, H. C. M., Hoenderdos, T. W., Romunde, L. K. J., Hop, W. C. J., Mallee, C., Terwiel, J. P., & Hekster, G. B. (1991). Controlled trial of hypnotherapy in the treatment of refractory fibromyalgia. *Journal of Rheumatology, 18,* 72–75.

Haber, C. H., Nitkin, R., & Shenker, I. R. (1979). Adverse reactions to hypnotherapy in obese adolescents: A developmental viewpoint. *Psychiatric Quarterly, 51,* 55–63.

H'ajek, P., Jakoubek, B., & Radil, T. (1990). Gradual increase in cutaneous threshold induced by repeated hypnosis of healthy individuals and patients with atopic eczema. *Perceptual and Motor Skills, 70,* 549–550.

Halama, P. (1989). Die Veranderung der corticalen Durchblutung vor und in Hypnose. *Experimentelle und Klinische Hypnose, 5,* 19–26.

Hall, H. R. (1982–1983). Hypnosis and the immune system: A review with implications for cancer and the psychology of healing. *American Journal of Clinical Hypnosis, 25,* 92–103.

Hall, H. R., Longos, S., & Dixon, R. H. (1981, October). *Hypnosis and the immune system: The effect of hypnosis on T and B cell function.* Paper presented at the annual meeting of the Society for Clinical and Experimental Hypnosis, Portland, OR.

Halliday, A. M., & Mason, A. A. (1964a). Cortical evoked potentials during hypnotic anaesthesia. *Electroencephalography and Clinical Neurophysiology, 16,* 312–314.

Halliday, A. M., & Mason, A. A. (1964b). The effects of hypnotic anesthesia on cortical responses. *Journal of Neurology, Neurosurgery and Psychiatry, 27,* 300–312.

Ham, M. W., & Spanos, N. P. (1974). Suggested auditory and visual hallucinations in task-motivated and hypnotic subjects. *American Journal of Clinical Hypnosis, 17,* 94–101.

Ham, M. W., Spanos, N. P., & Barber, T. X. (1976). Suggestibility in hospitalized schizophrenics. *Journal of Abnormal Psychology, 85,* 550–557.

Hammer, A. G., Walker, W., & Diment, A. D. (1978). A nonsuggested effect of trance induction. In F. H. Frankel & H. S. Zamansky (Eds.), *Hypnosis at its bicentennial: Selected papers* (pp. 91–100). New York: Plenum.

Hardy, J. D., Wolff, H. G., & Goodell, H. (1952). *Pain sensations and reactions.* Baltimore: Williams & Wilkins.

Hayward, J. N., Smith, N. E., & Stewart, D. G. (1966). Temporal gradients between arterial blood and brain in the monkey. *Proceedings of the Society for Experimental Biology and Medicine, 121,* 547–551.

Hargreaves, D., & Bolton, W. (1972). Selecting creativity tests for use in research. *British Journal of Psychology, 63,* 451–462.

Harrow, M. (1976). Primitive drive dominated thinking: Relationship to acute schizophrenia and sociopathy. *Journal of Personality Assessment, 40,* 31–41.

Hart, B. (1927). The concept of dissociation. *British Journal of Medical Psychology, 6,* 241–256.

Hart, B. (1929). *Psychopathology* (2nd ed.). Cambridge, England: Cambridge University Press.

Harter, S. (1977). A cognitive-developmental approach to children's expression of conflicting feelings and a technique to facilitate such expression in play therapy. *Journal of Consulting and Clinical Psychology, 45,* 417–432.

Harter, S. (1983). Children's understanding of multiple emotions: A cognitive-developmental approach. In W. F. Overton (Ed.), *The relationship between social and cognition development.* Hillsdale, NJ: Lawrence Erlbaum.

Harter, S. (1986). Cognitive-developmental process in the integration of concepts about emotions and the self. *Social Cognition, 4,* 119–151.

Harter, S., & Buddin, B. J. (1987). Children's understanding of the simultaneity of two emotions: A five-stage developmental acquisition sequence. *Developmental Psychology, 23,* 388–399.

Hartland, J. (1965). The value of "ego-strengthening" procedures prior to direct symptom-removal under hypnosis, *American Journal of Clinical Hypnosis, 8,* 89–93.

Hartmann, H. (1958). *Ego psychology and the problem of adaptation* (D. Rapaport, Trans.) New York: International Universities Press. (Original work published 1939)

Harvey, R. F., Hinton, R. A., Gunary, R. M., & Barry, R. E. (1989). Individual and group therapy in treatment of refractory irritable bowel syndrome. *Lancet, i*, 424–425.

Hathaway, S., & McKinley, J. (1967). *The Minnesota Multiphasic Personality Inventory manual.* New York: Psychological Corporation.

Hays, W. L. (1963). *Statistics for psychologists.* New York: Holt, Rinehart & Winston.

Hebb, D. O. (1949). *The organization of behavior.* New York: Wiley.

Hebb, D. O. (1975). Science and the world of imagination. *Canadian Psychological Review, 16*, 4–11.

Hebert, R., & Lehmann, D. (1979). Theta bursts: An EEG pattern in normal subjects practicing the transmeditational technique. *Electroencephalography and Clinical Neurophysiology, 42*, 397–405.

Heckhausen, H., & Beckmann, J. (1990). Intentional action and action slips. *Psychology Review, 97*, 36–48.

Hellige, J. B. (1990). Hemispheric asymmetry. *Annual Review of Psychology, 41*, 55–80.

Hennessey, B. A., & Amabile, T. M. (1988). The conditions of environment. In R. J. Sternberg (Ed.), *The nature of creativity: Contemporary psychological perspectives* (pp. 11–38). Cambridge, England: Cambridge University Press.

Hernandez-Peon, R., & Donoso, M. (1959). Influence of attention and suggestion upon subcortical evoked electric activity in the human brain. In L. Van Bogaert & J. Radermecker (Eds.), *First International Congress of Neurological Sciences* (Vol. 3, pp. 385–396). Oxford: Pergamon Press.

Herrmann, W. M. (1982). Development and critical evaluation of an objective procedure for the electroencephalographic classification of psychotropic drugs. In W. M. Herrmann (Ed.), *Electroencephalography in drug research* (pp. 249–351). Stuttgart: Gustav Fischer.

Heyneman, N. E. (1990). The role of imagery in hypnosis: An information processing approach. *International Journal of Clinical and Experimental Hypnosis, 38*, 39–59.

Hilgard, E. R. (1965a). *Hypnotic susceptibility.* New York: Harcourt, Brace & World.

Hilgard, E. R. (1965b). Posthypnotic amnesia: Experiments and theory. *International Journal of Clinical and Experiemntal Hypnosis, 15*, 104–111.

Hilgard, E. R. (1967). Individual differences in hypnotizability. In J. E. Gordon (Ed.), *Handbook of clinical and experimental hypnosis* (pp. 391–443). New York: Macmillan.

Hilgard, E. R. (1969). Pain as a puzzle for psychology and physiology. *American Psychologist, 24*, 103–113.

Hilgard, E. R. (1971a). Hypnosis: Its place in psychology. *Scientia, 65*, 369–389.

Hilgard, E. R. (1971b). Hypnotic phenomena: The struggle for scientific acceptance. *American Psychologist, 59*, 567–577.

Hilgard, E. R. (1973a). Dissociation revisited. In M. Henle, J. Jaynes, & J. Sullivan (Eds.), *Historical conceptions of psychology* (pp. 205–219). New York: Springer.

Hilgard, E. R. (1973b). A neodissociation interpretation of pain reduction in hypnosis. *Psychological Review, 80*, 396–411.

Hilgard, E. R. (1973c). The domain of hypnosis, with some comments on alternative paradigms. *American Psychologist, 28*, 972–982.

Hilgard, E. R. (1974). Toward a neo-dissociation theory: Multiple cognitive controls in human functioning. *Perspectives in Biology and Medicine, 17,* 301–316.

Hilgard, E. R. (1975, October). *The Stanford Hypnotic Susceptibility Scales: What they measure.* Paper presented at the annual meeting of the Society for Clinical and Experimental Hypnosis, Chicago.

Hilgard, E. R. (1977a). *Divided consciousness: Multiple controls in human thought and action.* New York: Wiley.

Hilgard, E. R. (1977b). The problem of divided consciousness: A neodissociation interpretation. *Annals of the New York Academy of Sciences, 296,* 48–59.

Hilgard, E. R. (1977c). Controversies over consciousness and the rise of cognitive psychology. *Australian Psychologist, 12,* 7–26.

Hilgard, E. R. (1978–1979). The Stanford Hypnotic Susceptibility Scales as related to other measures of hypnotic responsiveness. *American Journal of Clinical Hypnosis, 21,* 68–82.

Hilgard, E. R. (1979a). Divided consciousness in hypnosis: The implications of the hidden observer. In E. Fromm & R. E. Shor (Eds.), *Hypnosis: Developments in research and new perspectives* (2nd ed., pp. 45–79). New York: Aldine.

Hilgard, E. R. (1979b). Consciousness and control: Lessons from hypnosis. *Australian Journal of Clinical and Experimental Hypnosis, 7,* 107–115.

Hilgard, E. R. (1979c). *A saga of hypnosis: Two decades of the Stanford Laboratory of Hypnosis Research 1957–1979.* Unpublished manuscript, Stanford University.

Hilgard, E. R. (1981). Imagery and imagination in American psychology. *Journal of Mental Imagery, 5,* 5–66.

Hilgard, E. R. (1986). *Divided consciousness: Multiple controls in human thought and action* (rev. ed.). New York: Wiley.

Hilgard, E. R. (1987). Research advances in hypnosis: Issues and methods. *International Journal of Clinical and Experimental Hypnosis, 35,* 248–264.

Hilgard, E. R. (1990). [Conversation hour at the 41st Annual Meeting of the Society for Clinical and Experimental Hypnosis, Tucson, AZ].

Hilgard, E. R. (1991). A neodissociation interpretation of hypnosis. In S. J. Lynn & J. W. Rhue (Eds.), *Theories of hypnosis: Current models and perspectives* (pp. 83–104). New York: Guilford Press.

Hilgard, E. R., & Cooper, L. M. (1965). Spontaneous and suggested posthypnotic amnesia. *International Journal of Clinical and Experimental Hypnosis, 13,* 261–273.

Hilgard, E. R., Crawford, H. J., Bowers, P. G., & Kihlstrom, J. F. (1979). A tailored SHSS:C, permitting user modification for special purposes. *International Journal of Clinical and Experimental Hypnosis, 27,* 125–133.

Hilgard, E. R., Crawford, H. J., & Wert, A. (1979). The Stanford Hypnotic Arm Levitation Induction and Test (SHALIT): A six-minute hypnotic induction and measurement scale. *International Journal of Clinical and Experimental Hypnosis, 27,* 111–124.

Hilgard, E. R., & Hilgard, J. R. (1975) *Hypnosis in the relief of pain.* Los Altos, CA: William Kaufmann.

Hilgard, E. R., & Hilgard, J. R. (1983). *Hypnosis in the relief of pain* (2nd ed.). Los Altos, CA: William Kaufmann.

Hilgard, E. R., Hilgard, J. R., Macdonald, H., Morgan, A. H., & Johnson, L. S. (1978). Covert pain in hypnotic analgesia: Its reality as tested by the real–simulator design. *Journal of Abnormal Psychology, 87,* 239–246.

Hilgard, E. R., Morgan, A. H., & Macdonald, H. (1975). Pain and dissociation in the cold pressor test: A study of hypnotic analgesia with "hidden reports" through automatic key-pressing and automatic talking. *Journal of Abnormal Psychology, 84,* 280–289.

Hilgard, E. R., Morgan, A. H., & Prytulak, S. (1968). The psychophysics of the kinesthetic aftereffect in the Petrie block experiment. *Perception and Psychophysics, 4,* 129–132.

Hilgard, E. R., & Tart, C. T. (1966). Responsiveness to suggestions following waking and imagination instructions and following induction of hypnosis. *Journal of Abnormal Psychology, 71,* 196–208.

Hilgard, E. R., Weitzenhoffer, A., Landes, J., & Moore, R. K. (1961). The distribution of susceptibility to hypnosis in a student population: A study using the Stanford Hypnotic Susceptiblity Scale. *Psychological Monographs, 75* (8, Whole No. 512).

Hilgard, J. R. (1965). Personality and hypnotizability: Inferences from case studies. In E. R. Hilgard, *Hypnotic susceptibility* (pp. 343–374). New York: Harcourt, Brace & World.

Hilgard, J. R. (1970). *Personality and hypnosis: A study of imaginative involvement.* Chicago: University of Chicago Press.

Hilgard, J. R. (1974a). Imaginative involvement: Some characteristics of the highly hypnotizable and the nonhypnotizable. *International Journal of Clinical and Experimental Hypnosis, 22,* 138–156.

Hilgard, J. R. (1974b). Sequelae to hypnosis. *International Journal of Clinical and Experimental Hypnosis, 22,* 281–298.

Hilgard, J.R. (1979a). Imaginative and sensory-affective involvements in everyday life and in hypnosis. In E. Fromm & R. E. Shor (Eds.), *Hypnosis: Developments in research and new perspectives* (2nd ed., pp. 483–517). New York: Aldine.

Hilgard, J. R. (1979b). *Personality and hypnosis: A study of imaginative involvement* (2nd ed.). Chicago: University of Chicago Press.

Hilgard, J. R., Hilgard, E. R., & Newman, M. (1961). Sequelae to hypnotic induction with special reference to earlier chemical anesthesia. *Journal of Nervous and Mental Disease, 133,* 461–478.

Hilgard, J. R., & LeBaron, S. (1982). Relief of anxiety and pain in children and adolescents with cancer: Quantitative measures and clinical observations. *International Journal of Clinical and Experimental Hypnosis, 30,* 417–442.

Hilgard, J. R., & LeBaron, S. (1984). *Hypnotherapy of pain in children with cancer.* Los Altos, CA: William Kaufmann.

Hockenberry-Eaton, M. J. & Cotanch, P. H. (1989). Evaluation of a child's perceived self-competence during treatment for cancer. *Journal of Pediatric Oncology Nursing, 6*(3), 55–62.

Hodge, J. R. (1988). Can hypnosis help psychosis? *American Journal of Clinical Hypnosis, 30,* 248–256.

Hogan, M., MacDonald, J., & Olness, K. (1984). Voluntary control of auditory evoked responses by children with and without hypnosis. *American Journal of Clinical Hypnosis, 27,* 91–94.

Holroyd, J. (1980). Hypnosis treatment for smoking: An evaluative review. *International Journal of Clinical and Experimental Hypnosis, 28,* 341–357.

Holroyd, J. (1985–1986). Hypnosis applications in psychological research. *Imagination, Cognition and Personality, 5,* 103–115.

Holroyd, J. (1991). The uncertain relationship between hypnotizability and smoking treatment outcome. *International Journal of Clinical and Experimental Hypnosis, 34*, 93–102.

Holt, R. R. (1963). *Manual for the scoring of primary process manifestations in Rorschach responses* (9th ed.). New York: Research Center for Mental Health, New York University. (Mimeograph)

Holt, R. R. (1965). Ego autonomy re-evaluated. *International Journal of Psycho-Analysis, 46*, 151–167.

Holt, R. R. (1967). The development of the primary process: A structural view. In R. R. Holt (Ed.), Motives and thought: Psychoanalytic essays in honor of David Rapaport. *Psychological Issues, 5* (Monograph No. 18/19), 345–383. New York: International Universities Press.

Holt, R. R. (1969). Artistic creativity and Rorschach measures of adaptive regression. In B. Klopfer (Ed.), *Developments in the Rorschach technique* (Vol. III, pp. 263–320). Yonkers, NY: World.

Holt, R. R., & Havel, J. (1960). A method for assessing primary and secondary process in the Rorschach. In M. A. Rickers-Ovsiankina (Ed.), *Rorschach psychology* (pp. 263–315). New York: Wiley.

Holtzman, W. H., Thorpe, J. S., Swartz, J. D., & Herron, E. W. (1961). *Inkblot perception and personality: Holtzman Inkblot Technique*. Austin: University of Texas Press.

Horowitz, M. J., Wilner, N., & Alvarez, W. (1979) Impact of Events Scale: A measure of subjective stress. *Psychosomatic Medicine, 41*, 209–218.

Horwitz, L., Allen, J. G., Colson, D. B., Frieswyk, S. H., Gabbard, G. O., Coyne, L., & Newsom, G. E. (1991). Psychotherapy of borderline patients at the Menninger Foundation: Expressive compared with supportive interventions and the therapeutic alliance. In L. E. Beutler & M. Crago (Eds.), *Psychotherapy research* (pp. 48–55). Washington, DC: American Psychological Association Press.

Houle, M., McGrath, P. A., Moran, G., & Garrett, O. J. (1988). The efficacy of hypnosis- and relaxation-induced analgesia on two dimensions of pain for cold pressor and electrical tooth pulp stimulation. *Pain, 33*, 241–251.

Howard, M. L., & Coe, W. C. (1980). The effects of context and subjects' perceived control in breaching posthypnotic amnesia. *Journal of Personality, 48*, 342–359.

Hoyt, I. R., Nadon, R., Register, P. A., Chorny, J., Fleeson, W., Grigorian, E. M., Otto, L., & Kihlstrom, J. F. (1989). Daydreaming, absorption, and hypnotizability. *International Journal of Clinical and Experimental Hypnosis, 37*, 332–342.

Huba, G. J., Singer, J. L., Aneshensel, C. S., & Antrobus, J. S. (1982). *Short Imaginal Processes Inventory*. Port Huron, MI: Research Psychologists Press.

Huesman, L. R., Gruder, C. L., & Dorst, G. (1987). A process model of posthypnotic amnesia. *Cognitive Psychology, 19*, 33–62.

Huff, K., & Council, J. (1987, August). *Fantasy proneness and psychological coping*. Paper presented at the meeting of the American Psychological Association, New York.

Hugdahl, K. (Ed.). (1988). *Handbook of dichotic listening: Theory, methods and research*. New York: Wiley.

Hughes, D. (1988). *Factors related to heart rate change for high and low hypnotizables* during imagery. Unpublished doctoral dissertation, University of Waterloo, Waterloo, Ontario, Canada.

Hull, C. L. (1933). *Hypnosis and suggestibility: An experimental approach.* New York: Appleton-Century Crofts.

Hull, C. L. (1934). The concept of the habit-family hierarchy and maze learning. *Psychological Review, 41,* 33–54.

Hull, C. L. (1968). *Hypnosis and suggestibility: An experimental approach.* New York: Appleton-Century-Crofts. (Original work published 1933)

Huse, B. (1930). Does the hypnotic trance favor the recall of faint memories? *Journal of Experimental Psychology, 13,* 519–529.

Hyman, G. J., Stanley, R. O., Burrows, G. D., & Horne, D. J. (1986). Treatment effectiveness of hypnosis and behavior therapy in smoking cessation: A methodological refinement. *Addictive Behavior, 11*(4), 335–365.

Isaacs, P. (1982). *Hypnotic responsiveness and dimensions of imagery and thinking style.* Unpublished doctoral dissertation, University of Waterloo, Waterloo, Ontario, Canada.

Isaacson, R. L. (1982). *The limbic system.* New York: Plenum Press.

Isaksen, S. G. (1987). Introduction: An orientation to the frontiers of creativity research. In S. G. Isaksen (Ed.), *Frontiers of creativity research* (pp. 1–26). Buffalo, NY: Bearly Limited.

Jackson, D. N. (1974). *The Personality Research Form manual.* Goshen, NY: Research Psychology Press.

Jackson, J., & Sheehan, P. W. (1986). Imaginative capacity and individual differences in hypnotic responsivity. *Australian Journal of Clinical and Experimental Hypnosis, 14,* 139–152.

Jackson, L. M., & Gorassini, D. R. (1989). Artifact in the hypnosis–creativity relationship. *Journal of General Psychology, 116,* 333–344.

Jackson, S. W. (1969). The history of Freud's concepts of regression. *Journal of the American Psychoanalytic Association, 17,* 743–784.

Jacobs, G. D., & Lubar, J. F. (1989). Spectral analysis of the central nervous system effects of the relaxation response elicited by autogenic training. *Behavioral Medicine, 16,* 125–132.

Jacobson, E. (1954). The self and the object world. *Psychoanalytic Study of the Child, 9,* 75–129.

James, W. (1890). *Principles of psychology* (2 vols.). New York: Holt.

James, W. (1935). *The varieties of religious experience.* New York: Longmans, Green. (Original work published 1902)

James, W. (1979). *The will to believe and other essays in popular philosophy.* Cambridge, MA: Harvard University Press. (Original work published 1896)

James, W. (1981). Principles of psychology (3 vols.). In F. Burkhardt (Ed.), *The works of William James.* Cambridge, MA: Harvard University Press. (Original work published 1890)

Janet, P. (1889). *L'automatisme psychologique.* Paris: Felix Alcan.

Janet, P. (1901). *The mental state of hystericals* (C. R. Carson, Trans.). New York: Putnam.

Janet, P. (1907). *The major symptoms of hysteria.* New York: Macmillan.

Janet, P. (1925). *Psychological healing: A historical and clinical study* (E. Paul & C. Paul, Trans.). New York: Macmillan. (Original work published 1919)

Jeffrey, L. K., & Jeffrey, T. B. (1988). Exclusion therapy in smoking cessation, *International Journal of Clinical & Experimental Hypnosis, 36*(2), 70–74.

Jeffrey, T. B., Jeffrey, L. K., Greuling, J. W., & Gentry, W. R. (1985). Evaluation of a brief group treatment package including hypnotic induction for maintenance of smoking cessation: A brief communication. *International Journal of Clinical and Experimental Hypnosis, 33*, 95–98.

Jeness, A. (1944). Hypnotism. In J. M. Hunt (Ed.), *Personality and the behavior disorders* (pp. 466–502). New York: Ronald Press.

John, R., Hollander, B., & Perry, C. (1983). Hypnotizability and phobic behavior: Further supporting data. *Journal of Abnormal Psychology, 92*, 390–392.

Johnson, L. S. (1981). Current research in self-hypnotic phenomenology: The Chicago paradigm. *International Journal of Clinical and Experimental Hypnosis, 29*, 247–258.

Johnson, L. S., Dawson, S. L., Clark, J. L., & Sikorsky, C. (1983). Self-hypnosis versus heterohypnosis: Order effects and sex differences in behavioral and experiential impact. *International Journal of Clinical and Experimental Hypnosis, 31*, 139–154.

Johnson, L. S., & Weight, D. G. (1976). Self-hypnosis versus heterohypnosis: Experiential and behavioral comparisons. *Journal of Abnormal Psychology, 85*, 523–526.

Johnson, L. S., & Weise, K. F. (1979). Live versus tape-recorded assessments of hypnotic responsiveness in pain control patients. *International Journal of Clinical and Experimental Hypnosis, 27*, 74–84.

Johnson, M. K. (1983). A multiple-entry, modular memory system. *Psychology of Learning and Motivation, 17*, 81–123.

Johnson, R. F. Q. (1989). Hypnosis, suggestion, and dermatological changes: A consideration of the production and diminution of dermatological entities. In N. P. Spanos & J. F. Chaves (Eds.), *Hypnosis: The cognitive–behavioral perspective* (pp. 297–312). Buffalo, NY: Prometheus Books.

Johnson, R. F. Q., & Barber, T. X. (1978) Hypnosis, suggestions and warts: An experimental investigation implicating the importance of "believed-in efficacy." *American Journal of Clinical Hypnosis, 20*, 165–174.

Johnston, J. C., Chajkowaski, J., DuBreuil, S. C., & Spanos, N. P. (1989). The effects of manipulated expectancies on behavioural and subjective indices of hypnotisability. *Australian Journal of Clinical and Experimental Hypnosis, 17*, 121–130.

Jones, W. D., & Flynn, D. M. (1989). Methodological and theoretical considerations in the study of "hypnotic" effects in perception. In N. P. Spanos & J. F. Chaves (Eds.), *Hypnosis: The cognitive–behavioral perspective* (pp. 149–174). Buffalo, NY: Prometheus Books.

Jutai, J., Gruzelier, J. H., Golds, J., & Thomas, M. (in press). An electrophysiological investigation of asymmetric hemispheric activation during hypnosis. *International Journal of Clinical and Experimental Hypnosis*.

Kagan, N., Krathwohl, D. R., & Miller, R. (1963). Simulated recall in therapy using video-tape: A case study. *Journal of Counselling Psychology, 16*, 309–313.

Kahn, S. P., Fromm, E., Lombard, L. S., & Sossi, M. (1989). The relation of self-reports of hypnotic depth in self-hypnosis to hypnotizability and imagery production. *International Journal of Clinical and Experimental Hypnosis, 37*, 290–304.

Kaltsounis, B. (1971). Instruments useful in studying creative behavior and creative talent: Part I. Commercially available instruments. *Journal of Creative Behavior, 5,* 117–126.

Kaltsounis, B. (1972). Instruments useful in studying creative behavior and creative talent: Part III. Non-commercially available instruments. *Journal of Creative Behavior, 6,* 268–274.

Kaltsounis, B., & Honeywell, L. (1980). Instruments useful in studying creative behavior and creative talent: Part IV. Non-commercially available instruments. *Journal of Creative Behavior, 14,* 56–67.

Karlin, R., Cohen, A., & Goldstein, L. (1982). *A shift to the right: Electroencephalographic changes from rest to hypnotic induction.* Unpublished manuscript.

Karlin, R., Morgan, D., & Goldstein, L. (1980). Hypnotic analgesia: A preliminary investigation of quantitated hemispheric electroencephalographic and attentional correlates. *Journal of Abnormal Psychology, 89,* 591–594.

Kasamatsu, A., & Hirai, T. (1969). An EEG study on the Zen meditation (Zazen). In C. T. Tart (Ed.), *Altered states of consciousness.* New York: Wiley.

Kassin, S. M., Ellsworth, P. C., & Smith, V. L. (1989). The "general acceptance" of psychological research on eyewitness testimony: A survey of the experts. *American Psychologist, 44,* 1089–1098.

Katsanis, J., Barnard, J., & Spanos, N. P. (1988–1989). Self-predictions, interpretational set and imagery vividness as determinants of hypnotic responding. *Imagination, Cognition and Personality, 8,* 63–77.

Katz, A. N. (1984). Creative styles: Relating tests of creativity to the work patterns of scientists. *Personality and Individual Differences, 5,* 281–292.

Katz, E., Kellerman, J., & Ellenberg, L. (1987). Hypnosis in reduction of acute pain and distress in children with cancer. *General Pediatric Psychology, 12,* 379–394.

Katz, N. (1978). Hypnotic inductions as training in self-control. *Cognitive Therapy and Research, 2,* 365–369.

Katz, N. (1979). Comparative efficacy of behavioral training, training plus relaxation, and a sleep/trance induction in increasing hypnotic susceptibility. *Journal of Consulting and Clinical Psychology, 47,* 119–127.

Kearns, J. S., & Zamansky, H. S. (1984). Synthetic versus analytic imaging ability as correlates of hypnotizability. *International Journal of Clinical and Experimental Hypnosis, 32,* 41–50.

Kelly, M. A., McKinty, H. R., & Carr, R. (1988). Utilization of hypnosis to promote compliance with routine dental flossing. *American Journal of Clinical Hypnosis, 31,* 57–60.

Kelly, S. F. (1984). Measured hypnotic response and phobic behavior: A brief communication. *International Journal of Clinical and Experimental Hypnosis, 32,* 1–5.

Kendler, K. S. (1983). Overview: A current perspective on twin studies of schizophrenia. *American Journal of Psychiatry, 140,* 1413–1425.

Kendler, K. S., & Robinette, C. D. (1983). Schizophrenia in the National Academy of Sciences National Research Council Twin Registry: A 16-year update. *American Journal of Psychiatry, 140,* 1551–1563.

Khatena, J. (1976). Major directions in creativity research. *Gifted Child Quarterly, 20,* 336–349.

Khatena, J. (1987). Research potential of imagery and creative imagination. In S. G. Isaksen (Ed.), *Frontiers of creativity research* (pp. 314–340). Buffalo, NY: Bearly Limited.

Kihlstrom, J. F. (1978). Context and cognition in posthypnotic amnesia. *International Journal of Clinical and Experimental Hypnosis, 26,* 246–267.

Kihlstrom, J. F. (1980). Posthypnotic amnesia for recently learned material: Interactions with "episodic" and "semantic" memory. *Cognitive Psychology, 12,* 227–251.

Kihlstrom, J. F. (1982). Hypnosis and the dissociation of memory, with special reference to posthypnotic amnesia. *Research Communications in Psychology, Psychiatry, and Behavior, 7,* 181–197.

Kihlstrom, J. F. (1983). Instructed forgetting: Hypnotic and nonhypnotic. *Journal of Experimental Psychology, 112,* 73–79.

Kihlstrom, J. F. (1984). Conscious, subconscious, unconscious: A cognitive perspective. In K. S. Bowers & D. Meichenbaum (Eds.), *The unconscious reconsidered* (pp. 149–211). New York: Wiley.

Kihlstrom, J. F. (1985a). Hypnosis. *Annual Review of Psychology, 36,* 385–418.

Kihlstrom, J. (1985b). Posthypnotic amnesia and the dissociation of memory. In G. Bower (Ed.), *The psychology of learning and motivation: Advances in theory and research* (pp. 131–178). New York: Academic Press.

Kihlstrom, J. F. (1987a). The cognitive unconscious. *Science, 237,* 1445–1452.

Kihlstrom, J. F. (1987b). Integrating personality and social psychology. *Journal of Personality and Social Psychology, 53,* 989–992.

Kihlstrom, J. F. (1990). The psychological unconscious. In L. A. Pervin (Ed.), *Handbook of personality: Theory and research* (pp. 445–464). New York: Guilford Press.

Kihlstrom, J. F., Brenneman, H. A., Pistole, D. D., & Shor, R. E. (1985). Hypnosis as a retrieval cue in posthypnotic amnesia. *Journal of Abnormal Psychology, 94,* 264–271.

Kihlstrom, J. F., Diaz, W. A., McClellan, G. E., Ruskin, P. M., Pistole, D. D., & Shor, R. E. (1980). Personality correlates of hypnotic susceptibility: Needs for achievement and autonomy, self-monitoring and masculinity–femininity. *American Journal of Clinical Hypnosis, 22,* 225–229.

Kihlstrom, J. F., Easton, R. D., & Shor, R. E. (1983). Spontaneous recovery of memory during posthypnotic amnesia. *International Journal of Clinical and Experimental Hypnosis, 31,* 309–323.

Kihlstrom, J. F., & Evans, F. J. (1979a). Memory retrieval processes during posthypnotic amnesia. In J. F. Kihlstrom & F. J. Evans (Eds.), *Functional disorders of memory.* Hillsdale, NJ: Erlbaum.

Kihlstrom, J. F., & Evans, F. J. (Eds.). (1979b). *Functional disorders of memory.* Hillsdale, NJ: Erlbaum.

Kihlstrom, J. F., Evans, F. J., Orne, E. C., & Orne, M. T. (1980). Attempting to breach posthypnotic amnesia. *Journal of Abnormal Psychology, 89,* 603–616.

Kihlstrom, J. F., Hoyt, I. P., Nadon, R., & Register, P. A. (1987, August). *Cognitive correlates of hypnotizability: A re-examination of context effects.* Paper presented at the meeting of the American Psychological Association, New York.

Kihlstrom, J. F., & McConkey, K. M. (1990). William James and hypnosis: A centennial reflection. *Psychological Science, 1,* 174–178.

Kihlstrom, J. F., Register, P. A., Hoyt, I. P., Albright, J. S., Grigorian, E. M., Heindel, W. C., & Morrison, C. R. (1989). Dispositional correlates of hypnosis: A phenomenological approach. *International Journal of Clinical and Experimental Hypnosis, 37,* 249–263.

Kihlstrom, J. F., & Wilson, L. (1984). Temporal organization of recall during posthypnotic amnesia. *Journal of Abnormal Psychology, 93,* 200–208.

Kinney, J. M., & Sachs, L. B. (1974). Increasing hypnotic susceptibility. *Journal of Abnormal Psychology, 83,* 145–150.

Kirsch, I. (1985). Response expectancy as a determinant of experience and behavior. *American Psychologist, 40,* 1189–1202.

Kirsch, I. (1990). *Changing expectations: A key to effective psychotherapy.* Pacific Grove, CA: Brooks/Cole.

Kirsch, I. (1991). The social learning theory of hypnosis. In S. J. Lynn & J. W. Rhue (Eds.), *Theories of hypnosis: Current models and perspectives* (pp. 439–465). New York: Guilford Press.

Kirsch, I., & Council, J. R. (1989). Response expectancy as a determinant of hypnotic behavior. In N. P. Spanos & J. F. Chaves (Eds.), *Hypnosis: The cognitive–behavioral perspective* (pp. 360–379). Buffalo, NY: Prometheus Books.

Kirsch, I., Council, J. R., & Mobayed, C. (1987). Imagery and response expectancy as determinants of hypnotic behavior. *British Journal of Experimental and Clinical Hypnosis, 4,* 25–31.

Kirsch, I., Council, J. R., & Wickless, C. (1990). Subjective scoring for the Harvard Group Scale of Hypnotic Susceptibility, Form A. *International Journal of Clinical and Experimental Hypnosis, 38,* 112–124.

Kirsch, I., Mobayed, C. P., Council, J. R., & Kenny, D. A. (1990, August). State of the state debate: Can experts detect hypnosis? In R. St. Jean (Chair), *Social and cognitive aspects of hypnosis: Papers honoring W. C. Coe.* Symposium presented at the meeting of the American Pyschological Association, Boston.

Kirsch, I., Silva, C. E., Carone, J. E., Johnston, J. D., & Simon, B. (1989). The surreptitious observation design: An experimental paradigm for distinguishing artifact from essence in hypnosis. *Journal of Abnormal Psychology, 98,* 132–136.

Kissin, B. (1986). *Psychobiology of human behavior: Vol. 1. Conscious and unconscious programs in the brain.* New York: Plenum.

Klatzky, R. L., & Erdelyi, M. H. (1985). The response criterion problem in tests of hypnosis and memory. *International Journal of Clinical and Experimental Hypnosis, 33,* 246–257.

Klein, K. B., & Spiegel, D. (1989). Modulation of gastric acid secretion by hypnosis. *Gastroenterology, 96,* 1383–1387.

Kleinman, M. J. & Russ, S. W. (1988). Primary process thinking and anxiety in children. *Journal of Personality Assessment, 52,* 254–262.

Klinger, B. I. (1970). Effect of peer model responsiveness and length of induction procedure on hypnotic responsiveness. *Journal of Abnormal Psychology, 75,* 15–18.

Klinger, E. (1971). *Structure and functions of fantasy.* New York: Wiley.

Klopfer, B., & Kelley, D. (1942). *The Rorschach technique.* Yonkers: World Book.

Kluft, R. P. (1984). An introduction to multiple personality disorder. *Psychiatric Clinics of North America, 14,* 21–24.

Kluft, R. P. (1985). Using hypnotic inquiry protocols to monitor treatment progress and stability in multiple personality disorder. *American Journal of Clinical Hypnosis, 28,* 63–75.

Kluft, R. P. (1987). An update on multiple personality disorder. *Hospital and Community Psychiatry, 38,* 363–373.

Knapp, T. J., Downs, D. L., & Alperson, J. R. (1976). Behavior therapy for insomnia: A review. *Behavior Therapy, 7,* 614–625.

Knox, V. J., Crutchfield, L., & Hilgard, E. R. (1975). The nature of task interference in hypnotic dissociation: An investigation of hypnotic behavior. *International Journal of Clinical and Experimental Hypnosis, 23,* 305–323.

Knox, V. J., Gekoski, W. L., Shum, K., & McLaughlin, D. M. (1981). Analgesia for experimentally induced pain: Multiple sessions of acupuncture compared to hypnosis in high- and low-susceptible subjects. *Journal of Abnormal Psychology, 90,* 28–34.

Knox, V. J., Morgan, A. H., & Hilgard, E. R. (1974). Pain and suffering in ischemia: The paradox of hypnotically suggested anesthesia as contradicted by reports from the "hidden observer." *Archives of General Psychiatry, 30,* 840–847.

Koestler, A. (1964). *The act of creation.* New York: Macmillan.

Kohen, D. (1985, August). *Relaxation/mental imagery (self hypnosis) in asthma: Experience with 23 children.* Paper presented at the annual meeting of the International Congress of Hypnosis and Psychosomatic Medicine, Toronto.

Kohut, H. (1966). Forms and transformations of narcissism. *Journal of the American Psychoanalytic Association, 14,* 243–272.

Kohut, H. (1971). *The analysis of the self: A systematic approach to the psychoanalytic treatment of narcissistic personality disorders.* New York: International Universities Press.

Kosslyn, S. M. (1987). Seeing and imagining in the cerebral hemispheres: A computational approach. *Psychological Review, 94,* 148–175.

Kosslyn, S. M., & Jolicoeur, P. (1981). A theory based approach to the study of individual differences in mental imagery. In R. Snow, P. Fredrico, & W. Montague (Eds.), *Aptitude, learning, and instruction: Cognitive processes analyses.* Hillsdale, NJ: Erlbaum.

Kraemer, H. C., & Thieman, S. T. (1987). *How many subjects?* Newbury Park, CA: Sage.

Kramer, E. (1966). Group induction of hypnosis with institutionalized patients. *International Journal of Clinical and Experimental Hypnosis, 14,* 243–246.

Kramer, E., & Brennan, E. P. (1964). Hypnotic susceptibility of schizophrenic patients. *Journal of Abnormal and Social Psychology, 69,* 657–659.

Krass, J., Kinoshita, S., & McConkey, K. M. (1988). Hypnotic memory and confident reporting. *Applied Cognitive Psychology, 2,* 35–51.

Kris, E. (1952). *Psychoanalytic explorations in art.* New York: International Universities Press. (Original work published 1934)

Kroger, R. O. (1988). The social nature of hypnosis: An ethogenic analysis of hypnotic pain reduction. *New Ideas in Psychology, 6,* 67–73.

Kubie, L. S., & Margolin, S. (1944). The process of hypnotism and the nature of the hypnotic state. *American Journal of Psychiatry, 100,* 611–622.

Kumar, V. K., & Pekala, R. J. (1988). Hypnotizability, absorption, and individual differences in phenomenological experience. *International Journal of Clinical and Experimental Hypnosis, 36,* 80–88.

Kumar, V. K., & Pekala, R. J. (1989). Variations in phenomenological experience as a function of hypnosis and hypnotic susceptibility: A replication. *British Journal of Experimental and Clinical Hypnosis, 6,* 17–22.

Kunzendorf, R. G., & Benoit, M. (1985–1986). Spontaneous posthypnotic amnesia and spontaneous rehypnotic recovery in repressors. *Imagination, Cognition and Personality, 5,* 303–310.

Labelle, L., Lamarche, M. C., & Laurence, J.-R. (1990). Potential jurors' opinions on the effects of hypnosis on eyewitness identification: A brief communication. *International Journal of Clinical and Experimental Hypnosis, 38,* 315–319.

Labelle, L., Laurence, J.-R., Nadon, R., & Perry, C. (1990). Hypnotizability, preference for an imagic cognitive style, and memory creation in hypnosis. *Journal of Abnormal Psychology, 99,* 222–228.

LaBriola, F., & Karlin, R. (1984, October). *Quantitated EEG changes from prehypnotic to hypnotic periods.* Paper presented at the annual meeting of the Society of Clinical and Experimental Hypnosis.

LaBriola, F., Karlin, R., & Goldstein, L. (1987). EEG laterality changes from prehypnotic to hypnotic periods. In B. Taneli, C. Perris, & D. Kemali (Eds.), *Advances in biological psychiatry: Vol.16. Neurophysiological correlates of relaxation and psychopathology* (pp. 1–5). Basel: Karger.

Lacey, J. (1967). Somatic response patterning and stress: Some revisions of activation theory. In M. H. Appley & R. Trumbell (Ed.), *Psychological stress* (pp. 14–37). New York: Appleton-Century-Crofts.

Lamas, J. R., del Valle-Inclan, F., Blanco, M. J. & Diaz, A. A. (1989) Spanish norms for the Harvard Group Scale of Hypnotic Susceptibility: Form A. *International Journal of Clinical and Experimental Hypnosis, 37,* 264–273.

Lang, W., Lang, M., Kornhuber, A., Diekmann, V., & Kornhuber, H. H. (1988). Event related EEG spectra in a concept formation task. *Human Neurobiology, 6,* 295–301.

Langer, J. (1970). Werner's comparative organismic theory. In P. H. Mussen (Ed.), *Carmichael's manual of child psychology* (3rd ed., Vol. 1, pp. 733–771). New York: Wiley.

Lankton, S., & Lankton, C. (1983). *The answer within: A clinical framework of Ericksonian therapy.* New York: Brunner/Mazel.

Larbig, W. (1989). Kultur under Schmerz: Untersuchungen zur netral-nervosen Schmerzverarbeitung: Emplirische Befunde und klinische Konsequenzen. *Psychomedicine, 1,* 17–26.

Larbig, W., Elbert, T., Lutzenberger, W., Rockstroh, B., Schneer, G., & Birbaumer, N. (1982). EEG and slow brain potentials during anticipation and control of painful stimulation. *Electroencephalography and Clinical Neurophysiology, 53,* 298–309.

Lassen, N. A., Ingvar, D. H., & Skinhoj, E. (1978). Brain function and blood flow. *Scientific American, 239,* 62–71.

Latimer, P. R. (1983). *Functional aspects of gastrointestinal disorders: A behavioral medicine approach.* New York: Springer.

Laurence, J.-R. (1979). *Cognitive patterns in hypnosis.* Unpublished honors thesis, Concordia University, Montréal, Québec, Canada.

Laurence, J.-R. (1984). Creation of memory in hypnotizable individuals. *Svensk Tidskrift för Hypnos, 11,* 154–157.

Laurence, J.-R. (1990). Comportement et expérience hypnotique: Un modèle synergique. *Phoenix, 11–12,* 106–120.

Laurence, J.-R., Nadon, R., Nogrady, H., & Perry, C. (1986). Duality, dissociation, and memory creation in highly hypnotizable subjects. *International Journal of Clinical and Experimental Hypnosis, 34,* 295–310.

Laurence, J.-R., & Perry, C. (1981). The "hidden observer" phenomenon in hypnosis: Some additional findings. *Journal of Abnormal Psychology, 90,* 334–344.

Laurence, J.-R., & Perry, C. (1982). Montréal norms of the Harvard Group Scale of Hypnotic Susceptibility: Form A. *International Journal of Clinical and Experimental Hypnosis, 30,* 167–176.

Laurence, J.-R., & Perry, C. (1983). Hypnotically created memory among highly hypnotizable subjects. *Science, 222,* 523–524.

Laurence, J.-R., & Perry, C. (1988). *Hypnosis, will, and memory: A psycho-legal history.* New York: Guilford Press.

Laurence, J.-R., Perry, C., & Kihlstrom, J. F. (1983). The "hidden observer" phenomenon in hypnosis: An experimental creation? *Journal of Personality and Social Psychology, 44,* 163–169.

Lavoie, G. (1990). Clinical hypnosis: A psychodynamic approach. In M. L. Fass & D. P. Brown (Eds.), *Creative mastery in hypnosis and hypoanalysis: A festschrift for Erika Fromm* (pp. 77–105). Hillsdale, NJ: Erlbaum.

Lavoie, G., & Elie, R. (1985). The clinical relevance of hypnotizability in psychosis: With reference to thinking processes and sample variances. In D. Wayman, P. Misra, M. Gibson, & M. Baker (Eds.), *Modern trends in hypnosis* (pp. 41–66). New York: Plenum Press.

Lazar, B. S., & Dempster, C. R. (1984). Operator variables in successful hypnotherapy. *International Journal of Clinical and Experimental Hypnosis, 32,* 28–40.

LeBaron, S., Zeltzer, L. K., & Fanurik, D. (1988). Imaginative ability and hypnotizability in childhood. *International Journal of Clinical and Experimental Hypnosis. 36,* 284–295.

LeCron, L. M. (1953). A method of measuring the depth of hypnosis, and the experience of nonvolition. *International Journal of Clinical and Experimental Hypnosis, 31,* 293–308.

Lee-Teng, E. (1965). Trance-susceptibility, induction-susceptibility, and acquiescence as factors in hypnotic performance. *Journal of Abnormal Psychology, 70,* 383–389.

Leonard, G., & Lindauer, M. S. (1973). Aesthetic participation and imagery arousal. *Perceptual and Motor Skills, 36,* 977–978.

Levin, L. A., & Harrison, R. H. (1976). Hypnosis and regression in the service of the ego. *International Journal of Clinical and Experimental Hypnosis, 24,* 400–418.

Levine, J. L., Kurtz, R. M., & Lauter, J. L. (1984). Hypnosis and its effects on left and right hemisphere activity. *Biological Psychiatry, 19,* 1461–1475.

Levitan, A. A. (1985). Hypnotic death rehearsal. *American Journal of Clinical Hypnosis, 27,* 211–215.

Levitt, E. E., & Brady, J. P. (1963). Psychophysiology of hypnosis. In J. M. Schneck (Ed.), *Hypnosis in modern medicine* (3rd ed., pp. 314–362). Springfield, IL: Charles C Thomas.

Levitt, E. E., & Brady, J. P. (1964). Expectation and performance in hypnotic phenomena. *Journal of Abnormal and Social Psychology, 69,* 572–574.

Levitt, E. E., & Chapman, R. H. (1979). Hypnosis as a research method. In E. Fromm & R. E. Shor (Eds.), *Hypnosis: Developments in research and new perspectives* (pp. 185–215). New York: Aldine.

Lewicki, P. (1986). *Social-cognitive psychology*. New York: Wiley.

Lewin, K. (1935). *A dynamic theory of personality*. New York: McGraw-Hill.

Liébeault, A. A. (1866). *Du sommeil et des états analogues surtout au point de vue du moral sur le physique*. Paris: V. Masson et Fils.

Lind, P. (1989). The use of hypnosis with strategic family therapy for the individual adolescent symptom-bearer: Applications and limitations. *Australian Journal of Clinical and Experimental Hypnosis, 17*, 71–77.

Locke, S. E., Ransil, B. J., Covino, N. A., Toczydlowski, J., Lohse, C. M., Dvorak, H. F., Arndt, K. A., & Frankel, F. H. (1987). Failure of hypnotic suggestion to alter immune response to delayed-type hypersensitivity antigens. *Annals of the New York Academy of Sciences, 496*, 745–749.

Loftus, E. F. (1979). *Eyewitness testimony*. Cambridge, MA: Harvard University Press.

Lombard, L. S., Kahn, S. P., & Fromm, E. (1990). The role of imagery in self-hypnosis: Its relationship to personality characteristics and gender. *International Journal of Clinical and Experimental Hypnosis, 38*, 25–38.

London, P., Cooper, L. M., & Engstrom, D. R. (1974). Increasing hypnotic susceptiblity by brain wave feeedback. *Journal of Abnormal Psychology, 83*, 554–560.

London, P., Hart, J. T., & Leibovitz, M. P. (1968). EEG alpha rhythms and susceptibility to hypnosis. *Nature, 219*, 71–72.

Loomis, A. L., Harvey, E. N., & Hobart, G. A. (1936). Electrical potentials during hypnosis. *Science, 83*, 239–241.

Loring, D. W., & Sheer, D. E. (1984). Laterality of 40 Hz EEG and EMG during cognitive performance. *Psychophysiology, 21*, 34–38.

Lubar, J. F., Gordon, D. M., Harrist, R. S., Nash, M. R., Mann, C. R., & Lacy, J. E. (1991). EEG correlates of hypnotic susceptibility based upon fast Fourier power spectral analysis. *Biofeedback and Self-Regulation, 16*, 75–85.

Lundholm, H. (1933). Laboratory neuroses. *Character and Personality, 2*, 127–133.

Lynch, J. J., Paskewitz, D. A., & Orne, M. T. (1974). Some factors in the feedback control of human alpha rhythm. *Psychosomatic Medicine, 36*, 399–410.

Lynn, S. J. (1990, October). *Subject factors*. Paper presented at the 41st Annual Meeting of the Society for Clinical and Experimental Hypnosis, Tucson, AZ.

Lynn, S. J., Green, J. P., Rhue, J. W., Mare, C., & Williams, B. (1990). *Fantasy proneness and hypnotizability: A stringent test*. Unpublished manuscript, Ohio University.

Lynn, S. J., Jacquith, L., Green, J. P., Mare, C., & Gasior, D. (1991). *Hypnosis and performance standards*. Unpublished manuscript, Ohio University.

Lynn, S. J., Milano, M., & Weekes, J. R. (1991). Hypnosis and pseudomemories: The effects of prehypnotic expectancies. *Journal of Abnormal Psychology, 60*, 318–326.

Lynn, S. J., Nash, M. R., Rhue, J. W., Frauman, D. C., & Stanley, S. (1983). Hypnosis and the experience of nonvolition. *International Journal of Clinical and Experimental Hypnosis, 31*, 293–308.

Lynn, S. J., Nash, M. R., Rhue, J. W., Frauman, D. C., & Sweeney, C. (1984). Nonvolition, expectancies, and hypnotic rapport. *Journal of Abnormal Psychology, 93*, 295–303.

Lynn, S. J., Neufeld, V., & Matyi, C. L. (1987). Inductions versus suggestions: Effects of direct and indirect wording on hypnotic responding and experience. *Journal of Abnormal Psychology, 96,* 76–79.

Lynn, S. J., Predieri, K., Green, J., Mare, C., & Williams, B. (1990, August). Bulimia and hypnosis. In J. R. Council (Chair), *Hypnosis and bulimia: Research and clinical perspectives.* Symposium conducted at the meeting of the American Psychological Association, New Orleans.

Lynn, S. J., & Rhue, J. W. (1986). The fantasy-prone person: Hypnosis, imagination, and creativity. *Journal of Personality and Social Psychology, 51,* 404–408.

Lynn, S. J., & Rhue, J. W. (1987). Hypnosis, imagination, and fantasy. *Journal of Mental Imagery, 11,* 101–111.

Lynn, S. J., & Rhue, J. W. (1988). Fantasy proneness: Hypnosis, developmental antecedents, and psychopathology. *American Psychologist, 43,* 35–44.

Lynn, S. J., & Rhue, J. W. (1991). An integrative model of hypnosis. In S. J. Lynn & J. W. Rhue (Eds.), *Theories of hypnosis: Current models and perspectives* (pp. 397–438). New York: Guilford Press.

Lynn, S. J., Rhue, J. W., & Weekes, J. R. (1989). Hypnosis and experienced nonvolition: A social-cognitive model. In N. P. Spanos & J. F. Chaves (Eds.), *Hypnosis: The cognitive–behavioral perspective* (pp. 78–109). Buffalo, NY: Prometheus Books.

Lynn, S. J., Rhue, J. W., & Weekes, J. R. (1990). Hypnotic involuntariness: A social cognitive analysis. *Psychological Review, 97,* 169–184.

Lynn, S. J., Snodgrass, M., Rhue, J. W., & Hardaway, R. (1987). Goal-directed fantasy, hypnotic susceptibility, and expectancies. *Journal of Personality and Social Psychology, 53,* 933–938.

Lynn, S. J., Weekes, J. R., & Milano, M. J. (1989). Reality versus suggestion: Pseudomemory in hypnotizable and simulating subjects. *Journal of Abnormal Psychology, 98,* 137–144.

Lyons, W. (1986). *The disappearance of introspection.* Cambridge, MA: Bradford.

Lytle, R. A., & Lundy, R. M. (1988). Hypnosis and the recall of visually presented material: A failure to replicate Stager and Lundy. *International Journal of Clinical and Experimental Hypnosis, 36,* 327–335.

MacKinnon, D. (1971). Creativity and transliminal experience. *Journal of Creative Behavior, 5,* 227–241.

MacLeod-Morgan, C. (1979). Hypnotic susceptibility, EEG theta and alpha waves, and hemispheric specificity. In G. D. Burrows, D. R. Collison, & L. Dennerstein (Eds.), *Hypnosis 1979* (pp. 181–188). Amsterdam: Elsevier/North-Holland.

MacLeod-Morgan, C. (1982). EEG lateralization in hypnosis: A preliminary report. *Australian Journal of Clinical and Experimental Hypnosis, 10,* 99–102.

MacLeod-Morgan, C., & Lack, L. (1982). Hemispheric specificity: A physiological concomitant of hypnotizability. *Psychophysiology, 19,* 687–690.

Madigan, C. O., & Elwood, A. (1983). *Brainstorms and thunderbolts.* New York: Macmillan.

Maher-Loughnan, G. P., MacDonald, N., Mason, A. A., & Fry, L. (1962). Controlled trial of hypnosis in the symptomatic treatment of asthma. *British Medical Journal, ii,* 371–376.

Malmo, R. B., Boag, T. J., & Raginsky, B. B. (1954). Electromyographic study of hypnotic deafness. *International Journal of Clinical and Experimental Hypnosis, 2,* 305–317.

Malone, M. D., Kurtz, R. M., & Strube, M. J. (1989). The effects of hypnotic suggestion on pain report. *American Journal of Clinical Hypnosis, 31,* 221–229.

Malott, J. M., Bourg, A. L., & Crawford, H. J. (1989). The effects of hypnosis upon cognitive responses to persuasive communication. *International Journal of Clinical and Experimental Hypnosis, 37,* 31–40.

Marcel, A. J. (1983). Conscious and unconscious perception: Experiments on visual masking and word recognition. *Cognitive Psychology, 15,* 197–237.

Margolis, J., & Margolis, C. G. (1979). The theory of hypnosis and the concept of persons. *Behaviorism, 7,* 97–111.

Marks, D. F. (1973). Visual imagery differences in the recall of pictures. *British Journal of Psychology, 64,* 17–24.

Marlatt, G. A., & Gordon, J. R. (Eds.). (1985). *Relapse prevention: Maintenance strategies in the treatment of addictive behaviors.* New York: Guilford Press.

Martindale, C. (1975). *The romantic progression: The psychology of literary history.* Washington, DC: Hemisphere.

Martindale, C., Covello, E., & West, A. (1986). Primary process cognition and hemispheric asymmetry. *Journal of Genetic Psychology, 147,* 79–87.

Martindale, C., & Greenough, J. (1973). The differential effect of increased arousal on creative and intellectual performance. *Journal of Genetic Psychology, 123,* 329–335.

Maslach, C., Marshall, G., & Zimbardo, P. G. (1972). Hypnotic control of peripheral skin temperature: A case report. *Psychophysiology, 9,* 600–605.

Masling, J. (1966). Role-related behavior of the subject and psychologist and its effects upon psychological data. *Nebraska Symposium on Motivation, 14,* 67–103.

Mathew, R. J., & Partain, C. L. (1985). Midsaggittal sections of cerebellar vermis and fourth ventricle obtained with magnetic resonance imaging of schizophrenic patients. *American Journal of Psychiatry, 142,* 970–971.

Matthews, W. J., Bennett, H., Bean, W., & Gallagher M. (1985). Indirect versus direct hypnotic suggestions—an initial investigation: A brief communication. *International Journal of Clinical and Experimental Hypnosis, 33,* 219–223.

Matthews, W. J., Kirsch, I., & Mosher, D. (1985). The "double" hypnotic induction: An initial empirical test. *Journal of Abnormal Psychology, 94,* 92–95.

McAleney, P. J., Barabasz, A. F., & Barabasz, M. (1990). Effects of flotation restricted environmental stimulation on intercollegiate tennis performance. *Perceptual and Motor Skills, 71,* 1023–1028.

McCann, T. E., & Sheehan, P. W. (1987). The breaching of pseudomemory under hypnotic instruction: Implications for original memory retrieval. *British Journal of Experimental and Clinical Hypnosis, 4,* 101–108.

McCann, T., & Sheehan, P. W. (1988). Hypnotically induced pseudomemories: Sampling their conditions among hypnotizable subjects. *Journal of Personality and Social Psychology, 54,* 339–346.

McConkey, K. M. (1984). The impact of an indirect suggestion. *International Journal of Clinical and Experimental Hypnosis, 32,* 307–314.

McConkey, K. M. (1986). Opinions about hypnosis and self-hypnosis before and after hypnotic testing. *International Journal of Clinical and Experimental Hypnosis, 34,* 311–319.

McConkey, K.M. (1988). A view from the laboratory on the forensic use of hypnosis. *Australian Journal of Clinical and Experimental Hypnosis, 16,* 71–81.

McConkey, K. M. (1991). The construction and resolution of experience and behavior in hypnosis. In S. J. Lynn & J. W. Rhue (Eds.), *Theories of hypnosis: Current models and perspectives* (pp. 542–563). New York: Guilford Press.

McConkey, K. M., Glisky, M. L., & Kihlstrom, J. F. (1989). Individual differences among hypnotic virtuosos: A case comparison. *Australian Journal of Clinical and Experimental Hypnosis, 17,* 131–140.

McConkey, K. M., & Jupp, J. J. (1985). Opinions about the forensic use of hypnosis. *Australian Psychologist, 20,* 283–291.

McConkey, K. M., & Jupp, J. J. (1986). A survey of opinions about hypnosis. *British Journal of Experimental and Clinical Hypnosis, 3,* 87–93.

McConkey, K. M., & Kinoshita, S. (1986). Creating memories and reports. *British Journal of Experimental and Clinical Hypnosis, 3,* 162–166.

McConkey, K. M., & Kinoshita, S. (1988). The influence of hypnosis on memory after one day and one week. *Journal of Abnormal Psychology, 97,* 48–53.

McConkey, K. M., Labelle, L., Bibb, B. C., & Bryant, R. A. (1990). Hypnosis and suggested pseudomemory: The relevance of test context. *Australian Journal of Psychology, 42,* 197–205.

McConkey, K. M., & Sheehan, P. W. (1980). Inconsistency in hypnotic age regression and cue structure as supplied by the hypnotist. *International Journal of Clinical and Experimental Hypnosis, 28,* 394–408.

McConkey, K. M., & Sheehan, P. W. (1981). The impact of videotape playback of hypnotic events on posthypnotic amnesia. *Journal of Abnormal Psychology, 90,* 46–54.

McConkey, K. M., & Sheehan, P. W. (in press). Ethical issues in forensic hypnosis. *Australian Psychologist.*

McConkey, K. M., Sheehan, P. W., & Cross, D. G. (1980). Posthypnotic amnesia: Seeing is not remembering. *British Journal of Social and Clinical Psychology, 19,* 99–107.

McCormack, K., & Gruzelier, J. H. (in press). Cerebral asymmetry and hypnosis: A signal detection analysis of divided visual field stimulation. *Journal of Abnormal Psychology.*

McDougall, W. (1926). *Outline of abnormal psychology,* New York: Scribner's.

McDougall, W. (1938). The relation between dissociation and repression. *British Journal of Medical Psychology, 17,* 141–157.

McGlashan, T. H., Evans, F. J., & Orne, M. T. (1969). The nature of hypnotic analgesia and placebo response to experimental pain. *Psychosomatic Medicine, 31,* 227–246.

McKelvie, S. J., & Pullara, M. (1988). Effects of hypnosis and level of processing on repeated recall of line drawings. *Journal of General Psychology, 115,* 315–329.

Mednick, S. A., & Mednick, M. T. (1967). *Examiners manual: Remote Associates Test.* Boston: Houghton Mifflin.

Meichenbaum, D. M. (1977). *Cognitive behavior modification: An integrative approach.* New York: Plenum.

Melei, J. P., & Hilgard, E. R. (1964). Attitudes toward hypnosis, self-predictions and hypnotic susceptibility. *International Journal of Clinical and Experimental Hypnosis, 12,* 99–108.

Mesmer, F. A. (1779). *Mémoire sur la découverte du magnétisme animal.* Paris: Didot le Jeune.

Mesmer, F. A. (1799). *Mémoire de F. A. Mesmer, docteur en médecine, sur ses découvertes.* Paris: Fuchs.

Mesmer, F. A. (1948). *Mesmerism by Dr. Mesmer* (G. Frankau, Ed.; V. R. Myers, Trans.). London: MacDonald. (Original work published 1779)

Messerschmidt, R. (1927–1928). A quantitative investigation of the alleged independent operation of conscious and subconscious processes. *Journal of Abnormal and Social Psychology, 22,* 325–340.

Mészáros, I., & Bányai, E. I. (1978). Electrophysiological characteristics of hypnosis. In K. Lissák (Ed.), *Neural and neurohumoral organization of motivated behavior* (pp. 173–187). Budapest: Akademiai Kiado.

Mészáros, I., Bányai, E. I., & Greguss, A. C. (1985). Evoked potential correlates of verbal versus imagery coding in hypnosis. In D. Waxman, P. C. Misra, M. Gibson, & M. A. Basker (Eds.), *Modern trends in hypnosis* (pp. 161–168). New York: Plenum Press.

Mészáros, I., Crawford, H. J., Szabó, C., Nagy-Kovács, A., & Révész, M. A. (1989). Hypnotic susceptibility and cerebral hemisphere preponderance. In V. Ghorghui, P. Netter, H. Eysenck, & R. Rosenthal (Eds.), *Suggestion and suggestibility: Theory and research* (pp. 191–203). Berlin: Springer-Verlag.

Mészáros, I., & Révész, Z. (1990, July). *Hemispheric EEG activity and hypnosis.* Paper presented at the 5th International Congress of Psychophysiology, Budapest.

Meyer, H. K., Diehl, B. J., Ulrich, P. T., & Meinig, G. (1989). Anderungen der regionalen kortikalen durchblutung unter hypnose. [Changes in the regional cortical blood flow during hypnosis]. *Zeitschrift für Psychosomatische Medizin und Psychoanalyse, 35,* 48–58.

Miller, G. A., Galanter, E., & Pribram, K. H. (1960). *Plans and the structure of behavior.* New York: Holt, Rinehart & Winston.

Miller, L. S., & Cross, H. J. (1985). Hypnotic susceptibility, hypnosis and EMG biofeedback in the reduction of frontalis muscle tension. *International Journal of Clinical and Experimental Hypnosis, 33,* 258–272.

Miller, M. E., & Bowers, K. S. (1986). Hypnotic analgesia and stress inoculation in the reduction of pain. *Journal of Abnormal Psychology, 95,* 6–14.

Miller, M. E., & Bowers, K. S. (1992). *Hypnotic analgesia: Dissociated experience or dissociated control?* Unpublished manuscript.

Miller, M. F., & Barabasz, M. (1990). Effects of restricted environmental stimulation on inversion perception. In J. Turner & T. Fine (Eds.), *Restricted environmental stimulation: Research and commentary.* Toledo, OH: MCOT Press.

Miller, M. F., Barabasz, A. F., & Barabasz, M. (1991). Effects of active alert and relaxation hypnotic inductions on cold pressor pain. *Journal of Abnormal Psychology, 100,* 223–226.

Miller, R. (1989). Cortico-hippocampal interplay: Self-organizing phase-locked loops for indexing memory. *Psychobiology, 17,* 115–128.

Miller, R. J., Hennessy, R. T., & Leibowitz, H. W. (1973). The effects of hypnotic ablation of the background on the magnitude of the Ponzo perspective illusion. *International Journal of Clinical and Experimental Hypnosis, 21,* 180–191.

Mingay, D. J. (1986). Hypnosis and memory for incidentally learned scenes. *British Journal of Experimental and Clinical Hypnosis, 3,* 173–183.

Mingay, D. J. (1987). The effect of hypnosis on eyewitness memory: Reconciling forensic claims and research findings. *Applied Psychology: An International Review, 36,* 163–183.

Mitchell, G. P., & Lundy, R. M. (1986). The effects of relaxation and imagery inductions on responses to suggestions. *International Journal of Clinical and Experimental Hypnosis, 34,* 98–109.

Mitchell, M. B. (1932). Retroactive inhibition and hypnosis. *Journal of General Psychology, 7,* 343–358.

Mizuki, Y., Tanaka, M., Isozaki, H., Nishijima, H., & Inanaga, K. (1980). Periodic appearance of theta rhythm in the frontal midline area during performance of a mental task. *Electroencephalography and Clinical Neurophysiology, 49,* 345–351.

Moll, A. (1982). *Hypnotism.* New York: Da Capo Press. (Original work published 1889)

Montgomery, I., Perkins, G., & Wise, D. (1975). A review of behavioral treatments for insomnia. *Journal of Behavior Therapy, 6,* 93–100.

Moore, R. K. (1964). Susceptibility to hypnosis and susceptibility to social influence. *Journal of Abnormal and Social Psychology, 68,* 282–294.

Moos, R. H. (1970). Differential effects of psychiatric settings on patient change. *Journal of Nervous and Mental Disease, 74,* 316–321.

Morgan, A. H. (1973). The heritability of hypnotic susceptibility in twins. *Journal of Abnormal Psychology, 82,* 55–61.

Morgan, A. H., & Hilgard, J. R. (1975). Stanford Hypnotic Clinical Scale (SHCS). In E. R. Hilgard & J. R. Hilgard, *Hypnosis in the relief of pain* (pp. 209–221). Los Altos, CA: William Kaufmann.

Morgan, A. H., & Hilgard, J. R. (1978–1979a). The Stanford Hypnotic Clinical Scale for adults. *American Journal of Clinical Hypnosis, 21,* 134–147

Morgan, A. H., & Hilgard, J. R. (1978–1979b). The Stanford Hypnotic Clinical Scale for children. *American Journal of Clinical Hypnosis, 21,* 148–169.

Morgan, A. H., Hilgard, E. R., & Davert, E. C. (1970). The heritability of hypnotic susceptibility in twins: A preliminary report. *Behavior Genetics, 1,* 213–224.

Morgan, A. H., Johnson, D. L., & Hilgard, E. R. (1974). The stability of hypnotic susceptibility: A longitudinal study. *International Journal of Clinical and Experimental Hypnosis, 22,* 249–257.

Morgan, A. H., Macdonald, H., & Hilgard, E. R. (1974). EEG alpha: Lateral asymmetry related to task, and hypnotizability. *Psychophysiology, 11,* 275–282.

Morgan, A. H., McDonald, P. J., & Macdonald, H. (1971). Differences in bilateral alpha activity as a function of experimental task, with a note on lateral eye movements and hypnotizability. *Neuropsychologia, 9,* 459–469.

Morrison, J. B. (1988). Chronic asthma and improvement with relaxation induced by hypnotherapy. *Journal of the Royal Society of Medicine, 81*(1), 701–704.

Mott, T. (1979). The clinical importance of hypnotizability. *American Journal of Clinical Hypnosis, 11,* 263–269.

Murphy, A. I., Lehrer, P. M., Karlin, R., Swartzman, L., Hochron, S., & McCann, B. (1989). Hypnotic susceptibility and its relationship to outcome in the behavioral treatment of asthma: Some preliminary data. *Psychological Reports, 65*(2), 691–698.

Nadon, R., D'Eon, J. L., McConkey, K. M., Laurence, J.-R., & Perry, C. (1988). Post-hypnotic amnesia, the hidden observer effect, and duality during hypnotic age regression. *International Journal of Clinical and Experimental Hypnosis,* *36,* 19–37.

Nadon, R., Hoyt, I. P., Register, P. A., & Kihlstrom, J. F. (1991). Absorption and hypnotizability: Context effects reexamined. *Journal of Personality and Social Psychology, 60,* 144–153.

Nadon, R., & Kihlstrom, J. F. (1987). Hypnosis, psi, and the psychology of anomalous experience. *Behavioral and Brain Sciences, 10,* 597–599.

Nadon, R., Laurence, J.-R., & Perry, C. (1987). Multiple predictors of hypnotic susceptibility. *Journal of Personality and Social Psychology, 53,* 948–960.

Nadon, R., Laurence, J.-R., & Perry, C. (1989). Interactionism: Cognition and context in hypnosis. *British Journal of Experimental and Clinical Hypnosis, 6,* 141–150.

Nadon, R., Laurence, J.-R., & Perry, C. (1991). The two disciplines of scientific hypnosis: A synergistic model. In S. J. Lynn & J. W. Rhue (Eds.), *Theories of hypnosis: Current models and perspectives* (pp. 485–519). New York: Guilford Press.

Nakagawa, Y. (1988). Continuous observation of daytime EEG patterns in normal subjects under restrained conditions while sitting in armchair or on stool: Part 2. Awake state. *Japanese Journal of Psychiatry and Neurology, 42,* 247–264.

Nash, J. (1983). Negative visual hallucination and concomitant changes in cortical event-related potentials (Doctoral dissertation, University of California at Santa Barbara). *Dissertation Abstracts International, 45*(2), 716B. (University Microfilms No. 84-11,224)

Nash, M. R. (1987). What, if anything, is regressed about hypnotic age regression? A review of the empirical literature. *Psychological Bulletin, 102,* 42–52.

Nash, M. R. (1988). Twenty years of scientific hypnosis in dentistry, medicine, and psychology: A brief communication. *International Journal of Clinical and Experimental Hypnosis, 36,* 198–205.

Nash, M. R. (1991). Hypnosis as a special case of psychological regression. In S. J. Lynn & J. W. Rhue (Eds.), *Theories of hypnosis: Current models and perspectives* (pp. 171–194). New York: Guilford Press.

Nash, M. R., Drake, S. D., Wiley, S., Khalsa, S., & Lynn, S. J. (1986). Accuracy of recall by hypnotically age-regressed subjects. *Journal of Abnormal Psychology, 95,* 298–300.

Nash, M. R., Johnson, L. S., & Tipton, R. D. (1979). Hypnotic age regression and the occurrence of transitional object relationships. *Journal of Abnormal Psychology, 88,* 547–555.

Nash, M. R., Lynn, S. J., & Stanley, S. (1984). The direct hypnotic suggestion of altered mind/body perception . *American Journal of Clinical Hypnosis, 27,* 95–102.

Nash, M. R., Lynn, S. J., Stanley, S., & Carlson, V. (1987). Subjectively complete hypnotic deafness and auditory priming. *International Journal of Clinical and Experimental Hypnosis, 35,* 32–40.

Nash, M. R., Lynn, S. J., Stanley, S., Frauman, D., & Rhue, J. (1985). Hypnotic age regression and the importance of assessing interpersonally relevant affect. *International Journal of Clinical and Experimental Hypnosis, 33,* 224–235.

Nash, M. R., & Spinler, D. (1989). Hypnosis and transference: A measure of archaic involvement with the hypnotist. *Journal of Clinical and Experimental Hypnosis, 37,* 129–144.

Nasrallah, H. A., & Coffman, J. A. (1985). Computerized tomagraphy in psychiatry. *Psychiatric Annals, 15,* 239–249.

Neisser, U. (1967). *Cognitive psychology.* New York: Appleton-Century-Crofts.

Neufeld, V., & Lynn, S. J. (1988). Single-session group self-hypnosis smoking cessation treatment: A brief communication. *International Journal of Clinical and Experimental Hypnosis, 36*(2), 75–79.

Neufeld, V., Lynn, S. J., Jacquith, L., Weekes, J. R., & Brentar, J. (1987). *Fantasy style, imagination and hypnosis.* Paper presented at the annual meeting of the Society for Clinical and Experimental Hypnosis, Asheville, NC.

Newell, A., & Simon, H. A. (1972). *Human problem solving.* Englewood Cliffs, NJ: Prentice-Hall.

Newman, M. (1971). Hypnotic handling of the chronic bleeder in extraction: A case report. *American Journal of Clincal Hypnosis, 14,* 126–127.

Nisbett, R., & Wilson, T. D. (1977). Telling more than we can know: Verbal reports on mental processes. *Psychological Review, 84,* 231–254.

Nogrady, H., McConkey, K. M., Laurence, J.-R., & Perry, C. (1983). Dissociation, duality, and demand characteristics in hypnosis. *Journal of Abnormal Psychology, 92,* 223–235.

Nogrady, H., McConkey, K. M., & Perry, C. (1985). Enhancing visual memory: Trying hypnosis, trying imagination, and trying again. *Journal of Abnormal Psychology, 94,* 195–204.

Nolan, R. P., & Spanos, N. P. (1987). Hypnotic analgesia and stress inoculation: A critical reexamination of Miller and Bowers. *Psychological Reports, 61,* 95–102.

Noll, R. B. (1988). Hypnotherapy of a child with warts. *Journal of Developmental and Behavioral Pediatrics, 9,* 89–91.

Nowlis, D. P., & Rhead, J. C. (1968). Relations of eyes-closed resting EEG alpha activity to hypnotic susceptibility. *Perceptual and Motor Skills, 27,* 1047–1050.

Oberlander, M. I., Gruenewald, D., & Fromm, E. (1970, September). *Content and structural characteristics of thought processes in hypnosis.* Paper presented at the meeting of the American Psychological Association, Miami Beach, FL.

Obrist, W. D., Thompson, H. K., Wang, H. S., & Wilkinson, W. E. (1975). Regional cerebral blood flow estimated by 133-xenon inhalation. *Stroke, 6,* 245–256.

Obstoj, J., & Sheehan, P. W. (1977). Aptitude for trance, task generalizability, and incongruity response in hypnosis. *Journal of Abnormal Psychology, 86,* 543–552.

O'Connell, D. N., & Orne, M. T. (1962). Bioelectric correlates of hypnosis: An experimental reevaluation. *Journal of Psychiatric Research, 1,* 201–213.

O'Connell, D. N., & Orne, M. T. (1968). Endosomatic electrodermal correlates of hypnotic depth and susceptibility. *Journal of Psychiatric Research, 6,* 1–12.

O'Connell, D. N., Orne, M. T., & Shor, R. E. (1966). A comparison of hypnotic susceptibility as assessed by diagnostic ratings and initial standardized test scores. *International Journal of Clinical and Experimental Hypnosis, 14,* 324–332.

Okhowat, V. O. (1985). An eclectic hypno-emotive approach to psychotherapy. *International Journal of Clinical and Experimental Hypnosis, 33,* 109–121.

Olesko, B., Arany, C., & Crawford, H. J. (1989, June). *Cold pressor pain in low and high hypnotizables: Hypnotic analgesia versus waking.* Paper presented at the 1st Annual Meeting of the American Psychological Society, Alexandria, VA.

Olness, K., Culbert, T., & Uden, D. (1989). Self-regulation of salivary immunoglobulin A by children. *Pediatrics, 83,* 66–71.

Olness, K., MacDonald, J. T., & Uden, D. L. (1987). Comparison of self-hypnosis and propranolol in the treatment of juvenile classic migraine. *Pediatrics, 79*(4), 593–597.

Olness, K., Wain, H. J., & Lorenz, N. G. (1980). A pilot study of blood endorphin levels in children using self-hypnosis to control pain. *Journal of Developmental and Behavioral Pediatrics, 4,* 187–188.

Omer, H. (1987). A hypnotic relaxation technique for the treatment of premature labor. *American Journal of Clinical Hypnosis, 29*(3), 206–213.

Omer, H., Friedlander, D., & Palti, Z. (1986). Hypnotic relaxation in the treatment of premature labor. *Psychosomatic Medicine, 48*(5), 351–361.

Orman, D. J. (1991) Reframing of an addiction via hypnotherapy: A case presentation. *American Journal of Clinical Hypnosis, 33,* 263–277.

Orne, M. T. (1951). The mechanisms of hypnotic age regression: An experimental study. *Journal of Abnormal and Social Psychology, 16,* 213–225.

Orne, M. T. (1959). The nature of hypnosis: Artifact and essence. *Journal of Abnormal and Social Psychology, 58,* 277–299.

Orne, M. T. (1962a). On the social psychology of the psychological experiment: With particular reference to demand characteristics and their implications. *American Psychologist, 17,* 776–783.

Orne, M. T. (1962b). Antisocial behavior and hypnosis: Problems of control and validation in empirical studies. In G. H. Estrabrooks (Ed.), *Hypnosis: Current problems* (pp. 137–192). New York: Harper & Row.

Orne, M. T. (1962c). Hypnotically induced hallucinations. In L. J. West (Ed.), *Hallucinations* (pp. 211–219). New York: Grune & Stratton.

Orne, M. T. (1965, September). *Demand characteristics and their implications for real life: The importance of quasi-controls.* Paper presented at the annual convention of the American Psychological Association, Chicago.

Orne, M. T. (1966). Hypnosis, motivation and compliance. *American Journal of Psychiatry, 122,* 721–726.

Orne, M. T. (1969). Demand characteristics and the concept of quasi-controls. In R. Rosenthal & R. L. Rosnow (Eds.), *Artifact in behavioral research* (pp. 143–179). New York: Academic Press.

Orne, M. T. (1970). Hypnosis, motivation and the ecological validity of the psychological experiment. *Nebraska Symposium on Motivation, 18,* 187–265.

Orne, M. T. (1971a), *Is hypnosis only an episode set?* Paper presented at the meeting of the American Psychological Association, Washington, DC.

Orne, M.T. (1971b). The simulation of hypnosis: Why, how and what it means. *International Journal of Clinical and Experimental Hypnosis, 19,* 183–210.

Orne, M. T. (1972). On the simulating subject as a quasi-control group in hypnosis research: What, why, and how. In E. Fromm & R. E. Shor (Eds.), *Hypnosis: Research developments and perspectives* (pp. 519–565). Chicago: Aldine-Atherton.

Orne, M. T. (1974). *On the concept of hypnotic depth.* Paper presented at the 18th International Conference of Applied Psychology, Montréal.

Orne, M. T. (1977). The construct of hypnosis: Implications of the definition for research and practice. *Annals of the New York Academy of Sciences, 296,* 14–33.

Orne, M. T. (1979a). On the simulating subject as a quasi-control group in hypnosis research: What, why, and how. In E. Fromm & R. E. Shor (Eds.), *Hypnosis: Developments in research and new perspectives* (2nd ed., pp. 519–566). New York: Aldine.

Orne, M. T. (1979b). The use and misuse of hypnosis in court. *International Journal of Clinical and Experimental Hypnosis, 27*, 311–341.

Orne, M. T. (1981). The significance of unwitting cues for experimental outcomes: Toward a pragmatic approach. *Annals of the New York Academy of Sciences, 364*, 152–159.

Orne, M. T., Dinges, D. F., & Orne, E. C. (1984). On the differential diagnosis of multiple personality in the forensic context. *International Journal of Clinical and Experimental Hypnosis, 32*, 118–169.

Orne, M. T., & Evans, F. (1965). Social control in the psychological experiment: Antisocial behavior and hypnosis. *Journal of Personality and Social Psychology, 1*, 189–200.

Orne, M. T., Hilgard, E. R., Spiegel, H., Spiegel, D., Crawford, H. J., Evans, F. J., Orne, E. C., & Frischholz, E. J. (1979). The relation between the Hypnotic Induction Profile and the Stanford Hypnotic Susceptibility Scales, Forms A and C. *International Journal of Clinical and Experimental Hypnosis, 27*, 85–102.

Orne, M. T., & Paskewitz, D. A. (1974). Aversive situational effects on alpha feedback training. *Science, 186*, 458–460.

Orne, M. T., & Scheibe, K. E. (1964). The contribution of nondeprivation factors in the production of sensory deprivation effects: The psychology of the panic button. *Journal of Abnormal and Social Psychology, 68*(1), 3–12.

Orne, M. T., Sheehan, P. W., & Evans, F. J. (1968). Occurrence of posthypnotic behavior outside the experimental setting. *Journal of Personality and Social Psychology, 9*, 189–196.

Orne, M. T., Soskis, D. A., Dinges, D. F., & Orne, E. C. (1984). Hypnotically induced testimony. In G. L. Wells & E. F. Loftus (Eds.), *Eyewitness testimony: Psychological perspectives* (pp. 171–213). New York: Cambridge University Press.

Orne, M. T., Whitehouse, W. G., Dinges, D. F., & Orne, E. C. (1988). Reconstructing memory through hypnosis: Forensic and clinical implications. In H. M. Pettinati (Ed.), *Hypnosis and memory* (pp. 21–63). New York: Guilford Press.

Orton, D. M., & Gruzelier, J. H. (1989). Adverse changes in mood and cognitive performance of house officers after night duty. *British Medical Journal, 298*, 21–23.

Owens, M. E., Bliss, E. L., Koester, P., & Jeppsen, E. A. (1989). Phobias and hypnotizability: A reexamination. *International Journal of Clinical and Experimental Hypnosis, 37*, 207–216.

Pagano, R. R., Akots, N. J., & Wall, T. W. (1988). Hypnosis, cerebral laterality and relaxation. *International Journal of Clinical and Experimental Hypnosis, 36*, 350–358.

Paivio, A. (1971). *Imagery and verbal processes.* New York: Holt.

Palmer, R. E. (1969). *Hermeneutics: Interpretation theory in Schleiermacher, Dilthey, Heidegger, and Gadamer.* Evanston, IL: Northwestern University Press.

Paskewitz, D. A. (1977). EEG alpha activity and its relationship to altered states of consciousness. *Annals of the New York Academy of Sciences, 296*, 151–164.

Patterson, D. R., Questad, K. A., & Boltwood, M. D. (1987). Hypnotherapy as a treatment for pain in patients with burns: Research and clinical considerations. *Journal of Burn Care and Rehabilitation, 8*, 263–268.

Pattie, F. A. (1935). A report of attempts to produce uniocular blindness by hypnotic suggestion. *British Journal of Medical Psychology, 15*, 230–241.

Paul, G. L. (1963). The production of blisters by hypnotic suggestion: Another look. *Psychosomatic Medicine, 25*, 233–244.

Paul, G. L. (1969). Physiological effects of relaxation training and hypnotic suggestion. *Journal of Abnormal Psychology, 74*, 425–437.

Pavlov, G. L. (1923). Physiological effects of relaxation training and hypnotic suggestion. *Journal of Abnormal Psychology, Scientific Monthly, 17*, 603–608.

Payne, D. G. (1987). Hypermnesia and reminiscence in recall: A historical and empirical review. *Psychological Bulletin, 101*, 5–27.

Pekala, R. J. (1991). Hypnotic types: Evidence from a cluster analysis of phenomenal experience. *Contemporary Hypnosis, 8*, 95–104.

Pekala, R. J., & Bieber, S. L. (1989–1990). Operationalizing pattern approaches to consciousness: An analysis of phenomenological patterns of consciousness among individuals of differing susceptibility. *Imagination, Cognition and Personality, 9*, 303–320.

Pekala, R. J., & Kumar, V. K. (1987–1988). Phenomenological variations in attention across low, medium, and high susceptible subjects. *Imagination, Cognition and Personality, 7*, 303–314.

Pekala, R. J., & Kumar, V. K. (1989). Phenomenological patterns of consciousness during hypnosis: Relevance to cognition and individual differences. *Australian Journal of Clinical and Experimental Hypnosis, 17*, 1–20.

Pekala, R. J., & Nagler, R. (1989). The assessment of hypnoidal states: Rationale and clinical applications. *American Journal of Clinical Hypnosis, 31*, 231–236.

Perkins, D. N. (1981). *The mind's best work.* Cambridge, MA: Harvard University Press.

Perlini, A. H., Lee, A., & Spanos, N. P. (1992). The relationship between imaginability and hypnotic susceptibility: Does context matter? *Contemporary Hypnosis, 9*, 35–41.

Perlini, A. H., & Spanos, N. P. (1991). EEG alpha methodologies and hypnotizability: A critical review. *Psychophysiology, 28*, 511–530.

Perry, C. (1973). Imagery, fantasy, and hypnotic susceptibility. *Journal of Personality and Social Psychology, 26*, 217–221.

Perry, C. (1977). Is hypnotizability modifiable? *International Journal of Clinical and Experimental Hypnosis, 25*, 125–146.

Perry, C. (1983). *Dissociative phenomena and hypnosis.* Invited address presented at the annual convention of the American Psychological Association, Anaheim, CA.

Perry, C., Gelfand, R., & Marcovitch, P. (1979). The relevance of hypnotic susceptibility in the clinical context. *Journal of Abnormal Psychology, 88*, 592–603.

Perry, C. & Laurence, J.-R. (1980). Hypnotic depth and hypnotic susceptibility: A replicated finding. *International Journal of Clinical and Experimental Hypnosis, 28*, 272–280.

Perry, C., & Laurence, J.-R. (1983a). Hypnosis, surgery, and mind–body interaction: An historical evaluation. *Canadian Journal of Behavioural Science, 15*, 351–372.

Perry, C., & Laurence, J.-R. (1983b). The enhancement of memory by hypnosis in the legal investigative situation. *Canadian Psychology, 24*, 155–167.

Perry, C., & Laurence, J.-R. (1984). Mental processing outside of awareness: The contributions of Freud and Janet. In K. S. Bowers & D. Meichenbaum (Eds.), *The unconscious reconsidered* (pp. 9–48). New York: Wiley.

Perry, C., & Laurence, J.-R. (1986) Social and psychological influences on hypnotic behavior. *Behavioral and Brain Sciences, 9*, 478–479.

Perry, C., Laurence, J.-R., D'Eon, J., & Tallant, B. (1988). Hypnotic age regression techniques in the elicitation of memories: Applied uses and abuses. In H. Pettinati (Ed.), *Hypnosis and memory* (pp. 128–154). New York: Guilford Press.

Perry, C., & Walsh, B. (1978). Inconsistencies and anomalies of response as a defining characteristic of hypnosis. *Journal of Abnormal Psychology, 87,* 575–577.

Perry, C., Wilder, S., & Appignanesi, A. (1973). Hypnotic susceptibility and performance in a battery of creativity measures. *American Journal of Clinical Hypnosis, 15*(3), 170–180.

Pervin, L. A. (Ed.). (1990). *Handbook of personality: Theory and research.* New York: Guilford Press.

Pessin, M., Plapp, J. N., & Stern, J. A. (1968). Effects of hypnosis induction and attention direction on electrodermal responses. *American Journal of Clinical Hypnosis, 10,* 198–206.

Peterfreund, E. (1978). Some critical comments on psychoanalytic conceptualizations of infancy. *International Journal of Psycho-Analysis, 59,* 427–441.

Pététin, J. H. D. (1787). *Mémoire sur la découverte des phénomènes que présentent la catalepsie et le somnambulisme.* Paris: Unknown publisher.

Pettinati, H. M. (Ed.). (1988). *Hypnosis and memory.* New York: Guilford Press.

Pettinati, H. M., Evans, F. J., Orne, E. C., & Orne, M. T. (1981). Restricted use of success cues in retrieval during posthypnotic amnesia. *Journal of Abnormal Psychology, 90,* 345–353.

Pettinati, H. M., Horne, R. L., & Staats, J. S. (1985). Hypnotizability in patients with anorexia nervosa and bulimia. *Archives of General Psychiatry, 42,* 1014–1016.

Pettinati, H. M., Kogan, L. G., Evans, F. J., Wade, J. H., Horne, R. L., & Staats, J. S. (1990). Hypnotizability of psychiatric inpatients according to two different scales. *American Journal of Psychiatry, 147,* 69–75.

Pettinati, H. M., & Wade, J. H. (1986). Hypnosis in the treatment of anorexic and bulimic patients. *Seminars in Adolescent Medicine, 2,* 75–79.

Piaget, J. (1973). *The child and reality: Problems of genetic psychology* (A. Rosin, Trans.). New York: Grossman.

Piccione, C., Hilgard, E. R., & Zimbardo, P. G. (1989). On the degree of stability of measured hypnotizability over a 25-year period. *Journal of Personality and Social Psychology, 56,* 289–295.

Pinizzotto, A. J. (1989). Memory and hypnosis: Implications for the use of forensic hypnosis. *Professional Psychology: Research and Practice, 20,* 322–328.

Platt, J. R. (1964). Strong inference. *Science, 146,* 347–353.

Polkinghorne, D. E. (1991). Two conflicting calls for methodological reform. *The Counseling Psychologist, 19,* 103–114.

Posner, M. I., & Petersen, S. E. (1990). The attention span of the brain. *Annual Review of Neuroscience, 13,* 23–42.

Posner, M. I., Petersen, S. E., Fox, P. T., & Raichle, M. E. (1988). Localization of cognitive operations in the human brain. *Science, 240,* 1627–1631.

Posner, M. J., & Snyder, C. (1975). Facilitation and inhibition in the processing of signals. In P. M. A. Rabitt & S. Dornic (Eds.), *Attention and performance* (Vol. 5). New York: Academic Press.

Prévost, M. (1973). *Janet, Freud et la psychologie clinique.* Paris: Petite Bibliothèque Payot.

Pribram, K. H. (1991). *Brain and perception: Holonomy and structure in figural processing.* Hillsdale, NJ: Erlbaum.

Pribram, K. H., & McGuinness, D. (in press). Attention and para-attentional processing: Event-related brain potentials as tests of a model. *Annals of the New York Academy of Sciences.*

Price, D. D., & Barber, J. (1987). An analysis of factors that contribute to the efficacy of hypnotic analgesia. *Journal of Abnormal Psychology, 96,* 46–51.

Priebe, F. A., & Wallace, B. (1986). Hypnotizability, imaging ability, and the detection of embedded objects. *International Journal of Clinical and Experimental Hypnosis, 34,* 320–329.

Prince, M. (1906). *The dissociation of a personality.* New York: Longmans, Green.

Prince, M. (1909). Experiments to determine co-conscious (subconscious) ideation. *Journal of Abnormal Psychology, 3,* 33–42.

Prince, M. (1914). *The unconscious.* New York: Macmillan.

Prince, M. (1939). *Clinical and experimental studies in personality* (2nd ed.). Cambridge, MA: Sci-Art.

Prior, A., Colgan, S. M., & Whorwell, P. J. (1990). Changes in rectal sensitivity after hypnotherapy in patients with irritable bowel syndrome. *Gut, 31,* 896–898.

Putnam, F. W. (1985). Dissociation as a response to extreme trauma. In R. P. Kluft (Ed.), *Childhood antecedents of multiple personality* (pp. 65–98). Washington, DC: American Psychiatric Press.

Putnam, F. W. (1989). *Diagnosis and treatment of multiple personality disorder.* New York: Guilford Press.

Putnam, W. H. (1979). Hypnosis and distortions in eyewitness memory. *International Journal of Clinical and Experimental Hypnosis, 28,* 437–448.

Puységur, A. M. J. Chastenet, Marquis de. (1784–1785). *Mémoires pour servir à l'histoire et l'établissement du magnétisme animal [Memoirs of the history and establishment of animal magnetism]* (2 vols). Paris: Cellot.

Radil, T., Snydrova, I., Hacik, L., Pfeiffer, J., & Votava, J. (1988). Attempts to influence movement disorders in hemiparetics. *Scandinavian Journal of Rehabilitation Medicine, 17*(Suppl.), 157–161.

Radtke, H. L. (1989). Hypnotic depth as social artifact. In N. P. Spanos & J. F. Chaves (Eds.), *Hypnosis: The cognitive–behavioral perspective* (pp. 64–75). Buffalo, NY: Prometheus Books.

Radtke, H. L., & Spanos, N. P. (1981). Temporal sequencing during posthypnotic amnesia: A methodological critique. *Journal of Abnormal Psychology, 90,* 476–485.

Radtke, H. L., & Stam, H. J. (1991). The relation between absorption, openness to experience, anhedonia, and hypnotic susceptibility. *International Journal of Clinical and Experimental Hypnosis, 34,* 39–56.

Radtke-Bodorik, H. L., Planas, M., & Spanos, N. P. (1980). Suggested amnesia, verbal inhibition, and disorganized recall for a long word list. *Canadian Journal of Behavioural Science, 12,* 87–97.

Raikov, V. L. (1976). The possibility of creativity in the active stage of hypnosis. *International Journal of Clinical and Experimental Hypnosis, 24*(3), 258–268.

Raikov, V. L. (1977). Theoretical analysis of deep hypnosis: Creative activity of hypnotized subjects into transformed self-consciousness. *American Journal of Clinical Hypnosis, 19*(4), 214–220.

Raikov, V. L. (1982). Hypnotic age regression to the neonatal period: Comparisons with role playing. *International Journal of Clinical and Experimental Hypnosis, 30,* 106–116.

Raikov, V. L. (1990, October). *Hypnosis and the creative process*. Paper presented at the 41st Annual Meeting of the Society for Clinical Experimental Hypnosis, Tucson, AZ.

Rapaport, D. (1950). On the psychoanalytic theory of thinking. *International Journal of Psycho-Analysis, 31,* 161–170.

Rapaport, D. (1967). Some metapsychological considerations concerning activity and passivity. In M. M. Gill (Ed.), *The collected papers of David Rapaport* (pp. 530–568). New York: Basic Books. (Original work published 1953)

Ratner, H., Gross, L., Casas, J., & Castells, S. (1990). A hypnotherapeutic approach to the improvement of compliance in adolescent diabetics. *American Journal of Clinical Hypnosis, 32*(3), 154–159.

Ravitz, L. J. (1950). Electrometric correlates of the hypnotic state. *Science, 112,* 341–351.

Raynaud, J., Michaux, D., Bleirad, G., Capderou, A., Bordachar, J., & Durand, J. (1984). Changes in rectal and mean skin temperature in responses to suggested heat during hypnosis in man. *Physiology and Behavior, 33,* 221–226.

Reeves, J. L., Redd, W. H., Storm, F. K., & Minagawa, R. Y. (1983). Hypnosis in the control of pain during hyperthermia treatment of cancer. In J. J. Bonica, U. Lindblom, & A. Iggo (Eds.), *Advances in pain research and therapy* (pp. 857–861). New York: Raven Press.

Register, P., & Kihlstrom, J.F. (1986). Finding the hypnotic virtuoso. *International Journal of Clinical and Experimental Hypnosis, 34,* 84–97.

Register, P. A., & Kihlstrom, J. F. (1987). Hypnotic effects on hypermnesia. *International Journal of Clinical and Experimental Hypnosis, 35,* 155–170.

Register, P. A., & Kihlstrom, J. F. (1988). Hypnosis and interrogative suggestibility. *Personality and Individual Differences, 9,* 549–558.

Relinger, H. (1984). Hypnotic hypermnesia: A critical review. *American Journal of Clincal Hypnosis, 26,* 212–225.

Reyher, J., & Smeltzer, W. (1968). Uncovering properties of visual imagery and verbal association. *Journal of Abnormal Psychology, 73,* 218–222.

Rhodes, M. (1961). An analysis of creativity. *Phi Delta Kappan, 42,* 305–310.

Rhue, J. W., & Lynn, S. J. (1987). Fantasy proneness: Developmental antecedents. *Journal of Personality, 55,* 121–137.

Rhue, J. W., & Lynn, S. J. (1989). Fantasy proneness, absorption, and hypnosis: A re-examination. *International Journal of Clinical and Experimental Hypnosis, 37,* 100–106.

Rhue, J. W., Lynn, S. J., Bukh, K., & Henry, S. (1991). *Fantasy proneness, hypnotizability and creativity.* Unpublished manuscript, Ohio University.

Rhue, J. W., Lynn, S. J., & Jacquith, L. (1989, August). *Context effects, hypnosis, and absorption: Effects of labelling and sensitization.* Paper presented at the 97th Annual Meeting of the American Psychological Association, New Orleans.

Richards, R., Kinney, D. K., Benet, M., & Merzel, A. P. C. (1988). Assessing everyday creativity: Characteristics of the Lifetime Creativity Scales and validation with three large samples. *Journal of Personality and Social Psychology, 54,* 476–485.

Richardson, A. (1969). *Mental imagery.* New York: Springer.

Richeport, M. M. (1988). Transcultural issues in Ericksonian hypnotherapy. *Ericksonian Monographs, 3,* 130–147.

Riecken, H. W. (1962). A program for research on experiments in social psychology. In N. F. Washburne (Ed.), *Decisions, values and groups* (Vol. 2, pp. 25–41). New York: Macmillan.

Risberg, J., Ali, Z., Wilson, E. M., Wills, E. L., & Halsey, J. H. (1975). Regional cerebral blood flow by 133 xenon inhalation: Preliminary evaluation of an initial slope index in patients with unstable flow compartments. *Stroke, 6,* 142–148.

Roberts, A. H., Kewman, D. G., & Macdonald, H. (1973). Voluntary control of skin temperature: Unilateral changes using hypnosis and feedback. *Journal of Abnormal Psychology, 82,* 163–168.

Roberts, A. H., Schuler, J., Bacon, J. G., Zimmerman, R. L., & Patterson, R. (1975). Individual differences and autonomic control: Absorption, hypnotic susceptibility, and the unilateral control of skin temperature. *Journal of Abnormal Psychology, 84,* 272–279.

Robertson, L. A., McInnis, K., & St. Jean, R. (in press). Modification of hypnotic susceptibility using the Carleton Skills Training Program: A replication. *Contemporary Hypnosis.*

Roche, S. M., & McConkey, K. M. (1990). Absorption: Nature, assessment, and correlates. *Journal of Personality and Social Psychology, 59,* 91–101.

Rogers, C. (1954). Towards a theory of creativity. *ETC: A Review of General Semantics, 11,* 249–260.

Rogers, R. (Ed.). (1988). *Clinical assessment of malingering and deception.* New York: Guilford Press.

Rogers, R. C. (1984). *40-Hz EEG correlates of automatic and effortful information processing.* Unpublished doctoral dissertation, University of Houston.

Rorschach, H. (1954). *Psychodiagnostic plates* (5th ed.). New York: Grune & Stratton.

Rosen, G. (1946). Mesmerism and surgery: A strange chapter in the history of anesthesia. *Journal of the History of Medicine,* October, 527–551.

Rosen, H. (1960). Hypnosis: Applications and misapplications. *Journal of the American Medical Association, 172,* 683–687.

Rosen, H., & Bartemeir, L. H. (1961). Hypnosis in medical practice. *Journal of the American Medical Association, 175,* 976–979.

Rosenberg, M. J. (1969). The conditions and consequences of evaluation apprehension. In R. Rosenthal & R. S. Rosnow (Eds.), *Artifact in behavioral research* (pp. 67–89). New York: Academic Press.

Rosenhan, D. L., & Tomkins, S. S. (1964). On preference for hypnosis and hypnotizability. *International Journal of Clinical and Experimental Hypnosis, 12,* 109–114.

Rosenzweig, S., & Sarason, S. (1942). An experimental study of the triadic hypothesis: Reaction to frustration, ego-defense, and hypnotizability. I. Correlational approach. *Character and Personality, 11,* 1–14.

Ross, C. A., & Norton, G. R. (1989). Effects of hypnosis on the features of multiple personality disorder. *American Journal of Clinical Hypnosis, 32*(2), 99–105.

Ross, C. A., Norton, G. R., & Fraser, G. A. (1989). Evidence against the introgenesis of multiple personality. *Dissociation, 2,* 61–65.

Ross, C. A., Norton, G. R., & Wozney, K. (1989). Multiple personality disorder: An analysis of 236 cases. *Canadian Journal of Psychiatry, 34*(5), 413–418.

Rossi, A. M., Sturrock, J. B., & Solomon, P. (1963). Suggestion effects on reported imagery in sensory deprivation. *Perceptual and Motor Skills, 16,* 39–45.

Rossi, E. L. (1986). *The psychobiology of mind–body healing: New concepts of therapeutic hypnosis.* New York: Norton.

Rossi, E. L. (1989). Mind–body healing, not suggestion, is the essence of hypnosis: Invited discussion of Cohen's "Clinical uses of measures of hypnotizability." *American Journal of Clinical Hypnosis, 32,* 14–15.

Rossi, E. L., & Cheek, D. B. (1988). *Mind–body therapy: Ideodynamic healing in hypnosis.* New York: Norton.

Rothenberg, A. (1976). Homospatial thinking in creativity. *Archives of General Psychiatry, 33,* 17–26.

Rothmar, E. E. (1986). *The relationship between hypnotic ability and heart rate responsiveness to imagery.* Unpublished doctoral dissertation, University of Waterloo, Waterloo, Ontario, Canada.

Rubinfine, D. L. (1981). Reconstruction revisited: The question of the reconstruction of mental functioning during the earliest months of life. In S. Tuttman, C. Kaye, & M. Zimmerman (Eds.). *Object and self: A developmental approach: Essays in honor of Edith Jacobson* (pp. 383–395). New York: International Universities Press.

Ruch, J. C. (1975). Self-hypnosis: The result of heterohypnosis or vice versa? *International Journal of Clinical and Experimental Hypnosis, 23,* 282–304.

Ruch, J. C., Morgan, A. H., & Hilgard, E. R. (1974). Measuring hypnotic responsiveness: A comparison of the Barber Suggestibility Scale and the Stanford Hypnotic Susceptibility Scale, Form A. *International Journal of Clinical and Experimental Hypnosis, 22,* 365–376.

Saavedra, R. L., & Miller, R. J. (1983). The influence of experimentally induced expectations on responses to the Harvard Group Scale of Hypnotic Susceptibility, Form A. *International Journal of Clinical and Experimental Hypnosis, 31,* 37–46.

Sabourin, M. E. (1982). Hypnosis and brain function: EEG correlates of state–trait differences. *Research Communications in Psychology, Psychiatry, and Behavior, 7,* 149–168.

Sabourin, M. E., Cutcomb, S. D., Crawford, H. J., & Pribram, K. H. (1990). EEG correlates of hypnotic susceptibility and hypnotic trance: Spectral analysis and coherence. *International Journal of Psychophysiology, 10,* 125–142.

Saccuzzo, D. P., Safran, D., Anderson, V., & McNeill, B. (1982). Visual information processing in high and low susceptible subjects. *International Journal of Clinical and Experimental Hypnosis, 30,* 32–44.

Sachs, L. B. (1971). Construing hypnosis as modifiable behavior. In A. Jacobs & L. B. Sachs (Eds.), *Psychology of private events* (pp. 65–71). New York: Academic Press.

Sachs, L. B., & Anderson, W. L. (1967). Modification of hypnotic susceptibility. *International Journal of Clinical and Experimental Hypnosis, 15,* 172–180.

Sackheim, H. A., Nordlie, J. W., & Gur, R. C. (1979). A model of hysterical and hypnotic blindness: Cognition, motivation, and awareness. *Journal of Abnormal Psychology, 88,* 474–489.

St. Jean, R., & Coe, W. C. (1981). Recall and recognition memory during posthypnotic amnesia: A failure to confirm the disrupted-search hypothesis and the memory disorganization hypothesis. *Journal of Abnormal Psychology, 90,* 231–241.

St. Jean, R., MacLeod, C., Coe, W. C., & Howard, M. L. (1982). Amnesia and hypnotic time estimation. *International Journal of Clinical and Experimental Hypnosis, 30,* 127–137.

St. Jean, R., & Robertson, L. (1986). Attentional versus absorptive processing in hypnotic time estimation. *Journal of Abnormal Psychology, 95,* 40–42.

Saletu, B. (1987). Brain function during hypnosis, acupuncture and transcendental meditation. In B. Taneli, C. Perris, & D. Kemali (Eds.), *Advances in biological psychiatry: Vol. 16. Neurophysiological correlates of relaxation and psychopathology* (pp. 18–40). Basel: Karger.

Salwen, R. S., Reznikoff, M., & Schwartz, F. (1989). Identity integration and ego pathology in disturbed adolescents. *Journal of ClinicalPsychology, 45,* 138–149.

Salzman, L. K. (1982). A clinical modification of the Experiential Analysis Technique. *Australian Journal of Clinical and Experimental Hypnosis, 10,* 43–55.

Sanders, B. L. (1979). *An examination of the relationship between hypnosis and functional brain asymmetry in dichotic listening tasks.* Unpublished doctoral dissertation, Georgia State University.

Sanders, G. S., & Simmons, W. L. (1983). Use of hypnosis to enhance eyewitness accuracy: Does it work? *Journal of Applied Psychology, 68,* 70–77.

Sanders, R. S., & Reyher, J. (1969). Sensory deprivation and the enhancement of hypnotic susceptibility. *Journal of Abnormal Psychology, 74,* 375–381.

Sanders, S. (1969). *The effect of hypnosis on visual imagery* (Doctoral dissertation, University of Kentucky, 1967). *Dissertation Abstracts International, 30,* 2936B. (University Microfilms No. 69-15, 484)

Sanders, S. (1976). Mutual group hypnosis as a catalyst in fostering creative problem-solving. *American Journal of Clinical Hypnosis, 19,* 62–66.

Sanders, S. (1978). Creative problem-solving and psychotherapy. *International Journal of Clinical and Experimental Hypnosis, 26,* 15–21.

Sanders, S. (1986). The Perceptual Alteration Scale: A scale measuring dissociation. *American Journal of Clinical Hypnosis, 29,* 95–102.

Sands, S. (1986). The use of hypnosis in establishing a holding environment to facilitate affect tolerance and integration in impulsive patients. *Psychiatry, 49,* 218–230.

Sarbin, T. R. (1950). Contributions to role-taking theory: I. Hypnotic behavior. *Psychological Review, 57,* 255–270.

Sarbin, T. R. (1956). Physiological effects of hypnotic stimulation. In R. M. Dorcus (Ed.), *Hypnosis and its therapeutic applications* (pp. 1–57). New York: McGraw-Hill.

Sarbin, T. R. (1962). Attempts to understand hypnotic phenomena. In L. Postman (Ed.), *Psychology in the making* (pp. 745–785). New York: Knopf.

Sarbin, T. R. (1972). Imagining as muted role-taking: A historical–linguistic analysis. In P. W. Sheehan (Ed.), *The function and nature of imagery* (pp. 333–354). New York: Academic Press.

Sarbin, T. R. (1984). Nonvolition in hypnosis: A semiotic analysis. *Psychological Record, 34,* 537–549.

Sarbin, T. R. (1989). The construction and reconstruction of hypnosis. In N. P. Spanos & J. F. Chaves (Eds.), *Hypnosis: The cognitive–behavioral perspective* (pp. 400–416). Buffalo, NY: Prometheus Books.

Sarbin, T. R., & Coe, W. C. (1972). *Hypnosis: A social psychological analysis of influence communication.* New York: Holt, Rinehart & Winston.

Sarbin, T. R., & Coe, W. C. (1979). Hypnosis and psychopathology: Replacing old myths with fresh metaphors. *Journal of Abnormal Psychology, 88,* 506–526.

Sarbin, T. R., & Juhasz, J. B. (1970). Toward a theory of imagination. *Journal of Personality, 38,* 52–76.

Sarbin, T. R., & Slagle, R. W. (1979). Hypnosis and psychophysiological outcomes. In E. Fromm & R. E. Shor (Eds.), *Hypnosis: Developments in research and new perspectives* (2nd ed., pp. 273–303). New York: Aldine.

Sarbini, J., & Silver, M. (1982). *Moralities of everyday life.* New York: Oxford University Press.

Scagnelli-Jobsis, J. (1982). Hypnosis with psychotic patients: A review of the literature and presentation of theoretical framework. *American Journal of Clinical Hypnosis, 25,* 33–45.

Schacter, D. L. (1977). EEG theta waves and psychological phenomena: A review and analysis. *Biological Psychology, 5,* 47–82.

Schafer, R. (1958). Regression in the service of the ego: The relevance of a psychoanalytic concept for personality assessment. In G. Lindzey (Ed.), *Assessment of human motives* (pp. 119–148). New York: Holt, Rinehart & Winston.

Scheflin, A. W., & Shapiro, J. L. (1989). *Trance on trial.* New York: Guilford Press.

Schumaker, J. F. (Ed.). (1991). *Human suggestibility: Advances in theory, research, and application.* New York: Routledge.

Schuyler, B. A., & Coe, W. C. (1981). A physiological investigation of volitional and nonvolitional experience during posthypnotic amnesia. *Journal of Personality and Social Psychology, 40,* 1160–1169.

Schuyler, B. A., & Coe, W. C. (1989). More on volitional experiences and breaching posthypnotic amnesia. *International Journal of Clinical and Experimental Hypnosis, 37,* 320–331.

Schwartz, F., & Lazar, Z. (1984). Contaminated thinking: A specimen of the primary process. *Psychoanalytic Psychology, 1,* 319–334.

Schwartz, G. E., Davidson, R. J., & Maer, F. (1975). Right hemisphere lateralization for emotion in the human brain: Interactions with cognition. *Science, 190,* 286–288.

Scott, M.J. (1960). *Hypnosis in skin and allergic diseases.* Springfield, IL: Charles C Thomas.

Sears, R. R. (1936). Functional abnormalities of memory with special reference to amnesia. *Psychological Bulletin, 33,* 229–274.

Segal, G., Huba, G. J., & Singer, J. L. (1980). *Drugs, daydreaming and personality: A study of college youth.* Hillsdale, NJ: Erlbaum.

Serafetinides, E. A. (1968). Electrophysiological responses to sensory stimulation under hypnosis. *American Journal of Psychiatry, 125,* 112–113.

Shagass, C., & Schwartz, M. (1964). Recovery functions of somatosensory peripheral nerve and cerebral evoked response in man. *Electroencephalography and Clinical Neurophysiology, 17,* 126–135.

Shapiro, J. L., & Diamond, M. J. (1972). Increases in hypnotizability as a function of encounter group training: Some confirming evidence. *Journal of Abnormal Psychology, 79,* 112–115.

Sharav, V., & Tal, M. (1989). Masseter inhibitory periods and sensations evoked by electrical tooth-pulp stimulation in subjects under hypnotic anesthesia. *Brain Research, 479,* 247–254.

Shaw, G. A., & Belmore, S. M. (1982–1983). Some relationships between imagery and creativity. *Imagination, Cognition and Personality, 2,* 115–123.

Shaw, G. A., & De Meers, S. T. (1986–1987). Relationships between imagery and creativity in high IQ children. *Imagination, Cognition and Personality, 6,* 247–262.

Sheehan, D. V., Latta, W. D., Regina, E. G., & Smith, G. M. (1979). Empirical assessment of Spiegel's Hypnotic Induction Profile and eye-roll hypothesis. *International Journal of Clinical and Experimental Hypnosis, 27,* 103–110.

Sheehan, P. W. (1967). A shortened form of Betts's questionnaire upon mental imagery. *Journal of Clinical Psychology, 23,* 386–389.

Sheehan, P. W. (1971a). A methodological analysis of the simulating technique. *International Journal of Clinical and Experimental Hypnosis, 19,* 83–99.

Sheehan, P. W. (1971b). Countering preconceptions about hypnosis: An objective index of involvement with the hypnotist [Monograph]. *Journal of Abnormal Psychology, 78,* 299–322.

Sheehan, P. W. (1977). Incongruity in trance behavior: A defining property of hypnosis? *Annals of the New York Academy of Sciences, 296,* 14–33.

Sheehan, P. W. (1979a). Hypnosis and the processes of imagination. In E. Fromm & R. E. Shor (Eds.), *Hypnosis: Developments in research and new perspectives* (2nd ed., pp. 381–411). New York: Aldine.

Sheehan, P. W. (1979b). Clinical and research hypnosis: Toward rapprochement. *Australian Journal of Clinical and Experimental Hypnosis, 7,* 135–146.

Sheehan, P. W. (1980). Factors influencing rapport in hypnosis. *Journal of Abnormal Psychology, 89,* 263–281.

Sheehan, P. W. (1982). Imagery and hypnosis: Forging a link, at least in part. *Research Communications in Psychology, Psychiatry, and Behavior, 7,* 257–272.

Sheehan, P. W. (1982–1983). Imaginative consciousness: Function, process and method. *Imagination, Cognition and Personality, 2,* 177–194.

Sheehan, P. W. (1988). Memory distortion in hypnosis. *International Journal of Clinical and Experimental Hypnosis, 36,* 296–311.

Sheehan, P. W. (1991). Hypnosis, context, and commitment. In S. J. Lynn & J. W. Rhue (Eds.), *Theories of hypnosis: Current models and perspectives* (pp. 520–541). New York: Guilford Press.

Sheehan, P. W., & Dolby, R. M. (1979). Motivated involvement of hypnosis: The illusion of clinical rapport through hypnotic dreams. *Journal of Abnormal Psychology, 88,* 573–583.

Sheehan, P. W., Donovan, P., & MacLeod, C. M. (1988). Strategy manipulation and the Stroop effect in hypnosis. *Journal of Abnormal Psychology, 97,* 455–460.

Sheehan, P. W., & Grigg, L. (1985). Hypnosis, memory and the acceptance of an implausible cognitive set. *British Journal of Experimental and Clinical Hypnosis, 3,* 5–12.

Sheehan, P. W., Grigg, L., & McCann, T. (1984). Memory distortion following exposure to false information in hypnosis. *Journal of Abnormal Psychology, 93,* 259–265.

Sheehan, P. W., & McConkey, K. M. (1979) Australian norms for the Harvard Group Scale of Hypnotic Susceptibility, Form A. *International Journal of Clinical and Experimental Hypnosis, 27,* 294–304.

Sheehan, P. W., & McConkey, K. M. (1982). *Hypnosis and experience: The exploration of phenomena and process.* Hillsdale, NJ: Erlbaum.

Sheehan, P. W., & McConkey, K. M. (in press). Forensic hypnosis: The application of ethical guidelines. In J. W. Rhue, S. J. Lynn, & I. Kirsch (Eds.), *Handbook of clinical hypnosis.* Washington, DC: American Psychological Association.

Sheehan, P. W., McConkey, J. M., & Cross, D. (1978). Experimental analysis of hypnosis: Some new observations on hypnotic phenomena. *Journal of Abnormal Psychology, 87*, 570–573.

Sheehan, P. W., & Orne, M. T. (1968). Some comments on the nature of posthypnotic behavior. *Journal of Nervous and Mental Disease, 146*, 209–220.

Sheehan, P. W., & Perry, C. (1976). *Methodologies of hypnosis: A critical appraisal of contemporary paradigms of hypnosis.* Hillsdale, NJ: Erlbaum.

Sheehan, P. W., & Statham, D. (1989). Hypnosis, the timing of its introduction, and acceptance of misleading information. *Journal of Abnormal Psychology, 98*, 170–176.

Sheehan, P. W., Statham, D., & Jamieson, G. A. (1991a). Pseudomemory effects over time in the hypnotic setting. *Journal of Abnormal Psychology, 100*, 39–44.

Sheehan, P. W., Statham, D., & Jamieson, G. A. (1991b). Pseudomemory effects and their relationship to level of susceptibility to hypnosis and state instructions. *Journal of Personality and Social Psychology, 60*, 130–137.

Sheehan, P. W., Statham, D., Jamieson, G. A., & Ferguson, S. R. (1991). Ambiguity in suggestion and the occurrence of pseudomemory in the hypnotic setting. *Australian Journal of Clinical and Experimental Hypnosis, 19*, 1–18.

Sheehan, P. W., & Tilden, J. (1983). Effects of suggestibility and hypnosis on accurate and distorted retrieval from memory. *Journal of Experimental Psychology: Learning, Memory, and Cognition, 9*, 283–293.

Sheehan, P. W., & Tilden, J. (1984). Real and simulated occurrences of memory distortion in hypnosis. *Journal of Abnormal Psychology, 93*, 47–57.

Sheehan, P. W., & Tilden, J. (1986). The consistency of occurrences of memory distortion following hypnotic induction. *International Journal of Clinical and Experimental Hypnosis, 34*, 122–137.

Sheer, D. E. (1970). Electrophysiological correlates of memory consolidation. In G. Unger (Ed.), *Molecular mechanisms in memory and learning* (pp. 177–211). New York: Plenum.

Sheer, D. E. (1976). Focused arousal, 40 Hz EEG. In R. M. Knight & D. J. Bakker (Eds.), *The neuropsychology of learning disorders* (pp. 71–87). Baltimore: University Park Press.

Sheer, D. E. (1984). Focused arousal, 40 Hz EEG and dysfunction. In T. Elbert, B. Rockstroh, W. Lutzenberg, & N. Birbaumer (Eds.), *Self-regulation of the brain and behavior* (pp. 63–84). Berlin: Springer-Verlag.

Sheer, D. E. (1989). Sensory and cognitive 40-Hz event-related potentials: Behavior correlates, brain function, and clinical applications. In E. Basar & T. H. Bullock (Eds.), *Brain dynamics 2* (pp. 339–374). Berlin: Springer-Verlag.

Sheikh, A. A., & Jordan, C. S. (1983). Clinical uses of mental imagery. In A. A. Sheikh (Ed.), *Imagery: Current theory, research, and application* (pp. 391–435). New York: Wiley.

Sherman, S. J., & Lynn, S. J. (1990). Social-psychological principles in Milton Erickson's psychotherapy. *British Journal of Experimental and Clinical Hypnosis, 7*, 37–46.

Shertzer, C. L., & Lookingbill, D. P. (1987). Effects of relaxation therapy and hypnotizability in chronic urticaria. *Archives of Dermatology, 123*, 913–916.

Shields, I. W., & Knox, V. J. (1986). Level of processing as a determinant of hypnotic hypermnesia. *Journal of Abnormal Psychology, 95*, 350–357.

Shiffrin, R., & Schneider, W. (1977). Controlled and automatic human information processing: II. Perceptual learning, automatic attending, and a general theory. *Psychological Review, 84,* 127–190.

Shor, R. E. (1959). Hypnosis and the concept of the generalized reality-orientation. *American Journal of Psychotherapy, 13,* 582–602.

Shor, R. E. (1960). The frequency of naturally occurring "hypnotic-like" experiences in the normal college population. *International Journal of Clinical and Experimental Hypnosis, 8,* 151–163.

Shor, R. E. (1962). Three dimensions of hypnotic depth, *International Journal of Clinical and Experimental Hypnosis, 10,* 23–38.

Shor, R. E. (1969). Hypnosis and the concept of the generalized reality-orientation. In C. E. Tart (Ed.), *Altered states of consciousness: A book of readings* (pp. 233–250). New York: Wiley. (Original work published 1959)

Shor, R. E. (1970). The three-factor theory of hypnosis as applied to the book-reading fantasy and to the concept of suggestion. *International Journal of Clinical and Experimental Hypnosis, 18,* 89–98.

Shor, R. E. (1971). Expectations of being influenced and hypnotic performance. *International Journal of Clinical and Experimental Hypnosis, 19,* 154–166.

Shor, R. E. (1979). A phenomenological method for the measurement of variables important to an understanding of the nature of hypnosis. In E. Fromm & R. E. Shor (Eds.), *Hypnosis: Developments in research and new perspectives* (2nd ed., pp. 105–135). New York: Aldine.

Shor, R. E., & Cobb, J. C. (1968). An exploratory study of hypnotic training using the concept of plateau responsiveness as a referent. *American Journal of Clinical Hypnosis, 10,* 178–193.

Shor, R. E., & Orne, E. C. (1962). *Harvard Group Scale of Hypnotic Susceptibility, Form A.* Palo Alto, CA: Consulting Psychologists Press.

Shor, R. E., & Orne, E. C. (1963). Norms on the Harvard Group Scale of Hypnotic Susceptibility: Form A. *International Journal of Clinical and Experimental Hypnosis, 11,* 39–47.

Shor, R. E., Orne, M. T., & O'Connell, D. N. (1962). Validation and cross-validation of a scale of self-reported personal experiences which predicts hypnotizability. *Journal of Psychology, 53,* 55–75.

Shor, R. E., Orne, M. T., & O'Connell, D. N. (1966). Psychological correlates of plateau hypnotizability in a special volunteer sample. *Journal of Personality and Social Psychology, 3,* 80–95.

Shor, R. E., Pistole, D. D., Easton, R. D., & Kihlstrom, J. F. (1984). Relation of predicted to actual hypnotic responsiveness, with special reference to posthypnotic amnesia. *International Journal of Clinical and Experimental Hypnosis, 32,* 376–387.

Shostrom, E. (1972). *Manual for the Personality Orientation Inventory (POI): An inventory for the measurement of self actualization.* San Diego: Educational and Industrial Testing Service.

Sidis, B. (Ed.). (1902). *Psychopathological researches: Studies in mental dissociation.* New York: Stechert.

Sigman, A., Phillips, K. C., & Clifford, B. (1985). Attentional concomitants of hypnotic susceptibility. *British Journal of Experimental and Clinical Hypnosis, 2,* 69–75.

Silber, S. (1980). Induction of hypnosis by poetic hypnogram. *American Journal of Clinical Hypnosis, 22,* 212–215.

Silva, C. E. (1990). *Response expectancy versus interpretational set as mediators of hypnotic response.* Unpublished doctoral dissertation, University of Connecticut.

Silva, C. E., & Kirsch, I. (1987). Breaching hypnotic amnesia by manipulating expectancy. *Journal of Abnormal Psychology, 96,* 325–329.

Silverman, L. H. (1965). Regression in the service of the ego: A case study. *Journal of Projective Techniques and Personality Assessment, 29,* 232–244.

Sinclair-Gieben, A. H. C., & Chalmers, D. (1959). Evaluation of treatment of warts by hypnosis. *Lancet, ii,* 480–482.

Singer, J. L. (1966). *Daydreaming: An introduction to the experimental study of inner experiences.* New York: Random House.

Singer, J. L. (1975a). *The inner world of daydreaming.* New York: Harper.

Singer, J. L. (1975b). Navigating the stream of consciousness: Research in daydreaming and related inner experience. *American Psychologist, 30,* 727–738.

Singer, J. L. (1978). The constructive potential of imagery and fantasy processes. In E. Witenberg (Ed.), *Recent developments in interpersonal psychoanalysis.* New York: Gardner Press.

Singer, J. L., & Antrobus, J. S. (1972). Daydreaming, imaginal processes and personality: A normative study. In P. W. Sheehan (Ed.), *The function and nature of imagery.* New York: Academic Press.

Singer, J. L., & Bonanno, G. A. (1990). Personality and private experience: Individual variations in consciousness and in attention to subjective phenomena. In L. Pervin (Ed.), *Handbook of personality: Theory and research* (pp. 419–439). New York: Guilford Press.

Singer, J. L., & Pope, K. S. (1981). Daydreaming and imagery skills as predisposing capacities for self-hypnosis. *International Journal of Clinical and Experimental Hypnosis, 29,* 271–281.

Siuta, J. (1989). Normative and psychometric characteristics of a Polish version of the Creative Imagination Scale. *International Journal of Clinical and Experimental Hypnosis, 35,* 51–58.

Smith, J. M., & Schaefer, C. E. (1969). Development of a creativity scale for the Adjective Check List. *Psychological Reports, 25,* 87–92.

Smith, M. C. (1983). Hypnotic memory enhancement of witnesses: Does it work? *Psychological Bulletin, 94,* 387–407.

Smith, M. S., Womack, W. M., & Chen, A. C. N. (1989). Hypnotizability does not predict outcome of behavioral treatment of pediatric headache. *American Journal of Clinical Hypnosis, 31,* 237–241.

Smith-Rosenberg, C. (1972). The hysterical woman: Some reflections on sex role conflict in 19th century America. *Social Research, 38,* 652–678.

Smyth, L. D., & Lowy, D. (1983). Auditory vigilance during hypnosis: A brief communication. *International Journal of Clinical and Experimental Hypnosis, 31,* 67–71.

Snodgrass, M. J., & Lynn, S. J. (1989). Music absorption and hypnotizability. *International Journal of Clinical and Experimental Hypnosis, 37,* 41–54.

Solomon, G. F., & Amkraut, A. A. (1981). Psychoneuroendocrinological effects on the immune response. *Annual Review of Microbiology, 35,* 155–184.

Somer, E. (1990). Brief simultaneous couple hypnotherapy with a rape victim and her spouse: A brief communication. *International Journal of Clinical and Experimental Hypnosis, 38,* 1–5.

Spanos, N. P. (1970). Barber's reconceptualization of hypnosis: An evaluation of criticisms. *Journal of Experimental Research in Personality, 4,* 241–258.

Spanos, N. P. (1971). Goal-directed fantasy and the performance of hypnotic test suggestions. *Psychiatry, 34,* 86–96.

Spanos, N. P. (1982a). A social psychological approach to hypnotic behavior. In G. Weary & H. L. Mirels (Eds.), *Integrations of clinical and social psychology* (pp. 231–271). New York: Oxford University Press.

Spanos, N. P. (1982b). Hypnotic behavior: A cognitive social psychological perspective. *Research Communications in Psychology, Psychiatry, and Behavior, 7,* 199–213.

Spanos, N. P. (1983). *The Carleton University Responsiveness to Suggestion Scale (Group Administration).* Unpublished manuscript, Carleton University, Ottawa, Ontario, Canada.

Spanos, N. P. (1986a). Hypnosis and the modification of hypnotic susceptibility: A social psychological perspective. In P. L. N. Naish (Ed.), *What is hypnosis? Current theories and research* (pp. 85–120). Philadelphia: Open University Press.

Spanos, N. P. (1986b). Hypnotic behavior: A social psychological interpretation of amnesia, analgesia, and "trance logic." *Behavioral and Brain Sciences, 9,* 449–467.

Spanos, N. P. (1986c). Hypnosis, nonvolitional responding, and multiple personality: A social psychological perspective. In B. Maher & W. Maher (Eds.), *Progress in experimental personality research* (Vol. 14, pp. 1–62). New York: Academic Press.

Spanos, N. P. (1987). Hypnotic behavior: Special process accounts are still not required. *Behavioral and Brain Sciences, 10,* 776–781.

Spanos, N. P. (1989). Experimental research on hypnotic analgesia. In N. P. Spanos & J. F. Chaves (Eds.), *Hypnosis: The cognitive–behavioral perspective* (pp. 206–240). Buffalo, NY: Prometheus Books.

Spanos, N. P. (1991). A sociocognitive approach to hypnosis. In S. J. Lynn & J. W. Rhue (Eds.), *Theories of hypnosis: Current models and perspectives* (pp. 324–361) New York: Guilford Press.

Spanos, N. P., & Barber, T. X. (1968). "Hypnotic" experiences as inferred from subjective reports: Auditory and visual hallucinations. *Journal of Experimental Research in Personality, 3,* 136–150.

Spanos, N. P., & Barber, T. X. (1972). Cognitive activity during "hypnotic" suggestibility: Goal-directed fantasy and the experience of nonvolition. *Journal of Personality, 40,* 510–524.

Spanos, N. P., & Barber, T. X. (1974). Toward a convergence in hypnosis research. *American Psychologist, 29,* 500–511.

Spanos, N. P., & Bodorik, H. L. (1977). Suggested amnesia and disorganized recall in hypnotic and task-motivated subjects. *Journal of Abnormal Psychology, 86,* 295–305.

Spanos, N. P., Brett, P. J., Menary, E. P., & Cross, W. P. (1987). A measure of attitudes toward hypnosis: Relationships with absorption and hypnotic susceptibility. *American Journal of Clinical Hypnosis, 30,* 139–150.

Spanos, N. P., Bridgeman, M., Stam, H. J., Gwynn, M. I., & Saad, C. I. (1982–1983). When seeing is not believing: The effects of contextual variables on the reports of hypnotic hallucinations. *Imagination, Cognition and Personality, 2,* 195–209.

Spanos, N. P., Burgess, C. A., Cocco, L., & Pinch, N. (1991). *Compliance, and response to difficult suggestions in highly hypnotizable subjects*. Unpublished manuscript, Carleton University, Ottawa, Ontario, Canada.

Spanos, N. P., Burgess, C. A., Cross, W. P., & McCleod, G. (1992). Hypnosis, compliance and suggested negative hallucinations. *Journal of Abnormal Psychology, 101*, 192–199.

Spanos, N. P., Burgess, C. A., & Perlini, A. H. (1992). Compliance and suggested deafness in hypnotic and nonhypnotic subjects. *Imagination, Cognition and Personality, 11*, 211–223.

Spanos, N. P., Burgess, C. A., Roncon, V., & Wallace-Capretta, S. (1991). *Surreptitiously observed hypnotizability in simulators, and in skill-trained and untrained high hypnotizables*. Unpublished manuscript, Carleton University, Ottawa, Ontario, Canada.

Spanos, N. P., & Chaves, J. F. (1989a). The cognitive–behavioral alternative in hypnosis research. In N. P. Spanos & J. F. Chaves (Eds.), *Hypnosis: The cognitive–behavioral perspective* (pp. 9–16). Buffalo, NY: Prometheus Books.

Spanos, N. P., & Chaves, J. F. (1989b). The cognitive–behavioral perspective: Synopsis and suggestions for research. In N. P. Spanos & J. F. Chaves (Eds.), *Hypnosis: The cognitive–behavioral perspective* (pp. 437–446). Buffalo, NY: Prometheus Books.

Spanos, N. P., & Chaves, J. F. (Eds.). (1989c). *Hypnosis: The cognitive–behavioral perspective*. Buffalo, NY: Prometheus Books.

Spanos, N. P., & Chaves, J. F. (1989d). Hypnotic analgesia and surgery: In defense of the social-psychological position. *British Journal of Experimental and Clinical Hypnosis, 6*, 131–139.

Spanos, N. P., Cobb, P. C., & Gorassini, D. R. (1985). Failing to resist hypnotic test suggestions: A strategy for self-presenting as deeply hypnotized. *Psychiatry, 48*, 282–292.

Spanos, N. P., Cross, W. P., Menary, E. P., Brett, P. J., & de Groh, M. (1987). Attitudinal and imaginal ability predictors of social cognitive skill-training enhancements in hypnotic susceptibility. *Personality and Social Psychology Bulletin, 13*, 379–398.

Spanos, N. P., Cross, W. P., Menary, E. P., & Smith, J. (1988). Long term effects of cognitive skill training for the enhancement of hypnotic susceptibility. *British Journal of Experimental and Clinical Hypnosis, 5*, 73–78.

Spanos, N. P., & de Groh, M. (1983). Structure of communication and reports of involuntariness by hypnotic and nonhypnotic subjects. *Perceptual and Motor Skills, 57*, 1179–1186.

Spanos, N. P., & de Groh, M. (1984). *Effects of active and passive wording of inattention strategies on response to suggestions for complete selective amnesia*. Unpublished manuscript, Carleton University, Ottawa, Ontario, Canada.

Spanos, N. P., de Groh, M. & de Groot, H. P. (1987). Skill training for enhancing hypnotic susceptibility and word list amnesia. *British Journal of Experimental and Clinical Hypnosis, 4*, 15–23.

Spanos, N. P., de Groot, H. P., & Gwynn, M. I. (1987). Trance logic as incomplete responding. *Journal of Personality and Social Psychology, 53*, 911–921.

Spanos, N. P., de Groot, H. P., Tiller, D. K., Weekes, J. R., & Bertrand, L. D. (1985). "Trance logic" duality and hidden observer responding in hypnotic, imagination control, and simulating subjects. *Journal of Abnormal Psychology, 94,* 611–623.

Spanos, N. P., & D'Eon, J. L. (1980). Hypnotic amnesia, disorganized recall, and inattention. *Journal of Abnormal Psychology, 89,* 744–750.

Spanos, N. P., DuBreuil, S. C. & Gabora, N. J. (1991). Four month followup of skill-training-induced enhancements in hypnotizability. *Contemporary Hypnosis, 8,* 25–32.

Spanos, N. P., & Flynn, D. M. (1989a). Simulation, compliance and skill training in the enhancement of hypnotizability. *British Journal of Experimental and Clinical Hypnosis, 6,* 1–8.

Spanos, N. P., & Flynn, D. M. (1989b). Compliance, imaginal correlates and skill training [Authors' reply to discussion commentary by E. R. Hilgard]. *British Journal of Experimental and Clinical Hypnosis, 6,* 12–15.

Spanos, N. P., Flynn, D. M., & Gabora, N. (1989). Suggested negative visual hallucinations in hypnotic subjects: When no means yes. *British Journal of Experimental and Clinical Hypnosis, 6,* 63–67.

Spanos, N. P., Flynn, D. M., & Gwynn, M. I. (1988). Contextual demands, negative hallucinations, and hidden observer responding: Three hidden observers observed. *British Journal of Experimental and Clinical Hypnosis, 5,* 5–10.

Spanos, N. P., Flynn, D. M., & Niles, J. (1989–1990). Rapport and cognitive skill training in the enhancement of hypnotizability. *Imagination, Cognition and Personality, 9,* 245–262.

Spanos, N. P., Gabora, N. J., Jarrett, L. E., & Gwynn, M. I. (1989). Contextual determinants of hypnotizability and of the relationships between hypnotizability scales. *Journal of Personality and Social Psychology, 57,* 271–278.

Spanos, N. P., & Gorassini, D. R. (1984). Structure of hypnotic test suggestions and attributions of responding involuntarily. *Journal of Personality and Social Psychology, 46,* 688–696.

Spanos, N. P., & Gottlieb, J. (1979). Demonic possession, mesmerism, and hysteria: A social psychological perspective on their historical interrelations. *Journal of Abnormal Psychology, 88,* 527–546.

Spanos, N. P., Gwynn, M. I., Comer, S. L., Baltruweit, W. J., & de Groh, M. (1989). Are hypnotically induced pseudomemories resistant to cross-examination? *Law and Human Behavior, 13,* 271–289.

Spanos, N. P., Gwynn, M. I., Della Malva, C. L., & Bertrand, L. D. (1988). Social psychological factors in the genesis of posthypnotic source amnesia. *Journal of Abnormal Psychology, 97,* 322–329.

Spanos, N. P., Gwynn, M. I., & Stam, H. J. (1983). Instructional demands and ratings of overt and hidden pain during hypnotic analgesia. *Journal of Abnormal Psychology, 92,* 479–488.

Spanos, N. P., Gwynn, M. I., & Terrade, K. (1989). Effects on mock jurors of experts favorable and unfavorable toward hypnotically elicited eyewitness testimony. *Journal of Applied Psychology, 74,* 922–926.

Spanos, N. P., & Ham, M. W. (1973). Cognitive activity in response to hypnotic suggestions: Goal-directed fantasy and selective amnesia. *American Journal of Clinical Hypnosis, 15,* 191–198.

Spanos, N. R., & Ham, M. W. (1975). Involvement in suggestion-related imaginings and the "hypnotic dream." *American Journal of Clinical Hypnosis, 18,* 43–51.

Spanos, N. P., Ham, M. W., & Barber, T. X. (1973). Suggested ("hypnotic") visual hallucinations: Experimental and phenomenological data. *Journal of Abnormal Psychology, 92,* 479–488.

Spanos, N. P., & Hewitt, E. C. (1980). The hidden observer in hypnotic analgesia: Discovery or experimental creation? *Journal of Personality and Social Psychology, 39,* 1201–1214.

Spanos, N., Hodgins, D. C., Stam, H. J., & Gwynn, M. I. (1984). Suffering for science: The effects of implicit social demands on response to experimentally induced pain. *Journal of Personality and Social Psychology, 46,* 1162–1172.

Spanos, N. P., Horton, C., & Chaves, J. R. (1975). The effects of two cognitive strategies on pain threshold. *Journal of Abnormal Psychology, 84,* 677–681.

Spanos, N. P., Jones, B., & Malfara, A. (1982). Hypnotic deafness: Now you hear it—now you still hear it. *Journal of Abnormal Psychology, 91,* 75–77.

Spanos, N. P., & Katsanis, J. (1989). Effects of instructional set on attributions of nonvolition during hypnotic and nonhypnotic analgesia. *Journal of Personality and Social Psychology, 56,* 182–188.

Spanos, N. P., Kennedy, S. K., & Gwynn, M. I. (1984). Moderating effects of contextual variables on the relationship between hypnotic susceptibility and suggested analgesia. *Journal of Abnormal Psychology, 93,* 285–294.

Spanos, N. P., Lush, N. I., & Gwynn, M. I. (1989). Cognitive skill training enhancements of hypnotizability: Generalization effects and trance logic responding. *Journal of Personality and Social Psychology, 56,* 795–804.

Spanos, N. P., Lush, N. I., Smith, J. E., & de Groh, M. M. (1986). Effects of two hypnotic induction procedures on overt and subjective response to two measures of hypnotic susceptibility. *Psychological Reports, 59,* 1227–1230.

Spanos, N. P., Mah, C. D., Pawlak, A. E., D'Eon, J. L., & Ritchie, G. (1980). *A multivariate and factor analytic study of hypnotic susceptibility.* Unpublished manuscript, Carleton University, Ottawa, Ontario, Canada.

Spanos, N. P., & McLean, J. (1986). Hypnotically created pseudomemories: Memory distortions or reporting biases? *British Journal of Experimental and Clinical Hypnosis, 3,* 155–159.

Spanos, N. P., McNeil, C., Gwynn, M. I., & Stam, H. J. (1984). Effects of suggestion and distraction on reported pain in subjects high and low on hypnotic susceptibility. *Journal of Abnormal Psychology, 93,* 277–284.

Spanos, N. P., & McPeake, J. D. (1974). Involvement in suggestion-related imaginings, experienced involuntariness and credibility assigned to imaginings in hypnotic subjects. *Journal of Abnormal Psychology, 83,* 687–690.

Spanos, N. P., & McPeake, J. D. (1975a). Involvement in everyday imaginative activities, attitudes toward hypnosis, and hypnotic suggestibility. *Journal of Personality and Social Psychology, 31,* 594–598.

Spanos, N. P., & McPeake, J. D. (1975b). The interaction of attitudes toward hypnosis and involvement in everyday imaginative activities on hypnotic susceptibility. *American Journal of Clinical Hypnosis, 17,* 247–252.

Spanos, N. P., & McPeake, J. D. (1977). Cognitive strategies, goal-directed fantasy, and response to suggestions in hypnotic subjects. *American Journal of Clinical Hypnosis, 20,* 114–123.

Spanos, N. P., McPeake, J. D., & Churchill, N. (1976). Relationships between imaginative ability variables and the Barber Suggestibility Scales. *American Journal of Clinical Hypnosis, 19,* 39–46.

Spanos, N. P., Menary, E., Gabora, N. J., DuBreuil, S. C., & Dewherst, B. (1991). Secondary identity enactments during hypnotic past-life regression: A sociocognitive perspective. *Journal of Personality and Social Psychology,*

Spanos, N. P., Mullens, D., & Rivers, S. M. (1979). The effects of suggestion structure and hypnotic vs. task-motivation instructions on response to hallucination suggestions. *Journal of Research on Personality, 13,* 59–70.

Spanos, N. P., Perlini, A. H., Patrick, L., Bell, S. & Gwynn, M. I. (1990). The role of compliance in hypnotic and nonhypnotic analgesia. *Journal of Research in Personality, 24,* 433–453.

Spanos, N. P., Perlini, A. H., & Robertson, L. A. (1989). Hypnosis, suggestion, and placebo in the reduction of experimental pain. *Journal of Abnormal Psychology, 98,* 285–293.

Spanos, N. P., & Radtke, H. L. (1982). Hypnotic amnesia as a strategic enactment: A cognitive social-psychological perspective. *Research Communications in Psychology, Psychiatry, and Behavior, 7,* 215–231.

Spanos, N. P., Radtke, H. L., & Bertrand, L. D. (1984). Hypnotic amnesia as a strategic enactment: Breaching amnesia in highly susceptible subjects. *Journal of Personality and Social Psychology, 47,* 1155–1169.

Spanos, N. P., Radtke, L. H., & Dubreuil, D. L. (1982). Episodic and semantic memory in posthypnotic amnesia: A reevaluation. *Journal of Personality and Social Psychology, 43,* 565–573.

Spanos, N. P., Radtke, H. L., Hodgins, D. C., Bertrand, L. D., Stam, H. J., & Dubreuil, D. L. (1983). The Carleton University Responsiveness to Suggestion Scale: Stability, reliability, and relationships with expectancy and "hypnotic experiences." *Psychological Reports, 53,* 555–563.

Spanos, N. P., Radtke, H. L., Hodgins, D. C., Bertrand, L. D., Stam, H. J., & Moretti, P. (1983). The Carleton University Responsiveness to Suggestion Scale: Relationship with other measures of hypnotic susceptibility, expectancies, and absorption. *Psychological Reports, 53,* 723–734.

Spanos, N. P., Radtke, H. L., Hodgins, D. C., Stam, H. J., & Bertrand, L. D. (1983). The Carleton University Responsiveness to Suggestion Scale: Normative data and psychometric properties. *Psychological Reports, 53,* 523–535.

Spanos, N. P., Radtke-Bodorik, H. L., Ferguson, J. D., & Jones, B. (1979). The effects of hypnotic susceptibility, suggestions for analgesia, and the utilization of cognitive strategies on the reduction of pain. *Journal of Abnormal Psychology, 88,* 282–292.

Spanos, N. P., Radtke-Bodorik, H. L., & Stam, H. J. (1980). Disorganized recall during suggested amnesia: Fact not artifact. *Journal of Abnormal Psychology, 89,* 1–19.

Spanos, N. P., Rivers, S. M., & Gottlieb, J. (1978). Hypnotic responsivity, meditation and laterality of eye-movements. *Journal of Abnormal Psychology, 87,* 566–569.

Spanos, N. P., Rivers, S., & Ross, S. (1977). Experienced involuntariness in response to hypnotic suggestions. In W. E. Edmonston, Jr. (Ed.), *Conceptual and investigative approaches to hypnosis and hypnotic phenomena. Annals of the New York Academy of Sciences, 296,* 208–221.

Spanos, N. P., Robertson, L. A., Menary, E. P., & Brett, P. J. (1986). Component analysis of cognitive skill training for the enhancement of hypnotic susceptibility. *Journal of Abnormal Psychology, 95,* 350–357.

Spanos, N. P., Robertson, L. A., Menary, E. P., Brett, P. J., & Smith, J. (1987). Effects of repeated baseline testing on cognitive-skill-training-induced increments in hypnotic susceptibility. *Journal of Personality and Social Psychology, 52*, 1230–1235.

Spanos, N. P., Salas, J., Bertrand, L. D., & Johnston, J. (1988–1989). Occurrence schemas, context ambiguity and hypnotic responding. *Imagination, Cognition and Personality, 8*, 235–247.

Spanos, N. P., Salas, J., Menary, E. P., & Brett, P. J. (1986). Comparison of overt and subjective responses to the Carleton University Responsiveness to Suggestion Scale and the Stanford Hypnotic Susceptibility Scale under conditions of group administration. *Psychological Reports, 58*, 847–856.

Spanos, N. P., Spillane, J., & McPeake, J. C. (1976). Suggestion elaborateness, goal-directed fantasy, and response to suggestion in hypnotic and task-motivated subjects. *American Journal of Clinical Hypnosis, 18*, 254–262.

Spanos, N. P., Stam, H. J., D'Eon, J. L., Pawlak, A. E., & Radtke-Bodorik, H. (1980). The effects of social psychological variables on hypnotic amnesia. *Journal of Personality and Social Psychology, 39*, 737–750.

Spanos, N. P., Steggles, S., Radtke-Bodorik, H. L., & Rivers, S. M. (1979). Nonanalytic attending, hypnotic susceptibility, and psychological well-being in trained meditators and nonmeditators. *Journal of Abnormal Psychology, 88*, 85–87.

Spanos, N. P., Stenstrom, R. J., & Johnston, J. C. (1988). Hypnosis, placebo and suggestion in the treatment of warts. *Psychosomatic Medicine, 50*, 245–260.

Spanos, N. P., Tkachyk, M. E., Bertrand, L. D., & Weekes, J. R. (1984). The dissipation hypothesis of hypnotic amnesia: More disconfirming evidence. *Psychological Reports, 55*, 191–196.

Spanos, N. P., Weekes, J. R., & de Groh, M. (1984). The "involuntary" countering of suggested requests: A test of the ideomotor hypothesis of hypnotic responsiveness. *British Journal of Experimental and Clinical Hypnosis, 1*, 3–11.

Spanos, N. P., Williams, V., & Gwynn, M. I. (1990). Effects of hypnotic, placebo, and salicylic acid treatments on wart regression. *Psychosomatic Medicine, 52*, 109–114.

Spellacy, F., & Wilkinson, R. (1987). Dichotic listening and hypnotizability: Variability in ear preference. *Perceptual and Motor Skills, 64*, 1279–1284.

Spence, D. P., & Holland, B. (1962). The restricting effects of awareness: A paradox and an explanation. *Journal of Abnormal and Social Psychology, 64*, 163–174.

Sperling, G. (1960). The information available in brief visual presentations. *Psychological Momographs, 74*(11, Whole No. 498).

Spiegel, D. (1986). Dissociating damage. *American Journal of Clinical Hypnosis, 29*, 123–131.

Spiegel, D. (1989). Cortical event-related evoked potential correlates of hypnotic hallucinations. In V. A. Gheorghiu, P. Netter, H. J. Eysenck, & R. Rosenthal (Eds.), *Suggestion and suggestibility: Theory and research* (pp. 183–189). Berlin: Springer–Verlag.

Spiegel, D., & Albert, L. H. (1983). Naloxone fails to reverse hypnotic alleviation of chronic pain. *Psychopharmacology, 81*, 140–143.

Spiegel, D., & Barabasz, A. F. (1987). Psychophysiology of hypnotic hallucinations. In R. G. Kunzendorf & A. A. Sheikh (Eds.), *Psychophysiology of mental imagery: Theory, research, and application* (pp. 133–145). New York: Baywood.

Spiegel, D., & Barabasz, A. F. (1988). Effects of hypnotic instructions on P300 event-related-potential amplitudes: Research and clinical applications. *American Journal of Clincal Hypnosis, 31*, 11–17.

Spiegel, D., & Bloom, J. R. (1983). Group therapy and hypnosis reduce metastatic breast carcinoma pain. *Psychosomatic Medicine, 45*, 333–339.

Spiegel, D., Bierre, P., & Rootenberg, J. (1989). Hypnotic alteration of somatosensory perception. *American Journal of Psychiatry, 146*, 749–754.

Spiegel, D., Bloom, J. R., Kraemer, H. C., & Gottheil, E. (1989). Effect of psychosocial treatment on survival of patients with metastatic breast cancer. *Lancet, ii*, 888–891.

Spiegel, D., Cutcomb, S., Ren, C., & Pribram, K. (1985). Hypnotic hallucination alters evoked potentials. *Journal of Abnormal Psychology, 94*, 249–255.

Spiegel, D., Detrick, K., & Frischholz, E. (1982). Hypnotizability and psychopathology. *American Journal of Psychiatry, 136*, 777–781.

Spiegel, D., Hunt, T., & Dondershine, H. E. (1988). Dissociation and hypnotizability in posttraumatic stress disorder. *American Journal of Psychiatry, 145*(3), 301–305.

Spiegel, H. (1970). A single treatment method to stop smoking using ancillary self-hypnosis. *International Journal of Clinical and Experimental Hypnosis, 4*, 235–250.

Spiegel, H. (1972). An eye-roll test for hypnotizability. *American Journal of Clinical Hypnosis, 15*, 25–28.

Spiegel, H. (1990, October). *Bio-psycho-social theory of hypnosis.* Paper presented at the 41st Annual Meeting of the Society for Clinical and Experimental Hypnosis. Tucson, AZ.

Spiegel, H., & Bridger, A. A. (1970). *Manual for the Hypnotic Induction Profile.* New York: Soni Medica.

Spiegel, H., & Spiegel, D. (1978). *Trance and treatment: Clinical uses of hypnosis.* New York: Basic Books.

Spinhoven, P. (1987). Hypnosis and behavior therapy: A review. *International Journal of Clinical and Experimental Hypnosis, 35*, 8–31.

Spinhoven, P. (1988). Similarities and dissimilarities in hypnotic and nonhypnotic procedures for headache control: A review. *American Journal of Clinical Hypnosis, 30*, 183–194.

Spinhoven, P., Baak, D., Van Dyck, R., & Vermeulen, P. (1988). The effectiveness of an authoritative versus permissive style of hypnotic communication. *Journal of Personality and Social Psychology, 36*, 182–191.

Spinhoven, P., & Linssen, A. C. (1989). Education and self-hypnosis in the management of low back pain: A component analysis. *British Journal of Clinical Psychology, 28*, 145–153.

Spitz, R. A. (1965). *The first year of life: A psychoanalytic study of normal and deviant development of object relations.* New York: International Universities Press.

Springer, C. J., Sachs, L. B., & Morrow, J. E. (1977). Group methods of increasing hypnotic susceptibility. *International Journal of Clinical and Experimental Hypnosis, 25*, 184–191.

Spydell, J. D., Ford, M. R., & Sheer, D. E. (1979). Task dependent cerebral lateralization of the 40–Hz EEG rhythm. *Psychophysiology, 16*, 347–350.

Spydell, J. D., & Sheer, D. E. (1982). Effect of problem solving on right and left hemisphere 40 Hz EEG activity. *Psychophysiology, 19*, 420–425.

Stager, G. L., & Lundy, R. M. (1985). Hypnosis and the learning and recall of visually presented material. *International Journal of Clinical and Experimental Hypnosis, 33*, 27–39.

Stalnaker, J. M., & Riddle, E. E. (1932). The effect of hypnosis on long-delayed recall. *Journal of General Psychology, 6*, 429–440.

Stam, H. J. (1989). From symptom relief to cure: Hypnotic interventions in cancer. In N. P. Spanos & J. F. Chaves (Eds.), *Hypnosis: The cognitive–behavioral perspective* (pp. 313–339). Buffalo, NY: Prometheus Books.

Stam, H. J., McGrath, P. A., & Brooke, R. I. (1984). The effects of a cognitive–behavioral treatment program on temporo-mandibular pain and dysfunction syndrome. *Psychosomatic Medicine, 46*, 534–545.

Stam, H. J., McGrath, P. A., Brooke, R. I., & Cosier, F. (1986). Hypnotizability and the treatment of chronic facial pain. *International Journal of Clinical and Experimental Hypnosis, 34*, 182–191.

Stam, H. J., Radtke-Bodorik, L., & Spanos, N. P. (1980). Repression and hypnotic amnesia: A failure to replicate and an alternative formulation. *Journal of Abnormal Psychology, 89*, 551–559.

Stam, H. J., & Spanos, N. P. (1980). Experimental designs, expectancy effects, and hypnotic analgesia. *Journal of Abnormal Psychology, 89*, 751–762.

Stanton, H. E. (1978). A one-session hypnotic approach to modifying smoking behavior. *International Journal of Clinical and Experimental Hypnosis, 26*, 22–24.

Stanton, H. E. (1987). Alcoholism and hypnosis: Three case studies. *Australian Journal of Clinical and Experimental Hypnosis, 15*, 39–46.

Stanton, H. E. (1989a). Hypnotic relaxation and the reduction of sleep onset insomnia. *International Journal of Psychosomatics, 36*(1–4), 64–68.

Stanton, H. E. (1989b). Hypnosis and rational–emotive therapy—a de-stressing combination: A brief communication. *International Journal of Clinical and Experimental Hypnosis, 37*, 95–99.

Starker, S. (1974a). Effects of hypnotic induction upon visual imagery. *Journal of Nervous and Mental Disease, 159*, 433–437.

Starker, S. (1974b). Persistence of a hypnotic dissociative reaction. *International Journal of Clinical and Experimental Hypnosis, 22*, 131–137.

Starker, S. (1978). Dreams and waking fantasy. In K. S. Pope & J. L. Singer (Eds.), *The stream of consciousness*. New York: Plenum.

Starr, F. H., & Tobin, J. P. (1970). The effects of expectancy and hypnotic induction procedure on suggestibility. *American Journal of Clinical Hypnosis, 12*, 261–267.

Stava, L. J., & Jaffa, M. (1988). Some operationalizations of the neodissociation concept and their relationship to hypnotic susceptibility. *Journal of Personality and Social Psychology, 54*, 989–996.

Steck, W. D. (1979). The clinical evaluation of pathologic hair loss. *Cutis, 24*, 293–301.

Stein, M. I. (1953). Creativity and culture. *Journal of Psychology, 36*, 311–322.

Stein, M. I. (1974). *Stimulating creativity: Vol. 1. Individual procedures*. New York: Academic Press.

Stephenson, J. B. P. (1978). Letter: Reversal of hypnosis-induced analgesia by naloxene. *Lancet*, No. 8097, 991–992.

Sterman, M. B. (1990, November). *Cognitive correlates of EEG brain imaging*. Paper presented at the Biobehavioral Sciences Colloquium, Department of Psychiatry and Biobehavioral Sciences, University of California, Los Angeles.

Stern, D. B., Spiegel, H., & Nee, J. C. M. (1978–1979). The Hypnotic Induction Profile: Normative observations, reliability and validity. *American Journal of Clinical Hypnosis, 21,* 109–133.

Stern, J. A., Brown, M., Ulett, A., & Sletten, I. (1977). A comparison of hypnosis, acupuncture, morphine, Valium, aspirin, and placebo in the management of experimentally induced pain. *Annals of the New York Academy of Sciences, 296,* 175–193.

Stern, J. A., Edmonston, W., Ulett, G. A., & Levitsky, A. (1963). Electrodermal measures in experimental amnesia. *Journal of Abnormal and Social Psychology, 67,* 397–401.

Sternberg, R. (Ed.). (1988). *The nature of creativity: Contemporary psychological perspectives.* Cambridge, England: Cambridge University Press.

Stevenson, J. (1976). The effect of posthypnotic dissociation on the performance of interfering tasks. *Journal of Abnormal Psychology, 85,* 398–407.

Stolar, D. S., & Fromm, E. (1974). Activity and passivity of the ego in relation to the superego. *International Review of Psychoanalysis, 1,* 297–311.

Stolorow, R. D., & Lachmann, F. M. (1980). *Psychoanalysis of developmental arrests: Theory and treatment.* New York: International Universities Press.

Stowell, H. (1984). Event related brain potentials and human pain: A first objective overview. *International Journal of Psychophysiology, 1,* 137–151.

Strauss, B. L. (1990, October). *Sequelae to clinical and experimental hypnosis.* Paper presented at the 41st Annual Meeting of the Society for Clinical and Experimental Hypnosis. Tucson, AZ.

Stroop, J. R. (1935). Studies of interference in serial verbal reactions. *Journal of Experimental Psychology, 18,* 643–662.

Stukát, K. G. (1958). *Suggestibility: A factorial and experimental analysis.* Stockholm: Almqvist & Wiksell.

Stunkard, A. J. (1977). Behavioral treatment of obesity: Failure to maintain. In R. B. Stuart (Ed.), *Behavioral self-management: Strategies, techniques and outcomes* (pp. 317–350). New York: Brunner/Mazel.

Suedfeld, P. (1980). *Restricted environmental stimulation.* New York: Wiley.

Suedfeld, P. (1990). Distress, no stress, anti-stress, eustress: Where does REST fit in? In J. W. Turner & T. Fine (Eds.), *Restricted environmental stimulation: Research and commentary* (pp. 2–10). Toledo, OH: MCOT Press.

Suedfeld, P., Landon, P. B., Epstein, Y. M., & Pargament, R. (1971). The role of experimenter and subject expectations in sensory deprivation. *Representative Research in Social Psychology, 2*(1), 21–27.

Suler, J. R. (1980). Primary process thinking and creativity. *Psychological Bulletin, 88,* 144–165.

Suler, J. R., & Rizziello, J. (1987). Imagery and verbal processes in creativity. *Journal of Creative Behavior, 21,* 1–6.

Suls, J., & Miller, R. L. (Eds.). (1977). *Social comparison processes: Theoretical and empirical perspectives.* Washington, DC: Hemisphere.

Surman, O. S., Gottlieb, S. K., Hackett, T. P., & Silverberg, E. L. (1973). Hypnosis in the treatment of warts. *Archives of General Psychiatry, 28,* 439–441.

Sutcliffe, J. P. (1960). "Credulous" and "skeptical" views of hypnotic phenomena: A review of certain evidence and methodology. *International Journal of Clinical and Experimental Hypnosis, 8,* 73–101.

Sutcliffe, J. P. (1961). "Credulous" and skeptical" views of hypnotic phenomena:

Experiments on esthesia, hallucination and delusion. *Journal of Abnormal and Social Psychology, 62,* 189–200.

Sutcliffe, J. P., & Jones, J. (1962). Personal identity, multiple personality, and hypnosis. *International Journal of Clinical and Experimental Hypnosis, 10,* 231–269.

Sutcliffe, J. P., Perry, C. W., & Sheehan, P. W. (1970). Relation of some aspects of imagery and fantasy to hypnotic susceptibility. *Journal of Abnormal Psychology, 76,* 279–287.

Sweeney, C. A., Lynn, S. J., & Bellezza, F. S. (1986). Hypnosis, hypnotizability, and imagery-mediated learning. *International Journal of Clinical and Experimental Hypnosis, 34,* 29–40.

Swirsky-Sacchetti, T., & Margolis, C. G. (1986). The effects of a comprehensive self-hypnosis training program in the use of Factor VIII in severe hemophilia. *International Journal of Clinical and Experimental Hypnosis, 34,* 71–83.

Szasz, T. S. (1967). *The myth of mental illness: Foundations for a theory of personal conduct.* New York: Hoeber & Harper.

Talbot, J. D., Marrett, S., Evans, A. C., Meyer, E., Bushnell, M. C., & Duncan, G. H. (1991). Multiple representations of pain in human cerebral cortex. *Science, 251,* 1355–1358.

Talone, J. M., Diamond, M. J., & Steadman, C. (1975). Modifying hypnotic performance by means of brief sensory experiences. *International Journal of Clinical and Experimental Hypnosis, 23,* 190–199.

Taneli, B., & Krahne, W. (1987). EEG changes of transcendental meditation practitioners. In B. Taneli, C. Perris, & D. Kemali (Eds.), *Advances in biological psychiatry: Vol. 16. Neurophysiological correlates of relaxation and psychopathology* (pp. 41–71). Basel: Karger.

Tart, C. T. (Ed.). (1969). *Altered states of consciousness: A book of readings.* New York: Wiley.

Tart, C. T. (1970a). Increases in hypnotizability resulting from a prolonged program for enhancing personal growth. *Journal of Abnormal Psychology, 75,* 260–266.

Tart, C. T. (1970b). Self-report scales of hypnotic depth. *International Journal of Clinical and Experimental Hypnosis, 18,* 105–125.

Tart, C. T. (1979). Measuring the depth of an altered state of consciousness, with particular reference to self-report scales of hypnotic depth. In E. Fromm & R. E. Shor (Eds.), *Hypnosis: Developments in research and new perspectives* (2nd ed., pp. 567–601). New York: Aldine.

Taylor, C. W. (1988). Various approaches to and definitions of creativity. In R. J. Sternberg (Ed.), *The nature of creativity: Contemporary psychological perspectives* (pp. 99–121). Cambridge, England: Cambridge University Press.

Taylor, W. S., & Martin, M. F. (1944). Multiple personality. *Journal of Abnormal and Social Psychology, 39,* 281–300.

Tebecis, A. K., & Provins, K. A. (1976). Further studies of physiological concomitants of hypnosis: Skin temperature, heart rate and skin resistance. *Biological Psychology, 4,* 249–258.

Tebecis, A. K., Provins, K. A., Farnbach, R. W., & Pentony, P. (1975). Hypnosis and the EEG: A quantitative investigation. *Journal of Nervous and Mental Disease, 161,* 1–17.

Teitel, B. (1961). Post-hypnotic psychosis and the law. In *Scientific papers of the One*

Hundred and Seventeenth Meeting of the American Psychiatric Association in summary form (pp. 108–110). Washington, DC: American Psychiatric Association.

Tellegen, A. (1978–1979). On measures and conceptions of hypnosis. *American Journal of Clinical Hypnosis, 21,* 219–236.

Tellegen, A. (1980). *The Differential Personality Questionnaire.* Unpublished test materials, University of Minnesota.

Tellegen, A. (1981). Practicing the two disciplines for relaxation and enlightenment: Comment on "Role of the feedback signal in electromyograph biofeedback: The relevance of attention" by Qualls and Sheehan. *Journal of Experimental Psychology: General, 110,* 217–226.

Tellegen, A. (1982). *Brief manual for the Differential Personality Questionnaire.* Unpublished manuscript, University of Minnesota.

Tellegen, A. (1987, October). *Discussion of symposium: Hypnosis and absorption.* Paper presented at the annual meeting of the Society for Clinical and Experimental Hypnosis, Los Angeles.

Tellegen, A., & Atkinson, G. (1974). Openness to absorbing and self-altering experiences ("absorption"), a trait related to hypnotic susceptibility. *Journal of Abnormal Psychology, 83,* 268–277.

Tellegen, A., & Atkinson, G. (1976). Complexity and measurement of hypnotic susceptibility: A comment on Coe and Sarbin's alternative interpretation. *Journal of Personality and Social Psychology, 33,* 142–148.

Tenenbaum, S. J., Kurtz, R. M., & Bienias, J. L. (1990). Hypnotic susceptibility and experimental pain reduction. *American Journal of Clinical Hypnosis, 33,* 40–49.

Teng, E. L. (1981). Dichotic ear difference is a poor index for functional asymmetry between the cerebral hemispheres. *Neuropsychologia, 19,* 235–240.

Theodor, L. H., & Mandelcorn, M. S. (1973). Hysterical blindness: A case report and study using a modern psychophysical technique. *Journal of Abnormal Psychology, 82,* 552–553.

Thigpen, C. H., & Cleckley, H. (1957). *The three faces of Eve.* New York: McGraw-Hill.

Thigpen, C. H., & Cleckley, H. (1984). On the incidence of multiple personality disorder. *International Journal of Clinical and Experimental Hypnosis, 32,* 63–66.

t'Hoen, P. (1978). Effects of hypnotizability and visualizing ability on imagery mediated learning. *International Journal of Clinical and Experimental Hypnosis, 26,* 45–54.

Thompson, C. K., Hall, H. R., & Sison, C. E. (1986). Effects of hypnosis and imagery training on naming behavior in aphasia. *Brain and Language, 28*(1), 141–153.

Thurstone, L. L. (1952). Creative talent. In L. L. Thurstone (Ed.), *Applications of psychology.* New York: Harper & Row.

Tolman, E. C. (1948). Cognitive maps in rats and men. *Psychological Review, 55,* 189–208.

Tolman, E. C. (1949). *Purposive behavior in animals and men.* Berkeley: University of California Press. (Original work published 1932)

Torrance, E. P. (1966). *Torrance Tests of Creative Thinking.* Lexington, MA: Personnel Press.

Torrance, E. P. (1974). *Torrance Tests of Creative Thinking: Norms—technical manual.* Lexington, MA: Personnel Press.

Torrance, E. P. (1988). The nature of creativity as manifest in testing. In R. Sternberg (Ed.), *The nature of creativity: Contemporary psychological perspectives* (pp. 43–75). Cambridge, England: Cambridge University Press.

Torrance, E. P. (1990). *Torrance Tests of Creative Thinking: Norms—technical manual* (rev. ed.). Lexington, MA: Personnel Press.

Tosi, D. J., Judah, S. M., & Murphy, M. A. (1989). The effects of a cognitive experiential therapy utilizing hypnosis, cognitive restructuring, and developmental staging on psychological factors associated with duodenal ulcer disease: A multivariate experimental study. *Journal of Cognitive Psychotherapy, 3,* 273–290.

Treffinger, D. J. (1987). Research on creativity assessment. In S. G. Isaksen (Ed.), *Frontiers of creativity research* (pp. 103–119). Buffalo, NY: Bearly Limited.

Tryk, H. E. (1968). Assessment in the study of creativity. In P. McReynolds (Ed.), *Advances in psychological assessment* (pp. 34–54). Palo Alto, CA: Science & Behavior Books.

Tukey, J. W. (1986). Data analysis and behavioral science, or learning to bear the quantitative man's burden by shunning badmandments. In L. V. Jones (Ed.), *The collected works of John W. Tukey* (Vol. 3, pp. 187–389). Monterey, CA: Brooks/Cole.

Turk, D., Meichenbaum, D. H., & Genest, M. (1983). *Pain and behavioral medicine: A cognitive–behavioral perspective.* New York: Guilford Press.

Turner, R. M., & DiTomasso, R. A. (1980). The behavioral treatment of insomnia: A review and methodological analysis of the evidence. *International Journal of Mental Health, 9,* 129–148.

Tuttman, S. (1982). Regression: Curative factor or impediment in dynamic psychotherapy? In S. Slipp (Ed.), *Curative factors in dynamic psychotherapy* (pp. 177–198). New York: McGraw-Hill.

Twemlow, S. W., Gabbard, G. O., & Jones, F. C. (1982). The out-of-body experience: A phenomenological typology based on questionaire responses. *American Journal of Psychiatry, 139,* 450–455.

Ulett, G. A., Akpinar, S., & Itil, T. M. (1972a). Quantitative EEG analysis during hypnosis. *Electroencephalography and Clinical Neurophysiology, 33,* 361–368.

Ulett, G. A., Akpinar, S., & Itil, T. M. (1972b). Hypnosis: Physiological and pharmacological reality. *American Journal of Psychiatry, 128,* 799–805.

Ullman, M. (1959). On the psyche and warts: I. Suggestion and warts: A review and comment. *Psychosomatic Medicine, 21,* 473–487.

Van Denberg, E. J., & Kurtz, R. M. (1989). Changes in body attitude as a function of posthypnotic suggestions. *International Journal of Clinical and Experimental Hypnosis, 37,* 15–30.

Van Der Does, A. J. W., Van Dyck, R., Spinhoven, P., & Kloosman A. (1989). The effectiveness of standardized versus individualized hypnotic suggestions: A brief communication. *International Journal of Clinical and Experimental Hypnosis, 37,* 1–5.

van Dyck, R., Zitman, F. G., Linssen, A. C., & Spinhoven, P. (1991). Autogenic training and future oriented hypnotic imagery in the treatment of tension headache: Outcome and process. *International Journal of Clinical and Experimental Hypnosis, 39*(1), 6–23.

Van Dyne, W. T., & Stava, L. J. (1981). Analysis of relationships among hypnotic susceptibility, personality type, and vividness of mental imagery. *Psychological Reports, 48,* 23–26.

Van Gorp, W. G., Meyer, R. G., & Dunbar, K. D. (1985). The efficacy of direct versus indirect hypnotic induction techniques on reduction of experimental pain. *International Journal of Clinical and Experimental Hypnosis, 33,* 319–328.

Venn, J. (1986). Hypnosis and Lamaze method—an exploratory study: A brief communication. *International Journal of Clinical and Experimental Hypnosis, 35,* 79–82.

Vickery, A. R., & Kirsch, I. (1985, August). Expectancy and skill-training in the modification of hypnotizability. In S. J. Lynn (Chair), *Modifying hypnotizability.* Symposium conducted at the meeting of the American Psychological Association, Los Angeles.

Vickery, A. R., Kirsch, I., Council, J. R., & Sirkin, M. I. (1985). Cognitive skill and traditional trance hypnotic inductions: A within-subject comparison. *Journal of Consulting and Clinical Psychology, 53,* 131–133.

Vingoe, F. J., & Kramer, E. (1966). Hypnotic susceptibility of hospitalized psychotic patients: A pilot study. *International Journal of Clinical and Experimental Hypnosis, 14,* 47–54.

Vogel, W., & Broverman, D. M. (1964). Relationship between EEG and test intelligence: A critical review. *Psychological Bulletin, 62,* 132–144.

Vogel, W., Broverman, D. M., & Klaiber, E. L. (1968). EEG and mental abilities. *Electroencephalography and Clinical Neurophysiology, 24,* 166–175.

Wadden, T. A., & Anderton, C. H. (1982). The clinical use of hypnosis. *Psychological Bulletin, 91,* 215–243.

Wagaman, J., Barabasz, A. F., & Barabasz, M. (1991). Flotation REST and imagery in the improvement of collegiate basketball performance. *Perceptual and Motor Skills, 72,* 112–122.

Wagner, M. T., & Khanna, P. (1986). A neuropsychological model of hypnosis. *International Journal of Psychosomatics, 33,* 26–28.

Wagstaff, G. F. (1981a). *Hypnosis, compliance and belief.* New York: St. Martin's Press.

Wagstaff, G. F. (1981b). *The validity of posthypnotic amnesia.* Paper presented to the Experimental Psychology Society, Liverpool, England.

Wagstaff, G. F. (1982). Hypnosis and recognition of a face. *Perceptual and Motor Skills, 55,* 816–818.

Wagstaff, G. F. (1984). The enhancement of witness memory by 'hypnosis': A review and methodological critique of the experimental literature. *British Journal of Experimental and Clinical Hypnosis, 2,* 3–12.

Wagstaff, G. F. (1986). Hypnosis as compliance and belief: A socio-cognitive view. In P. L. N. Naish (Ed.), *What is hypnosis? Current theories and research* (pp. 59–84). Philadelphia: Open University Press.

Wagstaff, G. F. (1989). Forensic aspects of hypnosis. In N. P. Spanos & J. F. Chaves (Eds.), *Hypnosis: The cognitive–behavioral perspective* (pp. 340–357). Buffalo, NY: Prometheus Books.

Wagstaff, G. F. (1991). Compliance, belief, and semantics in hypnosis: A nonstate, sociocognitive perspective. In S. J. Lynn & J. W. Rhue (Eds.), *Theories of hypnosis: Current models and perspectives* (pp. 362–396). New York: Guilford Press.

Walker, L. G., Dawson, A. A., Pollet, S. M., Ratcliffe, M. A., & Hamilton, L. (1988).

Hypnotherapy for chemotherapy side effects. *British Journal of Experimental and Clinical Hypnosis, 5*(2), 79–82.

Walker, N. S., Garrett, J. B., & Wallace, B. (1976). Restoration of eidetic imagery via hypnotic age regression: A preliminary report. *Journal of Abnormal Psychology, 85*, 335–337.

Wall, V.J., & Womack, W. (1989). Hypnotic versus active cognitive strategies for alleviation of procedural distress in pediatric oncology patients. *American Journal of Clinical Hypnosis, 31*(3), 181–189.

Wallace, B. (1978). Restoration of eidetic imagery via hypnotic age regression: More evidence. *Journal of Abnormal Psychology, 87*, 673–675.

Wallace, B. (1986). Latency and frequency reports to the Necker Cube illusion: Effects of hypnotic susceptibility and mental arithmetic. *Journal of General Psychology, 113*, 187–194.

Wallace, B. (1988). Hypnotic susceptibility, visual distraction, and reports of Necker cube apparent reversals. *Journal of General Psychology, 115*, 389–396.

Wallace, B. (1990a). Imagery vividness, hypnotic susceptibility, and the perception of fragmented stimuli. *Journal of Personality and Social Psychology, 58*, 354–359.

Wallace, B. (1990b). Hypnotizability and the modification of cognitive search strategies. *International Journal of Clinical and Experimental Hypnosis, 38*, 60–69.

Wallace, B., & Garrett, J. B. (1973). Hypnotic susceptibility and autokinetic movement frequency. *Perceptual and Motor Skills, 36*, 1054.

Wallace, B., & Patterson, S. L. (1984). Hypnotic susceptibility and performance on various attention-specific cognitive tasks. *Journal of Personality and Social Psychology, 47*, 175–181.

Wallace, T., Benson, H., & Wilson, A. (1977). A wakeful hypometabolic state. *American Journal of Physiology, 221*, 795–799.

Wallas, G. (1926). *The art of thought.* New York: Franklin Watts.

Warrington, E. K. (1984). *Recognition Memory Test manual.* Windsor, UK: NFER-Nelson.

Watkins, J. G. (1986). *Hypnotherapeutic techniques.* New York: Irvington.

Watterson, J. M. (1991, October). *Hypnosis: Controlling or controlled by attention?* Paper presented at the annual meeting of the Society for Clinical and Experimental Hypnosis, New Orleans.

Weber, S. J., & Cook, T. D. (1972). Subject effects in laboratory research: An examination of subject roles, demand characteristics and valid inference. *Psychological Bulletin, 77*(4), 273–295.

Weisberg, R. W. (1986). *Creativity: Genius and other myths.* New York: W. H. Freeman.

Weitzenhoffer, A. M. (1953). *Hypnotism: An objective study in suggestibility.* New York: Wiley.

Weitzenhoffer, A. M. (1957). *General techniques of hypnotism.* New York: Grune & Stratton.

Weitzenhoffer, A. M. (1974). When is an "instruction" an instruction? *International Journal of Clinical and Experimental Hypnosis, 22*, 258–269.

Weitzenhoffer, A. M. (1978a). Hypnotism and altered states of consciousness. In A. A. Sugarman & R. E. Tarter (Eds.), *Expanding dimensions of consciousness* (pp. 183–225). New York: Springer.

Weitzenhoffer, A. M. (1978b). What did he (Bernheim) say? In F. H. Frankel & H. S. Zamansky (Eds.), *Hypnosis at its bicentennial* (pp. 47–56). New York: Plenum.

Weitzenhoffer, A. M. (1980). Hypnotic susceptibility revisited. *American Journal of Clinical Hypnosis, 22*, 130–146.

Weitzenhoffer, A. M. (1989). *The practice of hypnotism: Vol. 1. Traditional and semi-traditional techniques and phenomenology.* New York: Wiley.

Weitzenhoffer, A. M., Gough, P. B., & Landes, J. (1959). A study of the Braid effect: Hypnosis by visual fixation. *Journal of Psychology, 47*, 67–80.

Weitzenhoffer, A. M., & Hilgard, E. R. (1959). *Stanford Hypnotic Susceptibility Scale, Forms A and B.* Palo Alto, CA: Consulting Psychologists Press.

Weitzenhoffer, A. M., & Hilgard, E. R. (1962). *Stanford Hypnotic Susceptibility Scale, Form C.* Palo Alto, CA: Consulting Psychologists Press.

Weitzenhoffer, A. M., & Hilgard, E. R. (1967). *Revised Stanford Profile Scales of Hypnotic Susceptibility, Forms I and II.* Palo Alto, CA: Consulting Psychologists Press.

Weitzenhoffer, A. M., & Sjoberg, B. M. (1961). Suggestibility with and without "induction of hypnosis." *Journal of Nervous and Mental Disease, 132*, 205–220.

Welsh, G. S., & Barron, G. (1963). *Barron–Welsh Art Scale.* Palo Alto, CA: Consulting Psychologists Press.

Werner, H. (1948). *Comparative psychology of mental development.* Chicago: Follett.

West, A. N., & Martindale, C. (1988). Primary process content in paranoid schizophrenic speech. *Journal of Genetic Psychology, 149*, 547–553.

West, A. N., Martindale, C., Hines, D., & Roth, W. T. (1983). Marjuana-induced primary process content in the TAT. *Journal of Personality Assessment, 47*, 466–467.

West, J. V., Baugh, V. S., & Baugh, A. P. (1963). Rorschach and Draw-A-Person responses of hypnotized and nonhypnotized subjects. *Psychiatric Quarterly, 37*, 123–127.

West, L. J. (1960). Psychophysiology of hypnosis. *Journal of the American Medical Association, 172*, 672–675.

Westin, D. (1989). Are "primitive" object relations really preoedipal? *American Journal of Orthopsychiatry, 59*, 331–345.

White, K., Sheehan, P. W., & Ashton, R. (1977). Imagery assessment: A survey of self-report measures. *Journal of Mental Imagery, 1*, 145–170.

White, R. W. (1941). A preface to a theory of hypnotism. *Journal of Abnormal and Social Psychology, 36*, 477–505.

White, R. W., Fox, G. F., & Harris, W. W. (1940). Hypnotic hypermnesia for recently learned material. *Journal of Abnormal and Social Psychology, 35*, 88–103.

White, R. W., & Shevach, B. J. (1942). Hypnosis and the concept of dissociation. *Journal of Abnormal and Social Psychology, 7*, 309–328.

Whitehouse, W. G., Dinges, D. F., Orne, E. C., & Orne, M. T. (1988). Hypnotic hypermnesia: Enhanced memory accessibility or report bias? *Journal of Abnormal Psychology, 97*, 289–295.

Whorwell, P. J., Prior, A., & Colgan, S. M. (1987). Hypnotherapy in severe irritable bowel syndrome: Further experience. *Gut, 28*, 423–425.

Whorwell, P. J., Prior, A., & Faragher, E. B. (1984). Controlled trial of hypnotherapy in the treatment of severe refractory irritable bowel syndrome. *Lancet, ii*, 1232–1234.

Wickless, C., & Kirsch, I. (1989). The effects of verbal and experiential expectancy manipulations on hypnotic susceptibility. *Journal of Personality and Social Psychology, 57*, 762–768.

Wickless, C., Kirsch, I., & Moffitt, K. (1991, October). *Are the effects of environmental enhancement due to detection?* Paper presented at the meeting of the Society for Clinical and Experimental Hypnosis, New Orleans.

Wickramasekera, I. (1969). The effects of sensory restriction on susceptibility to hypnosis: A hypothesis, some preliminary data, and theoretical speculation. *International Journal of Clinical and Experimental Hypnosis, 17,* 217–224.

Wickramasekera, I. (1970). Effects of sensory restriction on susceptibility to hypnosis: A hypothesis and more preliminary data. *Journal of Abnormal Psychology, 76,* 69–75.

Wickramasekera, I. (1973). Effects of electromyographic feedback on hypnotic susceptibility: More preliminary data. *Journal of Abnormal Psychology, 82,* 74–77.

Williams, J. M., & Hall, D. W. (1988). Use of single session hypnosis for smoking cessation. *Addictive Behaviors, 13*(2), 205–208.

Williamsen, J. A., Johnson, H. J., & Ericksen, C. W. (1965). Some characteristics of post-hypnotic amnesia. *Journal of Abnormal Psychology, 70,* 123–131.

Willis, W. D. (1985). *The pain system: The neural basis of nociceptive transmission in the mammalian nervous system.* Basel: Karger.

Wilson, D. L. (1967). The role of confirmation of expectancies in hypnotic induction. *Dissertation Abstracts, 28,* 4787B. (University Microfilms No. 66-6781)

Wilson, L., & Kihlstrom, J. F. (1986). Subjective and categorical organization of recall during posthypnotic amnesia. *Journal of Abnormal Psychology, 95,* 264–273.

Wilson, L., Greene, E., & Loftus, E. F. (1986). Beliefs about forensic hypnosis. *International Journal of Clinical and Experimental Hypnosis, 34,* 110–121.

Wilson, N. J. (1968). Neurophysiologic alterations with hypnosis. *Diseases of the Nervous System, 29,* 618–620.

Wilson, S. C., & Barber, T. X. (1978). The Creative Imagination Scale as a measure of hypnotic responsiveness: Applications to experimental and clinical hypnosis. *American Journal of Clinical Hypnosis, 20,* 235–249.

Wilson, S. C., & Barber, T. X. (1981). Vivid fantasy and hallucinatory abilities in the life histories of excellent hypnotic subjects ("somnambules"): Preliminary report with female subjects. In E. Klinger (Ed.), *Imagery: Vol. 2. Concepts, results, and applications* (pp. 133–152). New York: Plenum Press.

Wilson, S. C., & Barber, T. X. (1983a). The fantasy-prone personality: Implications for understanding imagery, hypnosis, and parapsychological phenomena. In A. A. Sheikh (Ed.), *Imagery: Current theory, research, and application* (pp. 340–387). New York: Wiley

Wilson, S. C., & Barber, T. X. (1983b). *Inventory of Childhood Memories and Imaginings.* Framingham, MA: Cushing Hospital.

Wineburg, E. N., & Straker, N. (1973). An episode of acute, self-limiting depersonalization following a first session of hypnosis. *American Journal of Psychiatry, 130,* 98–100.

Wiseman, R. J., & Reyher, J. (1973). Hypnotically induced dreams using the Rorschach inkblots as stimuli: A test of Freud's theory of dreams. *Journal of Personality and Social Psychology, 27,* 329–336.

Woody, E. Z., Bowers, K. S., & Oakman, J. M. (1990, October 20). *Absorption and dissociation as correlates of hypnotic ability: Implications of context effects.* Paper presented at the 41st Annual Meeting of the Society for Clinical and Experimental Hypnosis, Tucson, AZ.

Woody, R. H., Krathwohl, D. R., Kagan, N., & Farquhar, W. W. (1965). Stimulated recall in psychotherapy using hypnosis and videotape. *American Journal of Clinical Hypnosis, 7,* 234–241.

Wright, L., Schaffer, A. B., & Solomons, J. G. (1979). *Encyclopedia of pediatric psychology.* Baltimore: University Park Press.

Yamamoto, S., & Matsuoka, S. (1990). Topographic EEG study of visual display terminal (VDT) performance with special reference to frontal midline theta waves. *Brain Topography, 2,* 257–267.

Yanchar, R. J., & Johnson, H. J. (1981). Absorption and attitudes toward hypnosis: A moderator analysis. *International Journal of Clinical and Experimental Hypnosis, 29,* 375–382.

Yapko, M. D. (1990). *Trancework: An introduction to the practice of clinical hypnosis* (2nd ed.). New York: Brunner/Mazel.

Yarnell, T. D. (1971). A common item creativity scale for the Adjective Check List. *Psychological Reports, 29,* 466.

Yuille, J. C., & Kim, C. K. (1987). A field study of the forensic use of hypnosis. *Canadian Journal of Behavioural Science, 19,* 418–429.

Yuille, J. C., & McEwan, N. H. (1985). Use of hypnosis as an aid to eyewitness memory. *Journal of Applied Psychology, 70,* 389–400.

Zachariae, R., & Bjerring, P. (1990). The effect of hypnotically induced analgesia on flare reaction of the cutaneous histamine prick test. *Archives of Dermatological Research, 282,* 539–543.

Zachariae, R., Bjerring, P., & Arendt-Nielsen, L. (1989). Modulation of type I immediate and type IV delayed immunoreactivity using direct suggestion and guided imagery during hypnosis. *Allergy, 44*(8), 537–542.

Zaidel, E., Clarke, J. M., & Suyenobu, B. (1990). Hemispheric independence: A paradigm case for cognitive neuroscience. In A. B. Scheibel & A. F. Wechsler (Eds.), *Neurobiology of higher cognitive function* (pp. 297–355). New York: Guilford Press.

Zakrzewski, K., & Szelenberger, W. (1981). Visual evoked potentials in hypnosis: A longitudinal approach. *International Journal of Clinical and Experimental Hypnosis, 29,* 77–86.

Zamansky, H. S. (1977). Suggestion and countersuggestion in hypnotic behavior. *Journal of Abnormal Psychology, 86,* 346–351.

Zamansky, H. S., & Bartis, S. P. (1984). Hypnosis as dissociation: Methodological considerations and preliminary findings. *American Journal of Clinical Hypnosis, 26,* 246–251.

Zamansky, H. S., & Bartis, S. P. (1985). The dissociation of an experience: The hidden observer observed. *Journal of Abnormal Psychology, 94,* 243–248.

Zamansky, H. S., & Clark, L. E. (1986). Cognitive competition and hypnotic behavior: Whither absorption? *International Journal of Clinical and Experimental Hypnosis, 34,* 205–214.

Zamansky, H. S., Scharf, B., & Brightbill, R. (1964). The effect of expectancy for hypnosis on prehypnotic performance. *Journal of Personality, 32,* 236–248.

Zeig, J. (1978). Tympanic temperature, hypnosis and laterality (Doctoral dissertation, Georgia State University). *Dissertation Abstracts International, 39*(1), 423B–424B. (University Microfilms No. 78-10,179)

Zelig, M., & Beidleman, W. B. (1981). The investigative use of hypnosis: A word of caution. *International Journal of Clinical and Experimental Hypnosis, 29,* 401–412.

Zeltzer, L. K., Fanurik, D., & LeBaron, S. (1989). The cold pressor pain paradigm in children feasibility of an intervention model (Part II). *Pain, 37,* 305–313.

Zeltzer, L. K., & LeBaron, S. (1982). Hypnosis and nonhypnotic techniques for reduction of pain and anxiety during painful procedures in children and adolescents with cancer. *Journal of Pediatrics, 101,* 1032–1035.

Zimbardo, P. G., Cohen, A., Weisenberg, M. D., Dworkin, L., & Firestone, I. (1969). The control of experimental pain. In P. G. Zimbardo (Ed.), *The cognitive control of motivation* (pp. 100–125). Glenview, IL: Scott, Foresman.

Zimbardo, P. G., Marshall, G., & Maslach, C. (1971). Liberating behavior from time-bound control: Expanding the present through hypnosis. *Journal of Applied Social Psychology, 1,* 305–323.

Zimet, C. N., & Fine, H. J. (1965). Primary and secondary process thinking in two types of schizophrenia. *Journal of Projective Techniques and Personality Assessment, 28,* 93–99.

Zubek, J. P. (1969). *Sensory deprivation: Fifteen years of research.* New York: Appleton-Century-Crofts.

Author Index

Subject Index